Organ Metabolism
and
Nutrition

Organ Metabolism and Nutrition

Ideas for Future Critical Care

Editors

John M. Kinney, M.D.
*Visiting Professor and
    Physician
The Hirsch–Leibel
    Laboratories
The Rockefeller University
New York, New York*

Hugh N. Tucker, Ph.D.
*Vice President
Clintec Nutrition Company
Deerfield, Illinois*

RAVEN PRESS NEW YORK

Raven Press, Ltd., 1185 Avenue of the Americas, New York, New York 10036

Made in the United States of America

Library of Congress Cataloging-in-Publication Data

Organ metabolism and nutrition : ideas for future critical care /
editors, John M. Kinney, Hugh N. Tucker.
     p.   cm.
    "The Second Clintec International Horizons Conference was held in
Amsterdam on May 16–20, 1993"—Introd.
   Includes bibliographical references and index.
   ISBN 0-7817-0160-0
   1. Multiple organ failure—Pathophysiology—Congresses.
2. Metabolism—Congresses. 3. Nutrition—Congresses. 4. Critical
care medicine—Congresses. I. Kinney, John M. 1921–
II. Tucker, Hugh N. III. Clintec International Horizons Conference
(2nd : 1993 : Amsterdam, Netherlands)
   [DNLM: 1. Critical Care—congresses. 2. Nutrition—congresses.
3. Metabolism—congresses. 4. Multiple Organ Failure—
physiopathology—congresses. WB 400 068 1993]
RB150.M84074 1994
616'.028—dc20
DNLM/DLC
for Library of Congress   93-41120
                                              CIP

9 8 7 6 5 4 3 2 1

Contents

Part III. Gastrointestinal Function

Part IV. Hepatic Function

Part V. Pulmonary Function and Gas Exchange

Contributing Authors

Naji N. Abumrad, M.D.
Professor and Chairman
Department of Surgery
SUNY at Stony Brook
HSC T-19, Room 020
Stony Brook, New York 11794–8191

Raphael Alon, M.D.
Senior Surgeon
Department of Surgery "A"
Ichilov Hospital
Tel Aviv Medical Center
6, Rehov Weizman
Tel Aviv, Israel 64239

Simon P. Allison, M.D.
Consulting Physician
Department of Diabetes and
  Endocrinology
University Hospital
Nottingham NG7 2UH
United Kingdom

Okezie I. Aruoma, Ph.D.
Pharmacology Group
Kings College
University of London
Manresa Road
London SW3 6LX
United Kingdom

Alberto Battezzatti, M.D.
Research Fellow in Medicine
Department of Medicine
Instituto Scientifico San Raffaele
Via Olgettina, 60
Milan, 20132
Italy

Simon Bursztein, M.D.
Associate Professor
General Intensive Care
Israel Institute of Technology
Rambam Medical Center
31 096 Haifa
Israel

G.L. Carlson, M.D.
Lecturer in Surgery
University of Manchester Medical
  School
Oxford Road
Manchester M13 9PT
United Kingdom

Yvon A. Carpentier, M.D.
Professor of Surgery
L. Deloyers Laboratory for
  Experimental Surgery
Universite Libre de Bruxelles
40, Avenue J. Wybran
B-1070 Brussels
Belgium

Frank B. Cerra, M.D.
Professor of Surgery
Department of Surgery
University of Minnesota Hospital an
  Clinic
406 Harvard Street
Minneapolis, Minnesota 55455

Harvey R. Colten, M.D.
Professor and Chairman
Department of Pediatrics
Washington University School of
  Medicine
One Children's Place
St. Louis, Missouri 63110

Nicholas Croft, M.B.B.S.
Clinical Research Fellow
Department of Medicine
University of Edinburgh
Western General Hospital
Edinburgh EH4 2XU
United Kingdom

Luc A. Cynober, Ph.D.
Professor of Biochemistry
Departments of Biochemistry,
    Molecular Biology, and Nutrition
Laboratoire de Biochimie
29 Place H. Dunant, BP 38
Clermont-Ferrand 63000
France

Nicolaas E.P. Deutz, M.D.
Academical Hospital Maastricht
P. Debeylaan 25
NL-6229 HX Maastricht
The Netherlands

Charles A. Dinarello, M.D.
Professor of Medicine and Pediatrics
Department of Geographic Medicine
    and Infectious Diseases
New England Medical Center
750 Washington Street
Boston, Massachusetts 02111

D.Y. Dubois, M.D.
Scientific Collaborator
L. Deloyers Laboratory for
    Experimental Surgery
Universite Libre de Bruxelles
40, Avenue J. Wybran
B-1070 Brussels
Belgium

Terje Espevik, Ph.D.
Professor of Cell Biology
Institute of Cancer Research
University Medical Center
N-7005 Trondheim
Norway

Patricia J. Evans, Ph.D.
Pharmacology Group
Kings College
University of London
Manresa Road
London SW3 6LX
United Kingdom

Anne Ferguson, Ph.D.
Professor of Gastroenterology
Department of Medicine
University of Edinburgh
Western General Hospital
Edinburgh EH4 2XU
United Kingdom

George K. Grimble, Ph.D.
Director, Biochemical Research
Department of Gastroenterology and
    Nutrition
Central Middlesex Hospital
Acton Lane
London NW10 7NS
United Kingdom

Barry Halliwell, M.D.
Professor
Pharmacology Group
Kings College
University of London
Manresa Road
London SW3 6LX
United Kingdom

Dieter Häussinger, M.D.
Professor of Internal Medicine
Department of Internal Medicine
The University of Freiburg
Hugstetterstrasse 55
D-79106 Freiburg
Germany

Herbert B. Hechtman, M.D.
Professor of Surgery
Department of Surgical Oncology
Brigham and Women's Hospital
75 Francis Street
Boston, Massachusetts 02115

Harparkash Kaur, Ph.D.
Pharmacology Group
Kings College
University of London
Manresa Road
London SW3 6LX
United Kingdom

John M. Kinney, M.D.
Visiting Professor and Physician
The Hirsch-Leibel Laboratories
Rockefeller University
1230 York Avenue
New York, New York 10021-6399

Matthew J. Kluger, Ph.D.
Professor of Physiology
Director, Institute of Basic and
    Applied Medical Research
2425 Ridgecrest Drive, SE
Albuquerque, New Mexico 87108

John I. Lew, A.B.
Research Assistant
Harrison Department of Surgical
    Research
University of Pennsylvania Medical
    Center
Stemmler Hall
36th Street and Hamilton Walk
Philadelphia, Pennsylvania 19104

Nina-Beate Liabakk, Ph.D.
Scientist
Institute of Cancer Research
University Medical Center
N-7005 Trondheim
Norway

Roderick A. Little, Ph.D.
Director
Northwest Injury Research Centre
University of Manchester Medical
    School
Stopford Building, Oxford Road
Manchester M13 9PT
United Kingdom

Stephen F. Lowry, M.D.
Professor and Director
Laboratory of Surgical Metabolism
New York Hospital
Cornell University Medical Center
East 68th Street
New York, New York 10021

Dwight E. Matthews, Ph.D.
Associate Professor of Biochemistry
Department of Medicine
Cornell University Medical College
1300 York Avenue
New York, New York 10021

Laura McLintock, Ph.D.
Post Doctoral Research Fellow
Department of Medicine
University of Edinburgh
Western General Hospital
Edinburgh EH4 2XU
United Kingdom

Lyle L. Moldawer, Ph.D.
Associate Professor
Department of Surgery
University of Florida College of
    Medicine
1600 SW Archer Road
Gainesville, Florida 32610

Patricia E. Molina, M.D.
Assistant Professor
Department of Surgery
SUNY at Stony Brook
HSC T-19, Room 020
Stony Brook, New York 11794-8191

Ian Poxton, Ph.D.
Reader in Medical Microbiology
Department of Medical Microbiology
University of Edinburgh
Teviot Place
Edinburgh EH8 9AG
United Kingdom

Michael J. Rennie, Ph.D.
Professor
Department of Anatomy and
    Physiology
University of Dundee
Nethergate
Dundee DD1 4HN
Scotland

M. Richelle, M.Sc.
Scientific Collaborator
L. Deloyers Laboratory for
    Experimental Surgery
Universite Libre de Bruxelles
40, Avenue J. Wybran
B-1070 Brussels
Belgium

John L. Rombeau, M.D.
Associate Professor of Surgery
Department of Surgery
University of Pennsylvania Medical
Center
3400 Spruce Street
Philadelphia, Pennsylvania 19104

Jamal Sallam, M.S.
Research Fellow
Department of Medicine
University of Edinburgh
Western General Hospital
Edinburgh EH4 2XU
United Kingdom

Hans P. Sauerwein, M.D.
Professor in Clinical Nutrition
Department of Internal Medicine/
   Endocrinology
Academic Medical Center
Meibergdreef 9
1105 AZ Amsterdam
The Netherlands

David Shepro, Ph.D.
Professor of Biology
Biology Department
Boston University
2 Cummington Street
Boston, Massachusetts 02215

V.S. Siderova, M.D.
Scientific Collaborator
L. Deloyers Laboratory for
   Experimental Surgery
Universite Libre de Bruxelles
40, Avenue J. Wybran
B-1070 Brussels
Belgium

Ruth Simpson, M.D.
Surgical House Officer
University Hospital of South
   Manchester
Nell Lane
Didsbury
United Kingdom

Peter B. Soeters, M.D.
Professor of Surgery
Academical Hospital Maastricht
P. Debeylaan 25
NL-6229 HX Maastricht
The Netherlands

Anders Sundan, Ph.D.
Senior Scientist
Institute of Cancer Research
University Medical Center
N-7005 Trondheim
Norway

Jukka Takala, M.D.
Associate Professor of Anesthesiology
Director, Critical Care Research
   Program
Department of Intensive Care
Kuopio University Hospital
Post Office Box 1777
SF-70211 Kuopio
Finland

Hugh N. Tucker, Ph.D.
Vice President
Scientific and Medical Affairs
Clintech Nutrition Company
Three Parkway North
Suite 500
Deerfield, Illinois 60015

C.R. Valeri, M.D.
Professor of Medicine
Research Professor of Surgery
Director, Naval Blood Research
   Laboratory
Boston Unversity School of Medicine
615 Albany Street
Boston, Massachusetts 02118

Sander J.H. van Deventer, M.D.
Center for Hemostasis, Thrombosis,
   Atherosclerosis and Inflammation
   Research
Academic Medical Center
Meibergdreef 9
1105 AZ Amsterdam
The Netherlands

Anders Waage, M.D.
Senior Scientist
Institute of Cancer Research
University Medical Center
N-7005 Trondheim
Norway

Peter A. Ward, M.D.
Professor and Chairman
Department of Pathology
University of Michigan Medical
 School
M-5240 Medical Science I
1300 Catherine Road
Ann Arbor, Michigan 48109-0602

Jan Wernerman, M.D.
Associate Professor
Department of Anesthesiology and
 Intensive Care
Karolinska Institute
Huddinge University Hospital
S-141 86 Huddinge
Sweden

Steven H. Zeisel, M.D.
Professor and Chairman
Department of Nutrition
University of North Carolina
 at Chapel Hill
CB #7400
Chapel Hill, North Carolina 27599-7400

Preface

The evolving worldwide healthcare environment provided the stimulus for the subject matter considered for the second Clintec International Horizons Conference. *Organ Metabolism and Nutrition: Ideas for Future Critical Care* is intended to encourage interdisciplinary discussions relevant to current and developing issues within the critical care community and to forecast future trends in care. Clinical practice in the current hospital setting is being concentrated to provide care for only the most ill, or for procedures that due to complexity or patient condition cannot be performed by services outside the hospital. Any patient that can be cared for adequately in some less costly alternative site or at home is no longer seen in the hospital. While total hospital beds are decreasing in number, there is an increasing number of critical care beds, reflecting improved technology for maintaining the more critical patients and the demographic shifts to more elderly patients. These critical care units are being further fragmented into specialized critical care settings with the length of stay becoming shorter. Average length of stay in critical care units in the United States has now been reduced to approximately 6.2 days. This concentration in both time and severity highlights the necessity to understand the role of each therapeutic intervention and its outcome-related benefit.

Management of organ failure from hypoperfusion or sepsis—systemic inflammatory response syndrome—remains the key unresolved issue in critical care medicine, while the role of metabolic and nutrition adjunctive support in improvement of outcome and quality of care in these complex patients is poorly understood. The relationship of cytokines, cytokine agonists, growth factors, and other emerging biopharmaceuticals must be considered in perspective with the techniques and substrates for providing specific energy and nutrient requirements. Outcome benefit, survival gains, or other relevant clinical parameters with quantitative endpoints are needed to further the understanding of clinical nutrition in the critical care setting. It is in this environment that the conference agenda was developed.

This book represents the papers and discussions which transpired during the second conference held in Amsterdam from May 16 to May 20, 1993. Completed manuscripts were submitted prior to the conference and were provided to each of five session chairmen for critical review. Overview discussions from each session were constructed by the chairmen based on both their session's material and a synthesis of the subject matter from the other material presented over the 4-day conference.

The conference objective was to provide multidisciplinary researchers associated with divergent fields the opportunity to review their current research findings with each other. The interchange fosters creative thinking regarding possible new avenues for investigative programs. It is only through discussions such as these that new directions for improving the quality of critical patient care will emerge. Clintec International Inc. and Clintec Nutrition Companies worldwide are greatly appreciative of the continued efforts of Dr. John Kinney in constructing and chairing this conference series. His dedication and enthusiasm are exemplary in contributing to the understanding of altered metabolic processes of the critically ill. It is through his efforts that technical and clinical advances on the horizon can be incorporated more rapidly into improved patient care techniques.

Hugh N. Tucker, Ph.D.
Clintec Nutrition Company
Affiliated with Baxter Healthcare Corporation and Nestlé S.A.

Introduction

The objectives of the Clintec International Horizons Conferences are twofold: to summarize knowledge in selected areas of human metabolism and to highlight directions that hold special promise for advancing nutrition in future patient care. The application of these objectives to the care of the critically ill patient presents a special challenge.

Many advances have been made in the support of patients with failure of a single organ yet the mortality for multiple organ failure continues to exceed 90%. The title of this book, *Organ Metabolism and Nutrition: Ideas for Future Critical Care*, represents an interdisciplinary approach to mechanisms which may underlie this lethal problem. It examines organ metabolism and nutrition in the light of new knowledge of cell biology and searches for ways in which the failure of one organ may predispose to the failure of other organs. It explores how malnutrition may contribute to organ failure and whether selective use of nutrients may have importance for the support of individual organs.

The care of the critically ill patient as a discipline is relatively young. The concept can be traced back to shock wards used by the military in World War II, to the need for mechanical ventilation during the polio epidemics of the 1950s, and EKG monitoring during the 1960s plus the need for intensive care of postoperative patients beyond the time available in the postanesthesia recovery room. Formal intensive care units began to appear by 1970, often under the supervision of anesthesiologists for surgical patients, while cardiac, pulmonary, and neonatal units usually functioned within their own services. Because of the complex nature of the patients requiring intensive care, these units were sometimes referred to as the "hospital's hospital."

It is interesting that intensive care units and total parenteral nutrition were both introduced during the turbulent 1960s. Their early growth, however, had little in common. Most attention in the intensive care unit was directed toward treating shock and the artificial support of vital organs. Nutritional care of patients in the intensive care unit was often of low priority. Only during the 1980s were guidelines sought for how nutrition could meet the quantitative needs inherent in the altered metabolism of the acutely ill patient.

Now, both the physicians involved in intensive care and those in clinical nutrition are more than ever in need of new understanding of how cellular mechanisms influence organ function, yet the cell biologist or other laboratory scientist frequently has too many demands on his or her time to interact with physicians and discuss how new biological concepts might influence future clinical care.

The Second Clintec International Horizons Conference was held in Amsterdam between May 16 and 20, 1993. This book represents the five subject areas that were presented and discussed at that conference. Each section combines chapters by laboratory investigators with those by clinical scientists. The chairman of each session was invited to write an overview presenting a personal perspective on the present status and important trends in that particular area.

The various scientific disciplines represented in this book reflect Clintec's dedication to encouraging communication between laboratory and clinical investigators in the search for concepts, which are only now emerging from the laboratory and may influence care of the critically ill patient in future years.

John M. Kinney M.D.

Organ Metabolism and Nutrition:
Ideas for Future Critical Care, edited by
J. M. Kinney and H. N. Tucker.
Raven Press, Ltd., New York © 1994.

1

Substrate Kinetics and Catabolic Hormones

Dwight E. Matthews and Alberto Battezzati

Department of Medicine, Cornell University Medical College, New York, New York 10021; and Department of Medicine, Istituto Scientifico San Raffaele, Milano 20132, Italy

Over 70 years ago Sir David Cuthbertson demonstrated that an injury, such as a long-bone fracture, causes wasting of body N through increased production of urea and that it is *the injury per se* which induces the wasting of N, rather than another associated factor, such as enforced bed rest (1). Trauma and sepsis produce a hypermetabolic state of increased energy expenditure and net loss of protein with increased urinary nitrogen (N) excretion and a negative N balance. Cumulative N loss is generally proportional to the severity of the injury, and there is often hyperglycemia and resistance to insulin.

The primary sources of fuel in the body are sugar and fat. Storage of carbohydrate as glycogen accounts for only enough energy for the body to withstand a brief fast. Over 80% of the body's energy reserve is in fat. However, critical tissues such as the brain cannot utilize fat directly. Therefore, the body must continue to provide the brain with glucose after glycogen supplies have been depleted in fasting. This glucose comes primarily from amino acids via gluconeogenesis. These amino acids come from catabolizing muscle protein. While the muscle protein pool may be large and, therefore, capable of providing the necessary energy, muscle function also depends on maintenance of the protein pool. Conservation of protein is also very important for the maintenance of immune and liver function. Protein is so important to body function that a cumulative loss of ≈25% of body protein mass will cause death due to depressed cardiopulmonary and immune function. To withstand simple starvation, the body adapts to utilizing fat instead of carbohydrate/protein. The brain uses ketone bodies, which are produced by the liver via conversion of fatty acids. Using fat and sparing protein allows us to survive weeks of starvation. However, in stress and trauma these adaptive mechanisms do not function the same to protect the body's protein stores with the onset of a hypermetabolic state. This may in part be due to the body's need to continue providing glucose as a fuel for white cells and injured tissues. The net effect is a loss of protein, which may be of little consequence to a patient with a self-limited disease or with adequate body stores of energy and protein but can be life threatening to a patient who is already nutritionally depleted or has a prolonged hypermetabolic episode.

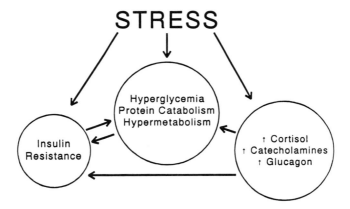

FIG. 1. Stress and trauma induces a hypercatabolic state of nitrogen loss and increased energy expenditure. In part this occurs via stress-induced increases in the "stress" hormones, through insulin resistance, and via other mechanisms such as cytokine pathways, which have not been fully elucidated.

Although the effects of stress (e.g., increased energy expenditure, increased N loss) are well documented, what factors specifically produce the response are not. Figure 1 illustrates some of the variables involved and their interrelationships. The concentrations of several endocrine hormones are altered in trauma and sepsis (2,3), and, as will be discussed, the hormones regulate many aspects of carbohydrate, fat, and amino acid metabolism. Therefore, it is only natural to assume that the endocrine hormones may be the primary mediators of the metabolic effects of stress and trauma. Only recently have investigators begun to elucidate the role of nonhormonal factors, such as cytokines, arachidonic acid derivatives (such as prostaglandins), and nitric oxide, and how they may be responsible for the hypermetabolic state seen in stress (4–7). Exposure of macrophages and circulating white blood cells in the body to endotoxin and other foreign materials induces the release of a cascade of cytokine factors that in turn promote the release of other factors. The regulation of these factors and their metabolic effects is only just beginning to be understood and will be discussed by other authors in this text.

The effect of endocrine hormones on metabolism has been studied in a variety of settings: in animals, animal tissue preparations, and in humans both healthy and critically ill. The effect of individual hormones upon protein and energy metabolism *in humans* is shown in Table 1 (8–33). The data presented are a composite of a variety of studies in normal humans who received infusions of the individual hormones at high physiologic levels often seen in stress and trauma. The rapidity of metabolic response is indicated in Table 1 under the column "speed of metabolic response." The metabolic response to a change in hormone concentrations varies from seconds to hours. Thyroid and the sex hormones produce a metabolic response that requires hours to evolve. Growth hormone and cortisol induce effects that can be seen in a period of 6 to 12 hours. Insulin and glucagon produce metabolic effects in minutes,

TABLE 1. *Effect of individual hormones on protein and energy metabolism in humans.*

| Hormone | Speed of metabolic response | Effect of increasing hormone concentration on | | | | References |
		Protein breakdown	Protein synthesis	Net N loss	Metabolic rate	
Thyroid	−	↑	−	↑	↑ ↑	(8,9)
Androgens	−	−	↑	↓	↑	(10,11)
Growth hormone	+	−	↑	↑	↑	(12–15)
Cortisol	+	↑	−	↑	↑ ↑	(16–20)
Glucagon	+ +	↑	−	↑	↑	(21–23)
Insulin	+ +	↓ ↓	−	↓		(24–29)
Epinephrine	+ + +	(↓)	(↑)	−	↑ ↑	(30–33)

Data are from studies in which healthy subjects have been infused with individual hormone to concentrations seen in stress. The speed of metabolic response to an increase in hormone concentration ranges from days (−), to hours (+), to minutes (+ +). The effects of glucagon are seen under conditions in which insulin is also suppressed and glucose and amino acid concentrations are rising. Therefore, the metabolic effects shown for glucagon may be exaggerated from that which glucagon actually produces in stress. Epinephrine's effect on protein metabolism is transient, as indicated by "( )".

while the catecholamines (epinephrine and norepinephrine) will cause metabolic changes in seconds.

The hormones shown in Table 2 have important effects on protein and energy metabolism, yet few of these hormones are altered significantly over the time course of the hypermetabolic response seen in injury and stress. For example, there is little change in thyroid status or sex hormone concentrations, indicating that these hormones are unlikely to play an important role in the stress response. Jeevanandam et al. (34) have recently shown that growth hormone may be either depressed or elevated postinjury, depending on the age and health of the patient and whether nutritional support is being given. However, cortisol, glucagon, insulin, and the catecholamines are all elevated. Epinephrine is well documented to increase energy expenditure, and together with cortisol and glucagon is probably responsible for the changes seen in glucose metabolism. Insulin is increased in stress because the stress hormones induce hyperglycemia. Because blood sugar does not return to normal with the hyperinsulinemia, the body is termed to be "insulin resistant." This insulin resistance is largely attributable to cortisol hormone (35). Cortisol is the prominent hormone whose time

TABLE 2. *Changes in hormone concentrations in stress and trauma in humans.*

Thyroid	No change or slight depression
Androgens/estrogens	No change or slight depression
Growth hormone	Slight change
Cortisol	Increased
Glucagon	Increased
Insulin	Increased but resistance occurs
Catecholamines	Increased

course remains elevated the longest in injury. In terms of protein metabolism the picture is less clear, but much of the metabolic effects of injury can be assigned to cortisol.

INSULIN

Insulin is also considered an "anabolic" hormone. However, in contrast to growth hormone, insulin acts by suppressing proteolysis (Table 3) and has very little effect on protein synthesis in humans. Insulin in physiologic amounts will suppress proteolysis by 25% or more (24,25,29,36,37). The insulin-induced reduction in proteolysis also causes a proportional fall in the concentrations of most amino acids. The suppression of leucine appearance from proteolysis and of plasma leucine in response to increasing concentrations of insulin are shown in Fig. 2. It is interesting to note that the half-maximal response of insulin on suppression of proteolysis is at 30 μU/ml (29), which is in the middle of the physiological range of insulin concentration. The results shown in Fig. 2 are based on measurement of whole-body leucine kinetics. These measurements have been repeated in other reports with both leucine and phenylalanine tracers. Many of the measurements were performed at a standard insulin infusion rate of 1 mU/kg/min, which produces an approximate insulin concentration of 100 μU/ml in plasma. The suppression of protein breakdown is a common finding in these reports (Table 3). The response of protein synthesis has been more difficult to show. Clearly, when amino acid concentrations fall due to reduced proteolysis, either amino acid oxidation or protein synthesis must be reduced to match and, therefore, stabilize amino acid concentrations. The whole-body tracer measurements indicate that insulin reduces proteolysis and (secondarily) protein synthesis. There is not a dramatic change in amino acid oxidation. Considering that amino acid oxidation is only ≈20% of proteolysis in the postabsorptive state, amino acid oxidation

TABLE 3. *Effect of insulin on protein metabolism: studies of whole body amino acid kinetics.*

| | | Suppression of proteolysis (% from basal) with infusion of: | | |
Study	Tracers used	Insulin	Insulin with amino acid replacement	References
Fukagawa et al. (1985)	^{13}C-leucine	−26		(29)
Castellino et al. (1987)	^{14}C-leucine	−40	−65	(36)
Flakoll et al. (1989)	^{14}C-leucine	−17	−55	(37)
Tessari et al. (1991)	^{14}C-leucine	−13		(25)
	^{3}H-phenylalanine	−22		
Heslin et al. (1992)	^{14}C-leucine		−17	(24)

Studies performed with an insulin infusion rate necessary to produce a plasma insulin concentration of ≈100 μU/ml. In some cases amino acids were also infused to restore some amino acid concentrations to basal values.

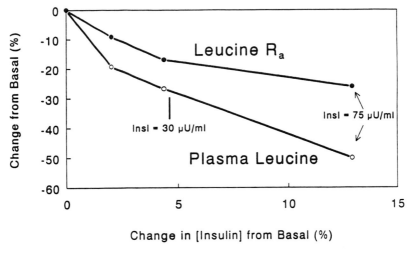

FIG. 2. Relative change in leucine R_a and plasma leucine concentration in postabsorptive adult men infused with varying amounts of insulin. Data adapted from ref. (29). The half-maximal response of insulin suppression of leucine R_a occurred at a plasma insulin concentration of ≈ 30 µU/ml. The insulin data are given as the relative increase from basal except where indicated ("Insl = ").

would have to be reduced to zero to begin to compensate for the reduction in proteolysis. Therefore, it is not surprising to see that the prominent response is a reduction in protein synthesis to compensate for the reduction in protein breakdown.

An alternative approach in humans to the whole body tracer methodology is to measure the balance of an essential amino acid tracer across forearm or leg. If the essential amino acid is not metabolized by muscle, these measurements will determine the net utilization of tracer by muscle for protein synthesis and the rate of proteolysis (38). This approach has been used with several variations by several groups, as shown in Table 4 (24,25,27,39). The most interesting is the Gelfand and Barrett report (27) in which the insulin was administered directly into the brachial artery to elevate insulin in the arm locally without producing systemic effects. They found a 40% reduction in proteolysis but without a concomitant drop in protein synthesis. Because this was a local infusion of insulin, systemic amino acid concentrations did not fall, and the effect of insulin on muscle was studied without a drop in amino acid concentrations. Because many reactions of amino acid metabolism are a function of amino acid concentrations, some of the effect of insulin on amino acid metabolism may occur through the reduction of amino acid concentrations per se. The data of Gelfand and Barrett demonstrate no fall in protein synthesis, but they also demonstrate no enhancement in protein synthesis. Other workers have also infused humans with insulin and variable amounts of an amino acid solution to maintain amino acid concentrations (Tables 3 and 4). Two studies found a further reduction in protein breakdown when amino acid concentrations were maintained (36,37), indicating that the full effect of insulin on proteolysis could only be seen with concomitant

TABLE 4. *Effect of insulin on protein metabolism: studies of forearm or leg amino acid kinetics.*

Study	Tracers used	Suppression of proteolysis (% from basal) with infusion of:		Changes in protein synthesis (% from basal) with infusion of:		Refs
		Insulin	Insulin while maintaining amino acid concentrations	Insulin	Insulin while maintaining amino acid concentrations	
Gelfand et al. (1987)	^{3}H-phenylalanine		−42		0	(27)
Denne et al. (1991)	^{2}H-phenylalanine	−41		−21		(39)
Tessari et al. (1992)	^{14}C-leucine	−26				(25)
	^{3}H-phenylalanine	−23		−7		
Heslin et al. (1992)	^{14}C-leucine	−37				(24)

infusion of amino acids. Protein synthesis was increased with infusion of amino acids but was not returned to basal values.

The information in humans to date indicates a significant role for insulin in the suppression of proteolysis with little direct effect on protein synthesis. However, it should be kept in mind what a physiologically significant change in protein metabolism is. In Fig. 2, insulin is shown suppressing protein breakdown by ≈25%. Increasing insulin concentration does not dramatically increase the suppression in proteolysis. In contrast, insulin greatly increases the utilization of glucose (Fig. 3). The

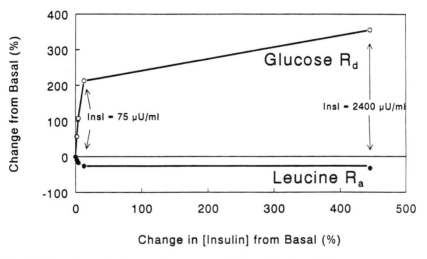

FIG. 3. Relative change in glucose disappearance (R_d) and leucine R_a in postabsorptive adult men infused with varying amounts of insulin. Data adapted from Fukagawa et al. (29). The maximal response of insulin enhancement of glucose disposal was several-fold greater than the corresponding suppression of leucine R_a. The insulin data are given as the relative increase from basal except where indicated ("Insl =").

increase in glucose disposal with insulin infusion is a >200% increase compared with a suppression of proteolysis of only 25%. The endocrine hormones almost always produce a considerably greater effect on glucose and fat metabolism compared with protein metabolism. A change of >10% in protein turnover is a large physiologic change compared with changes seen in glucose and fat metabolism.

GLUCAGON

The hormone glucagon and its role in contròlling protein metabolism has been controversial (40–42). Studies have clearly shown that elevation of glucagon (with insulin held at basal concentration via the somatostatin clamp) increases blood glucose concentration (43–45). The metabolic response to glucagon is transient, suggesting that glucagon is not important to long-term regulation of glucose metabolism. Glucagon stimulates liver glycogenolysis and gluconeogenesis (43,46,47). However, these effects wane with time. Glucagon's role in regulating protein metabolism has been studied in different ways to disassociate the response of insulin from the response of glucagon. When glucagon was infused in healthy subjects to elevate glucagon, while plasm insulin concentration was held constant via an infusion of somatostatin and basal insulin, neither proteolysis (measured from leucine and lysine kinetics) nor alanine flux changed (44). The conclusion of this study would be that glucagon has little effect on amino acid metabolism. When glucagon was infused to elevate glucagon and insulin was not replaced during an infusion of somatostatin, proteolysis increased with hyperglucagonemia (21). Proteolysis also increased in the control study of somatostatin infusion alone because insulin suppresses proteolysis and somatostatin reduced plasma concentration of insulin. However, proteolysis increased more than hyperglucagonemia than with hypoinsulinemia alone, indicating that glucagon increases proteolysis. This latter study also demonstrated an increase in energy expenditure with the glucagon infusion (22). These studies indicate the difficulty of studying the effect of one hormone (such as glucagon) when another related hormone (such as insulin) also produces profound effects on metabolism. Elevating glucagon concentration lowers the concentrations of mainly the gluconeogenic amino acids: alanine, glycine, glutamine, serine, proline, etc. (48). This drop in amino acids may occur via the glucagon-induced stimulation of hepatic gluconeogenesis. The concentrations of these amino acids would fall if uptake for gluconeogenesis occurred without an increase in the supply of these amino acids from other tissues, such as muscle. We postulate that glucagon effects primarily amino acid metabolism in the viscera and has little effect on muscle amino acid metabolism.

GROWTH HORMONE

Different studies have reported either increased (49–51), normal, or decreased (2,34) growth hormone concentrations following burn, sepsis, or trauma injury. These discrepancies may be due to differences in the type and severity of the insult or in the ages and nutritional status of the patients. In addition, the pulsatile secretion of growth hormone may have been either missed or have accentuated values when single daily measurements were made (52). The highest concentration of growth hormone is found immediately after injury with reduction to normal in the late (catabolic) phase of the stress response. Plasma growth hormone concentration increases with injury, while insulin-like growth factor I (IGF-I) concentration decreases. As the severity of the injury increases, growth hormone production is attenuated (53).

Clearly, growth hormone is a powerful anabolic and lipolytic hormone; children do not grow without growth hormone. In adults the effects of growth hormone are not so evident as in children, but the influence of growth hormone on metabolism and on body composition persist for the duration of our lives (54–56). Growth hormone induces changes in body composition that we consider anabolic: an accrual of muscle protein mass and a decrease in fat mass (54,55). However, the effect of growth hormone on body composition in grown adults, while significant, is not dramatic. The mechanism by which growth hormone increases body protein has been investigated in humans using several different protocols and techniques. Daily administration of growth hormone to healthy adults placed on total parenteral nutrition (TPN) for 6 days produced a shift from a negative to a positive N balance (57). Using [^{15}N]glycine to assess protein turnover, Manson et al. concluded that growth hormone produces its anabolic effect by specifically increasing protein synthesis without effecting protein breakdown (58). Horber and Haymond arrived at the same conclusion using [^{14}C]leucine to determine the effect of 6 days of growth hormone administration in normally fed adults (59). Fryburg et al. demonstrated direct effects of growth hormone on human skeletal muscle by infusing subjects intraarterially with growth hormone and measuring changes in amino acid kinetics across the forearm (13). Growth hormone stimulated amino acid tracer uptake but did not change the release of tracer from the forearm, indicating that growth hormone increased protein synthesis in the skeletal muscle without affecting protein breakdown. Another key point of this study was that the minimum time required to measure an effect after beginning infusion of growth hormone was 6 hours.

IGF-I and IGF-II are small peptides that are structurally related to insulin. IGF-I is thought to produce many of the growth promoting effects assigned to growth hormone. However, in terms of protein metabolism, the actions of growth hormone and IGF-I are distinctly different. Evidence to date in humans shows that growth hormone increases protein synthesis without significantly changing proteolysis. Studies in which IGF-I has been infused into humans and protein metabolism determined by using labeled leucine tracers (60,61) have produced differing results. In one case, 24-hour infusion of IGF-I produced marginal changes in protein kinetics, or even on blood glucose concentration (61). In the other study, Turkalj et al. demonstrated that IGF-I infusion decreases protein breakdown and amino acid oxidation but has little effect on protein synthesis (60). Turkalj et al. also demonstrated other similarities of IGF-I to insulin in that subjects infused with IGF-I needed to be infused with glucose to maintain euglycemia. Clearly the results of these studies show that these hormones produce different metabolic effects when administered to humans: growth hormone produces anabolic changes through increasing protein synthesis, while IGF-I and insulin decrease proteolysis.

Prominent effects of growth hormone administration are the induction of glucose intolerance and increased lipolysis (62–64). Growth hormone reduces the efficiency of glucose utilization, and elevating plasma growth hormone concentration impairs the normal disposal of an oral glucose load, despite an increase in the plasma insulin response (62). Other studies have shown that mild elevations of growth hormone impair insulin action on glucose disposal (65), suggesting that elevated growth hormone concentration could contribute to the observed insulin resistance seen in trauma. Insulin resistance is also induced by other catabolic hormones, in particular, cortisol. In contrast to cortisol, which induces a net loss of body protein, growth hormone promotes protein anabolism, even while it induces insulin resistance. Because the anabolic action of insulin is difficult to produce in trauma when there is resistance to insulin action, the hypothesis that growth hormone administration would be effective in counteracting the protein wasting of stress and trauma has been proposed. To support this hypothesis, the combined effect of glucocorticoids and growth hormone on protein metabolism has been studied in healthy volunteers receiving either one or both of the two hormones for 1 week (35,59). Both growth hormone and prednisone administration increased plasma glucose and induced insulin resistance. The effect of the two hormones together was additive on glucose (59). Prednisone administration caused an increased loss of protein by increasing proteolysis. Growth hormone decreased protein loss through a small increase in protein synthesis. Although growth hormone acts through a different mechanism on protein metabolism, adding growth hormone ameliorated the increased oxidation of protein caused by prednisone. This result occurred in part through an increase in protein synthesis and in part by a reduction of the proteolytic effects of prednisone (35). Studies such as these suggest that growth hormone administration may have a favorable impact on the catabolic derangements of stress.

EPINEPHRINE

The metabolic effects of the catecholamines have been well studied in endocrinology, metabolism, and cardiology. Here the primary effects sought have been counterregulation against hypoglycemia and maintenance of blood pressure. Both effects are acute, and, therefore, most of the studies of catecholamine action have been using short-duration infusions of higher doses of catecholamines. The details of the metabolic and physiologic effects of the catecholamines are discussed in most textbooks of endocrinology (e.g., (66)). In terms of stress and trauma, the prominent role of epinephrine is to increase resting energy expenditure (REE) (30,67–69). These studies have demonstrated that epinephrine increases REE both at elevations of epinephrine commonly seen with daily stress in normal life and under conditions commonly found in injury and trauma. This concentration of plasma epinephrine is clearly lower than those associated with the epinephrine response produced to counterregulate against hypoglycemia (66).

In comparing results of different studies where epinephrine has been measured, it must be kept in mind that there is a difference in epinephrine concentration between arterial and venous blood-draining tissue beds, such as the forearm (70). Many studies prior to the mid-1980s used peripheral venous sampling of blood (e.g., (66,71,72)). Because of tissue clearance of epinephrine, venous concentrations are approximately half those measured with arterial sampling (70). Matthews et al. (30) have also shown that the heated-hand vein technique is effective in reproducing arterial concentrations via "arterialized"-venous sampling. An example of the differences in epinephrine concentration as a function of sampling site is shown in Fig. 4. These differences must be kept in mind when comparing results among studies.

Epinephrine increases REE in a dose-dependent manner, as illustrated in Fig. 5. In contrast, the effect of epinephrine on glucose production is transient (71,73), although blood glucose concentration remains elevated with epinephrine infusion duration (Fig. 6). Epinephrine initially acts to increase glucose production through glycogenolysis and secondarily through increasing gluconeogenesis (74). At the same time, resistance to peripheral tissue utilization of glucose develops, keeping blood glucose concentration elevated even though the initial burst of glucose production has subsided. Epinephrine has been shown to have a potent effect on lipolysis (72). As with REE and glucose metabolism, increasing doses of epinephrine increase lipolysis in a dose-dependent fashion. In fact, the stimulation of lipolysis, the increase in plasma free fatty acid (FFA), and the increase in glycerol concentration occur at plasma concentrations of epinephrine lower than that needed to increase glucose production (71) or REE (69,74). The epinephrine-induced stimulation of lipolysis also results in

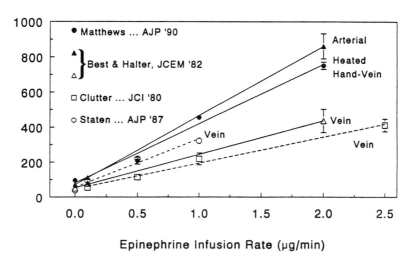

FIG. 4. Plasma epinephrine concentration measured as a function of epinephrine infusion rate and sampling site for venous *(open symbols)*, arterialized-venous heated "hand-vein" *(closed circles)* and arterial blood *(closed triangles)* samples. Figure taken from Matthews et al. (30).

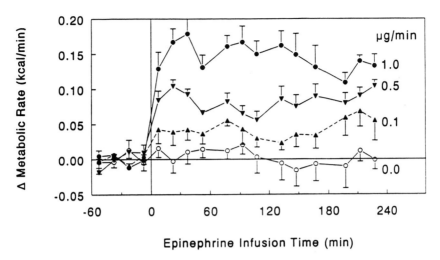

FIG. 5. Increase in REE (metabolic rate) with infusion of epinephrine. Epinephrine was infused at rates of 0, 0.1, 0.5, and 1.0 µg/min into healthy young adults as indicated in the figure. Metabolic rate increased with increasing epinephrine infusion. Figure adapted from Staten et al. (69).

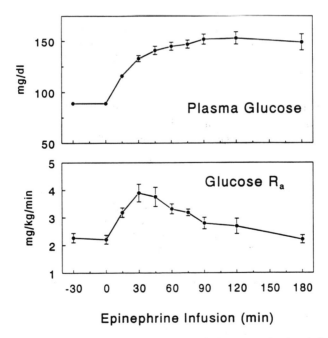

FIG. 6. Time course of blood glucose concentration and glucose production during infusion of epinephrine. Epinephrine was infused in healthy subjects from 0 to 180 min at 3.5 µg/min. Although glucose concentration remains high, the increase in glucose production is transient. Figure prepared from the data presented in Miles et al. (33).

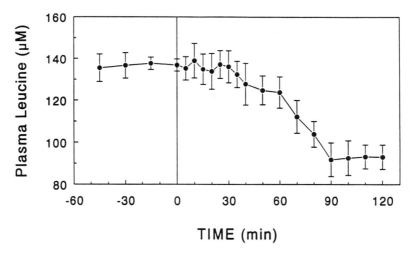

FIG. 7. Time course of plasma leucine before and after starting (time = 0 minutes) a 2-μg/min infusion of epinephrine in healthy normal postabsorptive adults.

an increase in ketone body production by the liver (75,76). As with glucose, however, the increase in lipolysis with epinephrine may be transient (72).

Infusion of epinephrine quickly causes the plasma levels of most amino acids to fall (77). For example, when normal subjects are infused with epinephrine at 2 μg/ min, plasma leucine concentration is reduced by >30%, reaching a new plateau within 90 minutes (Fig. 7). Infusing less epinephrine produces less suppression of amino acid concentrations (30). However, in contrast to insulin, the effect that epinephrine exerts on amino acid kinetics to reduce amino acid concentrations is transient. It is really not clear what the mechanism is by which epinephrine lowers amino acid concentrations. It must be either a decreased inflow of amino acids (reduced proteolysis) or an increased disposal (amino acid oxidation or protein synthesis). In vitro studies have not been very informative. The study of Miles et al. (33) suggests either an initial increase in disposal, a decrease in proteolysis, or both. Recent unpublished data from our laboratory tend to support the hypothesis that the primary event is amino acid removal, causing amino acid concentrations to fall. What is clear is that amino acid kinetics quickly return to normal while amino acid concentrations remain at the lower level (30). Because kinetics have returned to normal while amino acid concentrations remain low (30,31), it would appear that the primary effect of epinephrine on amino acid metabolism is to increase the metabolic efficiency of amino acid metabolism, i.e., to allow amino acid kinetics to operate normally at lower substrate concentrations. Clearly epinephrine does not cause a long-term increase in gluconeogenesis through amino acids because no net increase in protein catabolism can be found.

Although epinephrine blocks insulin secretion through alpha-adrenergic receptors and stimulates insulin secretion through beta-receptors, the changes seen in metabolic rate in response to epinephrine infusion have been shown to be independent of changes in insulin induced by epinephrine (78). Similar studies have been performed for glucose, FFA's, and ketone body metabolism. Epinephrine produces only transient increases in glucose production, lipolysis, and amino acid metabolism on the one hand, but increases REE for durations of at least 8 hours at physiologic concentrations of epinephrine (30,69) on the other hand. If epinephrine increases energy expenditure, one or more substrates must be used as a fuel. Epinephrine causes a dramatic transient increase in the respiratory quotient (RQ), indicating an initial glycogenolytic burst (69). However, this increase in RQ quickly subsides, leaving a hint that epinephrine may decrease RQ with time (69). Because any sustained increase in glucose production must be driven by increased gluconeogenesis and because no evidence exists that there is a significant increase in net amino acid catabolism (30), we do not feel that glucose contributes substantially to the increase in REE when epinephrine is elevated for a longer period. From the sustained concentrations of FFA and ketone bodies, we speculate that the primary fuel for the sustained, epinephrine-induced increase in REE is fat. What remains to be demonstrated is whether an elevation of epinephrine for 24 hours or longer will still elevate metabolic rate. There is a suggestion that epinephrine loses its effect of increasing energy expenditure with time (30).

CORTISOL

It has long been recognized that glucocorticoid excess causes wasting of lean body mass and accumulation of fat (79,80). Simmons et al. (19) determined the acute time course of cortisol action on protein metabolism in healthy postabsorptive adults. They demonstrated that elevating plasma cortisol into the high physiologic range commonly seen in stress (40 µg/dl) increased plasma leucine concentration by increasing leucine appearance rate (R_a) coming from proteolysis. They also noted a small increase in glucose concentration caused by a decreased utilization rather than increased R_a. The time course of this study appeared too short (8 hours) for the development of insulin resistance seen with hypercortisolemia. Hypercortisolemia induces a hyperglycemic state. In response, insulin concentration rises, yet the glucose concentration remains elevated, which is why cortisol is thought to induce a state of insulin resistance. Epinephrine exerts a direct effect on the β-cell to limit insulin secretion (75). The effect of cortisol comes by other means. When cortisol was infused into healthy subjects for longer periods of time (18), marked hyperglycemia was noticed by 12 hours and was sustained to the end of the infusion (64 hours). Insulin concentration climbed during the study, reaching a concentration of >20 µU/ml at the end. Hypercortisolemia increased both leucine and phenylalanine appearance rates by ≈15%. Because these studies were performed in the postabsorptive state, these increases in essential amino acid R_as reflect increased proteolysis. Cortisol induces even more dramatic increases in glutamine and alanine fluxes. These results suggest a dramatic outpouring of amino acid from muscle in the form of alanine and glutamine. Leg balance studies and muscle biopsies in dogs have confirmed cortisol's effect on reducing intracellular glutamine concentration and increasing efflux from muscle (20).

In a more recent study, Brillon et al. (81) addressed the question of the role of insulin in the production of the cortisol-induced increase in proteolysis. As discussed previously, insulin is a potent inhibitor of protein breakdown. Increasing plasma insulin concentration with cortisol infusion should reduce the response to cortisol in terms of protein breakdown, unless cortisol blocks the effects of insulin with respect to protein as it does with respect to glucose. The data in Fig. 8 show that infusing increasing doses of cortisol increases the rate of protein breakdown, as measured via phenylalanine R_a (81). Because the insulin concentration was also raised (from 9 to 15 μU/ml at the 200 μg/kg/h cortisol infusion rate), insulin should have suppressed proteolysis (e.g., as per Fig. 2). Therefore, normalizing insulin concentration with an infusion of somatostatin and basal replacement infusion of insulin and glucagon should have increased proteolysis and phenylalanine R_a. Because no elevation in phenylalanine R_a occurred with normalization of the insulin concentration, we conclude that cortisol induces an insulin-resistant state with respect to protein, as seen with glucose.

We (Brillon et al.) also measured REE in the subjects infused with cortisol in the aforementioned study (16). As illustrated in Fig. 9, infusing cortisol increased REE in a dose-dependent fashion. The increase in REE seen with cortisol infusion is of a similar magnitude to the increase in REE seen with similar physiologic elevations

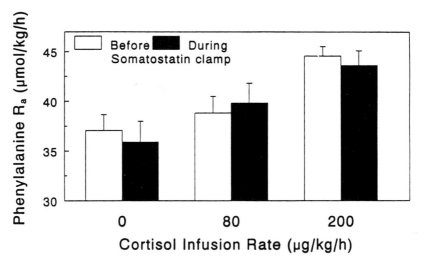

FIG. 8. Response of phenylalanine R_a to an overnight cortisol infusion into healthy adult men. Cortisol was infused for 14 hours. During the last 7 hours of cortisol infusion, phenylalanine flux was measured using ^{2}H-phenylalanine. During the last 3.5 hours, somatostatin with replacement amounts of insulin and glucagon were infused to normalize plasma insulin to basal postabsorptive concentration. Cortisol significantly increased phenylalanine R_a ($p < 0.001$). Reducing plasma insulin did not significantly alter phenylalanine R_a. Data adapted from Brillon et al. (81).

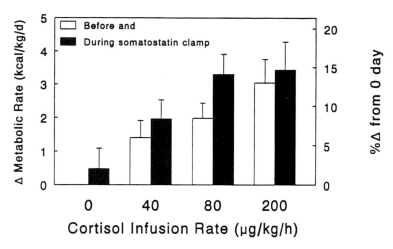

FIG. 9. Response of metabolic rate to an overnight cortisol infusion into healthy adult men. Cortisol was infused for 14 hours. During the last 7 hours of cortisol infusion, metabolic rate was measured. During the last 3.5 hours, somatostatin and replacement amounts of insulin and glucagon were infused to normalize plasma insulin to basal, postabsorptive concentration. The mean metabolic rate of the subjects was 23.4 ± 0.7 kcal/kg/d on the saline infusion day (0 μg/kg/h). The data are expressed as the difference from that day, paired for individual subjects. Cortisol significantly increased metabolic rate ($p < 0.001$) *(open bars)*. Reducing plasma insulin did not significantly alter metabolic rate *(shaded bars)*. Data adapted from Brillon et al. (16).

in epinephrine infusion (30,69). As in glucose and amino acids, when insulin concentration was reduced to normal, REE was not significantly altered. There was also an increase in FFA concentrations with cortisol infusion and a slight downward shift of the RQ. Both results indicate that the cortisol-induced increase in REE was fueled predominantly by fat (16). However, no increase in REE was found in subjects after treatment with prednisone for 9 days (35). It is possible that the effect of corticosteroids on energy expenditure wanes after several days or that prednisone does not produce the same metabolic effects as cortisol. The data in Fig. 9 suggest that cortisol is almost as potent as epinephrine in inducing an increase in energy expenditure. The data in Fig. 8 suggest that cortisol is almost as potent in increasing proteolysis as insulin is at suppressing it. These results indicate that cortisol may be the most important and potent of the endocrine hormones in generating the symptoms seen in stress and trauma.

Two studies have simulated the elevated hormonal pattern seen in stress and trauma in normal humans by infusing a combination of cortisol, glucagon, and catecholamines. Bessey et al. (68) infused a combination or individual stress hormones for 3 days into humans receiving normal foods as regular meals by mouth. They were able to demonstrate the characteristic insulin resistance, the increase in metabolic rate, and the increase in urinary N excretion seen in mild-to-moderate injury. Furthermore, they were able to attribute much of the observed effects to cortisol. Gelfand et al. (67) infused the stress hormones in combination or as cortisol alone in obese subjects receiving hypocaloric nutrition as intravenously infused dextrose. Either the combination of hormones or cortisol alone produced hyperglycemia, insulin resistance, and an increase in N loss. There was only a modest nonsignificant increase in energy expenditure. Although the metabolic response seen by Gelfand et al. was more modest than that found by Bessey et al., the subjects in the Gelfand study received inadequate caloric intake as an intravenous glucose infusion compared with a normal diet with adequate protein intake used by Bessey et al. This difference in nutritional intake may have been responsible for the differences in metabolic responses between the two studies. The conclusion of these two important studies was that the authors were able to simulate the hypermetabolic state of stress seen in injury and sepsis in normal subjects, but the response they found was much less than that seen in clinical patients, suggesting that other factors or combinations of factors (such as cytokines) were missing.

THERAPEUTIC USE OF HORMONES

If there is a beneficial side to the hypermetabolic response to stress, it must be the mobilization of fuel stores for those cells and tissues involved in the host-defense response and wound repair. White cells and cells involved in wound repair do not utilize fatty acids well and require glucose as energy substrate. After glycogen stores have been depleted within the first 24 hours postinjury, gluconeogenesis becomes the primary means of providing glucose. It is natural, therefore, that net protein catabolism must increase in order to supply amino acids to the liver for the liver to synthesize glucose. At the same time, the insulin resistance induced by the stress hormone response reduces the ability of insulin-sensitive tissues (e.g., muscle) to utilize glucose, thereby sparing the newly synthesized glucose for other tissues (3). However, protein is required for muscle function, and depletion of muscle protein cannot be maintained at an accelerated rate beyond several days. Nutritional support can provide the needed glucose calories and should resupply the lost amino acids, yet aggressive nutritional support does not prevent body protein loss in severe injury (82). Why does this occur *with* nutritional support? Are enough calories provided by the right source? Are specific amino acids needed in amounts greater than anticipated?

Insulin

Many metabolic actions elicited by insulin in normal physiology are anabolic, making insulin an ideal hormone to counteract the metabolic derangements during stress. Insulin reduces hyperglycemia by enhancing the rate of glucose uptake and oxidation in peripheral tissues and by reducing gluconeogenesis and glycogenolysis in the liver. Insulin greatly reduces protein breakdown and improves nitrogen balance. These effects of insulin should counteract the hyperglycemia, promote utilization of exogenous glucose, and reduce the accelerated protein catabolism seen in stress and trauma.

Unfortunately, insulin is much less effective during stress and trauma than it is under normal physiologic conditions. Plasma insulin is markedly elevated during stress, yet plasma glucose remains high, and body proteins are catabolized too rapidly (2). Hyperinsulinemia in stress probably develops in response to hyperglycemia, but the increased insulin secretion fails to return plasma glucose to a normal level. This phenomenon is the basis of the operative definition of insulin resistance (83). The reasons for which insulin resistance develops in stress and trauma and the role of insulin resistance in the metabolic derangements of stress and trauma are not clear. Both the hyperglycemia and the insulin resistance are likely caused by the increased concentrations of hormones that normally counteract the action of insulin. Cortisol is the most prominent hormone that causes insulin resistance, as outlined previously. One hypothesis is that a moderate degree of insulin resistance is beneficial for the injured organism (2). The stress hormones cortisol, epinephrine, and glucagon increase the production of glucose through gluconeogenesis. They also induce insulin resistance that limits the consumption of glucose by the "healthy" insulin-sensitive tissues. Therefore, more glucose is available for use by injured tissue and white cells, which do not depend on insulin for glucose utilization (2,84). The beneficial effect of this response is to provide more energy to the injured tissues; the negative effect is that body proteins are dissipated.

Because dissipation of protein stores cannot be indefinitely sustained, a major therapeutic benefit of administration of insulin is to promote utilization of glucose from *exogenous* sources and, by that, reduce protein catabolism for gluconeogenesis. To accomplish this goal, insulin must be administered to produce pharmacologic concentrations to overcome insulin resistance. The first goal of insulin therapy is to promote uptake of exogenous glucose and utilization by insulin-sensitive tissues. Because exogenous glucose is oxidized, endogenous glucose does not need to be produced and gluconeogenesis from amino acids is reduced, thus sparing the body proteins. In stress and trauma, glucose and protein metabolism are responsive to pharmacologic insulin concentrations. Insulin at high doses can overcome insulin resistance to achieve normoglycemia and inhibit protein catabolism after injury (85,86). After a major surgical stress, the insulin concentration required to achieve normoglycemia and a neutral nitrogen balance during the infusion of a TPN solution was increased approximately fourfold (87). Thus, if enough insulin and enough exogenous substrate are administered, insulin therapy can correct some of the metabolic derangements of stress and trauma. In clinical practice, insulin is customarily added to glucose solutions for infusion in trauma patients. However, insulin dosage is empirically adjusted for the endpoint of preventing hyperglycemia during glucose infusion rather than to improve the N balance. The latter goal requires administering more insulin and even more careful monitoring of the patients to prevent hypoglycemia. There is also the risk of development of respiratory and hepatic abnormalities with excessive infusion of glucose (88). Therefore, insulin with exogenous glucose administration may be effective in sparing protein, but a fine line exists between beneficial and harmful amounts of insulin and glucose delivery.

Growth Hormone

Growth hormone may be more useful than insulin in sparing protein by promoting protein anabolism. During the catabolic phase of stress, insulin resistance limits the anabolic effects of insulin. In contrast, under the same conditions where there is insulin resistance, growth hormone still exerts an anabolic effect. Insulin resistance in stress is due at least in part to the elevation of plasma cortisol, which is a powerful catabolic hormone. When growth hormone is administered to subjects already receiving cortisol, the positive effects of growth hormone are seen, and the catabolic effects of cortisol are reduced (35).

The goal of growth hormone administration to catabolic patients would be to reduce net protein utilization and amino acid oxidation by promoting protein synthesis. Several trials have demonstrated a beneficial effect of growth hormone administration on protein metabolism in injured, burned, or surgical patients (89–92). Two of those studies have focused on the effect of growth hormone on the metabolic efficacy of TPN in patients requiring parenteral feeding for gastrointestinal or pancreatic disease. Jiang et al. (89) administered growth hormone for 1 week to patients who, after surgery, received hypocaloric intravenous nutrition. They noted improved N retention and reduced weight loss in the growth hormone patients compared with patients receiving TPN alone. The improvement of N balance was attributed to increased protein synthesis. The study by Ziegler et al. confirmed that growth hormone improves N balance in stable patients with gastrointestinal/pancreatic disease receiving TPN (92). In another study, N excretion was reduced and protein synthesis was increased with growth hormone administration to patients during the catabolic phase of acute illness (sepsis and/or trauma) (91). At the same time, oxidation of fat was increased with the reduction in protein oxidation. Growth hormone administration in burned patients during the catabolic phase confirmed that growth hormone increases protein synthesis and improves N balance (90). These studies demonstrate use of an anabolic hormone to ameliorate the hypercatabolic state of stress and trauma. However, there appears to be attenuation of the anabolic effects of growth hormone therapy as the severity of the illness or injury increases. For this reason, an interest has developed in IGF-I as a therapeutic agent to produce a protein sparing effect without some of the complications of growth hormone. Unfortunately, our knowledge of the physiologic and metabolic effects of IGF-I administration to humans is lacking. Understanding the effects of IGF-I, both beneficial and detrimental, in normal humans is first required before therapeutic trials can be planned.

SUMMARY

The majority of the catabolic effects of stress (increased N loss and increased metabolic rate) can be attributed to alterations in the neuroendocrine hormonal axis (elevated cortisol, catecholamines, and glucagon—in decreasing order of importance). The "anabolic" hormones, insulin, and growth hormone are also often elevated in stress, but the body resists the effects of insulin. Insulin resistance for glucose as well as protein can be attributed to the elevations of the other stress hormones. However, it is difficult to mimic accurately normal stress response using an infusion of hormones alone, suggesting we are missing one or more important factors. The cytokine response may be the missing piece, but studies to date have been suggestive, not effective, in demonstrating in humans how the cytokines may be responsible.

ACKNOWLEDGMENTS

This work was supported in part by National Institutes of Health grants DK-38429 and RR-00047. Dr. Battezzati was a recipient of a grant from Istituto Scientifico San Raffaele, Milan, Italy.

REFERENCES

1. Cuthbertson DP. Observations on disturbance of metabolism produced by injury to the limbs. *Q J Med* 1932;25:233–246.
2. Frayn KN. Hormonal control of metabolism in trauma and sepsis. *Clin Endocrinol (Oxf)* 1986;24: 577–599.
3. Baue AE. Nutrition and metabolism in sepsis and multisystem organ failure. *Surg Clin North Am* 1991;71:549–565.
4. Cerami A. Inflammatory cytokines. *Clin Immunol Immunopathol* 1992;62:S3–S10.
5. Tracey KJ. TNF and other cytokines in the metabolism of septic shock and cachexia. *Clin Nutr* 1992;11:1–11.
6. Deitch EA. Multiple organ failure: pathophysiology and potential future therapy. *Ann Surg* 1992;216: 117–134.
7. Moncada S, Higgs EA. Endogenous nitric oxide: physiology, pathology and clinical relevance. *Eur J Clin Invest* 1991;21:361–374.
8. Lim VS, Tsalikian E, Flanigan MJ. Augmentation of protein degradation by L-triiodothyronine in uremia. *Metabolism* 1989;38:1210–1215.
9. Gelfand RA, Hutchinson-Williams KA, Bonde AA, et al. Catabolic effects of thyroid hormone excess: the contribution of adrenergic activity to hypermetabolism and protein breakdown. *Metabolism* 1987; 36:562–569.
10. Griggs RC, Kingston W, Jozefowicz RF, et al. Effect of testosterone on muscle mass and muscle protein synthesis. *J Appl Physiol* 1989;66:498–503.
11. Welle S, Jozefowicz R, Forbes G, Griggs RC. Effect of testosterone on metabolic rate and body composition in normal men and men with muscular dystrophy. *J Clin Endocrinol Metab* 1992;74: 332–335.
12. Fryburg DA, Louard RJ, Gerow KE, et al. Growth hormone stimulates skeletal muscle protein synthesis and antagonizes insulin's antiproteolytic action in humans. *Diabetes* 1992;41:424–429.
13. Fryburg DA, Gelfand RA, Barrett EJ. Growth hormone acutely stimulates forearm muscle protein synthesis in normal humans. *Am J Physiol* 1991;260:E499–E504.
14. Lundeberg S, Belfrage M, Wernerman J, et al. Growth hormone improves muscle protein metabolism and whole body nitrogen economy in man during a hyponitrogenous diet. *Metabolism* 1991;40: 315–322.
15. Fong Y, Rosenbaum M, Tracey KJ, et al. Recombinant growth hormone enhances muscle myosin heavy-chain mRNA accumulation and amino acid accrual in humans. *Proc Natl Acad Sci USA* 1989; 86:3371–3374.

16. Brillon DJ, Zheng B, Campbell RG, Matthews DE. Effect of cortisol and insulin on energy expenditure. *Clin Res* 1992;40:204A(abstr).
17. Beaufrere B. Horber FF, Schwenk WF, et al. Glucocorticosteroids increase leucine oxidation and impair leucine balance in humans. *Am J Physiol* 1989;257:E712–E721.
18. Darmaun D, Matthews DE, Bier DM. Physiological hypercortisolemia increases proteolysis, glutamine and alanine production. *Am J Physiol* 1988;255:E366–E373.
19. Simmons PS, Miles JM, Gerich JE, Haymond MW. Increased proteolysis: an effect of increases in plasma cortisol within the physiologic range. *J Clin Invest* 1984;73:412–420.
20. Muhlbacher F, Kapadia CR, Colpoys MF, et al. Effects of glucocorticoids on glutamine metabolism in skeletal muscle. *Am J Physiol* 1984;247:E75–E83.
21. Nair KS, Halliday D, Matthews DE, Welle SL. Hyperglucagonemia during insulin deficiency accelerates protein catabolism. *Am J Physiol* 1987;253:E208–E123.
22. Nair KS. Hyperglucagonemia increases resting metabolic rate in man during insulin deficiency. *J Clin Endocrinol Metab* 1987;63:896–901.
23. Pacy PJ, Cheng KN, Ford GC, Halliday D. Influence of glucagon on protein and leucine metabolism: a study in fasting man with induced insulin resistance. *Br J Surg* 1990;77:791–794.
24. Heslin MJ, Newman E, Wolf RF, et al. Effect of hyperinsulinemia on whole body and skeletal muscle leucine carbon kinetics in humans. *Am J Physiol* 1992;262:E911–E918.
25. Tessari P, Inchiostro S, Biolo G, et al. Effects of acute systemic hyperinsulinemia on forearm muscle proteolysis in healthy man. *J Clin Invest* 1991;88:27–33.
26. Frexes-Steed M, Lacy DB, Collins J, Abumrad NN. Role of leucine and other amino acids in regulating protein metabolism in vivo. *Am J Physiol* 1992;262:E925–E935.
27. Gelfand RA, Barrett EJ. Effect of physiologic hyperinsulinemia on skeletal muscle protein synthesis and breakdown in man. *J Clin Invest* 1987;80:1–6.
28. Tessari P, Trevisan R, Inchiostro S, et al. Dose-response curves of effects of insulin on leucine kinetics in humans. *Am J Physiol* 1986;251:E334–E342.
29. Fukagawa NK, Minaker KL, Rowe JW, et al. Insulin-mediated reduction of whole body protein breakdown: dose-response effects of leucine metabolism in postabsorptive men. *J Clin Invest* 1985; 76:2306–2311.
30. Matthews DE, Pesola G, Campbell RG. Effect of epinephrine upon amino acid and energy metabolism in humans. *Am J Physiol* 1990;258:E948–E956.
31. Castellino P, Luzi L, Del Prato S, DeFronzo RA. Dissociation of the effects of epinephrine and insulin on glucose and protein metabolism. *Am J Physiol* 1990;258:E117–E125.
32. Kraenzlin ME, Keller U, Keller A, et al. Elevation of plasma epinephrine concentrations inhibits proteolysis and leucine oxidation in man via β-adrenergic mechanisms. *J Clin Invest* 1989;84:388–393.
33. Miles JM, Nissen SL, Gerich JE, Haymond MW. Effects of epinephrine infusion on leucine and alanine kinetics in humans. *Am J Physiol* 1984;247:E166–E172.
34. Jeevanandam M, Ramias L, Shamos RF, Schiller WR. Decreased growth hormone levels in the catabolic phase of severe injury. *Surgery* 1992;111:495–502.
35. Horber FF, Marsh HM, Haymond MW. Differential effects of prednisone and growth hormone on fuel metabolism and insulin antagonism in humans. *Diabetes* 1991;40:141–149.
36. Castellino P, Luzi L, Simonson DC, et al. Effect of insulin and plasma amino acid concentrations on leucine metabolism in man: role of substrate availability on estimates of whole body protein synthesis. *J Clin Invest* 1987;80:1784–1793.
37. Flakoll PJ, Kulaylat M, Frexes-Steed M, et al. Amino acids augment insulin's suppression of whole-body proteolysis. *Am J Physiol* 1989;2570:E839–E847.
38. Barrett EJ, Revkin JH, Young LH, et al. An isotopic method for measurement of muscle protein synthesis and degradation in vivo. *Biochem J* 1987;245:223–228.
39. Denne SC, Liechty EA, Mei Liu Y, et al. Proteolysis in skeletal muscle and whole body in response to euglycemic hyperinsulinemia in normal adults. *Am J Physiol* 1991;261:E809–E814.
40. Batstone GF, Alberti KGMM, Hinks L, et al. Metabolic studies in subjects following thermal injury: intermediary metabolites, hormones and tissue oxygenation. *Burns* 1976;2:207–225.
41. Wilmore DW, Moylan JA, Pruitt BA, et al. Hyperglucagonaemia after burns. *Lancet* 1974;2:73–75.
42. Meguid MM, Brennan MF, Aoki TT, et al. Hormone-substrate interrelationships following trauma. *Arch Surg* 1974;109:776–783.
43. Lecavalier L, Bolli G, Gerich J. Glucagon-cortisol interactions on glucose turnover and lactate gluconeogenesis in normal humans. *Am J Physiol* 1990;258:E569–E574.
44. Couet C, Fukagawa NK, Matthews DE, et al. Plasma amino acid kinetics during acute states of glucagon deficiency and excess in healthy adults. *Am J Physiol* 1990;258:E78–E85.

45. Hartl WH, Miyoshi H, Jahoor F, et al. Bradykinin attenuates glucagon-induced leucine oxidation in humans. *Am J Physiol* 1990;259:E239–E245.
46. Cherrington AD, Williams PE, Shulman GI, Lacy WW. Differential time course of glucagon's effect on glycogenolysis and gluconeogenesis in the conscious dog. *Diabetes* 1981;30:180–187.
47. Lecavalier L, Bolli G, Cryer P, Gerich J. Contributions of gluconeogenesis and glycogenolysis during glucose counterregulation in normal humans. *Am J Physiol* 1989;256:E844–E851.
48. Wolfe BM, Culebras JM, Aoki TT, et al. The effects of glucagon on protein metabolism in normal man. *Surgery* 1979;86:248–257.
49. Wright PD, Johnston IDA. The effect of surgical operation on growth hormone levels in plasma. *Surgery* 1975;77:479–486.
50. Frayn KN, Price DA, Maycock PF, Carroll SM. Plasma somatomedin activity after injury in man and its relationship to other hormonal and metabolic changes. *Clin Endocrinol (Oxf)* 1984;20:179–187.
51. Göschke H, Bär E, Girard J, et al. Glucagon, insulin, cortisol, and growth hormone levels following major surgery: their relationship to glucose and free fatty acid elevations. *Horm Metab Res* 1978; 10:465–470.
52. Voerman HJ, Strack van Schijndel RJM, Groeneveld ABJ, et al. Pulsatile hormone secretion during severe sepsis: accuracy of different blood sampling regimens. *Metabolism* 1992;41:934–940.
53. Chwals WJ, Bistrian BR. Role of exogenous growth hormone and insulin-like growth factor I in malnutrition and acute metabolic stress: a hypothesis. *Crit Care Med* 1991;19:1317–1322.
54. Salomon F, Cuneo RC, Hesp R, Sönksen PH. The effects of treatment with recombinant human growth hormone on body composition and metabolism in adults with growth hormone deficiency. *N Engl J Med* 1989;321:1797–1803.
55. Jorgensen JOL, Thuesen L, Ingemann-Hansen T, et al. Beneficial effects of growth hormone treatment in GH-deficient adults. *Lancet* 1989;1221–1225.
56. Rudman D, Feller AG, Nagraj HS, et al. Effects of human growth hormone in men over 60 years old. *N Engl J Med* 1990;323:1–6.
57. Manson JM, Wilmore DW. Positive nitrogen balance with human growth hormone and hypocaloric intravenous feeding. *Surgery* 1986;100:188–197.
58. Manson JM, Smith RJ, Wilmore DW. Growth hormone stimulates protein synthesis during hypocaloric parenteral nutrition: role of hormonal substrate environment. *Ann Surg* 1988;208:136–142.
59. Horber FF, Haymond MW. Human growth hormone prevents the protein catabolic side effects of prednisone in humans. *J Clin Invest* 1990;86:265–272.
60. Turkalj I, Keller U, Ninnis R, et al. Effect of increasing doses of recombinant human insulin-like growth factor-I on glucose, lipid, and leucine metabolism in man. *J Clin Endocrinol Metab* 1992;75: 1186–1191.
61. Mauras N, Horber FF, Haymond MW. Low dose recombinant human insulin-like growth factor-I fails to affect protein anabolism but inhibits islet cell secretion in humans. *J Clin Endocrinol Metab* 1992;75:1192–1197.
62. Sherwin RS, Schulman GA, Hendler R, et al. Effect of growth hormone on oral glucose tolerance and circulating metabolic fuels in man. *Diabetologia* 1983;24:155–161.
63. Fong Y, Rosenbaum M, Hesse DG, et al. Influence of substrate background on peripheral tissue responses to growth hormone. *J Surg Res* 1988;44:702–708.
64. Moller N, Jorgensen JOL, Schmitz O, et al. Effects of a growth hormone pulse on total and forearm substrate fluxes in humans. *Am J Physiol* 1990;258:E86–E91.
65. Rizza RA, Mandarino LJ, Gerich JE. Effects of growth hormone on insulin action in man: mechanisms of insulin resistance, impaired suppression of glucose production, and impaired stimulation of glucose utilization. *Diabetes* 1982;31:663–669.
66. Cryer PE. Diseases of the sympathochromaffin system. In: Felig P, Baxter JD, Broadus AE, Frohman LA, eds. *Endocrinology and Metabolism.* 2nd ed. New York: McGraw-Hill, 1987;651–692.
67. Gelfand RA, Matthews DE, Bier DM, Sherwin RS. Role of counterregulatory hormones in the catabolic response to stress. *J Clin Invest* 1984;74:2238–2248.
68. Bessey PQ, Watters JM, Aoki TT, Wilmore DW. Combined hormonal infusion simulates the metabolic response to injury. *Ann Surg* 1984;200:264–281.
69. Staten MA, Matthews DE, Cryer PE, Bier DM. Physiologic increments in epinephrine stimulate metabolic rate in humans. *Am J Physiol* 1987;253:E322–E330.
70. Best JD, Halter JB. Release and clearance rates of epinephrine in man: importance of arterial measurements. *J Clin Endocrinol Metab* 1982;55:263–268.
71. Clutter WE, Bier DM, Shah SD, Cryer PE. Epinephrine plasma metabolic clearance rates and physiologic thresholds for metabolic and hemodynamic actions in man. *J Clin Invest* 1980;66:94–101.

72. Galster AD, Clutter WE, Cryer PE, et al. Epinephrine plasma thresholds for lipolytic effects in man: measurement of fatty acid transport with [1-^{13}C]palmitic acid. *J Clin Invest* 1981;67:1729–1738.
73. Rizza RA, Haymond M, Cryer P, Gerich J. Differential effects of epinephrine on glucose production and disposal in man. *Am J Physiol* 1979;237:E356–E362.
74. Clutter WE, Rizza RA, Gerich JE, Cryer PE. Regulation of glucose metabolism by sympathochromaffin catecholamines. *Diabetes Metab Rev* 1988;4:1–15.
75. Weiss M, Keller U, Stauffacher W. Effect of epinephrine and somatostatin-induced insulin deficiency on ketone body kinetics and lipolysis in man. *Diabetes* 1984;33:738–744.
76. Avogaro A, Cryer PE, Bier DM. Epinephrine's ketogenic effect on humans is mediated principally by lipolysis. *Am J Physiol* 1992;263:E250–E260.
77. Shamoon H, Jacob R, Sherwin RS. Epinephrine-induced hypoaminoacidemia in normal and diabetic human subjects: effect of beta blockade. *Diabetes* 1980;29:875–881.
78. Staten MA, Matthews DE, Cryer PE, Bier DM. Epinephrine's effect on metabolic rate is independent of changes in plasma insulin or glucagon. *Am J Physiol* 1989;257:E185–E192.
79. Sapir DG, Pozefsky T, Knochel JP, Walser M. The role of alanine and glutamine in steroid-induced nitrogen wasting in man. *Clin Sci Mol Med* 1977;53:215–220.
80. Roubenoff R, Roubenoff RA, Ward LM, Stevens MB. Catabolic effects of high-dose corticosteroids persist despite therapeutic benefit in rheumatoid arthritis. *Am J Clin Nutr* 1990;52:1113–1117.
81. Brillon DJ, Zheng B, Campbell RG, Matthews DE. Effect of cortisol and insulin on protein metabolism. *Diabetes* 1992;41:182A(abstr).
82. Wilmore DW. Catabolic illness: strategies for enhancing recovery. *N Engl J Med* 1991;325:695–702.
83. DeFronzo RA, Tobin JD, Andres R. Glucose clamp technique: a method for quantifying insulin secretion and resistance. *Am J Physiol* 1979;237:E214–E223.
84. Wilmore DW, Aulick LH. Metabolic changes in burned patients. *Surg Clin North Am* 1978;58:1173–1187.
85. Woolfson AMJ, Heatley RV, Allison SP. Insulin to inhibit protein catabolism after injury. *N Engl J Med* 1979;300:14–17.
86. Brooks DC, Bessey PQ, Black PR, et al. Insulin stimulates branched chain amino acid uptake and diminishes nitrogen flux from skeletal muscle of injured patients. *J Surg Res* 1986;40:395–405.
87. Brandi LS, Frediani M, Oleggini M, et al. Insulin resistance after surgery: normalization by insulin treatment. *Clin Sci* 1990;79:443–450.
88. Burke JF, Wolfe RR, Mullany CJ, et al. Glucose requirements following burn injury: parameters of optimal glucose infusion and possible hepatic and respiratory abnormalities following excessive glucose intake. *Ann Surg* 1979;190:274–285.
89. Jiang Z-M, He G-Z, Zhang S-Y, et al. Low-dose growth hormone and hypocaloric nutrition attenuate the protein-catabolic response after major operation. *Ann Surg* 1989;210:513–525.
90. Gore DC, Honeycutt D, Jahoor F, et al. Effect of exogenous growth hormone on whole-body and isolated-limb protein kinetics in burned patients. *Arch Surg* 1990;126:38–43.
91. Douglas RG, Humberstone DA, Haystead A, Shaw JHF. Metabolic effects of recombinant human growth hormone: isotopic studies in the postabsorptive state and during parenteral nutrition. *Br J Surg* 1990;77:785–790.
92. Ziegler TR, Rombeau JL, Young LS, et al. Recombinant human growth hormone enhances the metabolic efficacy of parenteral nutrition: a double-blind, randomized controlled study. *J Clin Endocrinol Metab* 1992;74:865–873.

Organ Metabolism and Nutrition:
Ideas for Future Critical Care, edited by
J. M. Kinney and H. N. Tucker.
Raven Press, Ltd., New York © 1994.

2

Human Skeletal and Cardiac Muscle Proteolysis: Evolving Concepts and Practical Applications

Michael J. Rennie

Department of Anatomy and Physiology, University of Dundee,
Dundee DD1 4HN, United Kingdom

The recognition of skeletal muscle as a tissue with roles as a store of fuel and amino acids and as a metabolic factory (1,2), in addition to its functions in locomotion and support of the body, has stimulated much scientific investigation. Information is now available about the extent of physiological and pathophysiological changes in the muscle mass (3), the net uptake or loss of amino acids from muscle (4), and the extent of intermediary amino acid metabolism, such as transamination and oxidation of branched-chain amino acids, glutamine synthesis, etc. (4–6), although much of the knowledge has been derived from work in animal rather than human muscle. We know much less about the processes that regulate the protein mass in muscle, i.e., protein synthesis and protein breakdown. Increasing efforts are now being made to apply appropriate methods to provide a description of what happens to protein synthesis in human skeletal muscle under a wide variety of physiologic and pathologic circumstances (7–13) (Fig. 1). When we turn to a consideration of protein breakdown in muscle and heart, however, it is apparent that not only is there less data available than for protein synthesis, but there is even less of a unifying theoretical framework within which to interpret the available information, especially in terms of its pathophysiologic relevance. There are few clear links between the results of different strands of work concerning, for example, activities of individual proteolytic enzymes, overall rates of protein breakdown, rates of breakdown of individual classes of proteins (e.g., myofibrillar proteins), and the exchange of amino acids or their tracers across limbs. As in other areas of physiology and pathophysiology, much of the basic work has been done in animals, and we still do not know to what extent this is directly applicable to the human circumstance. This chapter reviews the present status of the field to identify areas where there is a prospect of progress and to identify things we should be doing to foster such progress.

23

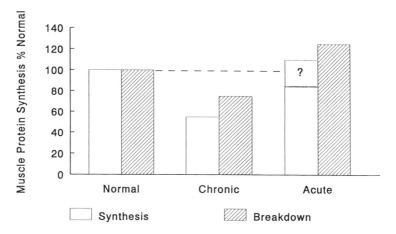

FIG. 1. Likely pattern of changes in muscle protein turnover in a variety of conditions causing chronic or acute muscle wasting. The box with the question mark signifies that we are uncertain whether protein synthesis falls or rises as a result of severe trauma, infection, or burns, but the likelihood is that, in trauma at least, it falls. There are insufficient data to allow certainty about the effects of infection or burn injury.

OVERVIEW OF THE MECHANISMS OF MUSCLE PROTEOLYSIS

Although protein breakdown is known to vary during muscle growth, as a result of a variety of nutritional and hormonal influences as well as during metabolic disease and following injury, knowledge of the mechanisms involved has accumulated slowly. It now seems reasonable, however, to conclude that muscle, like other mammalian tissues, contains a variety of proteolytic pathways, which probably have distinct physiological functions (14,15). For example, different cell components, such as the myofibrils or membrane proteins, may be degraded by mechanisms that are effectively independent of each other. This, of course, poses problems in understanding how such disparate processes are regulated to provide an overall and physiologically meaningful balance of amino acids contributing to the maintenance of the protein mass, or the supply of substrates for energy and protein metabolism in the rest of the body, as appropriate.

The lysosome is a major component of the proteolytic apparatus in most mammalian cells. This organelle has, enclosed within its membrane, the cathepsins, (acid proteases) plus a variety of other hydrolases. It appears to be important in the normal turnover of membrane proteins and receptor glycoproteins (a small portion only of the total cell protein mass) and may also become involved under conditions of nutritional deprivation in the proteolysis of cytoplasmic proteins. In liver and other tissues it is easy to identify and even isolate lysosomes, as well as the more voracious enlarged versions of them, the autophagic vacuoles, which arise under conditions that stimulate proteolysis, such a fall in availability of amino acids or insulin (16,17). In heart and skeletal muscle, direct morphological evidence of the involvement of lysosomes and autophagic vacuoles is harder to obtain, and such evidence as exists usually comes from experiments using inhibitors known to depress lysosomal activity in other tissues. For example, since the cathepsins work best at acid pH, if total proteolysis falls after the application of alkalizing reagents (e.g., weak bases, such as methylamine or chloraquine) or of specific inhibitors for cathepsins (such as leupeptin), the facts can be interpreted as indicating the involvement of lysosomal processes (15). Thus, rat and human muscle incubated in the absence of insulin shows an increase in net protein breakdown (15,18,19) which is proportional to the total lysosomal concentration (19) and is suppressible by the addition of chloraquine and methylamine or leupeptin (20). Experiments such as these have led to the conclusion that the muscle lysosomal apparatus makes little contribution to net proteolysis under optimal nutritional hormonal and mechanical conditions (15,21); furthermore, lysosomes are almost certainly *not* involved in the normal turnover of myofibrillar proteins (22,23), which comprise about two thirds of the total muscle protein.

Muscle also contains a variety of neutral calcium-dependent proteases, such as calpain I and calpain II. Although these can be stimulated by any circumstance that causes a substantial rise is sarcoplasmic calcium (to an extent normally only seen as a result of severe ischemia, anoxia, or inflammatory damage to muscle), they do not appear to be involved in the normal turnover of cellular protein (15,23). It seems, therefore, that the calcium-dependent proteases are probably only involved in end-stage proteolysis in damaged tissues (23,24).

Careful studies carried out by incubating muscle at resting length in a calcium-free medium with specific inhibitors of sarcoplasmic reticulum and mitochondrial calcium release have enabled cellular adenosine triphosphate (ATP) concentration to be depleted by anoxia without causing cell disruption (25,26). Such techniques have suggested that there is a component of overall muscle protein breakdown that is energy-dependent, the rate of which can be altered by nutritional and hormonal interventions (27,28). This process is likely to involve the soluble ATP-dependent, ubiquitin-requiring proteolytic pathway, which has been most fully described in reticulocytes and bacterial cells (29) but also exists in muscle (30). Its characteristic feature is the covalent linking (via an ATP-dependent process involving a number of distinct enzymatic steps) of the polypeptide ubiquitin to ε-amino groups on lysine residues in proteins destined for proteolysis. Once the protein has been "tagged" with ubiquitin, it may then be degraded by a complex of ubiquitin-conjugate degrading enzymes, which reside in the sarcoplasm. This process appears to be responsible for much of the basal protein breakdown in skeletal muscle, according to Kettelhut et al. (15).

In addition to the ATP-dependent ubiquitin pathway there appears to be another related ubiquitin-independent pathway that involves a large proteolytic complex (650 kd), christened the "proteasome" (31). The proteasome resembles nonlysosomal degradation pathways found in mitochondria and also in archaeobacteria to which mitochondria are evolutionarily related. The 650 kd proteasome has a multicatalytic function, which can apparently operate both independently of other proteolytic pathways as an ATP-dependent protease or as part of the ATP-dependent, ubiquitin-dependent pathway. In mammalian muscle, the large (1300 to 1500 kd) ubiquitin-dependent complex is formed by the ATP-dependent association of the proteasome with another ATP-dependent protease complex, multipain. Little is known about the physiological roles and mechanisms of these proteases in muscle, although it has been suggested that the proteasome is involved in antigen processing (32).

In agreement with the known higher rate of protein turnover in red muscle than in white muscle, both in animals (33) and humans (34,35), there appear to be greater amounts of lysosomal enzymes in red muscle; furthermore, more ubiquitin conjugates can be immunohistochemically localized to the Z-band (36) of red than white muscle. In the heart, the complexes are also found at Z-bands and at the intercalated discs (37). These facts suggest that the ubiquitin pathway may have an especially important function in controlling the macromolecular or even sarcomeric structure of skeletal and cardiac muscle.

METHODS APPROPRIATE TO THE STUDY OF PROTEIN BREAKDOWN IN VIVO AND IN VITRO

Much of our understanding of the biochemistry of protein breakdown has been obtained in cell-free homogenates of bacteria, reticulocytes, hepatocytes, and other mammalian cells (29,38) and then applied to the study of heart and skeletal muscle. Studies of the physiology and pathophysiology of muscle proteolysis have usually been carried out using whole incubated muscles (39) or isolated perfused systems (40), and results are rarest of all from in vivo studies (41,42). There are a limited number of approaches available for the study of protein breakdown in skeletal muscle, of whatever preparation, and each has advantages and disadvantages.

Estimation of Protein Breakdown from Changes in Protein Concentration

Information about individual protein components can often be obtained by using the approach of Schimke and colleagues, who showed that imposing a square wave stimulus often caused an induction of some protein component, which showed an exponential rise to a new plateau concentration (38,43). An examination of the kinetics shows that the rate of approach to the plateau depends only on the rate of breakdown of the protein. Schimke used this technique to investigate whether the rate of breakdown after induction was different to that before induction by following the time course of the decay back to the unstimulated state after removal of the stimulus. If the fall in the concentration of the component had the same kinetics as its rise, then obviously protein breakdown before and after application of the stimulus must have been the same. However, if protein breakdown fell more rapidly, then obviously during stimulation protein breakdown must have been depressed below its normal state. (The rates of synthesis in the basal state and after induction can be calculated because the rate of protein synthesis is simply the steady-state concentration of protein multiplied by the fractional breakdown rate.) One of the problems with this method is the uncheckable assumption that the rates of synthesis and breakdown remain constant during the periods of measurement.

Although this method has produced some valuable information for particular enzymes (see [43] for review), it appears not to have been used widely for muscle. This approach can certainly be used in tissue culture and even in vivo in certain circumstances (e.g., to look at the effects of exercise training on cytochrome oxidase activity) (44). It has not, so far as I am aware, been applied to studies of hormonal or nutritional intervention or indeed to the effects of injury on animal muscle; nor has it been applied to the study of human muscle, although with current biopsy techniques, (45) it ought to be feasible.

Breakdown Rate Measured by Efflux of Non-metabolizable Amino Acids

Some mature proteins contain unique amino acids produced by the post-translational modification of an amino acid residue; when the protein is broken down, the amino acid cannot be incorporated since there is no corresponding tRNA, and the amino acid is, therefore, lost from the tissue without further modification. Examples of such amino acids are hydroxyproline (produced by the hydroxylation of proline residues in collagen) and 3-methylhistidine, which is formed by the methylation of histidine residues in actin in all muscles and of myosin in white muscles (46). Obviously, measurement of rate of the release from tissues of hydroxyproline or 3-methylhistidine allows the specific quantitation of the rates of collagen and myofibrillar protein breakdown. There seems to be no work in which hydroxyproline A-V differences have been measured across limbs in humans, but 3-methylhistidine has been so measured (47–50) and produced valuable information. These methods can also be applied in tissue culture and in studies of perfused or isolated incubated muscles (23,51).

Amino acids that are involved in protein turnover but not in muscle intermediary metabolism, such as tyrosine, are also useful. If cycloheximide is used to block protein synthesis, tyrosine release will provide a measure of the average rate of breakdown for all protein in the tissue (23) or for particular proteolytic processes if others are specifically blocked (15). Strictly speaking, this is, of course, only applicable in vitro, but the measurement of tyrosine efflux in vivo is not worthless because it represents the net balance of protein synthesis and breakdown. Comparison of its efflux with changes in 3-methylhistidine efflux have been useful in dissecting out some of the physiological and pathophysiological influences on muscle protein breakdown (52,53).

Loss of Label from Previously Labelled Protein

In principle the method is simple: If a protein can be labelled by a pulse of isotope, then the breakdown rate can be determined from the rate of loss of label; if both the fractional and total labelling of the protein are known, then protein synthesis can be calculated in addition (43). Furthermore, given the controversy over the past five years (e.g. 11,13,126) concerning the correct assignment of labelling to that part of the free amino acid pool, which is the precursor for protein synthesis, a major advantage of the decay curve method is that it avoids this problem. In practice, the method can only be applied if it is possible to obtain a pure protein, and there is no reutilization of label, and the total amount of the protein in the tissue of interest is known. For certain muscle proteins, such as actin and myosin, it is not too difficult to obtain pure proteins by simple extraction methods, and other interesting proteins also may be obtainable in a sufficient pure state by using immunological techniques. However, the problems associated with recycling of amino acid label are such that no technique has been able to eliminate it completely, although the use of label delivered as carbonate comes close to doing so. Swick and Ipp (54) showed that when ^{14}C carbonate was fed to rats, labelled carbon appeared in the alpha-carboxyl groups of glutamate, glycine, serine, and glutamine and into both carboxyl groups of aspartate as a result of metabolic exchange, mainly in the liver. On breakdown from protein, any labelled amino acids should be rapidly diluted by *de novo* synthesis of such amino acids so that reutilization would be minimized. The reutilization of bicarbonate-delivered label approaches zero for aspartate and glutamate. Since muscle has a much narrower repertoire of amino acid metabolism, it was not surprising that Manchester and Young could show that in isolated incubated diaphragm only glutamate and aspartate became labelled (55). When Waterlow et al. applied the $^{14}CO_3^-$ technique in studies of rat skeletal muscle in vivo, (43) he found rates of synthesis of muscle proteins which agreed closely with those obtained by infusion of glycine or lysine. Special modifications of the method include the labelling of 3-methylhistidine with labelled methionine, and this method has been used in animals (56) but, so far as I know, never in people.

Measurements of decay rates have to be made over long periods of time, much longer than those necessary for measurement of amino acid incorporation, and ideally a period of at least one half-life is necessary to observe a sufficiently large change. For many structural muscle proteins, this is a long period; since myofibrillar protein turnover in man is ~1% to 2%/day, the half-life is of the order of 1 to 2 months. The method is, therefore, only practically applicable to studies of such proteins during long-term interventions, or for shorter periods to studies of proteins which turn over quickly in intact muscle or in systems which generally show fast turnover, such as cultured cells. Immunochemical methods to isolate specific individual proteins will obviously facilitate the preparation of pure identifiable proteins, but the immunoreactivity of a protein may alter within its lifetime, especially once it has been partially processed for protein breakdown, and this may introduce artifacts.

Of course, when dealing with a whole human being, the only way in which a decay curve for a labelled protein could be obtained would be by repeated biopsy sampling of tissues. Although this is possible for muscle and skin, it obviously poses a considerable limitation. Theoretically, this technique could be modified to limit the number of biopsies required to a minimum of two by using the carbonate labelling method with, for example, ^{13}C and ^{18}O. The technique would be to give a sufficient dose of [^{13}C]carbonate to allow the labelling of aspartate and glutamate in muscle and then, at some time later, to give more carbonate, but this time labelled with ^{18}O, followed within a few hours by a biopsy. Aspartate and glutamate isolated from a given protein, by preparative HPLC or GC (57), would be assayed for ^{13}C and ^{18}O. If it is assumed that for any given protein, the synthesis rate remained constant between the two injections, then depending on which isotope was given second, its isotope ratio would be a measure of the initial incorporation rate (the synthesis rate), and the ratio of the first and second labels would be a measure of the decay rate and, thus, of the breakdown rate. Ideally two biopsies would be needed—one to establish the basal labelling with ^{13}C and ^{18}O of glutamate and aspartate and one to establish the labelling ratios after the second dose of label. However, if sufficient labelled carbonate were given (which would be expensive for ^{18}O-labelled carbonate because it will exchange into the large water pool of the body), and the interindividual variation in basal ^{18}O and ^{13}C labelling was sufficiently small, then only a single biopsy would be required. A similar approach could be used with ^{13}C- and ^{2}H-labelled methionine (labelled on the methyl group) or proline to label 3-methylhistidine in actin and hydroxyproline in collagen. This method depends crucially on obtaining pure samples of a given protein; if a heterogeneous mixture of proteins is mistakenly analyzed, then the decay curve would be multiexponential, the log decay curve would not be linear, and measurement at a single point would be meaningless. Thus, there may be justification for taking additional biopsies to ensure that the protein is, in fact, sufficiently pure, i.e., shows a monoexponential loss of label.

Isotope Dilution Methods

Protein breakdown results in the release of amino acid from the protein pool. If a free amino acid of known, labelling is introduced into the free pool, then the extent of protein breakdown can be estimated by the extent of the dilution of the tracer by amino acids entering from protein breakdown. This is the basis of the method that has been used to determine protein turnover in organs for which access to the arterial supply and the venous drainage can be conveniently obtained—in man, the forearm and the heart (9,58–60). The technique has been used widely in perfused animal preparations of liver, muscle, and gastrointestine and, theoretically, could be used more widely in man, as long as appropriate amino acid tracers are used. The key criterion is that the amino acid should not undergo intermediary metabolism, though of course it should participate in protein turnover! For muscle, phenylalanine is a good tracer if it is labelled on the carbon chain (using ^{13}C or ^{14}C) or if one of the hydrogens on a carbon is labelled (with ^{2}H or ^{3}H). However, use of the ^{15}N-labelled phenylalanine is *not* ideal because there is a certain amount of transaminase L and K in skeletal muscle (61), which causes transfer (and therefore loss) of the ^{15}N label from phenylalanine to other amino acids, probably resulting in an overestimation of breakdown, and because of the algebra involved, of synthesis (59). The technique also can be used with ^{13}C- or ^{14}C-labelled, branched-chain amino acids, as long as the extent of transamination and oxidation is measured as the appearance of the labelled α-ketoacid and CO_2 (59,62). Other suitable, possible, non-metabolizable tracer amino acids for use in muscle include lysine, threonine, serine, glycine, cysteine, tryptophan, tyrosine, and histidine, with methionine and arginine possibly excluded because of metabolism in accessory tissues. In fact, apart from tyrosine, none of these candidates appears to have been used, probably because of a combination of measurement difficulties and large intramuscular pool sizes, which buffer the true protein turnover rates.

PHYSIOLOGY OF MUSCLE PROTEIN BREAKDOWN

As far as possible, the original work cited in support of the statements describing the normal physiology of proteolysis is drawn from studies in people, but, inevitably, citations to animal work predominate.

Changes during Normal Growth and during Hypertrophy

During normal growth (43,63), rehabilitation from malnutrition, and the muscle growth associated with weight lifting or weight bearing (64), the muscle protein breakdown rate changes in a way that appears to be adapted to the rate of protein synthesis (43); i.e., net accretion of tissue is associated with rises in both. Marked changes occur during postnatal growth, with the turnover rate falling from a high value at birth to a much lower one in mature animals and in adults. Protein breakdown in adult muscle shows little further fall after maturity, if 3-methylhistidine excretion data are to be believed (46,65–67) (but see [68] for criticisms of the urinary 3-methylhistidine method). Nevertheless, some recent work concerning rates of muscle protein synthesis measured by using [^{13}C]leucine incorporation in the elderly suggests that the protein synthetic rate in muscle is depressed as aging proceeds (S. R. Welle, personal communication), and it seems likely that muscle turnover in people generally falls with aging at the very least because of the loss of type I muscle fibers and ribosomal capacity (69,70). The rapid rise in human muscle protein synthesis shortly after a bout of weight lifting (71) suggests that, in human beings also, muscle hypertrophy is accompanied by an increase in the rate of protein breakdown, or the rate of muscle accretion would be much higher than is observed in practice (72).

Effect of Nutritional State

Starvation appears to be associated with an acute, short-term rise in muscle protein breakdown (9,73,74) (Fig. 2) followed by a longer term fall, which may be adaptive to the fall in protein synthesis that also generally accompanies starvation (28,63,75). In other words, muscle protein turnover seems to be depressed to the lowest possible state consistent with continued contractile activity and survival; during end-stage starvation, muscle protein breakdown probably rises uncontrollably (76).

The concentrations in muscle of mRNA for ubiquitin and the concentration of

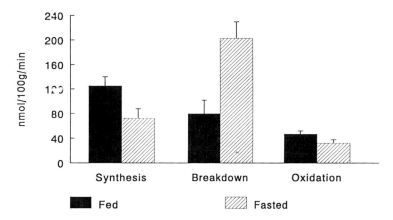

FIG. 2. Effects of concurrent feeding or fasting (12 to 18 hours) on muscle protein turnover measured by using the human forearm preparation. (From Rennie MJ. Metabolic insights from the use of stable isotopes in nutritional studies. *Clin Nutr* 1986;5:1–7. Used with permission.)

ubiquitinylated protein increase coordinately in muscle from short-term starved animals (15), and the changes parallel increases in the rate of ATP-dependent protein breakdown (18,34). It appears that myofibrillar protein breakdown cannot be suppressed by provision of sufficient energy alone, although sarcoplasmic protein can be; to suppress all muscle proteolysis sufficient energy and protein must be given (77). In malnutrition caused by consumption of a low protein diet, protein breakdown also falls (28), and the fall can be reversed by provision of an energy deficient but protein-adequate diet (42,43,63).

Kettelhut et al. (15) have suggested that, in rats at least, the reduction in protein breakdown during long-term starvation is due to a coordinate reduction of both the intralysosomal and nonlysosomal proteolytic systems, including ATP-dependent proteolysis. Furthermore, by using polyclonal antibodies to a peptide sequence which apparently targets proteins to lysosomes, it is possible to match increased lysosomal activity during starvation with depletion of proteins containing these sequences in liver and heart but *not* in skeletal muscle (78), which further supports the idea. Oddly, the capacity for neutral calcium-dependent proteolysis (in particular the activity of the calpains) increases during saturation at a time when overall proteolysis has decreased (27,28).

Variation in the availability of amino acids per se appears to have very little direct influence on muscle protein breakdown in any muscle preparation in vitro (79) or in vivo (80,81) (Fig. 3), suggesting that the effects seen in re-fed fasted rats in vivo (77) are having their effects via insulin or some other mediator. It is particularly noteworthy that although in the 1980s there was a lot of interest in the possibility that leucine or its transamination product α-ketoisocaproate might reduce muscle protein breakdown, and although such results can be seen reproducibly in healthy animal muscles in vitro (82,83) it has proved difficult to demonstrate any effects in vivo (84), espe-

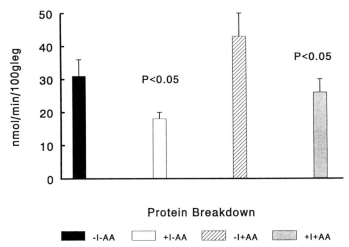

FIG. 3. Demonstration of lack of effect of amino acids on protein breakdown, but stimulation of protein synthesis in human leg investigated by the [^{13}C]leucine exchange method. (From Bennet WM et al. The effect of amino acid infusion on leg protein turnover assessed by L-[^{15}N]phenylalanine and L-[1-^{13}C]leucine exchange. *Eur J Clin Invest* 1990;20:41–50. Used with permission.

cially in people (85). And the evidence of any effect of leucine or alpha-ketoisoca-proate on muscle protein breakdown in humans is very limited (86). Also, even in isolated incubated muscle, no effects on either protein synthesis or breakdown can be shown in tissue from septic rats (87). It has been claimed that infusion of branched-chain amino acid decreases muscle protein breakdown in man when estimated by the phenylalanine and leucine tracer exchange methods (88), but the data presented are not unequivocal, and the absolute rates of proteolysis in the control condition do not match well the previously published data from the same group (58). Although amino acids appear to have little direct effect in suppressing protein breakdown in muscle, leucine may augment the effect of insulin in doing so (89). There are one or two reports that glutamine may suppress protein breakdown in cultured muscle cells and in perfused muscle tissue (90,91), but there is no evidence as yet to suggest that it has an inhibitory effect on protein breakdown in human muscle, and we have seen no such effects in man despite observing a significant stimulatory effect on muscle protein synthesis.

It seems likely that most of the changes that occur as a result of starvation are due to alterations in the availability of hormones (and possibly other mediators such as neurotransmitters and paracrine agents) and in the relative activity of muscle receptors for them. Of course without substrates for energy and protein synthesis, any hormonal or other mediator effect would be impossible. It seems, nevertheless, that the direct effects are small.

Other Possible Metabolic Effects in Regulating Muscle Protein Breakdown

Effects of variation in the availability of glucose, lactate, β-hydroxybutarate, fatty acids, and other substrates appear to be very minor at least, as far as skeletal muscle is concerned. The effect of insulin in suppressing proteolysis in heart and skeletal muscle may require the presence of glucose (15), and ketone bodies are reported to have an effect in suppressing proteolysis in muscle (92). There appear to be no direct effects of free fatty acids in suppressing muscle proteolysis. Oxidation of leucine may, to some extent, be inhibited by free fatty acids (93), but these effects are hardly likely to have a direct anabolic effect or to influence protein breakdown.

Effects of Hormones on Muscle Protein Breakdown

Insulin

Insulin has a profound inhibitory effect on muscle protein breakdown. The antiproteolytic effect of insulin is one of the earliest of its metabolic effects to be documented (94,95) and can be seen in a wide variety of preparations of animal and human skeletal and cardiac muscle (18,40,58,96–98) (Fig. 4).

Insulin reduces autophagic vacuole formation in the liver, and that the sensitivity of protein breakdown to inhibitors of lysosomal function is lessened by the addition of insulin suggests that insulin acts to inhibit the lysosomal processes in muscle as well (18). However, insulin appears *not* to have any effect on hydrolysis of skeletal muscle or cardiac myofibrillar proteins as judged by the production of 3-methylhistidine (24,51,98), strengthening the suggestion that its actions are confined to the fast turning-over proteins degraded by the lysosomal proteases. The sulphonylurea compound glyburide appears to act rather like insulin in inhibiting muscle proteolysis, but, unlike insulin, it does not stimulate protein synthesis (99).

Growth Hormone and Insulin-like Growth Factor I

There has been recent substantial interest in the possible anabolic effects of growth hormone in adults, and it appears that many of these effects are mediated via the

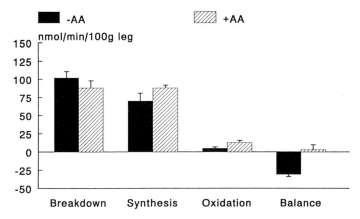

FIG. 4. Effect of insulin and amino acids on leg protein turnover indicated by phenylalanine exchange in diabetic subjects. (From Bennet WM et al. Effects of insulin and amino acids on leg protein turnover in IDDM patients. *Diabetes* 1991;40:499–508. Used with permission.)

insulin-like growth factors (IGF-I and IGF-II). IGF-I is synthesized in the liver and other tissues (including muscle) in response to growth hormone availability, and its rate of production depends not only on growth hormone but also on other metabolic features, such as dietary energy and protein intake, diabetes, and availability of other pituitary hormones.

Growth hormone itself appears to have no effect in depressing muscle protein breakdown, according to the results of studies involving leucine and phenylalanine tracer exchange across human muscle (100,101). However, somewhat surprisingly, growth hormone apparently antagonizes the antiproteolytic effect of insulin in the human forearm (101).

IGF-I has, as its name suggests, insulin-like effects on protein breakdown, which are apparent at high concentration when it probably acts via the insulin receptor. Such effects can be seen in primary muscle cultures (102) and in incubated rat soleus and extensor digitalis longus (EDL) muscles, the extent and characteristics of the inhibition being entirely insulin-like (15). Nevertheless, in diabetic rats, treatment with recombinant IGF-I had no or little effect on muscle protein breakdown, although insulin had a rapid inhibitory effect (103). Also, despite the persistence of IGF-I receptors in muscles, IGF-I seems to be unable to ameliorate protein breakdown in muscle of growth-retarded rats or in rats on a low-protein diet (104,105).

Glucocorticoids

Large doses of glucocorticoids increase protein breakdown, and this can be seen not only in isolated incubated muscles (106) and in perfused animal preparations (106) but also in animals and patients in vivo (107–109). The effect seems mainly to be due to a stimulation of myofibrillar protein breakdown although nonmyofibrillar proteolysis is stimulated to some extent (15,106,110). The corticosteroid receptor blocker, RU 38486, can completely abolish the effects of corticosterone on myofibrillar protein breakdown in appropriately treated rats in vivo (110). The effects of submaximal doses of glucocorticoids depend to some extent on nutritional status because insulin and the glucocorticoids antagonize each other's actions, so the effect of glucocorticoids in stimulating protein breakdown is ameliorated in the fed state (107,111). Oddly, there appears to be tachyphylaxis of protein breakdown to corticosteroids in otherwise healthy animals because the stimulation is diminished after a few days of treatment (106,108,109). It appears that in the fed state in vivo, prolonged corticosteroid treatment is antagonized by increased insulin secretion, but the effect only ameliorates the nonmyofibrillar proteolysis, and myofibrillar proteolysis is independent not only of insulin but also of thyroid hormone status, which therefore cannot explain the tachyphylaxis. Thus, a circumstance that causes a prolonged elevation of glucocorticoids will inevitably promote the loss of muscle protein through a suppression of protein synthesis, nonmyofibrillar proteolysis in the fed state, and more marked effects in the fasted state.

The effects of anabolic steroids on muscle protein breakdown have not been investigated in detail. However, it appears that any effects on muscle protein deposition are more likely to be effects on protein synthesis (12,112) than on breakdown because trenbolone acetate appears to have no effect on protein breakdown in growing cattle (113).

Thyroid Hormones

Thyroid hormones have a marked effect on protein turnover, which can be partially deduced from the phenomenology of parallel depression of protein turnover and of thyroid hormone status during starvation (41). Thyroid hormones stimulate protein breakdown, and that a depression of 3-methylhistidine excretion can be seen in starved and hypothyroid animals and patients strongly suggests that thyroid hormones stimulate nonlysosomal pathways of proteolysis (15,66). However, thyroid hormones also cause an increase in muscle lysosomal protease activity (15), and hypophysectomy decreases all pathways of proteolysis except the Ca^+-dependent ones (15). In untreated hypothyroid patients, muscle protein breakdown measured as 3-methylhistidine release is depressed; it is elevated in hyperthyroid patients (114).

It may also be that the thyroid hormones are involved in setting the level of sensitivity to other hormones. Such a mechanism would provide a useful adaptive advantage in modulating the responses of different classes of muscle proteins to short- and long-term fasting.

Adrenergic Agents

It has been known for some years that (perhaps unexpectedly, given their fight-or-flight role) catecholamines have an anabolic effect in muscle, but the mechanisms are not well understood. The nature of the effects are particularly paradoxical when it is realized that to obtain the full-blown "injury response profile" of muscle and plasma amino acids and a decrease in ribosomal capacity, adrenaline infusion is necessary in conjunction with infusion of other counterregulatory hormones, e.g., glucocorticoids and glucagon (115–118). It may be that in vivo the responses are partly the result of interaction via presently unknown signals between nonmuscle tissues and organs and muscle, but, in isolated muscle, glucagon has no effect until extremely high pathophysiological concentrations are applied (119). The synergism of the so-called triple-hormone response remains unexplained.

In fact, a survey of the literature shows that although the anabolic effect of catecholamines can now be generally accepted as being mediated via stimulation of beta-receptors, the mechanisms involved are still far from clear because some authors find effects on synthesis only, others find effects on breakdown, and some find effects on both. Clenbuterol, a nontypical β_2-agonist which causes preferential deposition of nutrient as lean tissue in farm animals (and judging by its popularity with body builders, also works to promote human skeletal muscle growth), is said by some workers to have an anabolic effect apparently independent of any inhibitory effects on acid, neutral, or alkaline proteinases (120), suggesting that the anabolism is entirely dependent on the stimulation of muscle protein synthesis. However, the beta-agonist cimaterol inhibits protein breakdown in isolated chick extensor digitorum communis muscles without affecting protein synthesis (121), and metaproterenol, a mixed beta-agonist, is reported to decrease muscle protein breakdown without increasing muscle protein synthesis (122). One possibility which should be explored is that different beta-agonists have different specific effects on myofibrillar and soluble protein synthesis and breakdown. Such a possibility is strengthened by the observation that beta$_2$-agonists decrease release of 3-methylhistidine and beta$_2$-antagonists inhibit such effects of clenbuterol (123).

EFFECTS OF INJURY, CANCER, AND INFECTION

Chronic Muscle Wasting

By and large, it appears that in a wide variety of chronic muscle wasting conditions, including cirrhosis, malnutrition, many slow growing cancers, chronic cardiac failure and chronic obstructive pulmonary disease, and some primary and endocrine myopathies, muscle protein breakdown, far from being elevated, may actually be depressed, in line with a general decrease in protein turnover. The evidence has been discussed in previous reviews (52,124–126) and will not be further rehearsed here, except to say that the changes seem to be similar to those observed in the models of energy and protein malnutrition previously discussed, which may suggest a common mechanism (a fall in ATP-dependent proteolysis?) between these responses.

Effects of Contractile Activity and Immobilization on Muscle Protein Breakdown

A number of workers have demonstrated that muscles kept at resting length, in vitro, show a lower rate of net loss of protein than those allowed to lie flaccid (15,21,127). Because it is a matter of common observation that muscle bulk depends on continued use, it is no surprise that weight lifting or weight bearing at high fractions of maximal voluntary contraction causes growth of muscle. Both in animals and man there appear to be increases in muscle protein synthesis that are sufficiently large that concomitant increases in muscle protein breakdown would be possible, and indeed likely, given that the rate of increase of muscle bulk is relatively modest (128) (Fig. 5). Contractile activity at lower proportions of maximal strength, i.e., those that can be sustained for long periods of time at power outputs below the maximal oxygen consumption, causes modification of muscle composition, chiefly alterations in myosin ATPase and the concentration of mitochondria (129). Exercise of this type appears to decrease muscle protein synthesis during the exercise bout and seems not to stimulate muscle protein breakdown (130–132). After exercise,

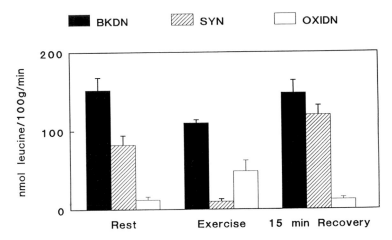

FIG. 5. Effect of isometric exercise on muscle protein turnover in normal healthy subjects. (From Rennie, MJ et al. Amino acid and protein metabolism during exercise. In: Devlin J, Horton ES, Vranic M (eds). *Diabetes Mellitus and Exercise.* London: Smith-Gordon, 1992.)

protein breakdown probably rises, and if there is some remodelling, then this must involve myofibrillar protein breakdown as well. Nevertheless, in studies of tyrosine and 3-methylhistidine release from isolated incubated muscles prepared from rats that were exercised on a treadmill (133), it appeared that there was no increase in myofibrillar protein breakdown, but total protein breakdown was elevated, suggesting that sarcoplasmic protein degradation was increased. Furthermore, the lysosomal inhibitor chloroquine has no effect on protein breakdown, suggesting that some nonlysosomal pathway is stimulated. However, such a pathway cannot be the one that is normally responsible for myofibrillar protein breakdown, for obvious reasons.

Studies in immobilized patients suggest that muscle protein turnover falls as a result of immobilization and rises again following remobilization and regrowth (Table 1). Certainly wasting occurs as a result of long-term immobilization, and the principal factor appears to be a fall of protein synthesis below the rate of muscle protein breakdown (134–136). A similar interpretation can be reached from the consideration of the literature concerning casting in animals. However, hypokinesia as a result of hindlimb suspension may involve an increase in muscle protein breakdown (137).

Denervation and Surgical and Thermal Injuries

The muscle atrophy induced by denervation appears to be due to a fall in protein synthesis plus increases in protein breakdown involving nearly all the degradative pathways, including the calcium-dependent pathways as well as the nonlysosomal, energy-dependent pathways (24,74,138). The clinical definition of denervation injury should probably be widened to include not only direct damage to muscle or nerves

TABLE 1. *Effect of immobilization on quadriceps protein turnover.*

	Control leg	Immobilized leg	Δ	
Synthesis (% day^{-1})	1.50 ± 0.50	1.00 ± 0.57	−30%	$p < 0.05$
Wasting (%/day^{-1})	0	0.31 ± 0.05	—	—
Calculated breakdown (%/day^{-1})	1.50 ± 0.50	1.31 ± 0.55	−12%	$p < 0.05$

From Rennie MJ. Metabolic insights from the use of stable isotopes in nutritional studies. *Clin Nutr* 1986;5:1–7.

Patients were studied after 35 days with one leg immobilized after a fracture. [I-^{13}C]leucine was infused for 7 hours to label muscle protein, analyzed after needle biopsy. Protein synthesis was calculated by reference to blood α-ketoisocaproate labelling. Protein breakdown was estimated by measurement of fiber area loss of muscle, using control leg remained in base state and from muscle protein concentration ($n = 6$, mean ± SD).

but also local secondary nerve damage of unknown etiology, as seems to occur in long-term intensive care patients, especially those with multiple organ failure according to the characteristic patterns of fiber loss and grouping observed (139).

Thermal and surgical traumas appear to have different effects on muscle protein breakdown in animal muscle; aseptic thermal trauma increased myofibrillar and sarcoplasmic muscle protein breakdown by threefold, but surgical trauma alone apparently had no effect on protein breakdown (101). Unfortunately, although it seems highly likely that burn injury in patients also involves decreases in muscle protein synthesis and increases in muscle (sarcoplasmic and myofibrillar) protein breakdown (140,141), the requisite measurements, e.g., using tracer incorporation or tracer A-V flux measurements, have simply not been made. Surgery per se definitely decreases human muscle protein synthesis by an anesthesia-independent mechanism (142,143), but no reliable data exist concerning protein breakdown itself, i.e., obtained by tracer flux methods. Measurements using the limb, arteriovenous 3-methyl-histidine method suggest that uncomplicated elective surgery is associated with a depression of myofibrillar protein breakdown (144).

Sepsis

The idea that there are particular blood-borne factors which stimulate muscle protein breakdown in sepsis (145), in some cancers associated with rapid development of cachexia, and possibly in other conditions (e.g., pancreatitis) is an attractive one because the changes in the hormonal milieu and in muscle sensitivity to the hormones does not explain the pattern or the rapidity of the changes. There is clear evidence that, in sepsis, muscle protein breakdown is elevated, and this effect can be seen not only in animal models but also in patients if the correct indices (e.g., 3-methylhistidine production by muscle) are examined (49,50,146) (Table 2).

Although there does appear to be some evidence that a low molecular weight (~5 kd) polypeptide present in the blood of animals and patients suffering from sepsis

TABLE 2. *Blood flow, oxygen consumption, and exchange of tyrosine and 3-methylhistidine in legs of patients suffering from accidental trauma and sepsis (a) and patients undergoing elective surgery (b).*

	Day 0		Day 1		Day 3		Day 6	
	(a)	(b)	(a)	(b)	(a)	(b)	(a)	(b)
Blood flow ml min^{-1} (100 g)$^{-1}$	5.0±0.6*	2.9±0.3	4.4±0.6	3.3±0.6	3.4±0.6	2.8±0.3	4.6±1.0	2.7±0.4
Oxygen consumption μmol min^{-1} (100 g)$^{-1}$	10.1±1.2	7.0±1.4	8.8±1.5	8.4±1.3	8.7±1.4	6.5±0.8	8.2±1.2	6.4±1.6
Efflux of tyrosine nmol min^{-1} (100 g)$^{-1}$	48±19	22±5	52±12	46±10	46±7	44±9	55±12	24±9
Efflux of 3-methylhistidine nmol min^{-1} (100 g)$^{-1}$	3.5±1.3	1.9±0.3	2.4±0.7	1.0±0.3	1.5±0.3	1.2±0.3	4.5±1.9	1.7±0.4

* Data are expressed as mean ± SD. Patients on day 0 were either preoperative (surgery and trauma) or within ? days of development of sepsis.
From Rennie MJ. Muscle protein turnover and the wasting due to injury and disease. *Br Med Bull* 1985;41: ?57–264.

can increase muscle protein breakdown in isolated incubated muscles (53,145), the mechanism of such an effect and the exact nature of the polypeptide involved has been difficult to pin down. Endotoxin itself has no direct stimulatory effect on protein breakdown in isolated incubated muscles (15). It is clear that many of the responses to infection, such as fever, activation of T and B cells, stimulation of neutrophil and lymphocyte morphogenesis, and the production of acute phase proteins from the liver, can be linked to the release of cytokines such as interleukin-1 (IL-1) and tumor necrosis factor-α (TNFα) from macrophages (and other cells, such as endothelial cells). However, it now seems clear that TNF has no direct effect to increase protein breakdown in incubated muscle in vitro: Numbers of workers now agree that this is the case if pure recombinant TNF is used (53,147,148). Furthermore, although there was a lot of initial excitement at the suggestion that partially purified human IL-1 from activated monocytes could stimulate muscle protein breakdown without affecting muscle protein synthesis and that the mechanism of such an effect involved the activation of prostaglandin production (149,150); in fact, when purified IL-1 (either mouse or human in nature) was used, the effects were almost uniformly negative (15,53,147). Various other cytokines, such as epidermal thymocyte activating factor, eosinophil cytotoxicity enhancing factors, interferons α, β, and γ, and transforming growth factor β, also fail to elicit any response in vitro (15).

How is it possible to resolve the conundrum that, when the direct effect of cytokines in muscle is investigated, all the evidence suggests that cytokines have no involvement with the observed stimulation of muscle protein breakdown associated with sepsis? One possibility is that the cytokines are involved but in a complicated fashion that requires other factors present in vivo and absent in vitro.

Although administration of recombinant IL-1α and TNFα appears to have no effect when muscle protein breakdown is assayed in vitro 8 hours after injection to live animals (147,151), Hasselgren et al. reasoned that a longer period of exposure to elevated cytokine concentration might be required to observe possible changes (53,152). They carried out experiments in which rTNF was given to rats as three equal IP injections of 100 μg/kg over 16 hours, then observed that in muscles removed and incubated in vitro there was a substantial rise in 3-methylhistidine efflux, suggesting increased myofibrillar protein breakdown. The possible involvement of glucocorticoids in the response was strengthened by the observations that such TNF injections increased plasma corticosterone concentration but had no effect in adrenalectomized animals. Also, the glucocorticoid receptor blocker RU 38486 abolished the TNF-induced protein breakdown, despite the fact that plasma corticosterone concentration was elevated (153). In a similar series of experiments to investigate the involvement of IL-1, a similar protocol of administration of rIL-1 also increased myofibrillar protein breakdown, and the effect could be abolished by the administration of recombinant IL-1 receptor antagonist—but not by administration of RU 38486 (154,155). Thus, the effects of IL-1 do not appear to involve the glucocorticoids and, in the absence of good evidence of a direct effect of IL-1 on muscle, its actions remain mysterious (53).

Insulin appears to have a smaller inhibitory effect in suppressing proteolysis in denervated muscle than in muscle from normal animals, and it may be that there is resistance to the effects of these substances during various kinds of disease and injury, including sepsis (51,137). This reinforces the idea that much of the increase in protein breakdown seen under these conditions was due to stimulation of nonlysosomal proteolysis, probably involving increased breakdown of myofibrillar proteins.

Acidosis

A lowered pH is a common correlate of many diseases of metabolic or renal origin, e.g., diabetes and kidney failure. Acidosis in its own right appears to stimulate protein breakdown in the whole body (156), and there is some evidence that the effect is due to a stimulation of muscle proteolysis (157). Although the effects of acidosis in vivo can be ameliorated by adrenalectomy, suggesting the involvement of corticosteroids (157), in cultured BC3H1 myocytes (which do not share all the characteristics of skeletal muscle in vivo), extracellular acidification caused intracellular acidification that was insulin suppressible, but there were no clear permissive or stimulatory effects of corticosteroids (158). The fact that, in the cultured, muscle cell line, the induced proteolysis was entirely insulin suppressible suggests that neither myofibrillar protein breakdown nor the energy-dependent nonlysosomal pathways were involved because these are both insulin-insensitive. These results tend to suggest that acidosis causes an increase in the proteolysis of soluble sarcoplasmic proteins and that, in circumstances in which it occurs (such as diabetic ketoacidosis and renal disease), steps to control acidosis (e.g., by simple bicarbonate infusion) would be beneficial.

In renal patients, muscle protein synthetic capacity is depressed (159) and muscle protein breakdown is enhanced by hemodialysis (160), possibly as a result of interaction between the hemodialysis membranes and white blood cells. Regenerated cellulose membranes apparently cause a stimulation in 3-methylhistidine efflux from the legs of patients undergoing dialysis with these membranes (160).

PRACTICAL APPLICATIONS OF WHAT WE KNOW ABOUT MUSCLE PROTEIN TURNOVER

My personal view, which may not be shared by others, is that the practical clinical problems concerning muscle protein wasting can be defined by (a) how to dampen the florid wasting that occurs as a result of severe injury, sepsis, burns, etc.; and (b) how to stimulate muscle regrowth or replete previously malnourished patients.

A stimulation of muscle protein synthesis is likely to be appropriate under both circumstances. Repletion or rehabilitation of previously malnourished patients is likely to be successful using this approach, although, because the rate of muscle protein turnover is slow, with a half-time of 1 month at least, long periods of artificial feeding may be required to obtain a noticeable improvement. It is unlikely that recovery and rehabilitation will require any aggressive treatment to limit protein breakdown, and indeed remodelling probably requires an increase in protein turnover so that such an approach would be counterproductive.

The most difficult problem is limiting the protein wasting that occurs as a result of trauma, burns, and sepsis. We *still* have no firm indication of the phenomenology of protein synthesis during florid wasting. There is some evidence that whole-body protein synthesis is elevated during infection and burns, and protein synthesis in skeletal muscle *may* be elevated after burn injury (124), but no good data exist using incorporation methods for human muscle protein synthesis. If protein synthesis is elevated but is unable to match the known elevation of protein breakdown, then it seems senseless to attempt to elevate protein synthesis further, and the target must be the depression of muscle protein breakdown.

How exactly to do this is not clear. Growth hormone is unlikely to have any marked effect on muscle protein breakdown and indeed may actually inhibit the antiproteolytic effect of insulin (101). It may be that IGF-1 has an insulin-like effect (15) which would be beneficial, but this remains speculative at the moment. Use of corticosteroid receptor blockers may be a promising avenue for therapy, as with the use of various beta$_2$-agonists—as long as their effects are sufficiently specific not to interfere with cardiovascular regulation.

It may be that the severe disruption of protein metabolism seen in injury, infection, and burns is best tackled by action at the most proximal possible link in the chain between the initial injury and the loss due to muscle protein breakdown. This means that various antibody preparations against, e.g., endotoxin or TNF-α or IL-1 would be beneficial, but because cytokines themselves may have some beneficial effects which are important for survival, it could be argued that greater benefit is obtained by tackling a distal step, i.e., specifically targeting muscle protein breakdown. The answer to this conundrum must await further research, and most of this research must address some rather fundamental problems before we can expect any progress.

SUGGESTIONS FOR FUTURE RESEARCH

Because protein synthesis and protein breakdown are likely to be regulated in a coordinated fashion, it appears that we need to have a lot more information about what actually happens to muscle protein synthesis in the variety of circumstances in which our knowledge is presently very poor. First, we should try to find out what happens to muscle protein synthesis during severe injury, multiple organ failure, sepsis, and burns.

Secondly, we need to find out to what extent in humans proteolysis of membrane proteins, sarcoplasmic proteins, and myofibrillar proteins occur via different pathways, which pathways they are, and how they are regulated. We already have a lot of clues from animals and from work on the relative rates of efflux of, e.g., tyrosine and methylhistidine but this work needs to be expanded to include indices of degradative activity of the lysosomal and nonlysosomal processes as well as measurements of mRNA and antibody reactivity for the proteolytic enzymes involved.

There are a few other areas that are likely to be fruitful. One concerns the effects on protein turnover of dietary manipulation to alter the proportion of unsaturated fatty acids in plasma membranes. The other areas which seem likely to be worthy of investigation are the effects of nitric oxide on protein breakdown in muscle and the effects of free radicals generally. So far as I am aware, no thorough studies of these possibly important, end-stage mediators have been carried out.

ACKNOWLEDGMENTS

The research work in our laboratory has been generously funded by The Wellcome Trust, Action Research, UK Medical Research Council, The Rank Prize Funds, Arthritis and Rheumatism Council, Scottish Home and Health Department, and The University of Dundee. I am grateful to my colleagues for helpful criticism and advice and to my secretary, Dorothea Watt, for her almost superhuman tact and perseverance.

REFERENCES

1. Cahill GF. Starvation in man. *N Engl J Med* 1970;282:668–675.
2. Daniel PM, Pratt OE, Spargo E. The metabolic homeostatic role of muscle and its function as a store of protein. *Lancet* 1977;ii:446–448.

3. Stirewalt WS, Low RB, Slaiby JM. Insulin sensitivity and responsiveness of epitrochlearis and soleus muscles from fed and starved rats. *Biochem J* 1985;227:355–362.
4. Felig P. Amino acid metabolism in man. *Annu Rev Biochem* 1979;44:993–955.
5. Palmer TN, Caldecourt MA, Snell K, Sugden MC. Alanine and inter-organ relationships in branched-chain amino and 2-oxo acid metabolism. *Biosci Rep* 1985;5:1015–1033.
6. Goldberg AL, Chang TW. Regulation and significance of amino acid metabolism in skeletal muscle. *Fed Proc* 1978;37:2301–2307.
7. Halliday D, McKeran RO. Measurement of muscle protein synthetic rate from serial muscle biopsies and total body protein turnover in man by continuous intravenous infusion of L-[α-^{15}N]lysine. *Clin Sci* 1975;49:581–590.
8. Halliday D, Pacy PJ, Cheng KN, et al. Rate of protein synthesis in skeletal muscle of normal man and patients with muscular dystrophy: a reassessment. *Clin Sci* 1988;74:237–240.
9. Cheng KN, Dworzak F, Ford GC, et al. Direct determination of leucine metabolism and protein breakdown in humans using L-[1-^{13}C, ^{15}N]-leucine and the forearm model. *Eur J Clin Invest* 1985; 15:349–354.
10. Carraro F, Stuart CA, Hartl WH, et al. Effect of exercise and recovery on muscle protein synthesis in human subjects. *Am J Physiol* 1990;259:E470–E476.
11. Garlick PJ, Wernerman J, McNurlan MA, et al. Measurement of the rate of protein synthesis in muscle of postabsorptive young men by injection of a "flooding dose" of [1-^{13}C]leucine. *Clin Sci* 1989;77:329–336.
12. Griggs RC, Kingston W, Jozefowicz RF, et al. Effect of testosterone on muscle mass and muscle protein synthesis. *J Appl Physiol* 1989;66:E498–E503.
13. McNurlan MA, Essén P, Heys SD, et al. Measurement of protein synthesis in human skeletal muscle: further investigation of the flooding technique. *Clin Sci* 1991;81:557–564.
14. Millward DJ, Bates PC, Brown JG, et al. Protein degradation and the regulation of protein balance in muscle. In: Evered D, Whelan J (eds). *Protein Degradation in Health and Disease.* Amsterdam: Excerpta Medica, 1989;307–329.
15. Kettelhut IC, Wing SS, Goldberg AL. Endocrine regulation of protein breakdown in skeletal muscle. *Diabetes Metab Rev* 1988;4:751–772.
16. Mortimore GE, Wert JJ Jr, Adams CE. Modulation of the amino acid control of hepatic protein degradation by caloric deprivation. Two modes of alanine co-regulation. *J Biol Chem* 1988;263: 19545–19551.
17. Mortimore GE, Pösö AR, Kadowaki M, Wert JJ. Multiphasic control of hepatic protein degradation by regulatory amino acids. *J Biol Chem* 1987;262:16322–16327.
18. Jefferson LS, Li JB, Rannels SR. Regulation by insulin of amino acid release and protein turnover in the perfused rat hemicorpus. *J Biol Chem* 1977;252:1476–1483.
19. Lundholm K, Schersten T. Determination in vitro of the rate of protein synthesis and degradation in human skeletal muscle tissue. *Eur J Biochem* 1975;60:181–186.
20. Furuno K, Goldberg AL. The activation of protein degradation in muscle by Ca^{2+} or muscle injury does not involve a lysosomal mechanism. *Biochem J* 1986;237:859–864.
21. Hasselgren P-O, Hall-Angeras M, Angeras U, et al. Regulation of total and myofibrillar protein breakdown in rat extensor digitorum longus and soleus muscle incubated flaccid or at resting length. *Biochem J* 1990;267:37–44.
22. Lowell BB, Ruderman NB, Goodman MN. Evidence that lysosomes are not involved in the degradation of myofibrillar proteins in rat skeletal muscle. *Biochem J* 1986;234:237–240.
23. Goodman MJ. Differential effects of acute changes in cell Ca^{2+} concentration on myofibrillar and non-myofibrillar protein breakdown in the rat extensor digitorum longus muscle *in vitro. Biochem J* 1987;241:121–127.
24. Furuno K, Goodman MN, Goldberg AL. Role of different proteolytic systems in the degradation of muscle proteins during denervation atrophy. *J Biol Chem* 1990;265:8550–8557.
25. Simonson DC, Tambourlane WV, Sherwin RS, et al. Improved insulin sensitivity in patients with type 1 diabetes mellitus after CSII. *Diabetes* 1985;34(Suppl 3):80–86.
26. Hammarqvist F, Wernerman J, von der Decken A, Vinnars E. Alpha-ketoglutarate preserves protein synthesis and free glutamine in skeletal muscle after surgery. *Surgery* 1991;109:28–36.
27. Tawa NE Jr, Kettelhut IC, Goldberg AL. Dietary protein deficiency reduces lysosomal and non-lysosomal ATP-dependent proteolysis in muscle. *Am J Physiol* 1992;263:E326–E334.
28. Tawa NE Jr, Goldberg AL. Suppression of muscle protein turnover and amino acid degradation by dietary protein deficiency. *Am J Physiol* 1992;263:E317–E325.

29. Goldberg AL, St. John AC. Intracellular protein degradation in mammalian and bacterial cells: part 2. *Ann Rev Biochem* 1976;45:747–803.
30. Goldberg AL. ATP-dependent proteases in prokaryotic and eukaryotic cells. *Semin Cell Biol* 1990; 1:423–432.
31. Driscoll J, Goldberg AL. Skeletal muscle proteasome can degrade proteins in an ATP-dependent process that does not require ubiquitin. *Proc Natl Acad Sci USA* 1989;86:787–791.
32. Goldberg AL, Rock KL. Proteolysis, proteasomes and antigen presentation. *Nature* 1992;357: 375–379.
33. Goldberg AL. Protein synthesis in tonic and phasic skeletal muscles. *Nature* 1967;216:1219–1220.
34. Lundholm K, Schersten T. Incorporation of leucine into human skeletal muscle proteins: a study of tissue amino acid pools and their role in protein biosynthesis. *Acta Physiol Scand* 1975;93:433–441.
35. Lundholm K, Edström S, Ekman L, et al. Protein degradation in human skeletal-muscle tissue: the effect of insulin, leucine, amino acids and ions. *Clin Sci* 1981;60:319–326.
36. Riley DA, Bain JL, Ellis S, Haas AL. Quantitation and immunocytochemical localization of ubiquitin conjugates within rat red and white skeletal muscles. *J Histochem Cytochem* 1988;36:621–632.
37. Hilenski LL, Terracio L, Haas AL, Borg TK. Immunolocalization of ubiquitin conjugates at Z-bands and intercalated discs of rat cardiomyocytes *in vitro* and *in vivo*. *J Histochem Cytochem* 1992;40:1037–1042.
38. Schimke RT, Ganschow R, Doyle D, Arias IM. Regulation of protein turnover in mammalian tissues. *Fed Proc* 1968;27:1223–1230.
39. Goldberg AL, Martel SB, Kushmerick MJ. In vitro preparations of the diaphragm and other skeletal muscles. In: Hardman JG, O'Malley BW (eds). *Methods in Enzymology*, vol. 39. New York: Academic Press, 1975;82–94.
40. Jefferson LS, Rannels DE, Munger BL, Morgan HE. Insulin in the regulation of protein turnover in heart and skeletal muscle. *Fed Proc* 1974;33:1098–1114.
41. Millward DJ, Bates PC, Brown JG, et al. Physiological mechanisms for the regulation of protein balance in skeletal muscle. In: Kidman AD, Tomkins JK, Morris CA, Cooper NA (eds). *Molecular Pathology of Nerve and Muscle: Noxious Agents and Genetic Lesions*. Clifton, New Jersey: Humana Press, 1983;315–342.
42. Millward DJ, Waterlow JC. Effect of nutrition on protein turnover in skeletal muscle. *Fed Proc* 1978;37:2283–2290.
43. Waterlow JC, Garlick PJ, Millward DJ. *Protein Turnover in Mammalian Tissues and in the Whole Body*. Amsterdam: Elsevier–North Holland, 1978.
44. Booth FW, Thomason DB. Molecular and cellular adaptation of muscle in response to exercise: perspectives of various models. *Physiol Rev* 1991;71:541–585.
45. Dietrichson P, Coakley J, Smith PEM. Conchotome and needle percutaneous biopsy of skeletal muscle. *J Neurol Neurosurg Psychiatry* 1987;50:1461–1467.
46. Young VR, Munro HN. N^t-Methylhistidine (3-methylhistidine) and muscle protein turnover: an overview. *Fed Proc* 1978;37:2291–2300.
47. Rennie MJ, Bennegård C, Edén E, et al. Urinary excretion and efflux from the leg of 3-methylhistidine before and after major surgical operation. *Metabolism* 1984;33:250–256.
48. Rennie MJ, Smith K, Watt PW, et al. Methods of assessment of muscle protein turnover and their application to problems in clinical nutrition. *Rev Ital Nutr Parenter Enter* 1992;20:63–71.
49. Bennegård C, Edén E, Emery PW, et al. Efflux of 3-methylhistidine and tyrosine in severe trauma and in patients with septicaemia. *Clin Nutr* 1985;4:P65.
50. Sjölin J, Stjernström H, Friman G, et al. Total and net muscle protein breakdown in infection determined by amino acid effluxes. *Am J Physiol* 1990;258:E856–E863.
51. Hasselgren P-O, James JH, Benson DW, et al. Total and myofibrillar protein breakdown in different types of rat skeletal muscle: effects of sepsis and regulation by insulin. *Metabolism* 1989;38:634–640.
52. Rennie MJ, Emery PW, Edwards RHT, et al. Hypothesis: Depressed protein synthesis may be the dominant characteristic of muscle wasting. *Clin Physiol* 1983;3:387–398.
53. Hasselgren P-O, Fischer JE. Recent advances on the regulation of muscle protein metabolism in catabolic states. With special reference to the role of cytokines and glucocorticoids for protein breakdown during sepsis. *Rev Ital Nutr Parenter Enter* 1992;10:72–84.
54. Swick RW, Ip MM. Measurement of protein turnover in rat liver with [^{14}C]carbonate. *J Biol Chem* 1974;249:6836–6841.
55. Manchester KL, Young FG. Location of ^{14}C in protein from isolated rat diaphragm incubated in vitro with [^{14}C]amino acids and with $^{14}CO_2$. *Biochem J* 1959;72:136–141.

56. Millward DJ, Bates PC, Grimble GK, Brown JC. Quantitative importance of non–skeletal-muscle sources of N^t-methylhistidine in urine. *Biochem J* 1980;190:225–228.
57. Smith K, Scrimgeour CM, Bennet WM, Rennie MJ. Isolation of amino acids by preparative gas chromatography for quantification of carboxy carbon ^{13}C enrichment by isotope ratio mass spectrometry. *Biomed Environ Mass Spectrom* 1988;17:267–273.
58. Barrett EJ, Gelfand RA. The in vivo study of cardiac and skeletal muscle protein turnover. *Diabet Metab Rev* 1989;5:133–148.
59. Bennet WM, Connacher AA, Scrimgeour CS, et al. L-[^{15}N]Phenylalanine and L-[1-^{13}C]leucine leg exchange and plasma kinetics during amino acid infusion and euglycaemic hyperinsulinaemia; evidence for stimulation of muscle and whole body protein synthesis in man by insulin. *Proc Nutr Soc* 1990;49:179A.
60. Thompson GN, Pacy PJ, Merritt H, et al. Rapid measurement of whole-body and forearm protein turnover using a [^{2}H$_5$]phenylalanine model. *Am J Physiol* 1989;256:631–639.
61. Kletzien RF. Amino acid transport as a rate-limiting reaction in hepatic gluconeogenesis. *Fed Proc* 1986;45:2440–2441.
62. Gelfand RA, Glickman MG, Castellino P, et al. Measurement of L-[1-^{14}C]leucine kinetics in splanchnic and leg tissues in humans. Effect of amino acid infusion. *Diabetes* 1988;37:1365–1372.
63. Millward DJ. Protein turnover in cardiac and skeletal muscle during normal growth and hypertrophy. In: Wildenthal K (ed). *Degradative Processes in Skeletal and Cardiac Muscle*. Amsterdam: Elsevier/North Holland, 1980;161–200.
64. Laurent GJ, Sparrow MP, Millward DJ. Turnover of muscle protein in the fowl. Changes in rates of protein synthesis and breakdown during hypertrophy of the anterior and posterior latissimus dorsi muscles. *Biochem J* 1978;176:407–417.
65. Elia M, Carter A, Smith R. The 3-methylhistidine content of human tissues. *Br J Nutr* 1979;42:567–569.
66. Elia M, Carter A, Bacon S, et al. Clinical usefulness of urinary 3-methylhistidine excretion in indicating muscle protein breakdown. *Br Med J* 1981;282:351–354.
67. Meredith CN, Zackin MJ, Frontera WR, Evans WJ. Dietary protein requirements and body protein metabolism in endurance-trained men. *J Appl Physiol* 1989;66:2850–2856.
68. Rennie MJ, Millward DJ. 3-Methylhistidine excretion and the urinary 3-methylhistidine/creatinine ratio are poor indicators of skeletal muscle protein breakdown. *Clin Sci* 1983;65:217–225.
69. Aniansson A, Grimby G, Hedberg M, et al. Muscle function in old age. *Scand J Rehabil Med* 1978;6:43–49.
70. Forsberg AM, Nilsson E, Wernerman J, et al. Muscle composition in relation to age and sex. *Clin Sci* 1991;81:249–256.
71. Chesley A, MacDougall JD, Tarnopolsky MA, et al. Changes in human muscle protein synthesis following resistance exercise. *J Appl Physiol* 1992;73:1383–1388.
72. Tarnopolsky MA, MacDougall JD, Atkinson SA. Influence of protein intake and training status on nitrogen balance and lean body mass. *J Appl Physiol* 1988;64:187–193.
73. Cheng KN, Pacy PJ, Dworzak F, et al. Influence of fasting on leucine and muscle protein metabolism across the human forearm determined using L-[1-^{13}C, ^{15}N]leucine as the tracer. *Clin Sci* 1987;73:241–246.
74. Medina R, Wing SS, Haas A, Goldberg AL. Activation of the ubiquitin-ATP–dependent proteolytic system in skeletal muscle during fasting and denervation atrophy. *Biomed Biochim Acta* 1991;50:347–356.
75. Lowell BB, Goldman MN. Protein sparing in skeletal muscle during prolonged starvation. Dependence on lipid fuel availability. *Diabetes* 1987;36:14–19.
76. Emery PW, Cotellessa L, Holness M, et al. Different patterns of protein turnover in skeletal and gastrointestinal smooth muscle and the production of N^t-methylhistidine during fasting in the rat. *Biosci Rep* 1986;6:143–153.
77. Goodman MN, Gomez MDP. Decreased myofibrillar proteolysis after refeeding requires dietary proteins or amino acids. *Am J Physiol* 1987;253:E52–E58.
78. Wing SS, Chiang HL, Goldberg AL, Dice JF. Proteins containing peptide sequences related to Lys-Phe-Glu-Arg-Gln are selectively depleted in liver and heart, but not skeletal muscle, of fasted rats. *Biochem J* 1991;275:165–169.
79. Li JB, Jefferson LS. Influence of amino acid availability on protein turnover in perfused skeletal muscle. *Biochim Biophys Acta* 1978;544:351–359.
80. Tracey KJ, Legaspi A, Albert JD, et al. Protein and substrate metabolism during starvation and parenteral refeeding. *Clin Sci* 1988;74:123–132.

81. Bennet WM, Connacher AA, Scrimgeour CM, Rennie MJ. The effect of amino acid infusion on leg protein turnover assessed by L-[^{15}N]phenylalanine and L-[^{13}C]leucine exchange. *Eur J Clin Invest* 1990;20:37–46.

82. Buse MG, Reid SS. Leucine: a possible regulator of protein turnover in muscle. *J Clin Invest* 1975; 56:1250–1261.

83. Tischler ME, Desautels M, Goldberg AL. Does leucine, leucyl-tRNA, or some metabolite of leucine regulate protein synthesis and degradation in skeletal and cardiac muscle? *J Biol Chem* 1982;257: 1613–1621.

84. McNurlan MA, Fern EB, Garlick PJ. Failure of leucine to stimulate protein synthesis in vivo. *Biochem J* 1982;204:831–838.

85. Hammarqvist F, Wernerman J, von der Decken A, Vinnars E. The effects of branched chain amino-acids upon postoperative muscle protein synthesis and nitrogen balance. *Clin Nutr* 1988;7:171–175.

86. May ME, Buse MG. Effects of branched-chain amino acids on protein turnover. *Diabetes* 1989;5: 227–245.

87. Hasselgren P-O, James JH, Warner BW, et al. Protein synthesis and degradation in skeletal muscle from septic rats. *Arch Surg* 1988;123:640–644.

88. Louard RJ, Barrett EJ, Gelfand RA. Effect of infused branched-chain amino acids on muscle and whole-body amino acid metabolism in man. *Clin Sci* 1990;79:457–466.

89. Garlick PJ, Grant I. Amino acid infusion increases the sensitivity of muscle protein synthesis *in vivo* to insulin. *Biochem J* 1988;254:579–584.

90. Smith RJ, Larson S, Stred SE, Durschlag RP. Regulation of glutamine synthetase and glutaminase activities in cultured skeletal muscle cells. *J Cell Physiol* 1984;120:197–203.

91. MacLennan PA, Smith K, Weryk B, et al. Inhibition of protein breakdown by glutamine in perfused rat skeletal muscle. *FEBS Lett* 1988;237:133–136.

92. Thompson JR, Wu G. The effect of ketone bodies on nitrogen metabolism in skeletal muscle. *Comp Biochem Physiol [B]* 1991;100:209–216.

93. Beaufrere B, Tessari P, Cattalini M, et al. Apparent decreased oxidation and turnover of leucine during infusion of medium-chain triglycerides. *Am J Physiol* 1985;249:E175–E182.

94. Van Slyke DD, Meyer GM. The fate of protein digestion products in the body. III. The absorption of amino acids from the blood by the tissues. *J Biol Chem* 1913;16:197–212.

95. Lotspeich W. The role of insulin in the metabolism of amino acids. *J Biol Chem* 1949;179:175–180.

96. Smith OLK. Insulin inhibits protein degradation in skeletal muscles of eviscerated fasted rats. *Metabolism* 1988;37:976–981.

97. Smith OLK, Wong CY, Gelfand RA. Skeletal proteolysis in rats with acute streptozocin-induced diabetes. *Diabetes* 1989;38:1117–1122.

98. Smith DM, Sugden PH. Contrasting response of protein degradation to starvation and insulin as measured by release of N^t-methylhistidine or phenylalanine from the perfused rat heart. *Biochem J* 1986;237:391–395.

99. Gorray KC, Maimon J, Schneider BS. Studies of antiproteolytic effects of glyburide on rat L6 myoblasts: comparisons with insulin. *Metabolism* 1990;39:109–116.

100. Fryberg DA, Barrett EJ. Growth hormone acutely stimulates whole-body skeletal-muscle protein-synthesis in humans. *Metabolism* 1991;42:1223–1227.

101. Fryburg DA, Louard RJ, Gerow KE, et al. Growth hormone stimulates skeletal muscle protein synthesis and antagonizes insulin's antiproteolytic action in humans. *Diabetes* 1992;41:424–429.

102. Hembree JR, Hathaway MR, Dayton WR. Isolation and culture of fetal porcine myogenic cells and the effect of insulin, IGF-1 and sera on protein turnover in porcine myotube cultures. *J Anim Sci* 1991;69:3241–3250.

103. Tomas FM, Knowles SE, Owens PC, et al. Increased weight gain, nitrogen retention and muscle protein synthesis following treatment of diabetic rats with insulin-like growth factor (IGF)-I and des(1-3) IGF-I. *Biochem J* 1991;276:547–554.

104. Tomas FM, Knowles SE, Owens PC, et al. Effects of full-length and truncated insulin-like growth factor-I on nitrogen balance and muscle protein metabolism in nitrogen-restricted rats. *J Endocrinol* 1991;128:97–105.

105. Frampton RJ, Jonas HA, MacMahon RA, Larkins RG. Failure of IGF-1 to affect protein turnover in muscle from growth-retarded neonatal rats. *J Dev Physiol* 1990;13:125–133.

106. Kayali AG, Goodman MN, Lin J, Young VR. Insulin and thyroid hormone-independent adaptation of myofibrillar proteolysis to glucocorticoids. *Am J Physiol* 1990;259:E699–E705.

107. Odedra BR, Millward DJ. Effect of corticosterone treatment on muscle protein turnover in adrenalec-tomized rats and diabetic rats maintained on insulin. *Biochem J* 1982;204:663–672.

108. Odedra BR, Bates PC, Millward DJ. Time course of the effect of catabolic doses of corticosterose on protein turnover in rat skeletal muscle and liver. *Biochem J* 1983;214:617–627.
109. Tomas FM, Munro HN, Young VR. Effect of glucocorticoid administration on the rate of muscle protein breakdown in vivo in rats, as measured by urinary excretion of N^τ-methylhistidine. *Biochem J* 1979;178:139–146.
110. Hall-Angeras M, Hasselgren P-O, Angeras U, et al. Glucocorticoid receptor blocker RU 38486 decreased muscle protein breakdown in sepsis. *Surg Forum* 1990;XLI:26–27.
111. Millward DJ, Odedra B, Bates PC. The role of insulin, corticosterone and other factors in the acute recovery of muscle protein synthesis on refeeding food-deprived rats. *Biochem J* 1983;216:583–587.
112. Forbes GB. The effect of anabolic steroids on lean body mass: the dose response curve. *Metabolism* 1985;34:571–573.
113. Hayden JM, Bergen WG, Merkel RA. Skeletal muscle protein metabolism and serum growth hormone, insulin, and cortisol concentrations in growing steers implanted with estradiol-17 beta, trenbolone acetate, or estradiol-17 beta plus trenbolone acetate. *J Anim Sci* 1992;70:2109–2119.
114. Morrison WL, Gibson JNA, Jung RT, Rennie MJ. Skeletal muscle and whole body protein turnover in thyroid disease. *Eur J Clin Invest* 1988;18:62–68.
115. Gelfand RA, Matthews DE, Bier DM, Sherwin RS. Role of counterregulatory hormones in the catabolic response to stress. *J Clin Invest* 1984;74:2238–2248.
116. Horber FF, Horber-Feyder CM, Krayer S, et al. Plasma reciprocal pool specific activity predicts that of intracellular free leucine for protein synthesis. *Am J Physiol* 1989;257:E385–E399.
117. Wernerman J, Botta D, Hammarqvist F, et al. Stress hormones given to healthy volunteers alter the concentration and configuration of ribosomes in skeletal muscle, reflecting changes in protein synthesis. *Clin Sci* 1989;77:611–616.
118. Warner BW, Hasselgren P-O, Hummel RP, et al. Effect of catabolic hormone infusion on protein turnover and amino acid uptake in skeletal muscle. *Am J Surg* 1990;159:295–300.
119. Preedy VR, Garlick PJ. Inhibition of protein synthesis by glucagon in different rat muscles and protein fractions *in vivo* and in the perfused rat hemicorpus. *Biochem J* 1988;251:727–732.
120. Mantle D, Delday MI, Maltin CA. Effect of clenbuterol on protease activities and protein levels in rat muscle. *Muscle Nerve* 1992;15:471–478.
121. Rogers KL, Fagan JM. Effect of beta agonists on protein turnover in isolated chick skeletal and atrial muscle. *Proc Soc Exp Biol Med* 1991;197:482–485.
122. Martinez JA, Portillo MP, Larralde J. Anabolic actions of a mixed beta-adrenergic agonist on nitrogen retention and protein turnover. *Horm Metab Res* 1991;23:590–593.
123. Benson DW, Foley-Nelson T, Chance WT, et al. Decreased myofibrillar protein breakdown following treatment with Clenbuterol. *J Surg Res* 1991;50:1–5.
124. Rennie MJ. Muscle protein turnover and the wasting due to injury and disease. *Br Med Bull* 1985; 41:257–264.
125. Griggs RC, Rennie MJ. Muscle wasting in muscular dystrophy: decreased protein synthesis or increased degradation? *Ann Neurol* 1983;13:125–132.
126. Rennie MJ, Bennet WM, Smith K, et al. Muscle protein synthesis in man: new insights from use of the stable-isotope tracer technique. *Riv Ital Nutr Parenter Enter* 1989;7:121–126.
127. Seider MJ, Kapp R, Chen C-P, Booth FW. The effects of cutting or of stretching skeletal muscle in vitro on the rates of protein synthesis and degradation. *Biochem J* 1980;188:247–254.
128. Mudge GH, Mills RM, Taegtmeyer H, et al. Alterations of myocardial amino acid metabolism in chronic ischemic heart disease. *J Clin Invest* 1976;58:1185–1192.
129. Saltin B, Henriksson J, Nyggard E, Andersen P. Fiber types and metabolic potentials of skeletal muscles in sedentary man and endurance runners. *Ann NY Acad Sci* 1977;301:3–29.
130. Rennie MJ, Edwards RHT, Krywawych S, et al. Effect of exercise on protein turnover in man. *Clin Sci* 1981;61:627–639.
131. Rennie MJ, Willhoft NM, Ahmed A, et al. Amino acid and protein metabolism during exercise. In: Devlin J, Horton ES, Vranic M (eds). *Diabetes Mellitus and Exercise*. London: Smith-Gordon, 1993;139–150.
132. Bylund-Fellenius A-C, Ojamaa KM, Flaim KE, et al. Protein synthesis versus energy state in contracting muscle of perfused rat hindlimb. *Am J Physiol* 1984;246:E297–E305.
133. Kasperek GJ, Snider RD. Total and myofibrillar protein degradation in isolated soleus muscles after exercise. *Am J Physiol* 1989;257:E1–E5.
134. Gibson JNA, Halliday D, Morrison WL, et al. Decrease in human quadriceps muscle protein turnover consequent on leg immobilization. *Clin Sci* 1987;72:503–509.

135. Gibson JNA, Smith K, Rennie MJ. Prevention of disuse muscular atrophy by means of electrical stimulation: maintenance of protein synthesis. *Lancet* 1988;ii:767–770.
136. Gibson JNA, Morrison WL, Scrimgeour CM, et al. Effects of therapeutic percutaneous electrical stimulation of atrophic human quadriceps on muscle composition protein synthesis and contractile properties. *Eur J Clin Invest* 1989;19:206–212.
137. Tischler ME, Satarug S, Eisenfeld SH, et al. Insulin effects in denervated and non-weight-bearing rat soleus muscle. *Muscle Nerve* 1990;13:593–600.
138. Tischler ME, Rosenberg S, Satarug S, et al. Different mechanisms of increased proteolysis in atrophy induced by denervation or unweighting of rat soleus muscle. *Metabolism* 1990;39:756–763.
139. Coakley JH, Nagendran K, Honovar M. Preliminary observations on the neuromuscular abnormalities in patients with organ failure and sepsis. *Intens Care Med* 1993;19:323–328.
140. Shaw JHF, Wolfe RR. An integrated analysis of glucose, fat and protein metabolism in severely traumatized patients. *Ann Surg* 1989;209:63–72.
141. Shaw JHF, Wolfe RR. Metabolic intervention in surgical patients. *Ann Surg* 1988;207:274–282.
142. Petersson B, Wernerman J, Waller S-O, et al. Elective abdominal surgery depresses muscle protein synthesis and increases subjective fatigue: effects lasting more than 30 days. *Br J Surg* 1990;77: 796–800.
143. Essén P, McNurlan MA, Wernerman J, et al. Uncomplicated surgery, but not general anesthesia, decreases muscle protein synthesis. *Am J Physiol* 1992;262:E253–E260.
144. Stjernström H, Lund J, Wiklund L, et al. The influence of abdominal surgical trauma on the exchange of blood-borne amino acids in the human leg. *Clin Nutr* 1986;5:123–131.
145. Clowes GHA, George BC, Vilee CA, Saravis CA. Muscle proteolysis induced by a circulating peptide in patients with trauma and sepsis. *N Engl J Med* 1983;308:545–552.
146. Sjölin J, Stjernström H, Henneberg S, et al. Splanchnic and peripheral release of 3-methylhistidine in relation to its urinary excretion in human infection. *Metabolism* 1989;38:23–29.
147. Moldawer LL, Svaninger G, Gelin J, Lundholm KG. Interleukin-1 and tumor necrosis factor do not regulate protein balance in skeletal muscle. *Am J Physiol* 1987;253:C766–C773.
148. Mitchell LA, Norton LW. Effect of cancer plasma on skeletal muscle metabolism. *J Surg Res* 1989; 47:423–426.
149. Baracos V, Rodemann HP, Dinarello CA, Goldberg AL. Stimulation of muscle protein degradation and prostaglandin E_2 release by leukocytic pyrogen (interleukin-1). *N Engl J Med* 1983;308:553–558.
150. McEligott MA, Chaung LY, Baracos V, Gulve EA. Prostaglandin production in myotube cultures. Influence on protein turnover. *Biochem J* 1988;253:745–749.
151. Kettelhut IC, Goldberg AL. Tumor necrosis factor can induce fever in rats without activating protein breakdown in muscle or lipolysis in adipose tissue. *J Clin Invest* 1988;81:1384–1389.
152. Zamir O, Hasselgren P-O, Kunkel SL, et al. Evidence that tumor necrosis factor (TNF) participates in the regulation of muscle proteolysis during sepsis. *Arch Surg* 1992;127:170–174.
153. Hall-Angerås M, Angerås U, Zamir O, et al. Interaction between corticosterone and tumor necrosis factor stimulated protein breakdown in rat skeletal muscle, similar to sepsis. *Surgery* 1990–108: 460–466.
154. Zamir O, Hasselgren P-O, Von Allmen D, Fischer JE. The effect of interleukin-1α and the glucocorticoid receptor blocker RU 38486 on total and myofibrillar protein breakdown in skeletal muscle. *J Surg Res* 1991;50:579–583.
155. Zamir O, Hasselgren P-O, Von Allmen D, Fischer JE. In vivo administration of interleukin-1α induces muscle proteolysis in normal and adrenalectomized rats. *Metabolism* 1993;42:204–208.
156. Hara Y, May RC, Kelly RA, Mitch WE. Acidosis not azotemia stimulates branched-chain amino acid catabolism in uremic rats. *Kidney Int* 1987;32:808–814.
157. May RC, Kelly RA, Mitch WE. Metabolic acidosis stimulates protein degradation in rat muscle by a glucocorticoid-dependent mechanism. *J Clin Invest* 1986;77:614–621.
158. England BK, Chastain JL, Mitch WE. Abnormalities in protein synthesis and degradation induced by extracellular pH in BC3H1 myocytes. *Am J Physiol* 1991;260:C277–C282.
159. Lofberg E, Wernerman J, Noree LO, et al. Ribosome and free amino acid content in muscle during hemodialysis. *Kidney Int* 1991;39:984–989.
160. Gutierrez A, Bergström J, Alvestrand A. Protein catabolism in sham-hemodialysis: the effect of different membranes. *Clin Nephrol* 1992;38:20–29.

Organ Metabolism and Nutrition:
Ideas for Future Critical Care, edited by
J. M. Kinney and H. N. Tucker.
Raven Press, Ltd., New York © 1994.

3

Insulin Resistance and Tissue Fuels

Roderick A. Little and G. L. Carlson

*North Western Injury Research Centre, University of Manchester Medical School,
Manchester M13 9PT, United Kingdom*

Injury and sepsis are associated with a number of alterations in fuel substrate metabolism. Therapeutic intervention may complicate the interpretation of these metabolic alterations, but awareness of the changes in the utilization of fuel substrate is important for the clinician caring for such patients and has particular relevance to the nutritional support of the critically ill.

This chapter discusses the normal homeostatic processes that regulate the supply of fuel substrate to tissues, examines the alterations in fuel substrate utilization seen in injured and septic patients, and considers the possible mechanisms underlying these metabolic alterations.

FUEL SUBSTRATE METABOLISM IN HEALTH

If the healthy subject is to remain in energy balance, total daily consumption of fuel must equal energy expenditure. Under normal circumstances, these energy requirements are met by the consumption of a variety of simple and complex carbohydrates, lipids, and proteins. Fuel substrate is made available, however, after digestion and absorption by the gastrointestinal tract, and the principal fuels available to humans are, thus, simple carbohydrates (principally glucose), simple lipids (triacylglycerol), and amino acids. During a fast, fuel substrates are mobilized from body stores. After feeding, a shift away from the use of stored fuel substrate occurs, and recently available substrate is used preferentially. Substrate available in excess of immediate requirements is used to replenish stores depleted during the fasting state.

Before glucose can be stored as glycogen or lipid, or oxidized, it must enter cells. Glucose entry into many cells is limited by the availability of insulin. Although a degree of insulin-independent glucose uptake may occur in many tissues, and some tissues (notably brain, kidney tubules, intestinal mucosa, and red blood cells) do not require insulin for glucose uptake (1), the increase in plasma insulin concentration associated with the stimulatory effects of glucose and, to a lesser extent, certain amino acids on pancreatic β-cell function (2) results in ingested glucose being taken up into liver and skeletal muscle (for storage as glycogen) and adipose tissue (for storage as fat). In conditions of substrate availability, insulin enhances the the deposition of glucose as glycogen by increasing the activity of glycogen synthetase (3). Glucose oxidation is also enhanced—directly, as a result of the increased concentration of glucose within the cell, and indirectly, as a result of the effect of insulin on rate-limiting enzymes for glucose oxidation, such as glucokinase, phosphofructokinase, and pyruvate dehydrogenase (3). Insulin inhibits lipolysis in the fat depots and stimulates the production of fat as a result of increased activity of enzymes such as lipoprotein lipase. Since less acetyl coenzyme A (CoA) enters Kreb's cycle and a relative excess of three-carbon intermediates are available, because of increased glycolytic activity, ketone body formation is reduced. Insulin-mediated amino acid uptake into cells results in increased incorporation of amino acids into tissue protein and a concomitant reduction of amino acid flux out of cells (and, in particular, skeletal muscle). Administration of carbohydrate, therefore, reduces the need for catabolism of body protein reserves, and, in health, a reduction in gluconeogenesis and nitrogen-sparing are observed after the administration of even small amounts of glucose (4). In the fasting state, insulin remains low, and plasma concentrations of glucagon, growth hormone, and adrenaline rise. This hormonal environment encourages a series of catabolic adjustments that have the effect of mobilizing fuel substrate from body stores. The liver has a small (150 to 200 g) but highly mobile store of glycogen, which is available for distribution to tissues of the body that have a limited ability to use fuels other than glucose (e.g., the brain). A larger store of glycogen exists within skeletal muscle (500 g) but, because muscle cannot convert glucose-6-phosphate to glucose-1-phosphate, this glycogen is not directly available to other tissues of the body. In both tissues, increased activity of phosphorylase occurs as a result of increased glucagon and adrenaline (5). Increased phosphorylase activity leads to glycogenolysis within the liver and the formation of glucose-1-phosphate within the hepatocyte, which can then be dephosphorylated and exported into the blood for transport to the brain.

The reduction in the availability of glucose in the fasted state leads to an increase in the rate of lipolysis within the fat depots. This is determined principally by the stimulatory action of adrenaline and mediated by the effect of cyclic adenosine monophosphate (AMP) on hormone-sensitive lipase (6). Release of lipids from fat depots provides triglycerides, which can be used by many tissues, particularly in times of carbohydrate depletion, and enables the carbohydrate generated as a result of glycogenolysis to be consumed preferentially by the brain. Fasting also leads to mobilization of body protein reserves. Since the amount of liver glycogen is sufficient to provide glucose for only 24 hours, fasts of a greater duration begin to erode body protein reserves. Amino acids are used to generate glucose by hepatic gluconeogenesis. Lipid becomes increasingly important as the fundamental energy currency in the fasting state because the deficiency of insulin permits significant glucose uptake only in tissues that manifest insulin-independent glucose uptake. The accumulation of acetyl CoA as a result of a relative deficiency of three-carbon intermediates leads to the generation of ketone bodies such as β-hydroxybutyrate and acetoacetate, which also become increasingly important fuel substrates in a prolonged fast. The fat stores are progressively eroded with continuing starvation, and this results in further depletion of body protein stores. While the compensatory responses to fasting exhibit a subtle change from the physiologic to the pathologic as the duration of the fast increases, the present review will focus on the particular effects of injury and sepsis on the availability and utilization of fuel substrate.

FUEL SUBSTRATE METABOLISM IN SEPSIS AND AFTER INJURY

Fuel Mobilization

In the injured and/or septic patient, characteristic changes occur that result in the mobilization of substrate from tissue fuel stores. Under fasting conditions, the principle fuels mobilized from stores are glucose (from the glycogen stores) and triacylglycerol (from fat stores). While these fuels are important to the critically ill patient, protein stores are also mobilized, and this process results in muscle wasting (7).

The total glycogen stores of postabsorptive humans represent less than the daily energy requirements for the body as a whole. In contrast, the stores of triacylglycerol are sufficient, in theory, to provide fuel for up to 3 months in a normally nourished individual (8).

Glucose Mobilization

As already indicated, the least energetically expensive source of endogenous glucose is derived from the breakdown of glycogen (9). Significant reserves of glycogen occur in the liver and muscle. Direct measurement of hepatic glycogen content has largely been confined to patients undergoing elective abdominal surgery. Surgery leads to a marked and rapid decline in hepatic glycogen content, even in the fasting state (10–12). Animal studies have indicated that the effects of injury are potentiated by anesthesia (13). As indicated previously, a number of hormones appear to regulate hepatic glycogen content in health. The role of these hormones in the mobilization of hepatic glycogen after injury may be inferred by comparing the plasma concentrations of these hormones after injury with the concentrations required to promote glycogenolysis in healthy subjects.

The threshold for adrenaline-stimulated glucose entry into the circulation has been shown to be of the order of 1 nmol/l (14), which is within the range commonly encountered in injured patients (15). The action of adrenaline does not appear to be related to changes in plasma insulin or glucagon concentration, and the relative roles of glycogenolysis and gluconeogenesis in adrenaline-mediated entry of glucose into the circulation are unclear. Glycogenolysis has been shown to contribute significantly to the increase in plasma glucose observed after adrenaline infusion (16). The role of adrenaline in the mobilization of glucose reserves after injury is further supported by the observation that hyperglycemia after injury relates closely to plasma adrenaline concentration (17). Sympathetic nervous activation may also play a direct role in these responses because hepatic glycogenolysis occurs after direct stimulation of the hepatic sympathetic nerves (18).

Although glucagon secretion after injury is mediated, at least in part, by β-adreno-ceptors (19), peripheral plasma glucagon concentrations rise slowly after injury (20). Stimulation of hepatic glucose production appears to occur at glucagon concentrations as low as 300 pg/ml (21). These data were derived from studies of the effects of exogenous glucagon administration, however, and lower plasma concentrations of endogenous glucagon may be equally effective because portal venous glucagon concentrations are approximately double those seen in peripheral venous blood (22). In addition, some studies have indicated that hepatic glucagon clearance is increased in sepsis and trauma (23)—portal venous glucagon may thus show a greater and more rapid response. The major source of glucose release stimulated by glucagon appears to be glycogen (24). Plasma concentrations of adrenaline and glucagon after accidental injury are usually in excess of those required for glycogenolysis (15) (Fig. 1). Although the glycogen-mobilizing effect of both hormones appears to be transient (16,21,22), stimulation of glycogenolysis appears to occur if plasma glucagon concentration is progressively increased (21), which may occur after injury (25). Although cortisol appears to be primarily involved in gluconeogenesis, as opposed to glycogenolysis, adrenaline and glucagon-mediated hepatic glucose production is potentiated and pro-longed by cortisol (26). The relative contributions of glycogenolysis and gluconeogen-esis to this potentiation are unclear.

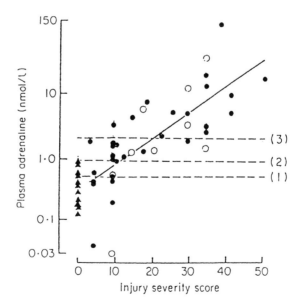

FIG. 1. Plasma adrenaline concentrations shortly (< 3 hours) after injury. Each point represents a separate patient. ▲, control; ●, injured; ○, injured; +, ethanol. Results are from Frayn et al. (17). *Dashed lines* represent threshold concentrations of adrenaline necessary for various metabolic effects, as determined by infusion into normal subjects (14): 1, stimulation of lipolysis; 2, elevation of plasma glucose and lactate concentrations; 3, suppression of plasma insulin concentration.

In comparison with hepatic glycogen, there is relatively little information regarding the effect of injury and sepsis on muscle glycogen content. Major and minor surgery appear to have little or no immediate effect on muscle glycogen content, although a gradual decline is seen several days postoperatively (27). Muscle glycogenolysis has, however, been reported in animal models of injury. Hindlimb ischemia leads to a rapid reduction in rat pectoralis muscle glycogen, and catecholamines appear to play a key role in this because the response is abolished after adrenal medullectomy (28). The type of injury may be of importance in the interpretation of these data, however, since a scald injury failed to affect muscle glycogen content in the fasted rat, although the capacity for glycogen synthesis after a glucose load was reduced (29). While other animal studies have supported these observations, hypothermia (which is associated with a hormonal response similar to injury) has been shown to lead to rapid muscle glycogenolysis in humans, indicated by the rapid efflux of glucose from the forearm (30). The validity of this assumption is supported by the observation that free glucose arises only from the branch points of the glycogen molecule (8% of the entire molecule); the rest of the glucose derived from muscle glycogenolysis is directed into glycolysis (31). The increased availability of glucose-6-phosphate within skeletal muscle, and its channelling into the glycolytic pathway may explain the accumulation of lactate after injury (32). Since muscle cannot export its glucose-6-phosphate directly, muscle glycogenolysis can only contribute to hyperglycemia indirectly, via lactate and pyruvate. This requires hepatic gluconeogenesis, which is characteristically unsuppressed by hyperglycemia in the critically ill patient (33). Adrenaline, glucagon, and cortisol appear to act synergistically to promote and maintain this process (26). The importance of hepatic gluconeogenesis is underlined by the continuation of markedly increased hepatic glucose production during the course of sepsis or injury (17,33–35), after hepatic glycogen might be expected to have been depleted, despite significant hyperglycemia, and even in the presence of intravenous glucose administration (33,36,37). This increased gluconeogenesis may relate to the increased availability of gluconeogenic substrate and/or the presence of the appropriate hormonal environment. The relative influences of the processes are difficult to separate. Lactate (from skeletal muscle and hypoxic tissue), pyruvate, alanine and glutamine (from muscle proteolysis), and glycerol (from adipose tissue lipolysis) may all compete for entry into the gluconeogenic pathway and maintain the increased hepatic production of glucose.

In burn injury, lactate appears to be quantitatively the most important gluconeogenic substrate (38). After accidental injury, the liver must accommodate the 40% increase in the rate of alanine appearance and the 100% increase in the rate of glycerol appearance and lactate availability (39). It is not entirely surprising that these markedly increased rates of three-carbon substrate delivery result in the increased hepatic production of glucose (40). This implies that the production of glucose is not geared to the body's ability to oxidize glucose or even the body's need for glucose, but simply relates to a disturbance in the normal mechanisms by which glucose requirements can be met by the mobilization of peripheral fuel substrate. Although this hypothesis appears reasonable, it should be noted, however, that, in circumstances in which insulin and glucagon levels have been clamped in such patients, a fall in hepatic glucose production is observed, despite the maintenance of increased rates of gluconeogenic substrate delivery (41). This suggests that the hormonal environment may be more important than the delivery of substrate in the maintenance of gluconeogenesis after injury.

Lipid Mobilization

Unlike glycogen, fat depots in normally nourished individuals are extensive, and it is difficult to ascertain the rate of lipid mobilization from the reduction in fat content. Turnover of free fatty acids (FFA) is, however, directly related to the plasma concentration of FFA, and this has been verified after limb ischemia (42), burns (43), and endotoxin administration (44). Although this may facilitate inferences regarding the effect of injury upon lipid mobilization, the effect of injury on FFA mobilization is still unclear. In the rat, limb ischemia leads to an increase in the FFA content of the epididymal fat pads (45). In the absence of hypovolemia, this rise is associated with a rise in plasma FFA concentration, but in shock, the delivery of FFA from the fat pads to the circulation is impaired as a result of the reduction in perfusion of the fat pads. Hypovolemia is associated with a fall in plasma FFA concentration toward that seen in controls (46). In contrast, scald injury appears to result in a fall in plasma FFA concentration, without accumulation of FFA in fat depots (43,47). The fall in plasma FFA concentration was associated with a rise in glycerol concentration, suggesting that the fall in FFA concentration was associated with reesterification. The interpretation of these effects is complicated by differences in the animal species and models of injury used. In the hindlimb ischemia model, for example, changes in plasma glycerol concentration were not observed (45,48). In the clinical situation, plasma concentrations of FFA and glycerol are raised within a few hours of injury. Studies of small groups of patients have shown these rises to be highly variable and unrelated to the severity of musculoskeletal injury (25) or burns (49,50). In a larger population of patients, however, FFA and glycerol concentrations were higher in patients with moderate than with minor injury, and the rise in FFA concentration correlated with the rise in glycerol concentration (15). In the most severely injured patients, FFA concentration was relatively low in comparison with glycerol concentration, suggesting either retention of FFA within the fat depots or increased reesterification in conditions in which lactate concentrations were particularly high.

In addition to oxidation of FFA via acetyl CoA, fat stores may also be mobilized to produce ketone bodies, which many tissues are capable of utilizing as fuel. There is evidence to suggest abnormalities of ketogenesis in the presence of sepsis and injury. In the ischemic limb injury model in the rat, the effect of injury appears to depend on nutritional status. In the postabsorptive period, circulating ketone body concentration and turnover increased (51). Liver ketone body content was raised relative to plasma FFA concentration (52), indicating that the increased ketone body concentration occurred as a result of hepatic diversion of FFA into ketogenesis, rather than simply as an effect related to increased availability of FFA. In contrast, after prolonged starvation, in the setting of accelerated ketogenesis, injury appears to reduce the concentration and turnover of ketone bodies (53). This suppression of ketogenesis has also been observed in experimental models of sepsis and appears to be related to a rise in plasma insulin concentration (54). A similar mechanism has been proposed to account for the suppression of ketogenesis seen in injured (55,56) and septic (57) patients.

Mobilization of Protein Stores

While negative nitrogen balance is an important aspect of the metabolic response to sepsis and injury, it should be noted that, in health, amino acids are not of particular importance as tissue fuel. Although the store of amino acids present within the protein of skeletal muscle becomes more important as a source of tissue fuel in injury and sepsis, it has been estimated that even under conditions of the most severe metabolic stress, the utilization of tissue protein stores only contributes up to 20% of the daily energy requirement (58).

Nevertheless, the wasting that accompanies critical illness as a result of the mobilization of tissue protein represents a considerable source of morbidity because it interferes with wound healing, ventilation, and rehabilitation (59). Trauma leads to characteristic changes in muscle amino acid concentrations: Decreases in muscle glutamine and basic amino acids are seen (60), while concentrations of branch-chain amino acids (BCAA) rise (61). Glutamine and alanine account for up to 45% of amino acid nitrogen released by skeletal muscle (62). These amino acids may act as tissue fuels directly or after deamination or be converted to glucose, or may be used either as fuels or incorporated into secretory proteins or structural proteins in the healing wound, white blood cells, kidney, gut mucosa, and acute phase proteins. The mechanisms for these responses and the factors that determine the partition of amino acids between the routes of disposal remain unclear. Although immobility, starvation, pyrexia, hypercortisolemia, and insulin resistance associated with other disease states (7,63–65) are associated with protein catabolism, negative nitrogen balance in these conditions seldom reaches the severity encountered in sepsis and trauma (66–68).

As in the case of glycogenolysis and gluconeogenesis, interest has centered on the possible role of counterregulatory hormones in the development of muscle protein catabolism. Cortisol has been shown to increase the rate of amino acid release from skeletal muscle, the rate of leucine oxidation within muscle, and the rate of hepatic gluconeogenesis, although its role in the protein catabolism of injury appears to be permissive (59). Glucagon has also been implicated in the proteolysis of trauma (69). Although combined infusion of cortisol, glucagon, and adrenaline into healthy subjects was associated with negative nitrogen balance (70), recent interest has been directed at the effect of cytokines such as interleukin (IL-1). Etiocholanolone injection (which induces IL-1 release) has been shown to lead to negative nitrogen balance (71), and incubation of skeletal muscle with IL-1 seems to induce proteolysis (72).

Prostaglandin E2 (PGE2) appears to act as a "second messenger" in this phenomenon, because incubation with IL-1 leads to an increase in PGE2 within muscle, and
the *in vitro* catabolic effect of IL-1 can be blocked by the administration of indomethacin (72). Unfortunately, IL-1 has not been found consistently in septic or injured
patients (73), and inhibitors of cyclooxygenase have not been shown to reduce the
nitrogen catabolism associated with experimental injury (74) or human sepsis (75).

Fuel Substrate Utilization

Injury and sepsis are associated with significant increases in resting energy expenditure (REE) (62,76) (Fig. 2). Indirect calorimetry has facilitated the measurement of
REE in injured and septic patients (77,78) and, when combined with measurement
of urinary nitrogen excretion, allows estimation of the relative contribution of glucose
and fat oxidation to energy production rate (79). We have already indicated that, in
stress, a series of pathophysiologic changes contribute to an increased availability
of glucose, fat, and amino acid fuel substrates. The following discussion reviews the
data relating to the oxidative and nonoxidative utilization of these fuel substrates in
critically ill patients.

Many studies have indicated a greater propensity for fat oxidation, compared with
glucose oxidation in injury and sepsis (80–85). In septic patients, glucose oxidation
rate and fat oxidation rate were negatively and positively related to the severity of
sepsis, respectively (82). Similarly, when indirect calorimetry was performed on
acutely injured patients, respiratory quotient (RQ) was shown to be low, indicating
preferential fat oxidation (86), and, in some cases, the amount of glucose oxidized

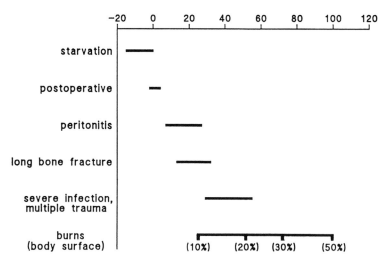

FIG. 2. Changes in resting metabolic rate during starvation and acute illness. Adapted from Wilmore (76).

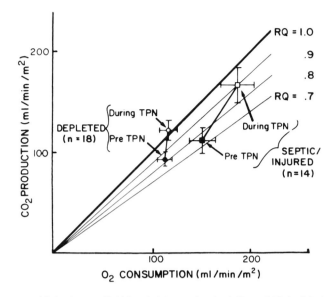

FIG. 3. Response, to high-glucose, lipid-free total parenteral nutrition, of 18 depleted and 14 septic/injured patients. Adapted from Askanazi et al. (81).

by the whole body was little more than that required by the brain (87). Although many of these reports have confirmed preferential fat oxidation, as suggested by a lower RQ, in the fasting state, the tendency for injured and septic patients to oxidize fat preferentially in the fed state is also supported by observations of the response of such patients to administration of intravenous glucose. Under normal circumstances, the administration of intravenous glucose to a fasting patient would be expected to result in a rise in RQ, indicating greater oxidation of glucose. As the rate of glucose administration increases, exceeding the energetic requirements of the patient, RQ typically rises above 1, indicating net lipid synthesis (88). This process is associated with a modest increase in REE, relating to the energetic requirements for the conversion of glucose to lipid. In contrast, injured and septic patients exhibit a smaller rise in RQ despite the administration of glucose, and RQ does not typically exceed 1 (81,83). Despite the absence of net lipogenesis, significantly greater increases in REE are observed when glucose is administered in excess of requirements (Fig. 3), and this response appears to be related to increased activity of the sympathetic nervous system, as indicated by an increase in the rate of urinary catecholamine excretion (81,89). The changes in the relative rates of fat and glucose oxidation associated with injury and sepsis must be interpreted in the light of the accompanying hypermetabolism. The absolute rate of glucose oxidation need not be reduced. There is evidence that glucose turnover may be increased after injury (90,91); however, the proportion of energy expenditure derived from the oxidation of glucose may be more important. It should also be noted that the rate of glucose clearance is not directly related to the rate of glucose oxidation (92). This implies that pathways of glucose disposal other than those directly related to oxidation may assume greater importance in stress, and it has been suggested that since lipogenesis appears to be negligible under these conditions, glycogen deposition may predominate (81). There is little direct evidence to support this claim, however, and we have previously shown that both glucose oxidation and storage are reduced in sepsis, and the proportion of glucose oxidized and stored were similar in septic and healthy subjects (Fig. 4). One might also expect that the hormonal environment encountered in the septic patient might be no more conducive to glycogen storage than to glucose oxidation.

The apparent preference of fat as a fuel substrate in the injured and septic patient is difficult to explain. Although some workers have claimed that insulin resistance (see below) is unlikely to contribute directly to defective glucose oxidation (40), it appears likely that insulin resistance might indirectly contribute to the observed pattern of fuel oxidation via a reduction in insulin-mediated entry of glucose into cells. Furthermore, impaired cellular glucose uptake may be compounded by defects in glycolytic pathways, which have been reported in sepsis (93,94). These defects appear to be unrelated to changes in counterregulatory hormones or insulin (94). Wilmore has stressed the importance of the "wound" as a metabolically active organ (95), and increased availability of glucose for the tissue of the wound can be regarded as a potential benefit of impaired glucose utilization by other body tissues. In addition, abnormalities of lipid mobilization might also directly influence glucose utilization. The ratio of glucose to fat oxidation appears to be related both to substrate availability and the hormonal milieu (96,97). Since the availability of glucose and fatty acids is

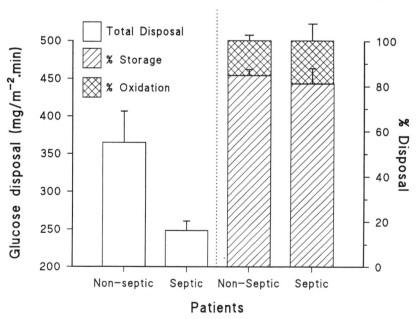

FIG. 4. Total, oxidative, and nonoxidative (percentage) glucose disposal in seven septic and seven nonseptic patients. Adapted from White et al. (83).

increased in stress, it has been suggested that the increase in fat metabolism may itself inhibit the oxidation of glucose (98). The effects of FFA on glucose utilization appear to be determined not only by plasma concentrations of FFA but also by the oxidative utilization of FFA. Increases in FFA oxidation impair glucose oxidation, and this leads to increases in the cytoplasmic concentration of acetyl CoA and citrate, which respectively inhibit the activity of the key glycolytic enzymes, pyruvate dehydrogenase and phosphofructokinase (98). These observations form the basis of Randle's "glucose/fatty acid cycle," which relates the increased availability and oxidation of FFA to impaired glucose oxidation and reduced responsiveness of muscle to insulin. The increase in sympathetic nervous system activity that characterizes sepsis and injury might indirectly impair glucose oxidation, via the effect of catecholamines on hormone sensitive lipase and the resulting increase in the availability of FFA. It is, therefore, pertinent to recognize that the administration of glucose in excess of the energetic requirements of the critically ill may lead to an increase in sympathetic nervous system activity (81,89). This may result in further lipid mobilization and oxidation, with a concomitant reduction in glucose utilization (99). This vicious cycle might result in a situation in which increasing glucose administration leads to a progressive reduction rather than a progressive increase in the percentage of energy derived from the oxidation of glucose.

Since insulin-mediated glucose uptake is responsible for glucose entry into the majority of tissues, it is understandable that early reports of hyperglycemia in injured and septic patients led investigators to conclude that, in stress states, the tissue of the body might be resistant to the effects of insulin.

INSULIN RESISTANCE IN SEPSIS AND INJURY

"Insulin resistance" implies that the normal anabolic effects of insulin are in abeyance in the injured, septic patient. Discussion of this phenomenon is complicated because insulin has a variety of anabolic effects, and it is important to be clear as to exactly what effect of insulin is attenuated when describing "insulin resistance." Although this might seem obvious, this approach has only rarely been adopted.

Clearly, the demonstration of an impaired response to insulin necessitates the demonstration of at least normal plasma concentrations of insulin in the presence of metabolic alterations that would normally be associated with absolute or relative insulin deficiency. Even this simple premise remains controversial: Some workers have shown that plasma insulin concentrations are markedly reduced acutely after injury (15), and then rise progressively, despite hyperglycemia, reaching a zenith 1 to 2 weeks after injury (84). Similar results have been reported after burns (100–102) and in septic patients (103). Unfortunately, other workers have reported normal or reduced basal plasma insulin concentrations in the same circumstances (83,104–106), and, furthermore, plasma insulin concentrations appear to depend on the cardiovascular status of septic patients. Septic shock rather than "high-flow" sepsis is associated with a reduction in plasma insulin concentrations (107), and hemodynamic variables are improved by the administration of high doses of exogenous insulin (108).

Even allowing for the decrease in plasma insulin observed in hypotensive septic patients, there are reports of increased (100) and decreased (49,106) insulin responses to a glucose load in stress. Some workers have described normal or elevated basal insulin concentrations but a reduction in peak stimulated concentrations (106), and increased splanchnic insulin release may occur despite a reduction in peripheral plasma concentrations in sepsis (109). These discrepancies may be explained in part by differences in the type and severity of disease in the patients and the adequacy of prior nutritional support and investigative protocols, but the lack of unequivocal data regarding the effect of injury and sepsis on plasma insulin concentration is a cause for concern. In addition, although many studies of the effects of sepsis and injury on plasma insulin concentration may be dismissed because they report static measurements rather than dynamic investigations of insulin responses to glucose administration, the use of the glucose clamp (110), which provides a dynamic index of the plasma insulin response to a glucose load, suffers the potential drawback of being nonphysiologic.

Before exploring the data relating to the presence or absence of insulin resistance, it is also important to note that in severe sepsis, increased glucose uptake has been shown to coexist with marked suppression of insulin secretion, suggesting that glucose metabolism can become dissociated from insulin secretion (104,105), that plasma insulin concentrations reliably reflect pancreatic secretion only if insulin clearance is unaltered, and that insulin clearance has been shown to increase in sepsis.

Insulin resistance has been defined as the "unresponsiveness of anabolic processes to the normal effects of insulin" (20). This definition implies enhanced hepatic glucose production despite high plasma glucose and insulin concentrations, together with a reduction in insulin-mediated glucose storage, increased lipid mobilisation and oxidation, and increased protein catabolism. What is the evidence to support these claims?

Glucose Metabolism

Early studies of glucose metabolism is burned (111) and injured (112) patients revealed that the hyperglycemia observed in such patients occurred despite increased plasma insulin concentrations and could not be overcome by the administration of large amounts of exogenous insulin. This "resistance" to the normal hypoglycemic effects of insulin appeared to be related directly to the severity of injury. As previously indicated, suppression of hepatic glucose production by insulin and glucose administration appears to be impaired in sepsis (33). However, isotopic studies suggest that glucose turnover is actually increased in stress (100,113). It has been suggested that this finding is not incompatible with insulin resistance, if, e.g., glucose oxidation alone were impaired, but glucose storage was increased (81). The results of glucose clamp studies do not support this explanation. In septic and normal subjects studied using the hyperglycemic glucose clamp technique, total glucose disposal was reduced and the relative rates of glucose storage and oxidation were preserved (83). Similar studies of injured patients using the euglycemic hyperinsulinemic clamp

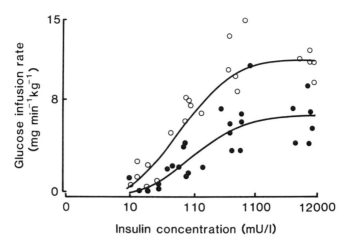

FIG. 5. Dose-response curves for the effect of insulin on whole-body glucose infusion rate necessary to maintain euglycemia in injured patients (•) and control subjects (○). Adapted from Henderson et al. (114).

technique have also demonstrated a reduction in whole-body and limb glucose uptake and, because a range of insulin concentrations were used, allowed the construction of dose-response curves (Fig. 5) for glucose disposal at different insulin concentrations, for normal and injured subjects (114). The dose-response curve in injured patients is shifted to the right, and the maximal response is reduced, indicating a postreceptor or a mixed postreceptor/receptor defect in insulin responsiveness. It is difficult to equate the evidence of increased glucose turnover with these findings. Furthermore, other studies have indicated that the increased glucose production and clearance can coexist with marked reductions in glucose-stimulated insulin secretion (106), which suggests either an *increased* sensitivity/responsiveness to insulin or a major role for non–insulin-dependent glucose uptake in sepsis. In this study, glucose clearance actually correlated negatively with plasma insulin concentrations, although it is interesting to note that plasma adrenaline concentrations were lower in septic than in control subjects, and the beta-adrenoceptor has been implicated in the pathogenesis of insulin resistance (115). Some studies have indicated that basal insulin concentrations exert an inhibitory effect on glucose production (41), which also fails to support the suggestion of insulin resistance. Although studies of fuel utilization in injured and septic patients suggest impairment of glucose oxidation, in keeping with the results of the clamp studies described above, when attempts have been made to relate glucose oxidation to plasma insulin concentration in injured patients, glucose oxidation was found to be appropriate to the elevated plasma insulin concentrations (116).

Although in general, glucose disposal appears to be either absolutely reduced, or reduced relative to glucose availability, it is difficult to reconcile these findings with the data suggesting increased glucose turnover, except to speculate that a significant proportion of the glucose turnover noted in isotopic studies relates to *futile cycling* of glucose, through lactate or glycerol.

Protein Metabolism

As indicated above, muscle wasting and protein catabolism characterize the metabolic state of the injured and septic patient. Insulin is generally believed to exert an anabolic effect on skeletal muscle (3). Studies of patients recovering from musculo-skeletal injury have demonstrated both temporal and quantitative correlations between hyperinsulinemia and urinary nitrogen excretion (84). This strongly suggests resistance of peripheral tissues (skeletal muscle) to the anabolic effects of insulin. Recent studies have failed to demonstrate insulin-dependent uptake of amino acids by skeletal muscle (117), and other studies in burned patients have indicated that although the hypoglycemic action of insulin was impaired (see above), hyperinsulinemia resulted in a reduction in the rate of leucine appearance (Ra) and oxidation, and a decrease in urea production (118). Despite the difference in hypoglycemic response, the effects of insulin on protein metabolism were almost identical in burned patients, compared with healthy controls. The use of somatostatin (which suppresses both endogenous insulin and glucagon secretion) has revealed that basal insulin levels in septic patients play a role in reducing the protein catabolism associated with sepsis (119). In this study, somatostatin administration resulted in a 52% reduction in plasma insulin concentrations and a 64% reduction in plasma glucagon concentrations. This reduction in insulin concentration, despite the simultaneous reduction of glucagon concentrations, was associated with a significant rise in leucine oxidation rate. Other studies have confirmed in vivo the preservation of insulin responsiveness in the anabolic regulation of protein metabolism, despite the presence of protein catabolism (120). These findings support the in vitro observation of normal rates of insulin-stimulated protein synthesis and inhibited protein breakdown at physiologic insulin concentrations in the soleus muscle of the burned rat (121).

Thus, although clinical experience suggests that muscle wasting is not readily prevented by the administration of glucose, insulin, or amino acids to septic or injured patients (122), there is little direct evidence to support the claim that the normal anabolic responses of protein metabolism to insulin are lost in injury or sepsis, which implies that factors other than insulin resistance play a role in the muscle wasting that accompany injury and sepsis.

Mechanisms of Insulin Resistance

Although insulin resistance may exist (at least in terms of the effect of insulin on glucose metabolism), the reasons for insulin resistance are unclear. Our incomplete knowledge of the cellular basis for the metabolic effects of insulin requires further studies of insulin resistance at the cellular level rather than at the whole-body or organ level before a clear understanding of the phenomenon of insulin resistance can be expected. Unfortunately, such studies will be difficult to conduct even in animal models of sepsis and injury. The relatively normal responses of tissues in vitro suggest that a circulating factor(s) mediate insulin resistance (123). Blood-borne agents have been shown to induce metabolic changes in isolated animal limbs that might be expected with insulin resistance, and the active moiety has been suggested to have a molecular weight of between 1,000 and 10,000 daltons (124). This agent has not, however, been identified, and thus far, interest has centered on the roles of counter-regulatory hormones and fatty acids in the pathogenesis of insulin resistance.

Infusions of glucagon, adrenaline, and cortisol into healthy human subjects appear to reproduce some features suggestive of insulin resistance (hyperglycemia and negative nitrogen balance), although the plasma concentration of counterregulatory hormones required appears to exceed those observed in sepsis (70). Cortisol, growth hormone, and adrenaline have been shown to induce insulin resistance associated with a postreceptor defect in the action of insulin (125). It should be noted, however, that this merely describes an abnormal pattern of the insulin dose-response curve and provides little or no information regarding the cellular mechanisms for the defect, which are likely to result from the combined interactions of hormones on enzymes systems that control metabolic pathways. Furthermore, in studies of insulin resistance associated with sepsis, the degree of insulin resistance, unlike the increase in the concentration of counterregulatory hormones, did not correlate with the severity of sepsis (83), which implies that other factors must have contributed.

As outlined earlier, sepsis and injury may be associated with increases in the rate of lipolysis, increased availability of lipid fuel substrate, and increased rates of fat oxidation. The increased mobilization and utilization of lipid have been suggested as a possible mechanism for insulin resistance (126). Increased delivery of fatty acids to the liver is known to lead indirectly to increased hepatic glucose production (127). Lipid is not itself converted to glucose, but the acetyl CoA and ATP resulting from increased fat oxidation appear to inhibit pyruvate dehydrogenase and supply the energy required for hepatic gluconeogenesis (126). Peripheral glucose utilization is also impaired by increased peripheral fat oxidation.

A final reason for insulin resistance relates to the demonstration of impaired glucose tolerance and insulin sensitivity in association with immobility (128). The underlying mechanisms for this response are unknown, but immobility is a feature common to all injured and septic patients and may explain the disturbances in glucose metabolism observed in surgical convalescence.

SUMMARY

Sepsis and injury are associated with fuel substrate mobilization and alterations in the oxidation of fuels. An inability to utilize glucose appears to coexist with an increase in the availability of glucose, lipid, and amino acid fuel substrate. This process is associated with the apparently purposeless consumption of body protein to provide glucose, which may be available in excess of the body's need for this fuel.

Some of the normal anabolic actions of insulin appear to be impaired in the setting of hypermetabolism and increased concentrations of counterregulatory hormones, although the relationship of these hormonal changes to the metabolic alterations is still incompletely understood.

Until a clearer understanding of the pathophysiology of these hormonal and metabolic alterations is available, attempts to provide rational and effective nutritional support to the critically ill patient are likely to be ineffective.

REFERENCES

1. Ganong WF. Endocrine functions of the pancreas and the regulation of carbohydrate metabolism. In: Ganong WF (ed). *Review of Medical Physiology*. Los Altos, California: Lange, 1977;251.
2. Kuhara T, Ikeda S, Ohneda A, Sasaki Y. Effects of intravenous infusion of 17 amino acids on the secretion of GH, glucagon and insulin in sheep. *Am J Physiol* 1991;260:E21–E26.
3. Devlin JJ, Horton ES. Hormone and nutrient interactions. In: Shils ME, Young VR (eds). *Modern Nutrition in Health and Disease*. Philadelpia: Lea and Febiger, 1988;570.
4. Long JM, Wilmore DW, Mason AD, Pruitt BA. Effect of carbohydrate and fat intake on nitrogen excretion during total intravenous feeding. *Ann Surg* 1977;185:417–422.
5. Barton RN. Neuroendocrine mobilisation of body fuels after injury. *Br Med Bull* 1985;41:218–225.
6. Hales CN, Luzio JP, Siddle K. Hormonal control of adipose-tissue lipolysis. *Biochem Soc Symp* 1978; 43:97–135.
7. Rennie MJ. Muscle protein turnover and the wasting due to injury and disease. *Br Med Bull* 1985; 41:257–264.
8. Cahill GF Jr. Starvation in man. *Clin Endocrinol Metab* 1976;5:397–415.
9. Flatt JP. The biochemistry of energy expenditure. In: Bray GA (ed). *Recent Advances in Obesity Research*. Washington, DC: Newman, 1977;211.
10. Annamunthodo H, Keating VJ, Patrick SJ. Liver glycogen alterations in anaesthesia and surgery. *Anaesthesia* 1958;13:429–433.
11. Sunzel H. Effects of surgical trauma on the liver glycogen in fasting and in glucose-fed patients. *Acta Chir Scand* 1963;125:118–128.
12. Hall GM, Traynor C, Paterson JL. Changes in liver glycogen and glycolytic intermediates during abdominal surgery in man. *Clin Sci* 1983;64:109–111.
13. Heath DF, Frayn KN, Rose JG. Effects of halothane on glucose metabolism after injury in the rat. *Br J Anaesth* 1978;50:899–904.
14. Clutter WE, Bier DM, Shah SD, Cryer PE. Epinephrine plasma metabolic clearance rates and physiological thresholds for metabolic and haemodynamic actions in man. *J Clin Invest* 1980;66:94–101.
15. Stoner HB, Frayn KN, Barton RN, et al. The relationships between plasma substrates and hormones and the severity of injury in 277 recently injured patients. *Clin Sci* 1979;95:93–104.
16. Sacca L, Vigorito C, Cicala M, et al. Role of gluconeogenesis in epinephrine-stimulated hepatic glucose production in humans. *Am J Physiol* 1983;245:E294–E302.
17. Frayn KN, Little RA, Maycock PF, Stoner HB. The relationship of plasma catecholamines to acute metabolic and hormonal responses to injury in man. *Circ Shock* 1985;16:229–240.
18. Hems DA, Whitton PD. Control of hepatic glycogenolysis. *Physiol Rev* 1980;60:1–50.
19. Rose JG, Heath DF. The effects of stress and injury on the activity of phosphoenolpyruvate carboxykinase in the liver of the rat. *Biochem J* 1986;233:239–244.
20. Frayn KN. Hormonal control of metabolism in trauma and sepsis. *Clin Endocrinol* 1986;24:577–599.
21. Fradkin J, Shamoon H, Felig P, Sherwin RS. Evidence for an important role of changes rather than absolute concentrations of glucagon in the regulation of glucose production in humans. *J Clin Endocrinol Metab* 1980;50:698–703.
22. Blackard WG, Nelson NC, Andrews SS. Portal and peripheral vein immunoreactive glucagon concentrations after arginine or glucose infusions. *Diabetes* 1974;23:199–202.
23. Zenser TV, Derubertis FR, Geroge DT, Rayfield EJ. Infection-induced hyperglucagonaemia and altered hepatic response to glucagon in the rat. *Am J Physiol* 1974;227:1299–1305.

24. Cherrington AD, Williams PE, Shulman GI, Lacy WW. Differential time course of glucagons' effect on glycogenolysis and gluconeogenesis in the conscious dog. *Diabetes* 1981;30:180–187.
25. Meguid MM, Brennan MF, Aoki TT, et al. Hormone-substrate interrelationships following trauma. *Arch Surg* 1974;109:776–783.
26. Shamoon H, Hendler R, Sherwin RS. Synergistic interactions among antiinsulin hormones in the pathogenesis of stress hyperglycaemia in humans. *J Clin Endocrinol Metab* 1981;52:1235–1241.
27. Bergstrom J, Castenfors H, Hultman E, Silander T. The effect of surgery upon muscle glycogen in man. *Acta Chir Scand* 1965;130:1–6.
28. Stoner HB. Studies on the mechanism of shock. The quantitative aspects of glycogen metabolism after limb ischaemia in the rat. *Br J Exp Pathol* 1958;39:635–661.
29. Hessman Y. Glycogen storage in rat liver and skeletal muscle in thermal trauma I. Effect of exogenous insulin. *Acta Chir Scand* 1975;141:385–392.
30. Stoner HB, Frayn KN, Barton RN, et al. Metabolic aspects of hypothermia in the elderly. *Clin Sci* 1980;59:19–27.
31. Wicklamyr M, Dietze G. On the mechanism of glucose release from the muscle of juvenile diabetics in acute insulin deficiency. *Eur J Clin Invest* 1978;8:81–86.
32. Daniel AM, Shizgal HM, Maclean LD. The anatomic and metabolic source of lactate in shock. *Surg Gynecol Obstet* 1978;147:697–700.
33. Long CL, Kinney JM, Geiger JW. Nonsuppressibility of gluconeogenesis by glucose in septic patients. *Metabolism* 1976;25:193–201.
34. Imamura M, Clowes GHA Jr, Blackburn GL, et al. Liver metabolism and gluconeogenesis in trauma and sepsis. *Surgery* 1975;77:868–880.
35. Wilmore DW, Goodwin CW, Aulick LH, et al. Effect of injury and infection on visceral metabolism. *Ann Surg* 1980;192:491–504.
36. Shaw JHF, Wolfe RR. Determination of glucose turnover and oxidation in normal volunteers and septic patients using stable and radioisotopes; the response to glucose infusion and total parenteral nutrition. *Aust NZ J Surg* 1986;56:785–791.
37. Wolfe RR. Burn trauma and increased glucose production. *Trauma* 1979;19:898–899.
38. Wolfe RR, Miller HI, Spitzer JJ. Glucose and lactate metabolism in burns and shock. *Am J Physiol* 1977;232:415–418.
39. Shaw JHF, Wolfe RR. An integrated analysis of glucose, fat and protein metabolism in severely traumatised patients; studies in the basal state and the response to intravenous nutrition. *Ann Surg* 1989;207:63–72.
40. Douglas RG, Shaw JHF. Metabolic response to sepsis and trauma. *Br J Surg* 1989;76:115–122.
41. Jahoor F, Herndon DN, Wolfe RR. Role of insulin and glucose in the response of glucose and alanine kinetics in burn injured patients. *J Clin Invest* 1986;78:807–814.
42. Heath DF, Stoner HB. Studies on the mechanism of shock. Non esterified fatty acid metabolism in normal and injured rats. *Br J Exp Pathol* 1968;49:160–169.
43. Robinson KM, Miller HI. Free fatty acid turnover and oxidation after burn shock in guinea pigs. *Circ Shock* 1981;8:283–290.
44. Romanosky AJ, Bagby GJ, Bockman EL, Spitzer JJ. Free fatty acid utilisation by skeletal muscle after endotoxin administration. *Am J Physiol* 1980;239:E391–E395.
45. Stoner HB, Matthews J. Studies on the mechanism of shock. Fat mobilisation after injury. *Br J Exp Pathol* 1962;43:556–563.
46. Stoner HB. Studies on the mechanism of shock. The effect of limb ischaemia on the non-esterified fatty acids of rat plasma. *Br J Exp Pathol* 1962;43:556–563.
47. Robinson KM, Miller HI. Adipose tissue and plasma free fatty acid and glycerol concentrations during burn shock in guinea pigs. *Proc Soc Exp Biol Med* 1980;165:375–379.
48. Matthews J. The effect of limb ischaemia on the serum glycerol concentration of the rat. *Experientia* 1965;21:611–612.
49. Allison SP, Hinton P, Chamberlain MJ. Intravenous glucose tolerance, insulin and free fatty acid levels in burned patients. *Lancet* 1968;2:1113–1116.
50. Birke G, Carlson LA, Liljedahl S-O. Lipid metabolism and trauma III. Plasma lipids and lipoproteins in burns. *Acta Med Scand* 1965;178:337–350.
51. Barton RN. The interconversion and disposal of ketone bodies in untreated and injured post-absorptive rats. *Biochem J* 1973;136:531–543.
52. Barton RN. Ketone body concentrations in liver and blood after limb ischaemia in the rat. *Clin Sci* 1971;40:463–477.

53. Barton RN. Effect of ischaemic limb injury on the rates of metabolism of ketone bodies in starved rats. *Biochem J* 1976;156:233–238.
54. Neufeld HA, Pace JG, Kaminski MV, et al. A probable endocrine basis for the depression of ketone bodies during infectious or inflammatory state in rats. *Endocrinology* 1980;107:596–601.
55. Williamson DH. Regulation of ketone body metabolism and the effects of injury. *Acta Chir Scand* 1981;Suppl 507:22–29.
56. Birkhahn RH, Long CL, Fitkin DL, et al. A comparison of the effects of skeletal trauma and surgery on the ketosis of starvation in man. *J Trauma* 1981;21:513–518.
57. Clowes GHA Jr, O'Donnell TF, Blackburn GL, Maki TN. Energy metabolism and proteolysis in traumatized and septic man. *Surg Clin North Am* 1976;56:1169–1184.
58. Long CL, Nelson KM, Akin JM, et al. A physiologic basis for the provision of fuel mixtures in normal and stressed patients. *J Trauma* 1990;30:1077–1085.
59. Ryan NT. Metabolic adaptations for energy production during trauma and sepsis. *Surg Clin North Am* 1976;56:1073–1090.
60. Askanazi J, Furst P, Michelsen CB, et al. Muscle and plasma amino acids after injury; hypocaloric glucose vs amino acid infusion. *Ann Surg* 1980;191:465–472.
61. Vinnars E, Bergstrom J, Furst P. Influence of the postoperative state on the intracellular free amino acids in human muscle tissue. *Ann Surg* 1975;182:665–671.
62. Arnold J, Little RA. Stress and metabolic response to trauma in critical illness. *Curr Anaesth* 1991; 2:139–148.
63. Bergstrom J. Muscle electrolytes in man. *Scand J Clin Lab Invest* 1962;14(Suppl 68):1–110.
64. Askanazi J, Elwyn DH, Kinney JM, et al. Muscle and plasma amino acids after injury: the role of inactivity. *Ann Surg* 1978;188:797–803.
65. Furst P, Bergstrom J, Chao I, et al. Influence of amino acid supply on nitrogen and amino acid metabolism in severe trauma. *Acta Chir Scand* 1979;494(Suppl):136–138.
66. Hassett J, Border JR. The metabolic response to trauma and sepsis. *World J Surg* 1983;7:125–131.
67. Kinney JM, Elwyn DH. Protein metabolism in the traumatised patient. *Acta Chir Scand* 1985; 522(Suppl):45–46.
68. Fleck A, Colley CM, Myers MA. Liver export proteins and trauma. *Br Med Bull* 1985;41:265–273.
69. Shaw JHF, Wolfe RR. Metabolic intervention in surgical patients: an assessment of the effects of somatostatin, ranitidine, naloxone, diclophenac, dipyramidole or salbutamol infusion on energy and protein kinetics in surgical patients using stable and radioisotopes. *Ann Surg* 1988;207:274–282.
70. Bessey PQ, Watters JM, Aoki TT, Wilmore DW. Combined hormonal infusion simulates the metabolic response to sepsis. *Ann Surg* 1984;200:264–281.
71. Watters JM, Bessey PQ, Dinarello CA, et al. The induction of interleukin-1 in humans and its metabolic effects. *Surgery* 1985;98:298–305.
72. Baracos V, Rodemann P, Dinarello CA, Goldberg AL. Stimulation of muscle protein degradation and prostaglandin E2 release by leucocyte pyrogen (IL-1). A mechanism for the increased degradation of muscle proteins during fever. *N Engl J Med* 1983;308:553–558.
73. Leinhardt DJ, Carlson GL, Lamb WR, et al. The cytokine response to abdominal sepsis. *Proc Nutr Soc* 1992;51:113A.
74. Clark AS, Kelly RA, Mitch WE. Systemic response to thermal injury in rats: accelerated protein degradation and altered glucose utilisation in muscle. *J Clin Invest* 1984;74:888–897.
75. Hasselgren P, Talamini M, Lofrance R, et al. Effect of indomethacin on proteolysis in septic muscle. *Ann Surg* 1985;202:557–562.
76. Wilmore DW. *The Metabolic Management of the Critically Ill.* New York: Plenum Publishing Co., 1977.
77. Kinney JM, Morgan AP, Dominguez FJ, Gildner KJ. A method for continuous measurement of gas exchange and expired radioactivity in acutely ill patients. *Metabolism* 1964;13:205–211.
78. Spencer JL, Zikria AB, Kinney JM, et al. A system for the continuous measurement of gas exchange and respiratory functions. *J Appl Physiol* 1972;33:523–528.
79. Ferrannini E. The theoretical bases of indirect calorimetry: a review. *Metabolism* 1988;37:287–301.
80. Jeevanandam M, Young DH, Schiller WR. Influence of parenteral nutrition on rates of net substrate oxidation in severe trauma patients. *Crit Care Med* 1990;18:467–473.
81. Askanazi J, Carpentier YA, Elwyn DH, et al. Influence of total parenteral nutrition on fuel utilisation in injury and sepsis. *Ann Surg* 1980;191:40–46.
82. Stoner HB, Little RA, Frayn KN, et al. The effect of sepsis on the oxidation of carbohydrate and fat. *Br J Surg* 1983;70:32–35.

83. White RH, Frayn KN, Little RA, et al. Hormonal and metabolic responses to glucose infusion in sepsis by the hyperglycaemic glucose clamp technique. *JPEN* 1987;11:345–353.
84. Frayn KN, Little RA, Stoner HB, Galasko CSB. Metabolic control in non-septic patients with musculoskeletal injuries. *Injury* 1984;16:73–79.
85. Giovannini I, Boldrini G, Castagneto M, et al. Respiratory quotient and patterns of substrate utilisation in human sepsis and trauma. *JPEN* 1983;7:226–230.
86. Little RA, Stoner HB, Frayn KN. Substrate oxidation shortly after accidental injury in man. *Clin Sci* 1981;61:789–791.
87. Frayn KN. Substrate turnover after injury. *Br Med Bull* 1985;41:232–239.
88. Kinney JM. The carbohydrate content of parenteral nutrition. In: Johnston IDA (Ed). *Advances in Clinical Nutrition*. Boston: MIT Press, 1983;283.
89. Nordenstrom J, Jeevanandam M, Elwyn DH, et al. Increasing glucose intake during total parenteral nutrition increases norepinephrine excretion in trauma and sepsis. *Clin Physiol* 1981;1:525–534.
90. Gump FE, Long CL, Geiger JW, Kinney JM. The significance of altered gluconeogenesis in surgical catabolism. *J Trauma* 1975;15:704–713.
91. Shaw JHF, Klein S, Wolfe RR. Assessment of alanine, urea and glucose interrelationships in normal subjects and in patients with sepsis with stable isotopic tracers. *Surgery* 1985;97:557–568.
92. Wolfe RR, O'Donnell TF, Stone MD, et al. Investigation of factors determining the optimal glucose infusion rate in total parenteral nutrition. *Metabolism* 1980;29:892–900.
93. Vary TC, Siegal JH, Wakatani T, et al. Effect of sepsis on activity of pyruvate dehydrogenase complex in skeletal muscle and liver. *Am J Physiol* 1986;13:634–640.
94. Arnold J, Hamer MJ, Irving MH. Hepatic phosphofructokinase-l-activity and fructose 2-6 biphosphate levels in patients with abdominal sepsis. *Clin Sci* 1991;80:213–217.
95. Wilmore DW, Aulick LH, Mason AD, Pruitt BA. Influence of the burn wound on local and systemic responses to injury. *Ann Surg* 1977;186:444–458.
96. Ruderman NB, Toews CJ, Shafrir E. Role of free fatty acids in glucose homeostasis. *Arch Intern Med* 1969;123:299–313.
97. Randle PJ, Garland PB, Hales CN, et al. Interactions of metabolism and the physiological role of insulin. *Recent Prog Horm Res* 1966;22:1–43.
98. Randle PJ, Garland PB, Hales CN, Newsholme EA. The glucose and fatty acid cycle; its role in insulin resistance and the metabolic disturbances of diabetes mellitus. *Lancet* 1963;1:785–789.
99. Steinberg D. Catecholamine stimulation of fat mobilization and its metabolic consequences. *Pharmacol Rev* 1966;18:217–235.
100. Wolfe RR, Durkot MJ, Allsop JR, Burke JF. Glucose metabolism in severely burned patients. *Metabolism* 1979;28:1031–1039.
101. Batstone GF, Alberti KGMM, Hinks L. Metabolic studies in subjects following thermal injury. Intermediary metabolites, hormones and tissue oxygenation. *Burns* 1976;2:207–225.
102. Shuck JM, Eaton RP, Shuck LW, et al. Dynamics of insulin and glucagon secretion in severely burned patients. *J Trauma* 1977;17:706–712.
103. Clowes GHA, Martin H, Walji S. Blood insulin responses to blood glucose levels in high output sepsis and septic shock. *Am J Surg* 1978;135:577–583.
104. Merrill GF, Spitzer JJ. Glucose and lactate kinetics in guinea pigs following E. coli endotoxin administration. *Circ Shock* 1978;5:11–21.
105. Witck-Janusek L, Filkins JP. Insulin-like action of endotoxin. Antagonism by steroidal and non-steroidal anti-inflammatory agents. *Circ Shock* 1981;8:573–583.
106. Dahn MS, Jacobs LA, Smith S, et al. The relationship of insulin production to glucose metabolism in severe sepsis. *Arch Surg* 1985;120:166–172.
107. Halter JD, Pflug AE. Relationship of impaired insulin secretion during surgical stress to anesthesia and catecholamine secretion. *J Clin Endocrinol Metab* 1980;51:1093–1098.
108. Clowes GHA, O'Donnell TF, Ryan NT, Blackburn GL. Energy metabolism in sepsis. Treatment based upon different patterns in shock and high output state. *Ann Surg* 1974;180:684–687.
109. Gump FE, Long C, Killian P, Kinney J. Studies of glucose intolerance in septic injured patients. *J Trauma* 1974;14:378–388.
110. DeFronzo RA, Tobin JD, Andres R. Glucose clamp technique; a method for quantifying insulin secretion and resistance. *Am J Physiol* 1979;237:E214–E223.
111. Evans EI, Butterfield WJH. The stress response in the severely burned. *Ann Surg* 1951;134:588–613.
112. Howard JM. Studies of the absorption and metabolism of glucose following injury. The systemic response to injury. *Ann Surg* 1955;141:321–326.

113. Long CL, Spencer JL, Kinney JM, Geiger JW. Carbohydrate metabolism in man: effect of elective operations and of major injury. *J Appl Physiol* 1971;31:110–116.
114. Henderson AA, Frayn KN, Galasko CSB, Little RA. Dose-response relationships for the effects of insulin on glucose and fat metabolism in injured patients and control subjects. *Clin Sci* 1991;80: 25–32.
115. Bessey PQ, Wilmore DW. β-adrenergic regulation of glucose disposal. A reciprocal relationship with insulin release. *J Surg Res* 1983;34:404–414.
116. Black PR, Brooks DC, Bessey PQ, et al. Mechanisms of insulin resistance following injury. *Ann Surg* 1982;196:420–435.
117. Tessari P, Inchiostro S, Biolo G, et al. Effects of acute systemic hyperinsulinaemia on forearm muscle proteolysis in healthy man. *J Clin Invest* 1991;88:27–33.
118. Jahoor F, Shangraw RE, Miyoshi H, et al. Role of insulin and glucose oxidation in mediating the protein catabolism of burns and sepsis. *Am J Physiol* 1989;257:E323–E331.
119. Zhang Z-J, Kunkel KR, Jahoor F, Wolfe RR. Role of basal insulin in the regulation of protein kinetics and energy metabolism in septic patients. *JPEN* 1991;15:394–399.
120. Brooks DC, Bessey PQ, Black PR. Insulin stimulates branched chain amino acid uptake and diminished nitrogen flux from skeletal muscle of injured patients. *J Surg Res* 1986;40:395–405.
121. Odessey R, Parr B. Effect of insulin and leucine on protein turnover in rat soleus muscle after burn injury. *Metabolism* 1982;31:82–86.
122. Cerra FB, Siegel JH, Coleman B, et al. Septic autocannibalism—a failure of exogenous nutritional support. *Ann Surg* 1980;192:570–580.
123. Frayn KN, le Marchand-Brustel Y, Freychet P. Studies on the mechanism of insulin resistance after injury in the mouse. *Diabetologia* 1978;14:337–341.
124. Clowes GHA, Geroge BC, Vilee CA, Saravis CA. Muscle proteolysis induced by a circulatory peptide in blood plasma of patients with sepsis and trauma. *N Engl J Med* 1983;30816:545–552.
125. Carlson GL, Little RA. The pathophysiology and pattern of the hormonal response to severe sepsis. In: Boles JM (ed). *Conséquences endocriniennes des états d'agression aiguë*. Paris: Arnette, 1992; 57.
126. Reaven GM. Role of insulin resistance in human disease. *Diabetes* 1988;37:1595–1607.
127. Groop LC, Bonadonna RC, DelPrato S, et al. Glucose and free fatty acid metabolism in non–insulin-dependent diabetes mellitus. *J Clin Invest* 1989;84:205–213.
128. Vernikos J. Metabolic and endocrine changes. In: Sandler H, Vernikos J. (eds). *Inactivity: Physiological effects*. Orlando: Academic Press, 1986;99.

*Organ Metabolism and Nutrition:
Ideas for Future Critical Care*, edited by
J. M. Kinney and H. N. Tucker.
Raven Press, Ltd., New York © 1994.

4

Hypothalamus, Glucopenia, and Fuel Mobilization

Patricia E. Molina and Naji N. Abumrad

Department of Surgery, SUNY at Stony Brook, Stony Brook, New York 11794

The role of the hypothalamus in orchestrating the neuroendocrine response to glucopenia has been suspected and supported by scientific findings dating back to the mid-1800s. Although sometimes controversial, the results of over 100 years of studies have led to substantial neurochemical and physiologic support of the importance of the hypothalamus in regulating energy metabolism. More recently, the scientific quest for accuracy has led to differentiation within the hypothalamus of what, at times, appears to be antagonistic functions of the different neuronal groupings. Sophisticated studies using localized stimulation of different areas in the CNS or their specific ablation have indicated that the control of glucose, protein, and fat metabolism may not occur at the same site and, furthermore, may not be mediated by the same neuropeptide or neurotransmitter. In this chapter, we discuss some of these results and present them in the context of what occurs during glucopenia. Some of the areas have been enriched by results from our laboratory during the past years. Others are presented as working hypotheses and reflect our speculations on how fuel mobilization is regulated during glucopenia.

THE HYPOTHALAMUS AS AN INTEGRATOR

The function of the hypothalamus as the integrative station for neural and hormonal regulation of peripheral metabolism has been supported by several studies (1). Plasma glucose concentrations have a significant correlation with hypothalamic neuronal activity (2), a mechanism whereby the brain is thought to modulate fuel mobilization. The hypothalamus is commonly divided into several nuclei arranged in three longitudinal zones, namely, a lateral, medial, and periventricular zone (3). The periventricular zone surrounds the third ventricle and is composed of the periventricular, suprachiasmatic, paraventricular, arcuate, and posterior nuclei of the hypothalamus. The medial is divided from the lateral zones by the fornix bundle. Many of the most conspicuous cell groups occupy the medial zone, among them the preoptic, anterior hypothalamic, ventromedial, dorsomedial, and premammillary nuclei. The lateral zone is traversed by massive longitudinal fibers of the medial forebrain bundle and includes the preoptic nucleus and the lateral hypothalamic area.

The ventromedial hypothalamus (VMH) and lateral hypothalamus (LH) have been areas of special focus in the study of the role of the CNS control of counterregulation and fuel mobilization. The LH and medial hypothalamus are considered to act reciprocally in neurometabolic influences in the liver and pancreas (4). Glucose-sensitive neurons, defined as those whose activity is decreased by direct application of glucose, constitute approximately 20% to 25% of the lateral and ventromedial hypothalamic neurons (5). Glucose-sensitive neurons in the LH decrease their activity in response to glucose application, and glucoreceptors of the VMH enhance their firing rate in response to glucose (1). Stimulation of the ventral part of the LH increases activity in the pancreatic vagus, which results in increased insulin release. Glucose sensors of the small intestine, portal vein, and liver also decrease firing when glucose is infused directly into the portal circulation or when glucose is applied directly. The presence of vagal intestinal glucoreceptors has been demonstrated, and their existence has also been linked to the splanchnic nerve. The presence of glucose sensors in the liver has been suggested by studies that show decreased firing in the vagus nerve after intraportal administration of glucose (6). This indicates that an increase in glucose concentration in the portal blood is relayed as a decrease in the rate of signals from the hepatoportal area to the hypothalamus via the vagus and the nucleus tractus solitarius (NTS) in the medulla oblongata (1). These changes in firing rate in glucose receptors are thought to be directly related to the activation of energy-dependent sodium pump because they can be blocked by ouabain (7). These glucoreceptors, connected to the vagus and the caudal portions of the NTS in the medulla oblongata, constitute a major afferent tract to the paraventricular, dorsomedial, and arcuate nuclei of the hypothalamus (8).

The fibers from the LH descend via the forebrain bundle and connect with the vagus of the medulla and form the LH-vagal circuit. This functional organization innervates several visceral organs mediating neural control of metabolism. Modulation of splanchnic viscera is not limited to vagus tone but is also influenced by sympathetic tone. Lesions of the ventrolateral hypothalamic area produce anorexia, wasting, and hypoinsulinemia. Thus, it is speculated that the decreased activity of the glucose sensitive neurons in the LH releases the inhibitory sympathetic tone on pancreatic insulin release. Part of these projections are noradrenergic and reach the parvicellular division of the hypothalamic nucleus. This division contains neurons that project directly to parasympathetic and sympathetic preganglionic cell groups in the brainstem and spinal cord as well as to the median eminence and posterior pituitary. The caudal part of the NTS also has projections that reach the ventromedial and posterior hypothalamic nuclei.

The VMH contains glucoreceptor neurons whose activity is enhanced by the direct application of glucose and that increase their discharge when glucose is applied to them. Electrical stimulation of the VMH is followed by a rapid rise in plasma glucose concentration. This response is not abolished by adrenalectomy, suggesting that this is a direct neural pathway for increasing hepatic glucose production (9). The axons extending from the VMH neurons project dorsocaudally to the locus ceruleus, central gray, and parabrachial nucleus. These last two areas project to the sympathetic motor neurons in the intermediolateral cell column of the spinal cord. The locus ceruleus and the parabrachial nucleus project to the NTS and the dorsal motor nucleus of the vagus. The NTS has direct connections with other nuclei within the hypothalamus.

The NTS contains glucose-sensitive neurons and is the first relay center for vagal visceral afferents. It has been reported that up to 27% of neurons tested from the NTS are glucose responding cells. This has been shown to be an intrinsic property of these neurons, the majority of which are located adjacent to the fourth ventricle (10). The site of glucoreceptors mediating the signals for a complete counterregulatory endocrine response, however, glucosensors do not appear to be located in a single brain structure. Differences in hypophyseal hormone release have been reported under conditions in which fructose is administered during generalized hypoglycemia. Because the ability of fructose to cross the blood-brain barrier (BBB) is limited, a differentiation has been proposed between the areas that are protected by the BBB versus those that are not. For example, stimuli for the release of growth hormone has been proposed to arise from areas protected by the BBB, and those for ACTH to be located both inside and outside the BBB (11). Furthermore, lesioning of the VMH fails to alter the characteristic hyperglycemic and insulinopenic response to the systemic administration of glucopenic doses of the glucose analog 2-DG (12). This suggests the existence and involvement of peripheral glucoreceptors in addition to those located in the VMH, for the effects of 2-DG. Alternatively, this could indicate the presence in the CNS of other glucosensitive areas besides the VMH. Thus, the involvement of multiple areas in the CNS during glucoregulation cannot be ruled out, and exclusivity of the VMH is not justified (13).

An integrated feedback loop of glucose control can be speculatively derived from this information. The lack of glucose in the periphery or in the CNS results in an increase in firing in the NTS and LH glucosensors. This results in increased firing from the LH, which increases sympathetic outflow through the splanchnic nerve and decreased parasympathetic activity. The CNS has sympathetic inhibitory tone upon insulin secretion, most probably to protect the CNS from hypoglycemia. During euglycemia, high CNS insulin and glucose favor glucose disposal. Thus, during euglycemia or hyperglycemia, the glucoreceptors in the VMH increase firing and release the inhibitory sympathetic tone on the pancreas, permitting an increase in insulin release. Thus, it is clear that glucose seems to provide a negative feedback signal sensed by the hypothalamic noradrenergic systems, which in turn appear to stimulate glucose output by a neural mechanism.

Not only have glucose-sensitive neurons been implicated in the CNS regulation of fuel mobilization during glucopenia, but the presence of insulin receptors in the CNS and brain insulinization have been postulated to contribute to metabolic control (8,14). Effects of insulin injected into the cerebrospinal fluid (CSF) include an increase in blood insulin levels mediated through the vagus, as well as generalized hypoglycemia (15). The glucose analog 2-DG is transported into the cell, phosphorylated but not metabolized further than the phosphohexose isomerase step (16). Thus, it is not recognized as a fuel source by the cell. The administration of intracerebroventricular (ICV) insulin following ICV 2-DG administration has been shown to counteract the hyperglycemic response to 2-DG. This has been considered as an indication that the effect of insulin concentration in the CNS is independent of insulin-stimulated glucose utilization beyond the phosphohexose isomerase step.

POSSIBLE NEUROENDOCRINE REGULATORS: NEUROTRANSMITTERS, HORMONES, OR PEPTIDES

Insulin-induced hypoglycemia normally evokes elevations in glucagon, epinephrine, norepinephrine, cortisol, growth hormone, and ACTH (17). The neurochemical basis for the CNS glucose counterregulation through adrenal catecholamine secretion is, as yet, vaguely defined. Although the activation of hypothalamic noradrenaline activity is associated with concurrent increases in plasma glucose concentration, several additional candidates have been considered to play an important role, and it appears that a sole player will not be the case. Peptides such as corticotropin-releasing factor (CRF), somatostatin, and thyrotropin-releasing factor (TRF), which are involved in the physiologic control of pituitary hormone secretion, are anatomically distributed in brain regions suspected of participating in the regulation of the autonomous nervous system (18). Neuroanatomic evidence exists suggesting neural peptidergic pathways connecting the brain stem and hypothalamic nuclei, which are capable of controlling and coordinating neuroendocrine and autonomic activities. Several neuropeptides, including bombesin, somatostatin, β-endorphin, TRH, and CRF, act within the brain to modify adrenal epinephrine secretion (19). When administered experimentally, these peptides have no effect peripherally but have been shown to produce CNS-mediated hyperglycemia and increased catecholamine release when given directly into the CNS.

Bombesin-like immunoreactivity has been demonstrated within the hypothalamus and the brain stem by both radioimmunoassay and immunocytochemistry (11). Injection of bombesin into the VMH results in marked hyperglycemia in the venous plasma. This effect is not limited to the VMH and was also seen on bombesin administration to the LH and appears to be mediated through the release of catecholamines and glucagon (20). Somatostatin has also been suggested as having an action on glucoregulation in the CNS (12). Although the site of action has not been extensively investigated, it is thought that somatostatin acts in the CNS by inhibiting CNS-mediated sympathetic outflow and inhibiting catecholamine elevation induced in various ways. Neuropeptide Y (NPY) containing neurons is mainly located in the arcuate nucleus of the hypothalamus with numerous fibers projecting to the paraventricular nuclei of the hypothalamus and thalamus (21). NPY can act both as a neurotransmitter and a hypophysiotrophic neurohormone. Neuropeptide Y has been shown to significantly increase plasma ACTH and cortisol concentrations, both of which are increased during periods of glucopenia (17). NPY activates the hypothalamic-pituitary-adrenal axis most probably at the level of the hypothalamus and/or pituitary levels because high concentrations of NPY-like immunoreactivity are detected in the hypothalamohypophyseal portal blood. These actions of ICV administration of NPY suggest its involvement in the multihormonal control of ACTH release. This is supported by the finding that immunoneutralization of NPY through the third ventricle, by ICV administration of NPY antibody, significantly inhibits the ACTH and cortisol release in response to hypoglycemia (22). Additionally, NPY may function as a sympathetic postganglionic neurotransmitter in the endocrine pancreas, so that, perhaps, its involvement in glucoregulation is not limited to its central actions on ACTH release (23).

Thyrotropin-releasing hormone is widely distributed in the central nervous system (24). It has been found to act in the brain by raising epinephrine and norepinephrine levels, which in turn are associated with an increase in plasma glucose (25). Pretreatment with hexamethonium (cholinergic ganglionic blockade) prior to the ICV administration of a TRH analog suppresses the response of plasma glucose, epinephrine, and norepinephrine (26). The response is also blunted by adrenalectomy. This suggests that TRH modulates glycemia through noradrenergic output from the CNS and that this results in sympathoadrenal activation and increased release of catecholamines, which are responsible for the hyperglycemic response. The site of action of TRH appears to be at the lateral hypothalamus, but is not limited to the area because hyperglycemic responses can also be evoked by its administration into the VMH and anterior hypothalamus. The antagonism of hyperglycemia by a cholinergic receptor blockade at the site of the hypothalamus suggests that, in the CNS, the TRH effects are mediated by cholinergic receptors. Its role during glucopenia has been stressed by the elevation of TRH secretion from intact isolated hypothalami in vitro as the glucose concentrations of the media are lowered (27). Moreover, the finding that antibody neutralization of CNS TRH delays recovery from the 2-DG–induced hyperglycemia indicates a role for TRH in restoring glycemia not only after glucopenia but also after hyperglycemic episodes (28).

In addition to the traditional elevations in norepinephrine described during glucopenia, we have provided evidence for elevations in ir-β-endorphins (29). These substances most likely act centrally as mediators of the counterregulatory response to glucopenia. β-Endorphin with its opiatelike activity has been demonstrated to have hyperglycemic effects similar to morphine (30). The site of action in the brain of β-endorphin–induced hyperglycemia is not clear since the direct administration of β-endorphins into the LH and VMH have not been shown to produce significant changes in glucose concentration. We have hypothesized that during situations of stress, such as glucopenia, control of fuel mobilization by endogenous opiates is an important regulatory mechanism. The hyperglycemic effects of ICV β-endorphins have been characterized in the conscious dog model. The mechanism for the hyperglycemia is thought to be the result of both an increase in glucose production and a late inhibition of glucose clearance through the stimulation of the sympathoadrenal axis as supported by 30-fold elevations in circulating plasma epinephrine and sixfold elevations in norepinephrine. Because no rise in glucagon was detected by the administration of β-endorphin, it appears that the hypothalamopancreatic axis was not directly stimulated and that the rises in plasma insulin are most probably secondary to the hyperglycemia. Cortisol and ACTH are also increased by the ICV administration of β-endorphins. In contrast, in the periphery, β-endorphin has been demonstrated to directly inhibit glucose production by the liver without producing changes in hormone concentrations. These appear to be independent effects from those produced in the CNS.

The involvement of the central endorphinergic system in control of fuel mobilization during glucopenia has been supported by our studies. Intracerebroventricular administration of β-endorphin in the dog results in significant elevations of plasma epinephrine, norepinephrine, cortisol and ACTH, and glucagon (23). Furthermore, ICV injection of naloxone, an effective central opiate blocker, prior to induction of hypoglycemia in dogs, blunted the rise in plasma β-endorphin, epinephrine, and norepinephrine without affecting the responses of glucagon and cortisol (31). Paradoxically, although pretreatment with naloxone has not been found to affect the hypoglycemic nadir, it did increase the rates of glucose utilization and production, which could well be the result of a diminished glucose-resistant state due to the lower epinephrine concentrations in dogs pretreated with naloxone (32). More recently, we have also shown plasma and CSF levels of endogenous opiates in response to insulin-induced hypoglycemia, and ongoing studies in our laboratory are suggestive of a regulatory role of these opiates in glucomodulation. Their exact mechanisms are, as yet, not understood but appear to involve the activation of CNS μ-receptors (Fig. 1).

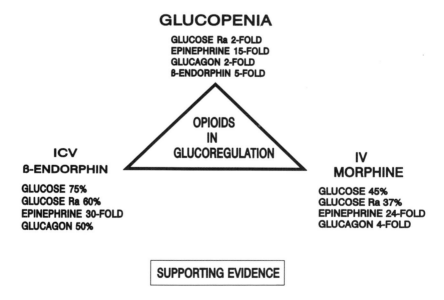

FIG. 1. Our laboratory has provided supporting evidence for a role of endogenous opioids in glucoregulation. This figure compares some of the metabolic and hormonal resulting from hypoglycemia, the intracerebroventricular (ICV) administration of β-endorphin and the intravenous (IV) administration of morphine. (Numbers indicate increases over basal).

The finding that endogenous morphine has been isolated from mammalian tissues, as well as the presence of receptors that specifically bind these substances in the CNS, suggests their modulatory functions under basal conditions as well as in situations of stress (33). Opiatelike substances and endogenous opioid peptides have been shown to exert indirect effects on pituitary secretory activity. The most probable area for action is the hypothalamus because this is an area where both the peptides and receptors are found. The hyperglycemic effects of morphine result from both a stimulation of glucose production and an inhibition of glucose clearance (34). These effects are mediated at the levels of the CNS because they can be reproduced by the ICV administration of small amounts of morphine that are not detected in the peripheral circulation. Their role is thought to be not only in maintenance of euglycemia but in counterregulation to a glucopenic insult, and our observations have provided supporting evidence for this concept. Additionally, naloxone has been shown to blunt the hyperglycemia and the increase in glucagon release in response to 2-DG. This indicates that endogenous opiates are involved in the glucose response to 2-DG.

The role of biogenic amines as modulators of neuroendocrine response to glucopenia is not only possible but very likely. Increases in catecholamines have been demonstrated after ICV administration of histamine. It has been described that the histamine content, histidine decarboxylase activity, and the turnover rate of histamine are highest in the hypothalamus (35). Studies suggest that histamine increases norepinephrine release in the paraventricular hypothalamic region of the conscious rat (36). This is abolished by bilateral adrenalectomy and by alpha- and beta-blockers administered systemically. This suggests that the stimulation of histamine receptors in the brain produces hyperglycemia through activation of the sympathoadrenomedullary axis (37). Thus, it is possible that the response to ICV administration of stressors such as 2-DG might result in increases in histamine release, which in turn stimulates a sympathoadrenal response (38). Histaminergic neurons appear to be involved in the regulation of CRF release from neurons within the paraventricular nucleus. Studies from our laboratory support the hypothesis that histamine may be involved in the counterregulatory response to glucopenia. Recent studies suggest that the injection of H_1- and H_2-blockers prior to the ICV administration of 2-DG results in a blunted and delayed hyperglycemic response when compared with animals injected with 2-DG alone. This might indicate that the immediate CNS activation of glycogenolysis is delayed by the absence of histamine.

NEURAL CONTROL OF COUNTERREGULATORY HORMONES

Glucose counterregulation involves a complex interaction between hormonal and nonhormonal factors. The hormonal contribution to restoration of plasma glucose concentrations during glucopenia is crucial and indispensable. Although the release and regulation of these hormones was traditionally considered to be exclusively mediated by substrate concentration, it is clear that hormonal and neural stimulation are also important controlling factors. The magnitude of the rise in counterregulatory

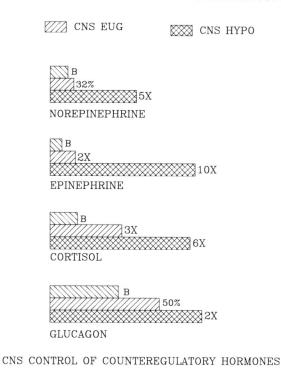

CNS CONTROL OF COUNTEREGULATORY HORMONES

FIG. 2.   The relative increases in hormone concentrations over basal values are depicted in this illustration. Note that the magnitude of the increase was greater as the result of generalized hypoglycemia (CNS HYPO) than that observed when CNS euglycemia was maintained (CNS EUG) for all hormones. X denotes -fold increase over basal.

hormones has been reported to be greater in dogs with generalized hypoglycemia than in those in whom the CNS was kept euglycemic (39) (Fig. 2). The temporal relationship and their relative contribution to restoring euglycemia has provided insight into the primary and secondary roles played by the hormonal milieu (10). It has been considered that glucagon plays a primary role and epinephrine a secondary role in glucose recovery from acute insulin-induced hypoglycemia in humans. A role for the immediate action of growth hormone, cortisol, or neurally released norepinephrine in acute hypoglycemic spells has not been supported, even though the long-term excess or deficiency of these factors may influence glucose counterregulation. Under conditions of normal glucagon release, plasma glucose recovery from insulin-induced hypoglycemia is normal despite epinephrine deficiency. However, it has been postulated that in the absence of glucagon release, there is augmented epinephrine release. This augmentation in the epinephrine response is then thought to partially compensate for the absence of glucagon, so that recovery from hypoglycemia, although attenuated, still occurs. Nevertheless, the counterregulatory effects of glucagon on hepatic glucose production are not transient and play a major role in glucose counterregulation (40). It seems that it is only in the absence of both glucagon and epinephrine that recovery from glucopenia fails to occur (41). Nevertheless, under conditions of prolonged hypoglycemia, the counterregulatory hormones can only account for a 50% contribution to glucose production. This further supports other, perhaps direct mechanisms of activation of glucose production (42) (Fig. 3).

The relative contribution of the counterregulatory response to restoring glycemic balance has been addressed in innovative protocols. Administration of 2-DG with somatostatin to prevent the rise in glucagon resulted in a rise in plasma glucose concentration that was 72% lower than when 2-DG was administered alone. This suggests that 28% of the 2-DG–induced rise in glucose is due to glucagon (43). Adrenalectomized animals had a significantly suppressed hyperglycemic response when compared to intact rats. These animals (adrenalectomy + 2-DG) showed a rise in insulin secretion due to the withdrawal of catecholamine inhibition of insulin release. To further dissect this, a group with adrenalectomy and somatostatin infusion (glucagon and insulin response to 2-DG was suppressed) showed a significant hyperglycemic response. This supports the importance of the direct neural stimulation of glucose production. Furthermore, it clearly supports the importance of the hormone-independent rise in glucose concentration in response to the CNS administration of 2-DG.

Glucagon release is increased by electrical stimulation of the splanchnic nerves (44), by epinephrine (from the adrenal medulla), and by norepinephrine released during sympathetic stimulation (34,45). Therefore, increased glucagon concentrations during hypoglycemia occur even in adrenalectomized animals and after section of splanchnic nerves. This release of glucagon in response to glucopenia can be blocked by atropine (inhibits acetylcholine [ACh]) pretreatment supporting vagus involvement in this response (46). Electrical stimulation of the VMH increases plasma glucagon, an effect that appears to be mediated through norepinephrine because noradrenergic neurones project intensively on the hypothalamus on their way to the preoptic area, and its injection into the VMH increases glucagon release; furthermore this effect is blocked by hexamethonium (ganglionic blocker). This effect, however, cannot be blocked by peripheral administration of phentolamine (α-adrenergic blockade), propranolol (β-blocker), or somatostatin infusion (inhibits glucagon and insulin release), indicating that it is a nonadrenergic, noncholinergic mechanism mediated through other unknown factors. On the other hand, administration of acetylcholine into the VMH induces selective release of glucagon through nicotinic (ACh) receptors, which is reduced by adrenalectomy, so that these effects are most likely mediated through sympathoadrenomedullary activity. It appears that there is some specificity for the control of glucagon release limited to the VMH because injection of norepinephrine into the LH elicits insulin release with no alterations in circulating glucagon levels. Glucopenia activates the three autonomic inputs to the pancreatic islet, parasympathetic nerves, circulating adrenal medullary epinephrine, and sympathetic nerves (47).

The adrenal medulla receives its main nerve supply from the greater and lesser splanchnic nerves (48). Adrenal medullary catecholamine secretion appears to be regulated by three distinct local mechanisms: adrenoreceptor-mediated, dihydropyridine-sensitive Ca^{2+} channel-mediated, and capsaicin-sensitive sensory nerve-mediated mechanisms. The activation of the sympathoadrenal system results in increases in adrenal catecholamine and pancreatic glucagon secretions, both of which

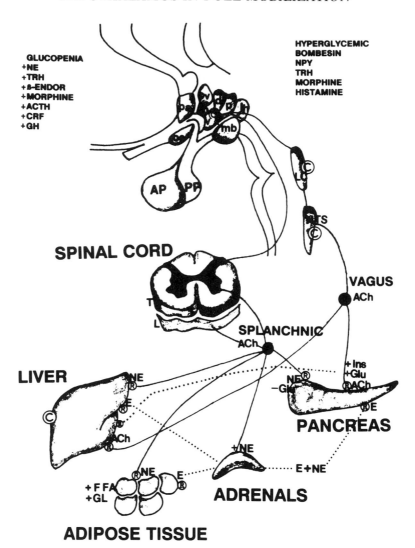

FIG. 3. Neural and hormonal connections between the CNS and periphery. *Solid lines* represent neural and *dotted lines* represent hormonal control. In the top left corner is a list of substances that are increased in response to glucopenia or 2-DG injection. On the top right corner is a list of substances that when administered into the third ventricle result in peripheral hyperglycemia. R, receptor; C, glucose sensitive neurons; E, epinephrine; NE, norepinephrine; ACh, acetylcholine; LC, locus ceruleus; NTS, nucleus tractus solitarius; oc, optic chiasm; AN, anterior nucleus; pa, preoptic area; pv, periventricular nuclei; d, dorsal nuclei; Lh, lateral hypothalamus; vm, ventromedial nucleus; Mb, mamillary body; an, anterior nucleus; p, posterior nucleus; AP, anterior pituitary; PP, posterior pituitary; T, thoracic; L, lumbar; FFA, free fatty acids; GL, glycerol; +, increases or stimulation; −, inhibition or decrease.

are significantly implicated in glucoregulatory mechanisms (47). The hypothalamic control of epinephrine release from the adrenal medulla in response to lack of metabolizable glucose is a well-accepted fact (48,49). The exact location of the sites of stimulus of catecholamine release have been the question of debate for some time (50,51). Their location in the caudal hindbrain and not in the hypothalamus have been supported by the lack of hyperglycemic response to the administration of 5-thioglucose into the lateral ventricles when the aqueduct is obstructed, but present when injected directly into the fourth ventricle.

Glucopenia stimulates ACTH secretion through a direct effect on the medial basal hypothalamus and not at the level of the adenohypophysis (52). ACTH is released as part of the proopiomelanocortin molecule (POMC), which, when processed, results in ACTH, melanin-stimulating hormone (MSH), and β-endorphin. Both β-endorphin and ACTH are thought to play major roles in the counterregulatory response to glucopenia. ACTH stimulates the release of cortisol from the adrenal cortex. Cortisol appears to play an important role in the stimulation of neurons via a direct neural connection to the medial basal hypothalamus (53). However, during prolonged hypoglycemia, there is a sustained increase in growth hormone levels, which can not be duplicated by growth hormone releasing hormone (GHRH) infusion (54,55). Thus, control of growth hormone release during hypoglycemia appears to be mediated not only by GHRH but by stimulation through other peptides and does not appear to have negative feedback inhibition on its own production (56). Growth hormone released during hypoglycemia stimulates lipolysis, providing glycerol, free fatty acids (FFA), and ketone bodies, thus contributing substrate for gluconeogenesis and facilitating glucose sparing for utilization by the brain. Lipolysis after growth hormone is not immediate and appears after a delay of about 2 hours; however, the effect persists for about 1 hour after the hormone has been removed. Lipolysis induced by growth hormone differs from that produced by catecholamines in time course and maximum response. In addition to its lipolytic effects, growth hormone is known to have insulin-antagonistic actions and to decrease peripheral glucose utilization. Thus, the role it plays during hypoglycemia may be twofold, providing increased amounts of glycerol as gluconeogenic substrate and at the same time as a glucose-sparing hormone.

FUEL MOBILIZATION DURING GLUCOPENIA: GLYCOGENOLYSIS AND GLUCONEOGENESIS

The initial rise in hepatic glucose production during counterregulation to hypoglycemia is mainly derived from glycogenolysis, but as glucopenia persists, the percent contribution from gluconeogenesis increases (57). Studies in which the hyperglycemic response to an ICV administration of neostigmine to fasted rats in blocked by 5,5-methoxyindole-2-carboxylic acid (MICA), an inhibitor of gluconeogenesis, indicate that although the hyperglycemic response in the fed state is the result of both glycogenolysis and gluconeogenesis, during the fasted state it is the result of an increase in gluconeogenesis (58). Although not considered rate limiting by some, a close correlation between the rate of glucose production and the flux of gluconeogenic substrates has been demonstrated (59). Precursor supply to maintain basal and accelerated hepatic glucose production is needed. The increased availability of gluconeogenic precursors as well as the increasing concentrations of counterregulatory hormones results in predominance of gluconeogenesis during the latter parts of glucoregulation, accounts for nearly 80% of overall hepatic glucose output, and is considered the predominant factor preventing further development of glucopenia (60).

Of the three main gluconeogenic substrates, lactate derived from the periphery, most likely as the result of increased muscle glycogenolysis, appears to account for most of the gluconeogenic precursor supply and its contribution to hepatic glucose production exceeds those of other substrates such as glycerol and alanine. Although it could be argued that the efficiency with which the liver converts glycerol and alanine into glucose is greater than that for lactate, we have provided evidence for a critical contribution of lactate as a gluconeogenic precursor. We have speculated that during prolonged periods of hypoglycemia, the overall contribution of lactate-derived carbons cannot be substituted by those of glycerol and/or alanine. An inhibition of net hepatic lactate uptake results in an inability to sustain the increased rates of hepatic glucose production observed during prolonged hypoglycemia (61).

There is increasing evidence that the stimulation of hepatic glucose production is affected not only by the counterregulatory hormones and substrate availability (62) but by direct hepatic neural stimulation as well (42,58,63). Three mechanisms have been described through which the sympathetic nervous system activates glycogenolysis: directly through hepatic innervation, secondary to the release of catecholamines from the adrenals, and in response to release of glucagon from the pancreas. Electrical stimulation of portal perivascular nerve bundles increases glucose and lactate release and stimulates phosphorylase-a activity, suggesting that hepatic glucose production is modulated predominantly by its own sympathetic nerve supply rather than by catecholamines and glucagon. These changes are not due to decreases in blood flow to the liver because vasoconstriction can be prevented pharmacologically without affecting the metabolic response. The activation of phosphorylase-a is mediated by an increase in the concentration of free Ca^{2+} in the cytosol, which is not limited to an increase in intracellular calcium mobilization but involves an increased flux from the extracellular space as well. The signal transduction mechanisms involved in the increase in intracellular calcium caused by the hormonal and the neural activation of phosphorylase can be differentiated from each other. The hormonal activation, i.e., that produced by catecholamines and glucagon, is mediated through a β-adrenergic mechanism involving cyclic AMP and activation of protein kinase and phosphorylase kinase. The activation resulting from splanchnic nerve stimulation is through the inactivation of phosphorylase phosphatase. Furthermore, electrical stimulation of the VMH has also been shown to activate phosphoenolpyruvate carboxykinase (PEPCK), a key gluconeogenic enzyme, and to suppress pyruvate kinase (PK). The activity of PEPCK, is increased in the fasted state in response to ICV neostigmine. This effect, however, is slow and probably plays a minor role under hypoglycemic conditions. Nevertheless, it is probable that this effect is synergistic with that of glucagon and catecholamines on the liver and complement each other in the glyco-genolytic and gluconeogenic effect on the liver during hypoglycemia.

The CNS control of glycogenolysis appears to be specific to the VMH because electrical stimulation of the VMH and splanchnic nerve and noradrenergic stimulation of the VMH result in glycogenolysis, while electrical stimulation of the LH and vagus and cholinergic stimulation of the LH activates glycogen synthase and promotes glycogenesis. Norepinephrine appears to be the neurotransmitter involved in glyco-gen mobilization from the liver because the response is stimulated by administration of norepinephrine into the VMH and is blocked by pretreatment with propranolol (β-blocker). This suggests that norepinephrine acts through a β-adrenergic receptor in the hypothalamus. The inhibition of the glycogenolytic response by peripheral administration of hexamethonium (competitive ganglionic cholinergic blockade) indi-cates that norepinephrine-sensitive neurons at the VMH act through peripheral sym-pathetic nerves. Furthermore, because adrenalectomy does not impair this response, the immediate glycogenolytic response is most likely directly neurally mediated. The participation of direct sympathetic nervous system innervation of the viscera is fur-ther demonstrated by the blockade of 2-DG–induced hyperglycemia by guanethidine (inhibition of adrenergic neurotransmitter release) (64). Thus, it appears that the early response to glucopenia is mediated by direct neural stimulation and that the increases in glucagon and catecholamine release are most probably involved in the prolonged sustainment of the hyperglycemic response to 2-DG. Thus, two distinct pathways for CNS counterregulation can be described: one directly through activation of hepatic enzymes that increase the release of glucose, "hypothalamo axis," and the other through the release of catecholamines and glucagon, hypothalamopancreatic and hy-pothalamonoradrenal axis. These latter ones appear to be more related with the prolongation and consolidation of the metabolic changes than with their initiation. Taken together, the evidence presented suggests that the VMH plays a role in the catabolic fuel mobilization while the LH has a more important role in an anabolic functions. The activation of liver glucose output by the CNS is thus the result of not only a direct neural input into the liver but also the indirect result of the stimulation of epinephrine release from the adrenals. This particular pathway appears to be me-diated by ACh since studies have shown that the ICV administration of carbachol (ACh-like nicotinic and muscarinic action) is accompanied by a marked increase in glucose production, increased plasma lactate concentrations, and incorporation of $^{14}CO_2$ into circulating glucose (65). These effects, which are abolished in adrenomed-ullated animals, appear to be the result of activation of cholinergic neurons in the CNS, a response that is in turn mediated by muscarinic receptors (stimulated by ACh) because ICV administration of neostigmine (an inhibitor of cholinesterase) produces hyperglycemia, elevated epinephrine, norepinephrine, and glucagon con-centrations in hepatic venous plasma.

LIPOLYSIS: FREE FATTY ACIDS AND GLYCEROL

Mobilization of FFA and glycerol from adipose tissue during glucopenia serves a dual function (66). It is one of the main mechanisms of supplying increasing amounts of gluconeogenic precursor to the liver for sustaining higher gluconeogenic rates and at the same time FFA decrease the utilization of glucose in the periphery, thus sparing it for use by the CNS. The FFA-mediated reduction of insulin-stimulated carbohydrate oxidation minimizes the irreversible loss of glucose carbons during hypoglycemia (67). Thus, catecholamine-induced elevations in FFA facilitate the recycling of glucose precursors by peripheral tissues and spares glucose carbons for oxidation by the brain (68). The logical sequence of events triggered during glucopenia is controlled by redundant and shared mechanisms. The hormones involved in lipid mobilization can be divided into three classes; pituitary peptide hormones, catecholamines, and norepinephrine directly released from the postganglionic sympathetic nerve endings. Due to the lack of glycerol kinase by adipose tissue, glycerol released during lipolysis is released into the circulation and directed to the liver where it contributes to gluconeogenesis. It is considered that during the late phase of hypoglycemia, the indirect effects of catecholamines on lipolysis account for at least 50% of the adrenergic contribution to increased hepatic glucose output and about 85% to the suppressed rates of glucose utilization. This underscores the importance of FFA mobilization in restoring euglycemia (69).

Few studies have focused on the participation of the CNS in the mobilization of FFA (69,70). However, the role in hypothalamic control of FFA mobilization during periods of glucopenia has recently been reexamined. Intracerebroventricular administration of minute amounts of 2-DG, which fail to produce hyperglycemia or to increase insulin, produced rapid increases in the concentrations of plasma FFA (71). A role for insulin-sensitive receptors in the preoptic area has been proposed to play a role in FFA mobilization because microinjections of insulin in this area rapidly reduced the elevated FFA levels of fasting rats (72,73). It appears that in contrast to chemoreceptors involved in glucose homeostasis, the chemoreceptors involved in FFA regulation are sensitive to insulin and that their activity is modulated by the rate of glucose utilization in the surrounding medium rather than by glucose concentrations (15). The persistence of the rise in plasma FFA in response to ICV 2-DG after adrenomedullation suggests that the mobilization of FFA results from a direct activation of sympathetic fibers of adipose tissue (74). The location for the FFA mobilizing structures is thought to be located within the ependymal lining of the ventricles or in the nervous tissue adjacent to the ventricular system. Lesions in the lateral hypothalamic areas and in the posterior hypothalamus have been shown to completely suppress the increase in plasma FFA induced by ICV 2-DG (74). A separation of hypothalamic elements, which may influence autonomic discharge to adipose tissue and to the liver, has been suggested because stimulation of the VMH produces rises in plasma glucose but not in FFA, whereas stimulation of the mammillary area results in higher FFA concentrations without a marked effect in plasma glucose (69). These findings would suggest specific localization for control of the two substrates in the CNS.

Electrical stimulation of the VMH increases plasma FFA and glycerol via sympathetic stimulation (73). Nevertheless, on some occasions electrical stimulation of the VMH has been shown to increase glycerol concentrations with no rise in FFA. This is suggestive of increased lipolysis in conjunction with reesterification. It is considered that the majority of the CNS effects on lipolysis are mediated by catecholamines because approximately 80% of the plasma glycerol elevation elicited by electrical stimulation of the VMH is abolished by adrenalectomy (75). However, even after adrenomedullation there is a small rise in the glycerol concentrations in plasma parallel to small rises in circulating norepinephrine, which most probably comes from sympathetic nerve endings. Furthermore, some studies suggest that the lipid mobilizing areas in the nervous system influence FFA mobilization through a direct activation of the sympathetic fibers of adipose tissue. This is supported by findings indicating that hypothalamic deafferentation in the rat impairs FFA mobilization in situations of stress that have been shown previously to be required for adequate lipid mobilizing response. Systematic studies of the hypothalamic areas involved in FFA mobilization suggest the presence of insulin-sensitive glucoreceptors in the preoptic area, which increase sympathetic outflow to adipose tissue and contribute to lipolysis. These localized areas when stimulated by direct application of insulin reduce the concentrations of plasma FFA and when stimulated with 2-DG increase circulating levels of FFA (15). Furthermore, ventromedial hypothalamic region lesioning reduces mobilization of FFA from adipose tissue depots in response to 2-DG (74). In contrast, adrenomedullectomy has no effect on the 2-DG lipid mobilizing response. This suggests that the ventromedial hypothalamic region may act as a modulator of peripheral efferent adrenergic activity, particularly that involved with regulating adipose tissue mobilization.

PROTEOLYSIS

Although the role of the CNS in control and regulation of carbohydrate metabolism has been described as early as 1890 by Claude Bernard (76), control of protein and amino acid metabolism by the brain has not been addressed extensively. This may be due to so much of glucose metabolism being localized in the liver in contrast to the wide array of tissues contributing to protein metabolism. Little is known about the hypothalamic control of protein metabolism. However, there is some evidence that direct neural input into the liver may modify the activity of enzymes involved in amino acid metabolism. Activity of tyrosine aminotransferase in rat liver is suppressed by sympathetic-adrenergic mechanisms and induced by the vagal-cholinergic system and after spinal cord transection. Furthermore, cholinergic stimulation of the LH results in activation of tyrosine aminotransferase, an effect that can be blocked by vagotomy.

The effects of glucopenia on protein and amino acid metabolism have been of special interest to our laboratory. Traditionally, increased fuel mobilization from the periphery to provide the liver with gluconeogenic substrates has been proposed to include mobilization of gluconeogenic amino acids from muscle to be shuttled to the liver and into gluconeogenesis. Alanine is the primary amino acid released by muscle and the primary gluconeogenic amino acid extracted by the liver during hypoglycemia (77). However, alanine comprises no more than 7% to 10% of the amino acid residues in skeletal muscle, and its release from the intracellular amino acid pool cannot explain the predominant contribution of alanine to total nitrogen released from muscle. It is estimated that only 30% of alanine released into the circulation proceeds from muscle protein breakdown and the rest proceeds from de novo synthesis in muscle by transamination of pyruvate. Nevertheless, its synthesis requires an appropriate source of amino groups that intuitively are derived from the branched-chain amino acids (valine, leucine, isoleucine) because they are predominantly catabolized in muscle rather than in liver. The efficiency of alanine incorporation into glucose has been utilized as an assessment of the gluconeogenic conversion rate, and the proportion of injected alanine recovered from glucose to similar to that of lactate, suggesting prompt incorporation of this amino acid into glucose (62).

Our laboratory has demonstrated that insulin-induced hypoglycemia (IIH) is characterized not only by the classically described glucose counterregulation of increased glycogenolysis, lipolysis, and gluconeogenesis but also by enhanced protein breakdown (78) (Fig. 4). Estimations of whole-body proteolysis using the isotopic dilution of leucine showed a marked increase in the rate of leucine appearance into the plasma compartment, followed by enhanced rates of amino acid oxidation, both suggestive of increased proteolysis. The primary site of this proteolytic response is not skeletal muscle but primarily the gastrointestinal tract, resulting in an increased net release of both essential and nonessential amino acids across the extrahepatic splanchnic tissues. During this process, the majority of amino acids released by the gut are taken up by the liver, but a significant component, specifically that of branched-chain amino

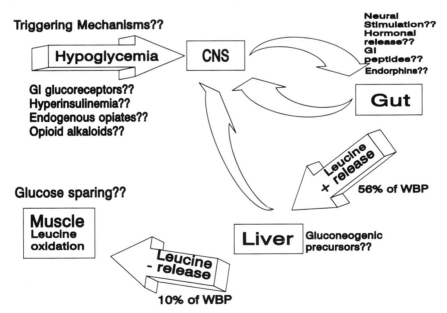

FIG. 4. This diagram summarizes some of our working hypothesis as well as some of the findings during hypoglycemia as they pertain to amino acid and protein metabolism. The *question marks* represent speculative pathways or mechanisms. WBP, whole-body proteolysis; GI, gastrointestinal; +release, greater release than during euglycemia; −release, drop in release from that during basal.

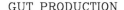

GUT PRODUCTION

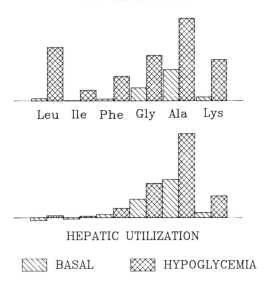

Leu Ile Phe Gly Ala Lys

HEPATIC UTILIZATION

BASAL   HYPOGLYCEMIA

FIG. 5. Amino acid production by the gut and utilization by the liver during euglycemia (basal) and experimental (hypoglycemia) are represented in this illustration. The net release of leucine by the gut is increased during hypoglycemia, but the net uptake by the liver is not significantly altered. In contrast, note the increase in liver utilization of gluconeogenic amino acids during hypoglycemia. The same amino acids are represented in the top and bottom panels. Calculation of amino acid production and utilization rates are based on arteriovenous differences and hepatic blood flow.

acids, is released into the systemic circulation and taken up by other organs, mainly skeletal muscle (Fig. 5). Contrary to what would be expected, net balance of leucine across the hindlimb tissues during hypoglycemia switched from neutral balance to a net uptake. The increase in net hindlimb uptake of branched-chain amino acids may help provide amino groups for pyruvate transamination and thus increased alanine release.

The role of neuroglucopenia in eliciting the proteolytic response to hypoglycemia has been demonstrated in dogs that have been subjected to peripheral hypoglycemia by intravenous infusions of insulin and allowed to either develop neuroglucopenia or be infused with glucose through the carotids and the vertebral arteries in order to maintain CNS euglycemia (39). Prevention of severe CNS glucopenia was associated with marked suppression of proteolysis and its rate of oxidation, in sharp contrast to that observed in the group in which generalized hypoglycemia is allowed to occur. This was the result of a nearly complete inhibition of proteolysis across the gastrointestinal tract as represented by gut leucine balance.

These studies also support the CNS control of counterregulatory hormones because neuroglucopenia was more effective in stimulating their release than was peripheral hypoglycemia. It is possible that the reduced release of glucagon and catecholamines during CNS euglycemia accounts for the lack of gut proteolysis observed in those studies (Fig. 6). However, it appears that the hormonal milieu is not completely responsible for the proteolytic response to glucopenia because the infusion of a combination of stress hormones fails to reproduce the proteolytic response to glucopenia. Determining the stimulus for enhanced protein catabolism during the hypoglycemia, or what it's localization in the brain might be, is a question that still needs to be addressed. Central administration of 2-DG into the third ventricle of overnight fasted dogs mimics the glucose metabolic response to hypoglycemia, the hormonal alterations, and the behavioral effects of IIH, but does not produce an increase in whole body proteolysis and or an increase in gut amino acid release (79). It is now known that various stressful stimuli trigger activation of the hypothalamic-pituitary-adrenal axis and sympathetic-adrenomedullary system and that there is also an overall enhancement of the activity of the central noradrenaline-containing neurons. These findings, taken with the differential activation of lipolysis and hyperglycemia by stimulating different areas in the CNS, indicate that fuel mobilization during glucopenia is the result of lack of glucose in multiple sites in the brain, and perhaps in the periphery as well.

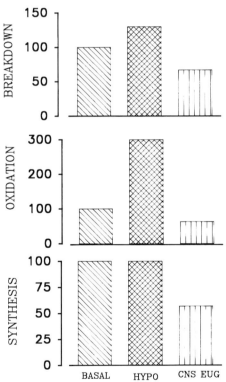

FIG. 6. This figure compares the rates of protein breakdown, oxidation, and synthesis during basal, insulin-induced hypoglycemia (HYPO) and during generalized hypoglycemia with CNS euglycemia (CNS EUG). The CNS is made euglycemic by the selective infusion of glucose to the brain, while hypoglycemia is maintained in the periphery. Changes are presented as percent difference from basal. These findings demonstrate that the proteolytic response during hypoglycemia is prevented if euglycemia is maintained.

The gut proteolytic response in response to glucopenia does not appear to play a major role in restoring glycemia, thus intuitively it can only result in deleterious consequences for the individual. Our results are supportive of a major role for the CNS in controlling this response. However, the determination of the contribution of hormonal, neural, opiate, and peptidergic changes accompanying glucopenia has only recently been initiated. Interestingly, it appears that neurocortisolemia prior to induction of hypoglycemia modulates the proteolytic response. This could indicate a protective role for cortisol in the CNS. Previously we have demonstrated a rise in cortisol levels in CSF during prolonged hypoglycemia. The role of this has been assumed to be that of a negative feedback inhibition of CRF and thus of ACTH. It is possible that it could also inhibit the triggering mechanism for the proteolytic response. The site of this inhibition or the possible neurotransmitter system involved in this response is the focus of future studies from our laboratory and cannot be discerned based on the available information.

We have presented an extensive and, we hope, comprehensive review of the different neural pathways and possible mechanisms involved in the regulation of fuel mobilization during glucopenia. These include central and integrative roles of the hypothalamus, existence of glucose-sensitive and glucoreceptor neurons in the central nervous system and in the periphery. When comparing the effects of neural and/or chemical stimulation of different areas of the CNS, it becomes apparent there is a high selectivity for the regulation of each of the substrate's metabolism, namely that the regulation of lipid, glucose, and protein metabolism, although interrelated and sometimes parallely stimulated, their individual modulation appears to have some selectivity. Thus, the localization, the neurotransmitter system involved, the second messenger system stimulated, and finally the afferent pathway through which the stimulus in conveyed are shared under some conditions but diverge under others. This makes generalization as to mechanisms of action of an insult such as glucopenia almost impossible, but is intriguing and exciting enough to stimulate speculative and innovative hypotheses. Much information has been collected since Claude Bernard first described glucosuria after puncture of the fourth ventricle in dogs. The availability of antibodies and antagonists to a variety of hormones, peptides, and neurotransmitters has allowed for a finer dissection of the possible mechanisms involved in the response to glucopenia. Finally, the importance of taking the information collected from several different species and discerning its integration and application to humans will be no lesser a task than that which investigators have set out to do by dissecting hypothalamic control of fuel mobilization during glucopenia.

ACKNOWLEDGMENT

This work was supported by Grants RO1 DK12562-03 RO1-DK.

REFERENCES

1. Shimizu N, Oomura Y, Novin D, et al. Functional correlations between lateral hypothalamic glucose-sensitive neurons and hepatic portal glucose-sensitive units in rat. *Brain Res* 1983;265:49–54.

2. Smythe GA, Grunstein HS, Bradshaw JE, et al. Relationships between the brain noradrenergic activity and blood glucose. *Nature* 1985;308:65–67.
3. Bleir R, Cohn P, Siggelkow IR. A cytoarchitectonic atlas of the hypothalamus and hypothalamic third ventricle of the rat. In: Morgane PJ, Panksepp J (eds). *Handbook of the Hypothalamus.* New York: Dekker, 1979;137:–220.
4. Shimazu T, Fukuda A, Ban T. Reciprocal influences of the ventromedial and lateral hypothalamic nuclei on blood glucose levels and liver glycogen content. *Nature* 1966;210:1178–1179.
5. Oomura Y, Ono T, Ooyama H, Wayner MJ. Glucose and osmosensitive neurones of the rat hypothalamus. *Nature* 1969;222:282–284.
6. Donovan CM, Halter JB, Bergman RN. Importance of hepatic glucoreceptors in sympathoadrenal response to hypoglycemia. *Diabetes* 1991;40:155–158.
7. Niijima A. Neural mechanisms in the control of blood glucose concentration. *J Nutr* 1989;119:833–840.
8. Schmitt M. Influences of hepatic portal receptors on hypothalamic feeding and satiety centers. *Am J Physiol* 1973;225:1089–1095.
9. Frohman LA, Bernardis LL. Effect of hypothalamic stimulation on plasma glucose, insulin, and glucagon levels. *Am J Physiol* 1971;221:1596–1603.
10. Mizuno Y, Oomura Y. Glucose responding neurons in the nucleus tractus solitarius of the rat: in vitro study. *Brain Res* 1984;307:109–116.
11. Vigas M, Tatar P, Jurcovicova J, Jezova D. Glucoreceptors located in different areas mediate the hypoglycemia-induced release of growth hormone, prolactin, and adrenocorticotropin in man. *Neuroendocrinology* 1990;51:365–368.
12. Panerai AE, Olgiati VR, Udeschini G, et al. Hyperglycemia and inhibition of insulin secretion by 2-deoxy-D-glucose in rats with hypothalamic lesions. *Pharmacol Res Commun* 1975;7:133–141.
13. Keller-Wood ME, Wade CE, Shinsako J, et al. Insulin-induced hypoglycemia in conscious dogs: effect of maintaining carotid arterial glucose levels on the adrenocorticotropin, epinephrine, and vasopressin responses. *Endocrinology* 1982;112:624–632.
14. Schwartz MW, Figlewicz DP, Baskin DG, et al. Insulin in the brain: a hormonal regulator of energy balance. *Endocrine Rev* 1992;13:387–414.
15. Szabo O, Szabo A. Studies on the nature and mode of action of the insulin-sensitive glucoregulator receptor in the central nervous system. *Diabetes* 1975;24:328–336.
16. Horton RW, Meldrum BS, Bachelard HS. Enzymic and cerebral metabolic effects of 2-deoxy-D-glucose. *J Neurochem* 1973;21:507–520.
17. Fish HR, Chernow B, O'Brian JT. Endocrine and neurophysiologic respones of the pituitary in insulin-induced hypoglycemia: a review. *Metabolism* 1986;35:763–780.
18. Emson PC. Peptides as neurotransmitter candidates in the mammalian CNS. *Prog Neurobiol* 1979; 13:61.
19. Brown MR, Fisher L. Brain peptide regulation of adrenal epinephrine secretion. *Am J Physiol* 1984; 247:E41–E46.
20. Iguchi A, Matsunaga H, Nomura T, et al. Glucoregulatory effects of intrahypothalamic injections of bombesin and other peptides. *Endocrinology* 1984;114:2242–2246.
21. Danger JM, Toon MC, Jenks BG, et al. Neuropeptide Y: localization in the central nervous system and neuroendocrine functions. *Fundam Clin Pharmacol* 1990;4:307–340.
22. Inui A, Inoue T, Nakajima M, et al. Brain neuropeptide Y in the control of adrenocorticotropic hormone secretion in the dog. *Brain Res* 1990;510:211–215.
23. Pilotte NS, Sharif NA, Burt DR. Characterization and autoradiographic localization of TRH receptors in sections of rat brain. *Brain Res* 1984;293:372–376.
24. Ahren B, Bottcher G, Kowalyk S, et al. Galanin is co-localized with noradrenaline and neuropeptide Y in dog pancreas and celiac ganglion. *Cell Tissue Res* 1990;261:49–58.
25. Kabayama Y, Kato Y, Tojo K, et al. Central effects of DN1417, a novel TRH analog, on plasma glucose and catecholamines in conscious rats. *Life Sci* 1985;36:1287–1294.
26. Shen DC, Lin MT, Shian LR. Thyrotropin-releasing hormone-induced hyperglycemia: possible involvement of cholinergic receptors in the lateral hypothalamus. *Neuroendocrinology* 1985;41:499–503.
27. Lewis BM, Dieguez C, Ham J, et al. Effects of glucose on thyrotropin-releasing hormone, growth hormone-releasing hormone, somatostatin and luteinizing hormone-releasing hormone release from rat hypothalamus in vitro. *J Neuroendocrinol* 1989;1:437–441.
28. Amir S, Jackson I. Immunological blockade of endogenous thyrotropin-releasing hormone impairs recovery from hyperglycemia in mice. *Brain Res* 1980;462:159–162.
29. Radosevich PM, Lacy DB, Brown LL, et al. Effects of insulin-induced hypoglycemia on plasma and

cerebrospinal fluid levels of ir-β-endorphins, ACTH, cortisol, norepinephrine, insulin and glucose in the conscious dog. *Brain Res* 1988;458:325–338.

30. Radosevich PM, Lacy DB, Brown LL, et al. Central effects of β-endorphins on glucose homeostasis in the conscious dog. *Am J Physiol* 1989;256:E322–E330.

31. Nash JA, Radosevich PM, Lacy DB, et al. Effects of naloxone on glucose homeostasis during insulin-induced hypoglycemia. *Am J Physiol* 1989;257:E367–E373.

32. Ipp E, Garberoglio C, Richter H, et al. Naloxone decreases centrally induced hyperglycemia in dogs. *Diabetes* 1981;33:619–621.

33. Donnerer J, Cardinale G, Coffey J, et al. Chemical characterization and regulation of endogenous morphine and codeine in the rat. *J Pharmacol Exp Ther* 1987;242:583–587.

34. Radosevich PM, Williams PE, Lacy DB, et al. Effects of morphine on glucose homeostasis in the conscious dog. *J Clin Invest* 1984;74:1473–1480.

35. Wada H, Watanabe T, Yamatodani A, et al. Physiological functions of histamine in the brain. In: Ganellin CR, Schwartz JC (eds). *Frontiers in histamine research*. Oxford: Pergamon Press, 1985; 225–235.

36. Knigge U, Matzen S, Warberg J. Histamine as a neuroendocrine regulator of the stress-induced release of peripheral catecholamines. *Endocrinology* 1990;126:1430–1434.

37. Nishibori M, Itoh Y, Oishi R, Saeki K. Effect of microinjection of histamine into the brain on plasma levels of epinephrine and glucose in freely moving rats. *Japan J Pharmacol* 1990;54:257–263.

38. Bealer SL. Histamine releases norepinephrine from the paraventricular nucleus/anterior hypothalamus region of the conscious rat. *J Pharmacol and Biophysics* 1993;264:734–738.

39. Hourani H, Lacy B, Tayeb KE, Abumrad NN. The role of central nervous system in modulating glucose and protein metabolism during insulin-induced hypoglycemia. *Brain Res* 1992;587:276–284.

40. De Feo P, Perriello G, Torlone E, et al. Evidence against important catecholamine compensation for absent glucagon counterregulation. *Am J Physiol* 1991;260:E203–E212.

41. Gerich J, Davis J, Lorenzi M, et al. Hormonal mechanisms of recovery from insulin-induced hypoglycemia in man. *J Physiol* 1979;236:E380–E385.

42. Frizzell RT, Hendrick GK, Brown LL, et al. Stimulation of glucose production through hormone secretion and other mechanisms during insulin-induced hypoglycemia. *Diabetes* 1988;37:1531–1541.

43. Ipp E, Piran H, Richter C, et al. Central control of peripheral circulating somatostatin in dogs: effect of 2-deoxy-glucose. *Am J Physiol* 1982;243:E213–E216.

44. Woods SC, Porte D. Neural control of the endocrine pancreas. *Physiol Rev* 1974;54:596–619.

45. Havel PJ, Taborsky GJ. The contribution of the autonomic nervous system to changes of glucagon and insulin secretion during hypoglycemic stress. *Endocrine Rev* 1989;10:332–350.

46. Havel PJ, Veith RC, Dunning BE, Taborsky GJ. Role for autonomic nervous system to increase pancreatic glucagon secretion during marked insulin-induced hypoglycemia in dogs. *Diabetes* 1991; 40:1107–1114.

47. Yamaguchi N. Sympathoadrenal system in neuroendocrine control of glucose: mechanisms involved in the liver, pancreas, and adrenal gland under hemorrhagic and hypoglycemic stress. *Can J Physiol Pharmacol* 1992;70:167–206.

48. Himsworth RL. Hypothalamic control of adrenaline secretion in response to insufficient glucose. *J Physiol* 1970;206:411–417.

49. Khalil Z, Marley PD, Livett BG. Elevation in plasma catecholamines in response to insulin stress is under both neuronal and nonneuronal control. *Endocrinology* 1986;119:159–167.

50. DiRocco R, Grill HJ. The forebrain is not essential for sympathoadrenal hyperglycemic response to glucoprivation. *Science* 1979;204:1112–1114.

51. Ritter RC, Slusser PG, Stone S. Glucoreceptors controlling feeding and blood glucose: location in the hindbrain. *Science* 1981;213:24–27.

52. Aizawa T, Yasuda N, Greer M. Hypoglycemia stimulates ACTH secretion through a direct effect on the basal hypothalamus. *Metabolism* 1991;30:996–1000.

53. Santiago JV, Clarke WL, Shah SD, Cryer PE. Epinephrine, norepinephrine, glucagon, and release in association with physiological decrements in the plasma glucose concentration in normal and diabetic man. *J Clin Endocrinol Metab* 1980;51:877–883.

54. De Feo P, Perriello G, Torlone E, et al. Demonstration of a role for growth hormone in glucose counterregulation. *Am J Physiol* 1989;256:E835–E843.

55. Gorin E, Tai L, Honeyman TW, Goodman HM. Evidence for a role of protein kinase C in the stimulation of kipolysis by growth hormone and isoproterenol. *Endocrinology* 1990;126:2973–2982.

56. Barbetti F, Crescenti C, Negri M, et al. Growth hormone does not inhibit its own secretion during prolongued hypoglycemia in man. *J Clin Endocrinol Metab* 1990;70:1371–1374.

57. Frizzell RT, Hendrick GK, Biggers DW, et al. Role of gluconeogenesis in sustaining glucose production during hypoglycemia caused by continuous insulin infusion in conscious dogs. *Diabetes* 1988; 37:749–759.
58. Iguchi A, Kunoh Y, Miura H, et al. Central nervous system control of glycogenolysis and gluconeogenesis in fed and fasted rat liver. *Metabolism* 1989;38:1216–1221.
59. Jahoor F, Peters EJ, Wolf RR. The relationship between the gluconeogenic substrate supply and glucose production in humans. *Am J Physiol* 1990;258:E288–E296.
60. Lecavalier L, Bolli G, Cryer P, Gerich J. Contributions of gluconeogenesis and glycogenolysis during glucose counterregulation in normal humans. *Am J Physiol* 1989;256:E844–E851.
61. Molina PE, Jabbour K, Williams PE, Abumrad NN. Ethanol modulates hepatic glucose production during indulin-induced hypoglycemia by inhibiting net hepatic lactate uptake. *Diabetes* 1992;41:163A.
62. Frizzell RT, Campbell PJ, Cherrington AD. Gluconeogenesis and hypoglycemia. *Diabetes Metab Rev* 1988;4:51–70.
63. Matsunaga H, Iguchi A, Yatomi A, et al. The relative importance of nervous system and hormones to the 2-deoxy-D-glucose-induced hyperglycemia in fed rats. *Endocrinology* 1989;124:1259–1264.
64. Storlien LH, Grunstein HS, Smythe GA. Guanethidine blocks the 2-deoxy-D-glucose-induced hypothalamic noradrenergic drive to hyperglycemia. *Brain Res* 1985;335:144–147.
65. Migliorini RH, Garofalo MA, Roselino JE, Kettelhut IC. Rapid activation of gluconeogenesis after intracerebroventricular carbachol. *Am J Physiol* 1989;257:E486–E490.
66. Fanelli CG, De Feo P, Porcellati F, et al. Adrenergic mechanisms contribute to the late phase of hypoglycemic glucose counterregulation in humans by stimulating lipolysis. *J Clin Invest* 1992;89: 2005–2013.
67. Caprio S, Gelfand RA, Tamborlane WV, Sherwin RS. Oxidative fuel metabolism during mild hypoglycemia: critical role of free fatty acids. *Am J Physiol* 1989;256:E413–E419.
68. Garber AJ, Cryer PE, Santiago JV, et al. The role of adrenergic mechanisms in the substrate and hormonal response to insulin-induced hypoglycemia in man. *J Clin Invest* 1976;58:7–15.
69. Barkai A, Allweis C. Effect of electrical stimulation of the hypothalamus on plasma levels of free fatty acids and glucose in rats. *Metabolism* 1972;21:921–927.
70. Paschoalini MA, Migliorini RH. Participation of the CNS in the control of FFA mobllization during fasting in rabbits. *Physiol Behav* 1990;47:461–465.
71. Coimbra CC, Gross JL, Migliorine RH. Intraventricular 2-deoxyglucose, glucose, insulin, and free fatty acid mobilization. *Am J Physiol* 1979;5:E317–E327.
72. Coimbra CC, Gross JL, Migliorine RH. Insulin-sensitive glucoreceptors in rat preoptic area that regulate FFA mobilization. *Am J Physiol* 1986;251:E703–E706.
73. Kumon A, Takahashi A, Hara T, Shimazu T. Mechanism of lipolysis induced by electrical stimulation of the hypothalamus in the rabbit. *J Lipid Res* 1976;17:551–558.
74. Nishizawa Y, Bray GA. Ventromedial hypothalamic lesions and the mobilization of fatty acids. *J Clin Invest* 1978;61:714–721.
75. Kumon A, Takahashi A, Kori-hara T. Epinephrine: a mediator of plasma glycerol elevation by hypothalamic stimulation. *Am J Physiol* 1977;233:E369–E373.
76. Bernard MC. Leçons surs la Physiologie et la Pathologie. In: Bernard MC, ed. *Systémè Nerveux.* Paris: Bailliere, 1858;349.
77. Felig P. The glucose-alanine cycle. *Metabolism* 1973;22:179–206.
78. Hourani H, Williams PE, Morris JA, et al. Effect of insulin-induced hypoglycemia on protein metabolism in vivo. *Am J Physiol* 1990;259:E342–E350.
79. Molina PE, ElTayeb K, Williams PE, Abumrad NN. Hormonal and metabolic effect of neuroglucopenia. *Brain Res* (in press).

Organ Metabolism and Nutrition:
Ideas for Future Critical Care, edited by
J. M. Kinney and H. N. Tucker.
Raven Press, Ltd., New York © 1994.

5

Fever: Metabolic Asset or Liability?

Matthew J. Kluger

Institute of Basic and Applied Medical Research, The Lovelace Institutes,
Albuquerque, New Mexico 87108

A fever is one of the most common host responses to infection, trauma, or injury. Fever, which is defined as "a regulated rise in body temperature," should not be confused with *hyperthermia* (1). During fever, the host behaves as if the temperature around which it is regulating, its thermoregulatory "set-point," were elevated. As such, during the rising phase of fever, the infected person will often shiver, increasing heat production, will be peripherally vasoconstricted, reducing heat loss, and will crawl under the covers or wear heavier clothing, which is a behavioral response that decreases heat loss. During hyperthermia, the core body temperature is above the thermoregulatory set-point, and the individual uses both physiologic and behavioral means to lower body temperature. This is what happens as a result of exercising, particularly in a warm environment or as a result of sitting in a sauna. When a fever "breaks," it is thought that the thermoregulatory set-point is returning to normal, and at this time the individual is hyperthermic. This is why the person will feel warm and will sweat as body temperature is returning to the prefebrile level.

A fever is an energetically costly process. Based on a Q_{10} of 2 to 3, for each 1°C elevation in body temperature, the metabolic rate of a febrile individual should increase about 13% (2). Of course, associated with most fevers is a decrease in overall activity, due in part to muscle aches, sleepiness, and loss of food appetite, and as a result, metabolic rate may not rise as much as predicted, simply based on the estimated effects of temperature on biochemical reaction rates.

Since 1974 it has been known that fever has had a long phylogenetic history (3). Fevers occur not only in infected endotherms (birds and mammals) but also in infected ectotherms (reptiles, amphibians, fishes, and even insects) (Table 1). As a result of the elevation in thermoregulatory set-point, the infected organism raises its body temperature by physiologic and behavioral means if it is an endotherm (e.g., shivers, seeks a warmer microclimate) and by behavioral means if it is an ectotherm.

WHAT CAUSES THE RISE IN THERMOREGULATORY SET-POINT?

Most evidence indicates that some exogenous stimulus (e.g., bacterial endotoxin, virus) causes the release of an endogenous pyrogen (EP) from macrophages. Endoge-

TABLE 1. *Development of fever in animals other than birds and mammals.*

	Activator of fever (exogenous pyrogen)	References
Reptiles		
Dipsosaurus dorsalis	Bacteria, EP	3,4
Iguana iguana	Bacteria	5
Crotaphytus collaris	Bacteria	6
Terrepene carolina	Bacteria	7
Chrysemys picta	Bacteria	7
Sauromalus obesus	Bacteria	8
Alligator mississippiensis	Bacteria	9
Callopistes maculatus	Bacteria	10
Amphibians		
Hyla cinerea	Bacteria	11
Rana pipiens	Bacteria	12
Rana catesbeiana	Bacteria	12
Rana esculenta	Bacteria, PGE_1, EP	13
Necturus maculosus	PGE_1	14
Bufo marinus	LPS	15
Fishes		
Micropterus salmoides	Bacteria	16
Lepomis macrochirus	Endotoxin, Bacteria	16
Carassius auratus	Endotoxin, Bacteria	16,17
Invertebrates		
Cambarus bartoni (crayfish)	Bacteria	18
Gromphadorhina portentosa (cockroach)	Endotoxin, Bacteria	19
Gryllus bimaculatus (cricket)	*Rickettesiella grylli*	20
Melanoplus sanguinipes (grasshopper)	*Nosema acridophagus*	21
Homarus americanus (lobster)	PGE_1	22
Penaeus duorarum (shrimp)	PGE_1	22
Limulus polyphemus (horseshoe crab)	PGE_1	22
Buthus occitanus (scorpion)	PGE_1	23
Androctonus australis (scorpion)	PGE_1	23
Onymacris plana (tenebrionid beetle)	Endotoxin	24
Nephelopsis obscrua (leech)	Endotoxin, PGE_1	25

nous pyrogen, a 15- to 25-kd protein, travels through the circulation to the brain, where in, or near, the anterior hypothalamus it causes a rise in thermoregulatory set-point, presumably by causing an increase in prostaglandin E_2. Shortly after the first cytokines were identified, most investigators working in the area of temperature regulation and fever concluded that the cytokine, interleukin-1 (IL-1), was the circulating EP. Interleukin-1, of which there are two forms—α and β–is thought to be responsible for numerous immune and nonimmune host-defense responses. There is, however, one problem with the oft-repeated statement that IL-1 is equivalent to EP—generally when either experimental animals or human beings are injected with fever-inducing doses of endotoxin, or other exogenous pyrogens, elevated concentrations of IL-1 are not detected in the circulation (1). In one study, when IL-1 concentrations have been claimed to rise, this rise in IL-1 actually occurred *after* the fever had developed. Often, whatever IL-1 is found in the circulation can only be shown to be biologically active after removing a larger molecular-weight inhibitor, or by extracting the plasma first with chloroform or other solvents. It is as though IL-1 evolved as a molecule that under normal circumstances was not designed to be a circulating mediator. Nevertheless, when rats are injected with neutralizing antiserum to IL-1β (but not to IL-1α) and then injected with endotoxin, the fevers are blocked almost 100%. These data are interpreted to support the following hypothesis: IL-1β is involved in the fever pathway, but it is not the circulating EP (1,26).

What, then, is the circulating EP? Many other cytokines have been discovered since the mid-1980s that are capable of producing fevers when injected into experimental animals or people (Table 2). Are all of these EPs? Not necessarily. In order for any of the cytokines listed in Table 2 to be an endogenous mediator of fever, it is critically important that the physiologic or pathophysiologic concentrations of these substances be sufficiently high to cause fever. Most of the cytokines listed in Table 2 were injected into people or experimental animals at pharmacologic doses. Since many cytokines stimulate the production and release of other cytokines (the so-called cytokine cascade), studies in which high doses of a cytokine are injected have little relevance to the in vivo changes in cytokine concentrations seen during infection. Which of the cytokines listed in Table 2 are the best candidates for the circulating EP?

Of all the cytokines listed in Table 2, the plasma concentration of IL-6 correlates best with the development of fever (27). There are also data implicating tumor necrosis factor (TNF) as a circulating pyrogen (28), but within the past couple of years some data have also been generated that support the hypothesis that endogenously produced TNF may actually lower febrile temperatures (see next section).

It may not even be necessary for there to be a circulating EP. There are considerable data that have shown that the central nervous system contains cells capable of making many of the cytokines listed in Table 2 as possible EPs. The anterior hypothalamus is an area that most investigators believe is critically involved in the development of fever, and in "push-pull" experiments, in which fluid bathing the anterior hypothalamus is collected in guinea pigs and rats injected with fever-inducing doses of endotoxin, there is an increase in both IL-6 and TNF (29,30). It may turn out that combinations of cytokines are responsible for raising the thermoregulatory

TABLE 2. *Cytokines that are capable of causing fever when injected into experimental animals or people.*

IL-1α and IL-1β
IL-2
IL-6
IL-8
Tumor necrosis factor α (TNFα)
Lymphotoxin (TNFβ)
Macrophage inflammatory protein-1 (MIP-1)
Interferons
Colony stimulating factors (CSF)

For detailed review, see Kluger (1).

set-point, and during different illnesses, different combinations are responsible for the characteristic pattern observed.

WHAT PREVENTS BODY TEMPERATURE FROM GETTING TOO HIGH?

Dubois noted that fevers seldom reached levels that caused direct harm to patients (31). We now know that during fever, not only are pyrogens being produced, which raise the thermoregulatory set-point, but so are many antipyretic substances or *endogenous cryogens* (ECs) (1). Two of these are peptides: arginine vasopressin (AVP) and α-melanocyte stimulating hormone (α-MSH). A third is glucocorticoids. As mentioned, it is possible that some cytokines, themselves, may exert antipyretic activity.

Arginine Vasopressin

Kasting et al. (32) and Cooper et al. (33) showed that microinjection of AVP into the septal region of sheep produced antipyresis to injections of bacterial pyrogens. In a variety of correlative studies, it has been shown that conditions that cause elevations in AVP are associated with reduced fevers (34,35) and those that cause decreased AVP are associated with enhanced fever (36), further supporting the hypothesis that AVP is an EC. In addition, studies that have relied on specific blockers or on specific antagonists to vasopressin receptors support the hypothesis that AVP is an EC. For example, Malkinson et al. (37) have shown that fevers induced by bacterial pyrogen are enhanced when AVP antiserum is perfused into the septum of rabbits.

There are at least two types of AVP receptors, V_1 (vasopressor) and V_2 (antidiuretic), and most evidence supports the hypothesis that AVP-induced antipyresis appears to work via the V_1 receptor (38,39). In an excellent review on the subject of AVP and its role in thermoregulation, Kasting (40) reported that administration of the V_1 receptor antagonist blocks the antipyretic effects of parenterally administered indomethacin. Similar data have been published by Alexander et al. (41). In this study, infusion of sodium salicylate into the ventral septal region of the rat brain led to suppresion of fever due to injection of prostaglandin E_1. Data were presented that supported the hypothesis that salicylate was producing its antipyresis via stimulation of AVP release or action. Fyda et al. (42) have shown that administration of an antipyretic drug (sodium salicylate) or AVP into the ventral septal area induces antipyresis in rats injected intracerebroventricularly (ICV) with PGE_1. These are intriguing findings because most investigators had concluded that the antipyretic action of salicylates and other antipyretic drugs was solely via inhibition of prostaglandin synthesis.

It is also possible that part of the antipyretic action of AVP may be via its induction of the release of α-MSH (see next section) from the hypothalamus (43). Recently, Christensen et al. (44) have shown that IL-1β is capable of facilitating the release of AVP from isolated superfused rat neurohypophysis. Thus, a putative EP (IL-1β) might induce the production of a centrally acting pyrogen (PGE) as well as a centrally acting cryogen (AVP). The AVP might then produce its antipyresis directly by acting on neurons in the forebrain or via the induction of α-MSH.

α-Melanocyte Stimulating Hormone

α-MSH is a 13–amino acid peptide often derived from the precursor proopiomelanocortin (POMC) molecule. It is found within the pituitary, as well as in other areas of the brain. Samson et al. (45) showed that following injection of EP into the lateral cerebral ventricles of rabbits, the concentration of α-MSH rose in the septal region. To determine whether α-MSH within the septal region could influence fever, Glyn-Ballinger et al. (46) injected rabbits intravenously (IV) with a mixture of EPs, followed by bilateral injections of α-MSH into the septal region. The results, which indicated that α-MSH attenuated fever, supported the hypothesis that α-MSH within the septum could be an endogenous antipyretic or EC.

Perhaps the strongest evidence that endogenously produced α-MSH has a role in limiting the magnitude and duration of fever comes from a study by Shih et al. (47) in which antiserum to α-MSH was injected ICV into rabbits. After 3 days of injection with antiserum or control serum, rabbits were injected IV with IL-1. The rabbits that received antiserum to α-MSH developed significantly larger fevers. More remarkable, however, was the duration of these fevers. In rabbits that received control serum, the fevers peaked within 1 to 2 hours and returned to baseline by 4 hours. In the rabbits that received antiserum to α-MSH, there was no evidence of defervescence at 9 hours postinjection.

α-MSH has also been found to have immunosuppressive properties. Intravenous injection of α-MSH has been shown to inhibit the synthesis of the acute phase protein, serum amyloid P, and the neutrophilia that occur in response to injection of purified human IL-1 in mice (48). α-MSH injected ICV also attenuates other acute phase responses initiated via the central nervous system. Dao et al. (49) have shown that ICV injection of EP in rabbits causes fever, and an increase in C-reactive protein and plasma leukocyte concentration. α-MSH injected ICV suppressed all of these responses. Opp et al. (50) showed that α-MSH also attenuated the IL-1–induced increase in non-REM sleep.

IL-1 and IL-2 have been shown to stimulate the production of mRNA of the POMC gene in primary cultures of pituitary cells and in the murine anterior pituitary cell line (AtT-20) (51). Thus, it is possible that during infection cytokines responsible for fever and other acute phase responses induce the synthesis of α-MSH, which then serves as a negative-feedback signal acting to attenuate this response.

Glucocorticoids

Although it has been known for several years that the addition of glucocorticoids such as cortisol or corticosterone to macrophages grown in vitro would result in a reduction in the concentrations of a variety of cytokines in the media, until recently there were no studies on the effects of physiologic levels of glucocorticoids on fever. Coelho et al. (52) have shown that adrenalectomized rats developed larger fevers in response to an injection of lipopolysaccharide (LPS). Morrow et al. (53) extended these observations by showing that administration of corticosterone to adrenalecto-mized rats led to an attenuation of LPS-induced fever only when the plasma levels of corticosterone were similar to that seen in sham-adrenalectomized rats during periods of stress. In other words, basal levels of corticosterone were not exerting a permissive effect on modulating LPS-induced fever. Rather, it was necessary for there to be an elevation in circulating levels of corticosterone to induce antipyresis. Experiments using the glucocorticoid (and progesterone) antagonist RU-38486 in-jected into different central nervous sites of intact rats have shown that the primary location of the negative feedback of glucocorticoids on LPS-induced fever is the anterior hypothalamus (54).

Tumor Necrosis Factor

As mentioned, although injection of TNF into experimental animals or human patients often results in fever, there are also data that support the hypothesis that endogenously produced TNF is an EC. Mathison et al. (55) have found that pre-treating rabbits with polyclonal antibody to TNF resulted in in vivo neutralization of TNF and led to significant protection against LPS-induced hypotension, fibrin deposition, and lethality. Despite this demonstration of the efficacy of their anti-serum, fever was not attenuated, and actually appeared to be significantly enhanced. We reported similar increased fevers in rats pretreated with antiserum to TNF in amounts that completely blocked the rise in plasma TNF (26,56). When rats injected with antiserum either intraparenterally (IP) or IV were then injected with LPS, the resultant fevers were significantly *enhanced*, rather than suppressed.

Further support for TNF being involved in lowering the body temperature of ill animals comes from a study by Smith and Kluger (57). In this study, rats were inoculated with an methylcholanthrene-induced (MCA) sarcoma. After about 2 weeks, body temperature of the tumor-bearing rats fell. This fall in body temperature was markedly attenuated by pretreatment of the rats with antiserum to TNF. In another study from my laboratory, Kozak et al. (58) has found that injection of mice with LPS results in a small fall in body temperature, followed by a fever that lasts about 24 hours. Injection of antiserum to TNF not only prevented the initial fall in body temperature, but resulted in a more rapid rise in body temperature.

IS FEVER BENEFICIAL OR HARMFUL?

Based on the previously mentioned description of *fever*, it is clear that fever is a regulated process for which there are mediators that elevate the thermoregulatory set-point and mediators that modulate this elevation. In this regard, fever can be considered an elegant homeostatic control system. By itself, this could form the basis for speculation that fever is an adaptive host response. For close to 2 decades, I have argued that fever is an adaptive response of the host, which evolved as one of many mechanisms to fight infection. Some of this was based on our observation that fever was a phylogenetically ancient phenomenon. Fever occurs in "cold-blooded" (ectothermic) organisms such as lizards (3), and this fever is associated with an increase in survival rate in these animals (59). In response to injection of live bacterial or even heat-killed bacteria, the lizards sought out a warmer microclimate, and their body temperatures rose. When lizards were given antipyretic drugs (i.e., sodium salicylate), their fevers fell, and this resulted in an increase in mortality rate (60). Since these initial studies, numerous other "lower" species have been shown to develop fevers when injected with exogenous pyrogens or infected with pathogens (see Table 1). In several of these animals, it has been found that fever resulted in enhanced survival rate during infection (reviewed in 1,61,62).

Many studies supporting the hypothesis that fever is beneficial were based on correlations between fever and mortality or morbidity. For example, New Zealand white rabbits respond to infection with *Pasteurella multocida* by developing large fevers. Most rabbits developed a fever of less than 2.25°C, and within this temperature range, there is an increase in survival rate as body temperature is elevated (63). However, a small number of animals developed fevers above 2.25°C and showed a decrease in survival rate.

Another correlation study was reported by Toms et al. (64). In this study, ferrets were infected with different strains of influenza viruses and the resultant fever was correlated with the presence of live viruses in their nasal passages. Groups of three to six nonimmune ferrets were inoculated intranasally with a constant dose of virus. At 4-hour intervals, the nasal passages were washed and the fluid was collected and assayed for the presence of live virus. Statistically significant ($p < 0.01$) negative correlations were found between the ferrets' rectal temperatures and the presence of live viruses in the nasal washes, suggesting that fever might lead to the inactivation of viruses. In vitro observations from this same laboratory, in which organ cultures of ferret nasal turbinates were grown in the presence of influenza virus, are consistent with the in vivo data previously described (65); i.e., an elevation in temperature decreased the replication of the viruses. Interestingly, the more virulent strain of virus was less sensitive to the effects of temperature.

In studies that have correlated body temperature of human subjects with survival rate, several investigators have found that fever is associated with better prognoses during bacterial infections (66–69). In one study, it was found that there was no correlation between fever and survival rate, but simply that hypothermia in adults or newborns was associated with higher mortality rate (70). Thus, overall, the results of correlation studies are generally consistent with the theory that fever has a beneficial function.

There have also been several studies in which a population of mammals has been infected with identical amounts of pathogens and the effects of antipyresis on mortality or morbidity were quantified. Van Miert et al. (71) studied the effects of flurbiprofen, a nonsteroidal antiinflammatory/antipyretic, on *Trypanosoma vivax* infection in goats. They found that this drug blocked the febrile responses during the acute phase of the infection. Sixteen of 17 nontreated goats had a mild infection. All five goats treated with an antipyretic dosage of flurbiprofen died.

Vaughn et al. (72) studied the effect of administration of an antipyretic drug directly into the preoptic-anterior hypothalamus of rabbits on mortality rate during infection of rabbits with *Pasteurella multocida*. The fevers in the rabbits infused with the antipyretic drug was reduced by about 50%. This group of infected rabbits had a significant increase in mortality compared to the group of infected rabbits infused with control solution.

Husseini et al. (73) investigated fever and influenza titers in ferrets infected with influenza. They studied the effects of suppression of fever using sodium salicylate on viral titers in nasal washes and found that treatment with the antipyretic drug resulted in attenuation of fever and an increased concentration of virus in washes, as well as an increase in the duration of illness.

Small et al. (74) investigated the effects of body temperature on bacterial growth rates in experimental pneumococcal infection in rabbits. Rabbits injected with *Streptococcus pneumoniae* intracisternally developed fevers averaging 1.5°C. To induce antipyresis, the rabbits were anesthetized with pentobarbital or urethane. Body temperature was controlled by varying ambient temperature. The growth rate of bacteria was significantly higher in anesthetized rabbits maintained at afebrile body temperatures. The correlation between changes in bacterial titer in the cerebrospinal fluid and body temperatures (from 38.5°C to 41°C) was -0.70 ($p < 0.001$), data supporting the hypothesis that elevated temperatures suppressed growth rate of the bacteria.

Kurosawa et al. (75) studied the effects of antipyretics in rinderpest infection (RPV) in rabbits. Rabbits were infected with the lapinized Nakamura III strain of RPV (L strain) and then treated with mefanamic acid, acetylsalicylic acid, or untreated. The antipyretic drugs led to varying amounts of reduction in body temperature. The antipyretic drug, mefanamic acid, was a more potent antipyretic than acetylsalicylic acid. Treatment with these drugs led to increased mortality rate and slower recovery among the survivors.

As mentioned, ectothermic vertebrates have also been used to study the role of fever in disease. Bernheim and Kluger (60) studied the effects of sodium salicylate–induced antipyresis on survival of the desert iguana. Lizards were injected with the live bacteria *(Aeromonas hydrophila)* along with a dose of sodium salicylate, which produced antipyresis in 7 of the 12 animals. All febrile lizards survived, while the afebrile lizards died. To determine whether the dose of sodium salicylate used in these experiments was toxic, eight lizards were injected with live bacteria and sodium salicylate and placed inside a constant temperature chamber. Their body temperatures were maintained at the febrile level by adjusting the chamber temperature to about 41°C during the day (about the average temperature selected by febrile lizards in the simulated natural environment) and at low temperatures at night (again, as in the simulated natural environment). Only one of these eight lizards died, indicating that the dose of sodium salicylate used in these experiments was not toxic. These data indicated to us that the administration of sodium salicylate to these infected lizards was harmful only when it resulted in a reduction in body temperature to the afebrile level. When sodium salicylate failed to produce antipyresis (as in the five lizards in the simulated desert environment or in the eight lizards maintained in the constant-temperature chamber), the survival in infected lizards was not adversely affected by the drug. Thus, the results of studies using antipyretic drugs to attenuate fever support the hypothesis that fever is a host-defense response.

An area that has received considerable attention is that of the febrile responses of newborns. It has been known for a long time that many newborn mammals have a labile body temperature during their first few days of life (76). Furthermore, in response to infection, newborn human infants (77) or other infant mammals such as rabbits (78) tend to have a limited febrile response. Satinoff et al. have shown, however, that newborn rabbits, although not raising their body temperature by physiologic means following an injection of endotoxin, will raise their body temperature by behavioral means (78). When injected with *Pseudomonas* endotoxins and allowed to select a range of environmental temperatures, these rabbits selected a warmer environmental temperature, resulting in an elevation in their body temperatures. Haahr and Mogensen (77) suggested that hyperthermia (or, more precisely, a rise in body temperature) during certain viral infections was beneficial to newborns. To support their claim, they cited several studies that demonstrated that elevations in body temperature during various viral infections have reduced the mortality rate in newborn mice, dogs, and human beings. For example, Teisner and Haahr (79) found that when 2- to 3-day-old mice were infected with Coxsackie virus and held at an environmental temperature of 34°C, they had a mean body temperature of 35.8°C, some 2°C to 3°C higher than control mice held at room temperature of 22°C to 24°C. Those mice that were held at 34°C had a considerably lower mortality rate than did the control mice. Carmichael et al. (80) reported similar findings for 2- to 5-day-old dog pups that were inoculated with canine herpesvirus. When the pups were held at an environmental temperature of 28°C to 30°C, they had a rectal temperature of about 35°C to 37°C; those held at an environmental temperature of 36.7°C to 37.7°C had a rectal temperature of 38.3°C to 39.4°C, approximately normal rectal temperatures for adult dogs. Following inoculation with herpesvirus, those dogs with the lower rectal temperatures died within 8 days, whereas those with the higher rectal temperatures survived 9 days or longer. The authors of this study concluded that the elevation of the body temperature to the adult level was beneficial to the infected pups. Based on these data, Haahr and Mogensen (77) suggested that one of the reasons that generalized herpes-simplex infections are greatly overrepresented in premature babies might be attributable to their restricted temperature regulation and poor febrile response.

Bell and Moore (81) have found that housing of mice in a warm ambient temperature (35°C) led to decreased mortality due to inoculation with rabies virus. The average body temperatures of mice in the warm environmental temperature was 2°C higher than those in the control environment (20°C).

As mentioned earlier, there have also been studies designed to investigate the role of fever using ectothermic species. For example, to investigate whether the rise in body temperature in the bacterially infected desert iguana had survival value, lizards were injected with live *Aeromonae hydrophila* and placed in incubators at Celsius temperatures of 34°, 36°, 38°, 40°, and 42° (59). Control lizards were inoculated with saline and then placed into the incubators. The relation between the lizards' temperatures and percentage survival following bacterial infection was highly significant ($p < 0.005$). Within 24 hours, approximately 50% of the lizards maintained at the afebrile temperature of 38°C were dead. However, lizards maintained at the febrile temperatures of 40°C and 42°C had only 14% and 0% mortality, respectively. Conversely, lizards maintained at 36°C and 34°C, temperatures that are hypothermic for this species of lizard, experienced mortalities of 66% and 75%, respectively. After 3½ days, all the lizards at 34°C were dead. After 7 days, the percentage mortalities were: 42°C, 25%; 40°C, 33%; 38°C and 36°C, 75%; and 34°C, 100%. In contrast, lizards injected with saline and maintained at 34°C, 38°C, and 42°C for 7 days experienced 0%, 0%, and 34% mortality, respectively. At the highest temperature tested, the pattern of deaths was similar for the controls and the infected lizards. Whereas most deaths occurred within 3½ days in infected lizards maintained at 34°C to 40°C, virtually all deaths at 42°C occurred after 3½ days. Apparently, maintenance at 42°C for a period exceeding 3½ days is harmful in itself. This suggests that the deaths at 42°C were not due to the bacterial infection, but to some undetermined adverse effect of long-term elevation in body temperature.

There have been several studies involving the effects of temperature on the mortality rate of fishes. One of these, by Covert and Reynolds (82), involved infecting goldfish with live *A. hydrophila* and monitoring their survival rate over a period of 3 days. These investigators had previously reported that several species of freshwater fishes developed fevers in response to injections with these bacteria. In their survival study, they infected goldfish and then held them at temperatures of 25.5°C, 28.0°C, or 30.5°C. These represented, respectively, hypothermic, normothermic, and febrile temperatures. Goldfish maintained at a febrile temperature of 30.5°C had a survival rate of 84%; those maintained at 28.0°C had a survival rate of 64%; those at 25.5°C had a survival rate of 24%. Another ten fish were injected with the same dose of live *A. hydrophila* and were allowed to thermoregulate in a shuttlebox. These fish developed a fever averaging almost 5°C and had a mean body temperature of 32.7°C. None of these fish died. Covert and Reynolds concluded that a fever in response to infection with *A. hydrophila* increases the survival rate of goldfish.

There have been several studies involving the effects of elevations in water (i.e., body) temperature on the mortality rate of various species of freshwater fishes infected with viruses. For example, Watson et al. (83) reported that sockeye salmon infected with sockeye salmon virus experienced fewer deaths when held at a water temperature of 20°C than when held at 15.5°C or lower. In 1970, Amend reported similar findings for sockeye salmon infected with hematopoietic necrosis virus (IHN) (84). The mortality rate of salmon held between 12°C and 16°C was about 66%, whereas for those held between 18°C and 20°C, it was only about 30%. Even when there was a delay of up to 24 hours before the infected fishes were placed in the warmer environment, there was still a substantial decrease in the mortality rate.

Similar results were reported for IHN-infected rainbow trout (85). One of the difficulties in interpreting these studies is that because it is unknown whether these fishes develop fevers in response to viral infections, it is unclear whether raising their body temperatures simulates hyperthermia or fever. If the former were the case, then the beneficial effects of raising the body temperatures of these fishes would simply be a form of fever therapy and, therefore, these results would not be applicable to a discussion of the role of naturally occurring fever in disease. Since several species of freshwater fishes develop fevers in response to bacterial infection, I believe that it is likely that, given the opportunity, the species of fishes used in the viral studies would also behaviorally select warmer environmental temperatures. If this turns out to be the case, then these results would support the thesis that fever has an adaptive function in fishes.

Louis et al. (20) infected crickets with the intracellular parasite *Rickettsiella grylli*. They reared the crickets at different ambient temperatures and found that those crickets reared at warmer temperatures (higher than 29°C) survived this infection. It should be noted that when these crickets were infected and allowed to select a preferred body temperature in a temperature gradient, they selected a temperature averaging 33.0°C. The average body temperature of noninfected crickets was 26.6°C.

Boorstein and Ewald (21) inoculated grasshoppers with the protozoan *Nosema acridophagus* and found that this resulted in an increase in preferred body temperature of about 6°C (to ca. 40°C). Maintenance of grasshoppers at febrile and afebrile temperatures demonstrated that fever enhanced both survival rate and growth. The maintenance of infected grasshoppers at febrile temperatures also increased fecundity, as quantified by numbers of eggs laid, compared to infected grasshoppers at afebrile temperatures.

In addition to the data described here, most of which support the hypothesis that fever is beneficial, there are numerous studies that have shown that various components of specific and nonspecific immunity are enhanced at febrile temperatures (see Table 3).

Despite the evidence that fever, an energetically costly process, has a long phylogenetic history, and considerable experimental data indicating that fever enhances specific components of host defenses, many physicians still think of fever as being harmful to their patients. Based on my reading of the literature, I believe that the probable explanation for why fever came to be thought of as a harmful side-effect of infection

TABLE 3. *Some effects of febrile temperatures on host-defense responses.*

Enhanced neutrophil migration
Increased production of antibacterial substances by neutrophils (e.g., superoxide anion)
Increased production of interferon
Increased antiviral and antitumor activity of interferon
Increased T-cell proliferation
Decreased growth of microorganisms in iron-poor environment

For more detailed information, see Kluger (1), Mackowiak (61), and Roberts (62).

is related to the association between fever and pain. Antipyretic drugs, by also being analgesics, reduce *both* the fever and the pain associated with infections. However, there are no data that show that fever, by itself, is painful. Clearly, people feel comfortable sitting in saunas or exercising at environmental temperatures that result in a 2°C, or even greater, rise in body temperature. No pain is associated with these rises in body temperature. The magnitude of a fever is most likely simply an indicator of the severity of an illness (and thus a crude indicator of the host's response to the particular pathogen). I contend that drugs that reduce fever are making the individual less uncomfortable and less irritable as a result of the analgesic (and perhaps antiinflammatory) effects of these drugs, and not based on their antipyretic properties.

In some clinical studies it has been argued that the administration of antipyretic drugs to patients appears to have little effect on the course of the disease. There are several possible explanations for these findings. Some studies do demonstrate that treatment with "antipyretic" drugs had no affect on duration of illness (86,87). However, in neither of these studies were temperature data presented. Were the doses of antipyretic drugs used high enough to actually induce lowering of body temperature? If so, why weren't these data presented? In one study (88), acetaminophen was administered to children with chickenpox, but the dose of this drug was stated as not being sufficiently high to produce antipyresis. To my knowledge, there have been no prospective studies to determine whether fever actually shortens or prolongs illness, with the possible exception of a recent correlative study by El-Radhi et al. (89). They have shown that in children with salmonella gastroenteritis there was a significant negative correlation between the magnitude of fever and the duration of bacterial excretion. The patients with presenting fevers ≥40°C had the shortest duration of salmonella excretion, followed by those patients with temperatures ranging from 38°C to 39.9°C. The children with the longest duration of salmonellosis had the lowest admitting temperatures, ≤37.9°C.

It is often stated that patients and professionals are alarmed by the threat of febrile convulsions or seizures. This fear is reinforced by the results of a recent survey conducted by May and Bauchner (90). They polled pediatricians and found that "seizures were cited 58% of the time as the most frequent complication of fever. . . ." I have discussed this issue with many pediatricians, including the senior author of the aforementioned survey, and have concluded that there are no data indicating that seizures associated with modest fevers are in any way related to the presence of fever. In fact, in one study it has been shown that the recurrence rate of febrile convulsions actually decreased ninefold in those children who had the highest temperatures during their "febrile" convulsions (91). Whether this means that high fever (>40°C) actually is protective during convulsions is unclear.

Antipyretic (analgesic/antiinflammatory) drugs have been used for centuries, probably to make patients feel more comfortable during infection. I contend that these drugs were used not to reduce fever but primarily to reduce the pain and discomfort produced by the same inflammatory substances that cause fever—prostaglandins. Why isn't the use of these drugs associated with a marked increase in mortality rate? I believe that the answer to this questions is relatively simple once one begins to think of the response to infection as following the same homeostatic rules that other physiologic systems obey. A disturbance to one component of a complex system induces feedback regulatory responses in other components of the system. Since there are numerous host defenses to infection, if one response is suppressed, the infected organism would presumably increase its other host-defense responses, and as a result, during most illnesses, the effects of suppressing fever may not be readily observed. However, during a life-threatening illness, the attenuation of fever *may* result in moving infected patients closer toward a critical point where they are unable to mount an adequate host response.

An important caveat to consider is that fever, which probably evolved as a general host-defense response, might not be beneficial during *all* infections. In some illnesses, the host responses to that illness can be so severe that it is the overzealous host defenses that *contribute* to the severity of the illness. This might be particularly true for those infections (or injuries) that lead to uncontrolled inflammation (e.g., during endotoxic shock) in which the fever may actually facilitate the inflammatory process.

REFERENCES

1. Kluger MJ. Fever: role of endogenous pyrogens and cryogens. *Physiol Rev* 1991;71:93–127.
2. Elia M. Organ and tissue contribution to metabolic rate. In: Kinney JM, Tucker HM (eds). *Energy Metabolism: Tissue Determinants and Cellular Corollaries.* New York: Raven Press, 1992;61–79.
3. Vaughn LK, Bernheim HA, Kluger MJ: Fever in the lizard *Dipsosaurus dorsalis. Nature.* 1974;252: 473–474.
4. Bernheim HA, Kluger MJ. Endogenous pyrogen-like substance produced by reptiles. *J Physiol (Lond)* 1977;267:659–666.
5. Kluger MJ. The evolution and adaptive value of fever. *Am Scientist* 1977;66:38–43.
6. Firth BT, Ralph CL, Boardman TJ. Independent effects of the pineal and a bacterial pyrogen in behavioural thermoregulation in lizards. *Nature* 1980;285:399–400.
7. Monagas WR, Gatten RE Jr. Behavioural fever in the turtles *Terrapene carolina* and *Chrysemys picta. J Therm Biol* 1983;8:285–288.
8. Muchlinski AE, Stoutenburgh RJ, Hogan JM. Fever response in laboratory-maintained and free-ranging chuckwallas (*Sauromalus obesus*). *Am J Physiol* 1989;257:R150–R155.
9. Lang JW. Crocodilian thermal selection. In: Webb GJW, Manolis SC, Whitehead PJ (eds): *Wildlife Management: Crocodiles and Alligators.* Surrey: Beatty and Sons, 1987;301–317.
10. Hallman GM, Ortega CE, Towner MC, Muchlinski AE. Effect of bacterial pyrogen on three lizard species. *Comp Biochem Physiol* 1990;96A:383–386.
11. Kluger MJ. Fever in the frog, *Hyla cinerea. J Thermal Biol* 1977;2:79–81.
12. Casterlin ME, Reynolds WW. Behavioral fever in anuran amphibian larvae. *Life Sci* 1977;20:593–596.
13. Myhre KM, Cabanac M, Myhre G. Fever and behavioural temperature regulation in the frog *Rana esculenta. Acta Physiol Scand* 1977;101:219–229.
14. Hutchison VH, Erskine DJ. Thermal selection and prostaglandin E_1 fever in the salamander *Necturus maculosus. Herpetologica* 1981;37:195–198.
15. Sherman E, Baldwin L, Fernandex G, Deurell E. Fever and thermal tolerance in the toad *Bufo marinus. J Thermal Biol* 1991;16:297–301.
16. Reynolds WW, Casterlin ME, Covert JB. Behavioural fever in teleost fishes. *Nature* 1976;259:41–42.
17. Reynolds WW, Casterlin ME, Covert JB. Febrile responses of bluegill (*Lepomis macrochirus*) to bacterial pyrogens. *J Thermal Biol* 1978;3:129–130.
18. Casterlin ME, Reynolds WW. Fever and antipyresis in the crayfish *Cambarus bartoni. J Physiol (Lond)* 1980;303:417–421.
19. Bronstein SM, Conner WE: Endotoxin-induced behavioural fever in the Madagascar cockroach, *Gromphadorhina portentosa. J Insect Physiol* 1984;30:327–330.

20. Louis C, Jourdan M, Cabanac M. Behavioral fever and therapy in a rickettsia-infected Orthoptera. *Am J Physiol* 1986;50:R991–R995.
21. Boorstein SM, Ewald PW. Costs and benefits of behavioral fever in *Melanoplus sanuinipes* infected by *Nosema acridophagus*. *Physiol Zool* 1987;60:586–595.
22. Casterlin ME, Reynolds WW. Fever induced in marine arthropods by prostagladin E_1. *Life Sci* 1979; 25:1601–1604.
23. Cabanac M, Guelte LL. Temperature regulation and prostaglandin E_1 fever in scorpions. *J Physiol (Lond)* 1980;303:365–370.
24. McClain E, Magnuson P, Warner SJ. Behavioural fever in a namib desert tenebrionid beetle, *Onymacris plana*. *J Insect Physiol* 1988;34:279–284.
25. Cabanac M. Fever in a leech. Thermal Physiology Symposium, Tromso, Norway. Satellite Symposium of XXXI International Physiological Congress, 1989; p. 6.
26. Long NC, Otterness I, Kunkel SL, et al. The roles of interleukin-1β and tumor necrosis factor in lipopolysaccharide-fever in the rat. *Am J Physiol* 1990;259:R724–R728.
27. Nijsten MWN, De Groot ER, Ten Duis HJ, et al. Serum levels of interleukin-6 and acute phase response. *Lancet* 1987;2:921.
28. Michie HR, Spriggs DR, Manogue KR, et al. Tumor necrosis factor and endotoxin induce similar metabolic responses in human beings. *Surgery* 1988;104:280–286.
29. Klir JJ, Roth J, Kluger MJ. Interleukin-6 (IL-6) and tumor necrosis factor (TNF) in hypothalamus of rats during lipopolysaccharide (LPS)-induced fever. *FASEB J* 1992;6(5):1522.
30. Roth J, Conn C, Kluger MJ, Zeisberger E. Release of interleukin-6 and tumor necrosis factor during lipopolysaccharide induced fever in guinea pigs. In: Lomax P, Schonbaum E (eds.): *Thermoregulation: The Pathophysiological Basis of Clinical Disorders*. 1992; 8th International Symposium on Pharmacology of Thermoregulation, Kananaskis, Canada. Basel: Karger, 1991;28–32.
31. Dubois EF. Why are fever temperatures over 106°F rare? *Am J Med Sci* 1949;217:361–368.
32. Kasting NW, Cooper KE, Veale WL. Antipyresis following perfusion of brain sites with vasopressin. *Experientia* 1979;35:208–209.
33. Cooper KE, Kasting NW, Lederis K, Veale WL. Evidence supporting a role for endogenous vasopressin in natural supression of fever in sheep. *J Physiol (Lond)* 1979;295:33–45.
34. Kasting NW. Potent physiological stimuli for vasopressin release, hypertonic saline and hemorrhage, cause antipyresis in the rat. *Regul Pept* 1986;15:293–300.
35. Kasting NW, Veale WL, Cooper KE, Lederis K. Effect of hemorrhage on fever: the putative role of vasopressin. *Can J Physiol Pharmacol* 1981;59:324–328.
36. Pittman QJ, Malkinson TJ, Kasting NW, Veale WL. Enhanced fever following castration: possible involvement of brain arginine vasopressin. *Am J Physiol* 1988;254:R513–R517.
37. Malkinson TJ, Bridge TE, Lederis K, Veale WL. Perfusion of the septum of the rabbit with vasopressin antiserum enhances endotoxin fever. *Peptides* 1987;8:385–389.
38. Kasting NW, Wilkinson MF. Vasopressin functions as an endogenous antipyretic in the newborn. *Biol Neonate* 1987;51:249–254.
39. Naylor AM, Gubitz GJ, Dinarello CA, Veale WL. Central effects of vasopressin and 1-desamino-8-D-arginine vasopressin (DDAVP) on interleukin-1 fever in the rat. *Brain Res* 1987;401:173–177.
40. Kasting NW. Criteria for establishing a physiological role for brain peptides. A case in point: the role of vasopressin in thermoregulation during fever and antipyresis. *Brain Res Rev* 1989;14:143–153.
41. Alexander SJ, Cooper KE, Veale WL. Sodium salicylate: alternate mechanism of central antipyretic action in the rat. *Pflugers Arch* 1989;413:451–455.
42. Fyda DM, Mathieson WB, Cooper KE, Veale WL. The effectiveness of arginine vasopressin and sodium salicylate as antipyretics in the Brattleboro rat. *Brain Res* 1990;512:243–247.
43. Bronstein DM, Akil H. In vitro release of hypothalamic β-endorphin (βE) by arginine vasopressin, corticotropin-releasing hormone and 5-hydroxytryptamine: evidence for release of opioid active and inactive βE forms. *Neuropeptides* 190;16:33–40.
44. Christensen JD, Hansen EW, Fjalland B. Interleukin-1β stimulates the release of vasopressin from rat neurohypophysis. *Eur J Pharmacol* 1989;171:233–235.
45. Samson WK, Lipton JM, Zimmer JA, Glyn JR. The effect of fever on central alpha-MSH concentrations in the rabbit. *Peptides* 1981;2:419–423.
46. Glyn-Ballinger JR, Bernadini GL, Lipton JM. α-MSH injected into the septal region reduces fever in rabbits. *Peptides* 1983;4:199–203.
47. Shih ST, Khorram O, Lipton JM, McCann SM. Central administration of α-MSH antiserum augments fever in the rabbit. *Am J Physiol* 1986;250:R803–R806.

48. Robertson BA, Gahring LC, Daynes RA. Neuropeptide regulation of interleukin-1 activities. Capacity of α-melanocyte stimulating hormone to inhibit interleukin-1-inducible responses in vivo and in vitro exhibits target cell selectivity. *Inflammation* 1986;10:371–385.
49. Dao TK, Bell RC, Feng J, et al. C-reactive protein, leukocytes, and fever after central IL 1 and α-MSH in aged rabbits. *Am J Physiol* 1988;254:R401–R409.
50. Opp MR, Obal F Jr, Krueger JM. Effects of alpha-MSH on sleep, behavior, and brain temperature: interactions with IL 1. *Am J Physiol* 1988;255:R914–R922.
51. Brown SL, Smith LR, Blalock JE. Interleukin 1 and interleukin 2 enhance proopiomelanocortin gene expression in pituitary cells. *J Immunol* 1987;139:3181–3183.
52. Coelho MM, Souza GEP, Pela IR. Endotoxin-induced fever is modulated by endogenous glucocorticoids in rats. *Am J Physiol* 1992;263:R423–R427.
53. Morrow LE, McClellan JL, Conn CA, Kluger MJ. Glucocorticoids alter fever and IL-6 responses to psychological stress and lipopolysaccharide. *Am J Physiol* 1993;264:R1010–R1016.
54. McClellan JL, Morrow LE, Klir JJ, Kluger MJ. The effects of glucocorticoid receptor antagonist RU38486 (RU386) on lipopolysaccharide (LPS) and stress-induced fever, plasma interleukin 6 (IL-6) and plasma corticosterone (CORT) in rats. *Exp Biol* 1993;7:A593.
55. Mathison JC, Wolfson E, Ulevitch RJ. Participation of tumor necrosis factor in the mediation of gram negative bacterial lipopolysaccharide-induced injury in rabbits. *J Clin Invest* 1988;81:1925–1937.
56. Long NC, Kunkel SL, Vander AJ, Kluger MJ. Antiserum against TNF enhances LPS fever in the rat. *Am J Physiol* 1990;258:R332–R337.
57. Smith BK, Kluger MJ. Anti-TNFα antibodies normalized body temperature and enhanced food intake in tumor-bearing rats. *Am J Physiol* 1992;(In Press).
58. Kozak W, Conn CA, Kluger MJ. Temperature responses of mice to endotoxin or polyinosinic:polycytidylic acid. *Soc Neuroscienc Abstracts* 1992;18:490.
59. Kluger MJ, Ringler DH, Anver MR. Fever and survival. *Science* 1975;188:166–168.
60. Bernheim HA, Kluger MJ. Fever: effect of drug-induced antipyresis on survival. *Science* 1976;193:237–239.
61. Mackowiak PA (ed). *Fever: Basic Mechanisms and Management.* New York: Raven Press, 1991.
62. Roberts NJ Jr: Impact of temperature elevation on immunologic defenses. *Rev Infect Dis* 1991;13:462–472.
63. Kluger MJ, Vaughn LK. Fever and survival in rabbits infected with *Pasteurella multocida. J Physiol (London)* 1978;282:243–251.
64. Toms GL, Davies JA, Woodward CG, et al. The relation of pyrexia and nasal inflammatory response to virus levels in nasal washings of ferrets infected with influenza viruses of differing virulence. *Br J Exp Pathol* 1977;58:444–458.
65. Sweet C, Cavanagh D, Collie MH, Smith H. Sensitivity to pyrexial temperatures: a factor contributing to the virulence differences between two clones of influenza virus. *Br J Exp Pathol* 1978;59:373–380.
66. Bryant RE, Hood AF, Hood CE, Loenig MG. Factors affecting mortality of gram-negative rod bacteremia. *Arch Intern Med.* 1971;127:120–128.
67. Weinstein MP, Iannin PB, Stratton CW, Eickhoff TC. Spontaneous bacterial peritonitis. A review of 28 cases with emphasis on improved survival and factors influencing prognosis. *Am J Med* 1978;64:592–598.
68. Hoefs J, Sapico FL, Canwati HN, Montgomerie JZ. The relationship of white blood cell (WBC) and pyrogenic response to survival in spontaneous bacterial peritonitis (SBP). *Gastroenterology* 1980;78:1308.
69. Mackowiak PA, Browne RH, Southern PM Jr, Smith JW. Polymicrobial sepsis: an analysis of 184 cases using log linear models. *Am J Med Sci* 1980;280:73–80.
70. DuPont HG, Spink WW. Infections due to gram-negative organisms: an analysis of 860 patients with bacteremia at the University of Minnesota Medical Center, 1958–1966. *Medicine* 1969;48:307–332.
71. Van Miert ASJPAM, Van Duin CTh, Busser FJM, et al. The effect of flurbiprofen, a potent non-steroidal anti-inflammatory agent, upon *Trypansosoma vivax* infection in goats. *J Vet Pharmacol Ther* 1978;1:69–76.
72. Vaughn LK, Veale WL, Cooper KE. Antipyresis: its effect on mortality rate of bacterially infected rabbits. *Brain Res Bull* 1980;5:69–73.
73. Husseini RH, Sweet C, Collie MH, Smith H. Elevation of nasal viral levels by suppression of fever in ferrets infected with influenza viruses of differing virulence. *J Infect Dis* 1982;145:520–524.
74. Small PM, Tauber MG, Hackbarth CJ, Sande MA. Influence of body temperature on bacterial growth rates in experimental pneumococcal meningitis in rabbits. *Infect Immun* 1986;52:484–487.

75. Kurosawa S, Kobune F, Okuyama K, Sugiura A. Effects of antipyretics in rinderpest virus infection in rabbits. *J Infect Dis* 1987;155:991–997.
76. Pembrey MS. The effect of variations in external temperature upon the output of carbonic acid and the temperature of young animals. *J Physiol (Lond)* 1895;18:364–379.
77. Haahr S, Mogensen S. Function of fever. *Lancet* 1977;2:613.
78. Satinoff E, McEwen GN Jr, Williams BA. Behavioral fever in newborn rabbits. *Science* 1976;193: 1139–1140.
79. Teisner B, Haahr S. Poililothermia and susceptibility of suckling mice to Coxsackie B_1 virus. *Nature* 1974;247:568.
80. Carmichael LE, Barnes FD, Percy DH. Temperature as a factor in resistance of young puppies. *J Infect Dis* 1969;120:669–678.
81. Bell JF, Moore GJ. Effects of high ambient temperature on various stages of rabies virus infection in mice. *Infect Immun* 1974;10:510–515.
82. Covert JB, Reynolds WW. Survival value of fever in fish. *Nature* 1977;267:43–45.
83. Watson SW, Guenther RW, Rucker RR. A virus disease of sockeye salmon: interim report. *US Fish Wildlife Serv Sci Rep Fish* 1954;138:36.
84. Amend DF. Control of infectious hematopoietic necrosis virus disease by elevating the water temperature. *J Fish Res Board Can* 1970;27:265–270.
85. Amend DF. Prevention and control of viral diseases of salmonids. *J Fish Res Board Can* 1976;33: 1059–1066.
86. Munzenberger PA, Robayo JR, del Valle J. Effect of antipyretics on the length of hospital stay of pediatric patients with bacterial infections. *J Hosp Pharmacol* 1981;38:861–863.
87. Kramer MS, Naimark LE, Roberts-Brauer R, et al. Risks and benefits of paracetamol antipyresis in young children with fever of presumed viral origin. *Lancet* 1991;337:591–594.
88. Doran TF, deAngelis C, Baumgartner RA, et al. Acetaminophen: more harm than good for chicken pox? *J Pediatr* 1989;114:1045–1048.
89. El-Radhi AS, Rostila T, Vesikari T. Association of high fever and short bacterial excretion after salmonellosis. *Arch Dis Child* 1992;67:531–532.
90. May A, Bauchner H. Fever phobia: the pediatricians contribution. *Pediatrics* 1992;90:851–854.
91. El-Radhi AS, Withana K, Banajeh S. Effect of fever on recurrence of febrile convulsions. *Arch Dis Child* 1989;64:869–870.

Overview: Substrate and Acute Catabolism

Simon P. Allison

Department of Diabetes and Endocrinology, University Hospital, Nottingham NG7 2UH, United Kingdom

The body fat of an average human contains enough fuel, theoretically, to last for 2 to 3 months. The stores of carbohydrate in the form of glycogen, however, contain enough fuel for only 24 hours. If fasting continues beyond that, then the demands of the glucose-requiring tissues, such as the wound, brain, white cells and gut, can only be met through the process of gluconeogenesis, largely from the breakdown of protein. In normal life, the pendulum swings gently between the fed and the fasted state, i.e., between storage and consumption, under the influence of small changes in insulin and its counterregulatory hormones adrenaline, glucagon, cortisol, and to some extent growth hormone. Considering the relative stores of carbohydrate and fat, it is hardly surprising that, during prolonged starvation, we derive 80% to 90% of our energy from fat, and that mechanisms have evolved, such as reduction in metabolic rate and adaptation of the brain, to use ketones, which allow conservation of protein and the body cell mass on which we depend for continuing function and survival. Graham Hill (1) has pointed to the correlation between reduction in total body protein and impairment of muscle and respiratory function. He showed that up to 20% of the body protein (correlating roughly with 15% weight loss), can be lost before serious changes in function are seen, but, after this point, there is a rapid deterioration in function that constitutes a threat to recovery. After injury, in contrast to starvation, the adaptations to conserve protein are lost and the process of gluconeogenesis from protein continues at an accelerated rate, posing a greater threat to the body cell mass. We are faced, therefore, with a paradox that, to have evolved at all, the metabolic response to injury must have had some survival value, yet when taken to extremes, it threatens the essential structure and function of the body.

As long ago as 1794, in his *Treatise on the Blood, Inflammation and Gunshot Wounds,* John Hunter described this paradox in the following words: "Impressions are capable of producing or increasing natural action and are then called stimuli. They are likewise capable of producing too much action, as well as depraved, unnatural or what we commonly call diseased actions." In order, therefore, to develop new and intelligent treatments of the acutely ill and injured, we must have a better understanding of the response to injury, its mechanism, and its purpose. This session is devoted to exploring these questions and how far the neuroendocrine response can explain the observed metabolic changes.

It is said that science is concerned with answering the question "How?" rather than "Why?" Intelligent therapeutics is, however, concerned with both questions because to confuse a purposeful symptom with the underlying disease, and by treatment try and oppose it, is a trap that physicians have fallen into for centuries and that still has its hold on our thinking. The giving of antipyretics, such as Aspirin, to children with fever, for example, is still a regular practice. In his paper on fever in this session, Dr. Kluger raises the question of not only how but also why, and presents impressive evidence showing that fever is a beneficial response, aiding recovery from infectious illness.

From the fourth century AD until the middle of the nineteenth century, the teachings of Galen dominated the practice of medicine. Diseases were thought to be due to an imbalance between the four humours of the body—blood, phlegm, and black and yellow bile. From these concepts grew the custom of bleeding, purging, and starving those who were suffering from fever, and it seems not unlikely that this treatment contributed to the mortality from infectious disease. In 1843 the Dublin physician, Dr. Robert Graves, famous for his description of thyrotoxicosis, began to question this conventional wisdom. During an epidemic of typhus fever, he abandoned bleeding and purging and gave his patients food and drink. A dramatic reduction in mortality followed. To colleagues who inquired about the secret of his success, he replied as follows: "You are not to permit your patient to encounter the terrible consequences, because he does not ask for nutriment. Gentlemen, these results are due to good feeding. When I am gone, you may be at a loss for an epitaph for me. I give it you in these words: He fed fevers."

Robert Graves had made the intellectual leap from trying to oppose fever to allowing it to take its course, giving the patients the substrate with which to meet its increased demands. The development of antipyretics such as Aspirin during the nineteenth century led to similar ways of thinking. It was easy to argue that, because recovery from illness was associated with a fall in fever, if one could reduce the fever by artificial means, the chances of recovery would be enhanced. If, as Dr. Kluger suggests, fever is a beneficial response, this form of treatment, which is still current today, is truly putting the cart before the horse.

The middle of the nineteenth century saw rapid developments in chemistry. Liebig described the methods for measuring urinary nitrogen excretion and showed that febrile illnesses were associated with an increased excretion of this element. In 1884, Müller described the use of antipyretics to reduce the nitrogen excretion associated with fever, linking together the inflammatory response to illness, fever, and the catabolic state, but again falling into the trap of treating the manifestations of disease rather than the underlying disease itself. The last 100 years has seen a gradual increase in our knowledge of the mechanism of inflammation and injury. Du Bois (2) described the metabolic consequences of fever. In the early 1930s, Cuthbertson (3) described the increased oxygen consumption and nitrogen excretion associated with injury. As techniques for the measurement of hormones developed between 1940 and 1970, the "jigsaw puzzle pieces" of the neuroendocrine response to injury fell into place. We have come a long way, therefore, in answering the question of how, although as the papers in this session show, we have a lot further to go. The answer to the question of why is still debated. The rational development of treatment in the future will depend on more detailed answers to these questions, and it is a tribute to the Organizers of this meeting that they have recognized this.

When considering the neuroendocrine and metabolic changes in sick patients, the predominant influence may be the severity of the injury or illness, but we must not forget other factors. Immobility of itself causes negative nitrogen balance (4), possibly by diminishing the mechanical stimulus to protein synthesis in muscle. It also increases insulin resistance. This is illustrated by the case of a young 70-kg insulin-dependent diabetic with an active job that involved carrying parcels up and down stairs at least 12 times a day. He was stable on an insulin dose of 40 units daily, but as soon as he was promoted and become desk-bound, using the elevator when he wished to go upstairs, his insulin requirements to maintain the same level of control rose to 144 units daily. He then, despite continuing the same job, made a conscious effort to use the stairs instead of the elevator at least four times a day and his insulin dosage was reduced to 90 units a day, again for the same level of control. This is not just an immediate insulin-like effect of exercise on glucose uptake in muscle, for the lowered insulin resistance induced by exercise may persist for 24 hours, inducing hypoglycaemia in the diabetic during rest 12 hours later. Starvation also causes negative nitrogen balance by a decrease in protein synthesis, but it may also create insulin resistance, possibly through the action of the Randle fatty-acid cycle. This is illustrated by the case of an insulin-dependent diabetic requiring total parenteral nutrition after a period of starvation. With a glucose infusion rate of 25 g/h, his initial insulin requirements to maintain normoglycaemia were 4 to 6 units per hour. This requirement fell gradually to 1.8 units an hour after 72 hours. Therefore, in devising strategies to counteract the wasting effects of illness, we need to consider early mobilization and adequate feeding, as well as means of manipulating the metabolic response to injury. Such strategies also need to take into account that the approach to the difference phases after injury will need to be designed (a) to allow survival during the shock phase when cardiorespiratory problems predominate, (b) to preserve body cell mass in the flow phase when aggressive proteolysis is occurring, and (c) to restore body tissues and their functions during the convalescent phase when the promotion of protein synthesis is the major challenge.

THE NEUROENDOCRINE AND METABOLIC RESPONSE TO INJURY

In his review of the work from his own department and that of others, Dr. Matthews discussed the evidence linking the neuroendocrine and metabolic changes after injury. After comparing the response to starvation and to injury (see previous section), he went on to consider the time relationship between changes in hormone levels and in metabolic events. He contrasted the immediate response in seconds to a change in catecholamine levels, the response in minutes to insulin and glucagon, in 6 to 12 hours to growth hormone and cortisol, and the even greater time to respond to a change in thyroid and sex hormones. He argued that the changes in thyroid and sex hormones may be of little importance in the immediate flow phase of injury, but I wonder whether this could be said of the more prolonged period of convalescence. Is the pattern of high reverse T3 and low T3 with low gonadal hormone levels associated with diminished protein synthesis in convalescence a necessary permissive effect or one that should be counteracted? Dr. Matthews also discussed the phenomenon that the metabolic response to a given level of hormone may wane with time. Although epinephrine increases resting energy expenditure in a dose-dependent manner, the effect of epinephrine on glucose production is transient, hyperglycemia being maintained by diminished glucose oxidation. The response to glucagon may also be transient. Many years ago, Francis Moore raised the question of why the increase in metabolic rate and the negative nitrogen balance after surgery continue for some time after the hormone levels have returned to normal. Dr. Matthews felt that this question could not be answered with certainty, although Dr. Wernerman referred to some of his own work showing that a few hours' exposure to increased levels of cortisol can result in several days of increased proteolysis, suggesting an initiating or inducing effect of neuroendocrine changes on metabolism.

Dr. Matthews went on to discuss the increase in catecholamines, glucagon and cortisol after injury and the decreased effectiveness of insulin favoring a rise in energy expenditure, in proteolysis and gluconeogenesis, and in lipolysis. He attributes insulin resistance largely to raised cortisol levels, which he also blames largely for protein catabolism, producing persuasive evidence for this view. This conclusion contrasts with old observations showing that, with hypophysectomy and adrenalectomy, a normal metabolic response to injury is seen on constant cortisone replacement (5). He discussed the triple hormone infusion studies of Bessey et al. (6), showing increased nitrogen losses blunted by previous administration of an hypocaloric diet, but concluded that the response is less than that seen in clinical situations. There must, therefore, be an additional mechanism to produce the extensive and prolonged response in injured subjects. Whether cytokines can explain the difference was debated, although disappointingly, no clear conclusion emerged. Michael Rennie quoted studies showing no effect of cytokines on proteolysis and suggested that there may be an interaction between cytokines and cortisol, enhancing the effect of the latter on proteolysis. Triple hormone infusions ignore the direct effect of the central nervous system; perhaps some of the hypothalamic mechanisms described by Dr. Abumrad (see next section) may also contribute to the metabolic response to injury. The benefit of the response was seen as a mobilization of fuel reserves to provide essential nutrients for white cells and the wound. Insulin resistance in muscle and liver may be a necessary mechanism to prevent consumption by these organs of the new glucose derived from protein. The short-term benefit of this response was emphasized because the capacity to endure the loss of total body protein is strictly limited (described previously). Our discussions came to the same conclusion as that of Robert Graves—that nutritional support can provide the substrates, although catabolism continues.

Dr. Little also discussed the relationship between hormonal and metabolic changes, but with particular emphasis on the role of insulin and the mechanisms of insulin resistance. He reviewed normal insulin physiology before discussing its central role in the response to sepsis and injury. Dr. Matthews cited studies showing that insulin inhibits protein catabolism from muscle with little effect on protein synthesis. The studies of Gelfand and Barrett (7), e.g., in which insulin was infused directly into the brachial artery, showed a 40% reduction in proteolysis but no change in protein synthesis. Whole-body studies, in which insulin causes a reduction in plasma amino acid levels, may show an actual reduction in protein synthesis, which is probably secondary to the reduction in amino acids. In contrast to Dr. Matthews, Dr. Little regarded the role of cortisol as being permissive and only one of many factors causing insulin resistance. He concluded, in essence, that it is a multifactorial phenomenon, the end result of a number of different mechanisms, including high levels of counter-regulatory hormones, high fatty acids, and other unidentified extra- and intracellular mechanisms. He described studies showing that the dose-response curve for glucose disposal at different insulin concentrations in injured patients is shifted to the right; the maximal response is also reduced, indicating resistance either at the insulin receptor on the cell or at a postreceptor defect in insulin responsiveness within the cell itself. This resistance is seen throughout the range of insulin concentration, arguing against the simple notion of a raised threshold.

Our own observations have shown that, in the acute phase of injury, there is a sympathetically mediated suppression of insulin release in response to glucose, and that this is followed by a period of insulin resistance in relation to both glucose and fat metabolism (8). We found, in response to glucose infusion, persistent glucose intolerance in the presence of higher than normal insulin levels, and also a diminished rate of reduction of fatty-acid levels in response to glucose infusion, indicating insulin resistance in relation to fat metabolism as well.

We then argued that, because the catabolic response to injury could not be reversed by feeding, perhaps protein catabolism could be blocked by insulin, while the substrates that would have been released from the patient's own cells could be provided by exogenous feeding of amino acids and an energy source (9). With a daily intravenous intake of 2,400 calories as glucose and 9.4 grams of nitrogen as amino acids, we compared the urinary urea excretion with glucose alone (to give serum insulin levels of approximately 80 mu/l) and to glucose and insulin (to give serum insulin levels of over 200 mu/l). In catabolic patients with an initially high urea excretion rate, there was up to 40% reduction in urea excretion at the higher levels of insulin, but in noncatabolic subjects, no effect was seen. When the same experiment was repeated, infusing 18.8 grams of nitrogen instead of 9.4 grams of nitrogen a day, the same phenomenon was seen, except that the relationship was shifted to the right, but not in parallel. In other words, the same percentage reduction in urea excretion was seen in the catabolic patients, but doubling the nitrogen intake produced no net increase in urea loss. In contrast, in the noncatabolic patients, the doubling of nitrogen intake was associated with a corresponding increase in urea excretion rate and no response to insulin. The catabolic patients, while retaining their response to insulin, appeared to be able to utilize the extra nitrogen, whereas patients with a lower protein turnover seemed unable to do so. Perhaps it is time to reconsider the possibility of a cocktail of anticatabolic and anabolic hormones, with a substrate combination of appropriate design, so that on the one hand the more destructive effects of the metabolic response to injury are blocked and on the other the substrate requirements are substituted by exogenous sources.

NEUROENDOCRINE MECHANISMS

The paper by Dr. Abumrad on the hypothalamus, glucopenia, and fuel mobilization was not, at first sight, directly relevant to the response to injury in which there is hyperglycemia. On the other hand, the response to injury is associated with alterations in the balance between anabolic and catabolic hormones controlled at hypothalamic level. Glucopenia provides a model allowing detailed analysis of these important hypothalamic mechanisms. Information gained from such studies may, therefore, have a very important bearing on understanding the modulation of fuel mobilization after injury. Dr. Abumrad described in some detail the anatomic and physiologic pathways within the hypothalamus, which, as well as controlling pituitary activity, is the central autonomic nucleus controlling the output of noradrenaline from the sympathetic nervous system and of adrenalin from the adrenal medulla. He concluded that peptides such as corticotropin-releasing factor, somatostatin, and thyrotropin-releasing factor influence autonomic as well as pituitary secretion. He also discussed the role of several other neuropeptides, including β-endorphin, which, while having no effect peripherally, can modify adrenal epinephrine secretion when given directly into the central nervous system. The proposal that endogenous opiates have an important role as mediators of the counterregulatory response to glucopenia is a novel and important idea and raises interesting possibilities for pharmacologic manipulation. He produced evidence showing that, in response to hypoglycaemia, the hypothalamus produces morphine and codeine as well as endorphins. These endogenous opiates have hyperglycemic effects through stimulation of glucose production and inhibition of glucose clearance, but exert their effects through the central nervous system rather than directly on peripheral tissues. The primary role of glucagon in the counterregulatory response to hypoglycaemia was described, and the secondary role of epinephrine acknowledged. We have carried out glucose infusion tests in normal and hypopituitary patients (10), showing that, despite failure of a rise in cortisol and growth hormone in the latter group, the rise in blood glucose when insulin infusion was stopped was identical in the two situations, except in long-standing insulin-dependent diabetics in whom glucagon and epinephrine responses are both blunted. Despite identical glucose curves, however, we found higher adrenaline and noradrenaline responses in the hypopituitary patients than in the normal subjects. The paper by Gerich et al. (11) was cited in support of the statement that "only in the absence of both glucagon and epinephrine does recovery from glucopenia fail to occur." Dr. Abumrad pointed out that, under conditions of prolonged hypoglycaemia, counterregulatory hormones cause only half the increase in glucose production, indicating other direct mechanisms of activation of glucose production. Following initial hepatic glycogenolysis, continuing glucopenia is opposed by an increase in gluconeogenesis from lactate and amino acids. Initial glycogenolysis is activated by the sympathetic nervous system acting on the liver, adrenals, and pancreas. The mobilization of fatty acids and glycerol may also have an important role because glycerol is a direct gluconeogenic precursor and fatty acids inhibit glucose utilization through the Randle cycle. He also contrasted the insulin-sensitive receptors in the hypothalamus that trigger lipolysis with those involved in glucose homeostasis, which are glucose rather than insulin sensitive.

The substantial body of information concerning the central control of glucose and fat metabolism is contrasted with the paucity of knowledge concerning the hypothalamic control of protein metabolism. As with the response to injury, hypoglycemia is not only associated with increased glycogenolysis, lipolysis, and gluconeogenesis, but also with enhanced protein breakdown. An exciting new observation is the finding that, in response to hypoglycemia, amino acids for gluconeogenesis are released from the gut not from muscle. This finding was discussed and two possible mechanism were considered. It seemed most likely that amino acids are derived from the digestion and absorption of cells shed from the tip of the mucosal villus, although the possibility of a labile pool of amino acids within the mucosa was suggested by Dr. Soeters. It is clear that, whatever the details of the mechanism, the amino acids are derived from the mucosal rather than the smooth-muscle layer of the gut wall. In elegant studies of peripheral hypoglycemia but central nervous euglycemia, they prove that these changes are centrally mediated, although the exact mechanisms involved are unclear. The applications of pure scientific research cannot always be foreseen, but these studies, particularly those relating to endogenous opiates, raise possibilities for manipulating metabolic responses by drugs that act through the central nervous system.

PROTEIN METABOLISM

An understanding of protein metabolism and its controlling mechanism is fundamental to the problem at issue in this session. Although diminished protein synthesis is a factor in moderate injury, excessive protein catabolism may dominate the picture in severe illness. Michael Rennie pointed out that our knowledge of the latter process is less detailed than that of the former, and that a better understanding of the factors that govern proteolysis is vital. He emphasized that most of the work has been done in animals and it is uncertain how much of this can be extrapolated to humans. He showed that the rates of turnover of proteins vary from tissue to tissue and between proteins within the same tissue. The methodology of study must, therefore, be appropriate to the proteins concerned. The efflux of methylhistidine, for example, is a reflection of muscle protein breakdown, whereas that of hydroxyproline is a reflection of collagen breakdown. He gave us a critical review of the methods of investigation of these processes and highlighted the correlation between breakdown and synthesis; e.g., the rapid rise in muscle protein synthesis shortly after weight lifting is associated with an increase in the rate of breakdown, although there may be net accretion of protein within the tissue. Similar effects are seen during normal growth and rehabilitation from malnutrition. In contrast, both synthesis and breakdown are reduced with long-term starvation. In discussing direct effects of other substrates, he argued that variations in the availability of glucose, lactate, β-hydroxybuterate, fatty acids, and other substrates have minor effects on protein turnover, although the suppression of proteolysis may require the presence of glucose. He highlighted the predominant role of insulin in suppressing proteolysis in skeletal muscle, although not in cardiac muscle, and the fact that, under appropriate conditions of amino acid supply, insulin may also stimulate protein synthesis. In contrast, growth hormone appears to have no effect on proteolysis, although it may promote protein synthesis. Glucocorticoids appear to have a particular effect on proteolysis of myofibrillar protein in skeletal muscle, an effect that is not antagonized by increased insulin secretion, which can only ameliorate nonfibrillar cytoplasmic proteolysis. Both anabolic steroids and thyroid hormones may have longer-term effects, possibly by setting the degree of sensitivity to other hormones.

Dr. Rennie then went on to discuss the effects of disease, reminding us that immobilization can cause muscle wasting, as can denervation. He contrasted the proteolytic response to severe injury with that due to surgical trauma alone, which appears to have a modest effect on protein breakdown, although protein synthesis may be reduced. He pointed out that the requisite measurements, using tracer incorporation, have not been made in order to allow us to understand the changes in protein turnover following severe injury. The contribution of cytokines to the changes in protein metabolism after simple injury is not clear. On the other hand, the changes in proteolysis with sepsis cannot be explained solely as a result of neuroendocrine changes, and other factors must be implicated. Cytokines are the obvious candidates, but when the direct effect of cytokines in muscle has been investigated, it has been difficult to find evidence of their involvement with the proteolysis of sepsis. He suggested the possibility that cytokines are involved, but in a complex interrelationship with other factors, e.g., hormones, which are present in vivo but not in vitro. He discussed, in particular, a possible interaction between cytokines, cortisol, and insulin resistance.

He crystallized the therapeutic problem of how to limit proteolysis while stimulating synthesis. In the depleted patient, or during convalescence from wasting illness, the devising of some means to stimulate protein synthesis may be more appropriate. Feeding alone, while important, takes an extremely long time to have its effect. In contrast, during the flow phase of severe injury, e.g., burns, there may even be an increase in protein synthesis that is outweighed by aggressive protein catabolism. Inhibition of protein catabolism may, therefore, be the goal of treatment. He considered that growth hormone is unlikely to be beneficial, and that IGF-I and corticosteroid receptor blockers hold promise. Other workers (12–20) have, however, shown that growth hormone improves nitrogen balance in surgical patients and that the addition of insulin to growth hormone in normal subjects causes a further increment in nitrogen gain. Curiously, Dr. Rennie did not mention insulin, whose effect has been demonstrated in this circumstance. He mentioned the possible role of cytokine blockers, but emphasized the importance of avoiding blockade of those mechanisms that may confer a net advantage in terms of survival, bringing us straight back to John Hunter! In Dr. Rennie's suggestions for future research, he highlighted the need for more studies on protein synthesis in severe disease and of the mechanism of proteolysis of different proteins within muscle tissue. Nonhormonal influences on protein breakdown, such as those of nitric oxide and of free radicals, need study, as do the effects of dietary manipulations.

FEVER

The final paper, by Dr. Kluger, brought us back to my introductory remarks, since it addressed the question of whether this and other responses to inflammation are assets or liabilities. It also acted as a bridge between this session on neuroendocrine changes and metabolism and the following session, which concerns cytokines. He showed that fever is not a wild and uncontrolled response to infection, but a change in thermoregulatory set-point with its own control mechanisms. The rise in certain cytokines increases fever, while simultaneously endogenous antipyretic factors are released, three of which are hormones, namely arginine vasopressin, alpha-melano-cyte stimulating hormone, and glucocorticoids. There may also be antipyretic cyto-kines. This provides yet another example of the close interrelationship between cyto-kines and hormones in the responses to acute illness. One cannot help seeing similarities between a reset of stimulating and inhibitory factors to achieve a new temperature set-point and those that reset metabolic balances after injury, e.g., the glucostat. Dr. Kluger then described persuasive evidence that, far from being harm-ful, fever is a closely regulated process that, in a wide range of studies in animals and humans, has been found to enhance survival. In his final paragraph, however, he brought us back again to the idea of John Hunter—that, although fever evolves as a beneficial host-defense response to most infections, it may occasionally be so severe as to be counterproductive.

SUMMARY

Papers presented during this session gave a thoughtful review of what is known about the neuroendocrine and metabolic responses to acute illness and highlighted the important gaps in our knowledge, which stand between us and better therapeutic strategies. It seems unlikely that any simplistic answer will emerge or that we shall discover some holy grail of metabolism that will lead us to a single therapeutic pana-cea. Although the neuroendocrine response to injury has a central role in mediating and permitting the response to injury, it is by no means the sole mechanism, and the interaction between hormone and cytokine responses may be another factor. Therapeutic strategies will need to have as their goal the preservation of essential protein structures. A deeper understanding of how these are broken down and synthesized under different conditions is essential to this objective. It is clear that there are differences between tissues and within a given tissue, which will necessitate a tailored and multicomponent approach. One could speculate, e.g., that whereas insulin may be used to inhibit muscle proteolysis, it might be combined with growth hormone to promote synthesis. A number of recent publications (12–20) provide some support for this notion. The provision of special substrates, such as glutamine, may have beneficial effects both on the gut and on muscle. Protein synthesis during convalescence may be stimulated by an appropriate combination of growth factors and substrates. The idea of manipulating metabolism through drugs that affect the central nervous system also opens a whole new field of therapeutic possibilities. Treatment not only must be selective, as between one tissue or another and between one circumstance and another, but also must be able to choose between responses that are an asset and those that are a liability.

CONCLUSIONS

The accelerated protein catabolism and gluconeogenesis of injury is, up to a point, an advantageous response to meet the metabolic demands of tissues such as the wound, white cells, the gut, and the brain. The paradox remains that, when the loss of total body protein exceeds 20%, function deteriorates rapidly and recovery is threatened. The therapeutic challenge is to oppose those aspects of the response that are a liability and avoid blocking those that may be necessary for survival. The neuroendocrine response plays a major role in mediating the metabolic changes, but cannot explain them all, and other factors such as cytokines may be involved. Because the normal action of insulin is to inhibit proteolysis, insulin resistance may be a major factor that allows proteolysis and gluconeogenesis to continue, and at the same time prevents the resultant glucose being consumed by liver and muscle, glucose; other important substrates can then be diverted to the wound, white cells, the gut, and the brain. The precise mechanism of insulin resistance is ill understood, although cortisol and other counterregulatory hormones may play an important role, as well as intracellular metabolic events such as the fatty-acid cycle. Other extracellular and intracellular influences must also be involved. It should be remembered that immobility and starvation both confer insulin resistance as well as enhance negative nitrogen balance.

The hypothalamus holds the key to the control of counterregulatory hormones through the pituitary and autonomic nervous system. The neurotransmitter control of these processes is complex, but new information is emerging that raises important therapeutic possibilities. In particular, the observations that endorphine and other endogenous opiates act on metabolism through the central nervous system constitute a new and important area of research. The finding that the gut is the main source of amino acids for gluconeogenesis in response to glucopenia is a novel and potentially important discovery.

The negative nitrogen balance of patients is a net result of changes in both protein synthesis and protein catabolism, which may vary in different degree between patients as well as during the time course of an illness in individual patients. Breakdown and synthesis rates are usually correlated, although one may outstrip the other during catabolic or anabolic states. Starvation, immobility, and uncomplicated trauma may give rise to diminished prote.. synthesis during the flow phase of injury. With major injury and sepsis, however, proteolysis predominates. During the convalescent phase of illness, the very slowness of protein synthesis limits the rate of restoration of lean body mass, even with optimal feeding. Since preservation of the protein mass must remain a major goal of patient management, a deeper understanding of these processes is necessary. In such research, the methodology is crucial and the role of basic science is fundamental to any future therapeutic advance. I, as a clinician, and our host, as a pharmaceutical company, naturally have a bias toward the therapeutic consequences of our discussions. It is clear that no single strategy will suffice and that treatment will have to be tailored to the individual patient and based on a very clear understanding of the hormonal, metabolic, and inflammatory processes that are taking place, which may change with time in the same patient. At the same time, we must not forget practical considerations, such as vigorous treatment of the underlying disorder to minimize the stimulus to the neuroendocrine response and also optimal feeding and early mobilization to promote protein synthesis. At all times, we should be wary of blocking any of the inflammatory responses in a blind hope of doing good. Better understanding should allow us to exploit that which is an asset while preventing those extremes of the response that are a liability.

REFERENCES

1. Hill GL. *Disorders of Nutrition and Metabolism in Clinical Surgery.* Edinburgh: Churchill Livingstone, 1992.
2. Du Bois EF. *Basal Metabolism in Health and Disease.* Philadelphia: Lea & Febiger, 1924.
3. Cuthbertson DP. Effect of injury on metabolism. *Biochem J* 1930;2:1244.
4. Schønheyder F, Heilskov NSC, Oleson K. Isotope studies on the mechanism of negative nitrogen balance produced by immobilization. *Scand J Clin Lab Invest* 1954;6:178–188.
5. Mason AS. Metabolic response to total adrenalectomy and hypophysectomy. *Lancet* 1955;2:632.
6. Bessey PQ, Watters JM, Aoki TT, Wilmore DW. Combined hormonal infusion simulates the metabolic response to injury. *Ann Surg* 1984;200:264–281.
7. Gelfand RA, Barrett EJ. Effect of physiologic hyperinsulinaemia on skeletal muscle protein synthesis and breakdown in man. *J Clin Invest* 1987;80:1–6.
8. Allison SP, Hinton P, Chamberlain MJ. Intravenous glucose tolerance, insulin and free fatty acid levels in burned patients. *Lancet* 1968;2:113.
9. Woolfson AMJ, Heatley RV, Allison SP. Insulin to reduce protein catabolism after injury. *N Engl J Med* 1979;300:14–17.
10. Newman GH, Macdonald IA, Allison SP. Testing the anterior pituitary hypoglycaemia produced by continuous intravenous insulin infusion. *Br Med J* 1983;287:571–574.
11. Gerich J, Davis J, Lorenzi M, et al. Hormonal mechanisms of recovery from insulin induced hypoglycaemia in man. *J Physiol* 1979;236:E380–E385.
12. Haymond HW, Horber FF, Manras N. Human growth hormone but not insulin-like growth factor I positively affects whole-body estimates of protein metabolism. *Horm Res* 1992;38(Suppl 1):73–75.
13. Haymond MW, Horber FF. The effects of human growth hormone and prednisolone on whole body estimates of protein metabolism. *Horm Res* 1992;38(Suppl 2):44–46.

14. Zeisel HJ, Willgerodt H, Richter I, et al. Stimulation of nitrogen and whole-body protein metabolism in growth hormone–deficient children by recombinant human growth hormone; relationship to growth. *Horm Res* 1992;37(Suppl 2):14–21.

15. Voerman HJ, van Schijndel RJ, Groeneveld AB, et al. Effects of recombinant human growth hormone in patients with severe sepsis. *Ann Surg* 1992;216:648–655.

16. Vara-Thorbeck R, Guerrero JA, Ruiz-Requena ME, et al. Effects of growth hormone in patients receiving total parenteral nutrition following major gastrointestinal surgery. *Hepatogastroenterology* 1992;39:270–272.

17. Hammarqvist F, Stromberg C, von der Deaken A, et al. Biosynthetic human growth hormone preserves both muscle protein synthesis and the decrease in muscle-free glutamine, and improves whole-body nitrogen economy after operation. *Ann Surg* 1992;216:184–191.

18. Wolf RF, Heslin MJ, Newman E, et al. Growth hormone and insulin combine to improve whole-body and skeletal muscle protein kinetics. *Surgery* 1992;112:284–291.

19. Fryburg DA, Louard RJ, Gerow KE, et al. Growth hormone stimulates skeletal muscle protein synthesis and antagonizes insulin's antiproteolytic action in humans. *Diabetes* 1992;41:424–429.

20. Bennett WM, Haymond MW. Growth hormone and lean tissue catabolism during long-term glucocorticoid treatment. *Clin Endocrinol* 1992;36:161–164.

Organ Metabolism and Nutrition:
Ideas for Future Critical Care, edited by
J. M. Kinney and H. N. Tucker.
Raven Press, Ltd., New York © 1994.

6

Interactions Among Proinflammatory Cytokines and the Classic Macro-Endocrine System in Sepsis and Inflammation

Lyle L. Moldawer and Stephen F. Lowry

Department of Surgery, University of Florida College of Medicine, Gainesville, Florida 32610; and Laboratory of Surgical Metabolism, New York Hospital, Cornell Medical Center, New York, New York 10021

It is now recognized that several of the metabolic responses to acute injury, infection, and inflammation result from the endogenous production of several proinflammatory cytokines, including interleukin-1 (IL-1), interleukin-6 (IL-6), and tumor necrosis factor-α (TNFα). These proteinaceous mediators are produced by inflammatory cells and represent a newly described cytokine network by which inflammatory cells communicate with somatic tissues the presence of inflammation. Unlike the classical macrohormone system, the cytokine network differs from classical macrohormones in several important regards. Firstly, cytokines principally act in a paracrine and autocrine nature, and the cells that produce these mediators are widely distributed throughout tissues and organ systems of the body. Secondly, several of these proinflammatory cytokines, including IL-1 and TNFα, show structural polymorphism with both cell-associated and secreted forms. Finally, there is considerable redundancy and overlap in biological activities among different classes of proinflammatory cytokines. Despite these fundamental differences between the cytokine network and the classic macrohormonal system, the two systems are tightly interrelated. The interactions among the proinflammatory cytokines and the glucocorticoid system has been most well-described. Not only do the cytokines IL-1 and TNFα induce the production of glucocorticoids involved in the stress response, but cytokines interact with glucocorticoids to regulate somatic tissue responses. This latter point has been best characterized in the liver where the proinflammatory cytokines IL-1, TNFα, and IL-6, in conjunction with cytokine-mediated production of cortisol, potentiate the uptake of amino acids, increase gluconeogenesis, and redirect hepatic protein synthesis to the production of acute phase reactants. However, increased production of cortisol serves to down-regulate the production of TNFα and IL-1, without affecting the induction of inhibitors of IL-1 and TNFα, IL-1 receptor antagonist (IL-1ra), and sTNFR, respectively. Whereas induction of proinflammatory cytokines is perhaps the initial event in the host response to infection and injury, their sustained production and actions on end tissues are modulated in part through the macroendocrine network.

The importance of proinflammatory cytokines in mediating the host responses to injury and infections is no longer a matter of general dispute. It is now recognized that many of both the beneficial and detrimental aspects of the host response to injury are modulated by the proinflammatory cytokines. For example, several independent research groups have demonstrated that passive immunization of animals with anti-TNFα antibodies (1,2), anti-TNF immunoadhesions (3,4), or IL-1 receptor antagonist (5–7) confers survival to otherwise lethal endotoxemia or bacteremia. In fact, several therapies aimed at blocking an endogenous TNFα and IL-1 response are currently in clinical trials for the treatment of patients with sepsis syndrome. Similarly, a consensus is developing that the continued production of the proinflammatory cytokines, TNFα, IL-1, IL-6, and interferon-γ, among others, contributes to the anorexia, lean tissue wasting, and hepatic acute phase protein responses seen in patients with ongoing inflammatory disease (8–10).

Despite an overwhelming amount of data to suggest that the inappropriate or exaggerated release of proinflammatory cytokines is pathogenic, there is convincing evidence that these cytokines also regulate beneficial host responses during nonlethal infections or injury (for review, see refs. 11,12). For example, the absence of endogenously produced TNFα or IL-1 is associated with inappropriate antimicrobial responses and increased mortality due to peritonitis (13), *Leishmaniasis, Listeriosis,* and cerebral malaria (14–16). This has led to the general conclusion that the actions of TNFα and IL-1 are two-sided and that pathologic reactions are associated with either deficient or excessive production.

It has only been recently recognized that the integrated cytokine response to infection and injury is complex, and that, ultimately, tissue responses depend not only on the absolute concentrations of IL-1 and TNFα, but also on the presence of cytokine inhibitors, antiinflammatory cytokines, and the number of cellular receptors. Furthermore, as this review documents, the actions of cytokines on end tissues are regulated, at least in part, through the release of several endocrine mediators, including ACTH, cortisol, insulin, glucagon, and growth hormone. Increased production of corticosteroids in response to proinflammatory cytokines also serves to down-regulate proinflammatory cytokine production.

A mild endotoxemia in either human volunteers or experimental animals results in the early synthesis and release of at least two proinflammatory cytokines (IL-1 and TNF) whose concentrations at the local site of tissue production are often greater than those in the plasma (17,18). This early release of proinflammatory cytokines into the local tissue milieu acts to initiate and orchestrate many of the beneficial responses aimed at improving antimicrobial function and reducing tissue damage. For example, local production of TNFα and IL-1 in the liver serves to induce hepatocyte and Kupffer cell IL-6 production (19,20), which, in combination with IL-1 and TNFα, reprioritizes hepatic metabolism to increase acute-phase protein synthesis and gluconeogenesis (21–23). At the site of tissue injury, local production of these proinflammatory cytokines provokes the release of additional mediators that serve to recruit and activate inflammatory cells via up-regulation of leukocyte and endothelial cell adhesion molecules (24). This also stimulates fibroblast proliferation (25) and increases local antimicrobial properties (26). In the spleen, locally produced IL-1 can serve as a comitogen (27) and an immune adjuvant, increase IL-2 receptor affinity and number (28), and increase macrophage bactericidal function (29). In the bone marrow, both IL-1 and TNFα can stimulate the synthesis of other hematopoietic regulators (30,31), promote the release of granulocytes (31) and redirect hematopoietic development along myeloid rather than erythroid pathways (32,33). All of these early responses mediated by TNFα and IL-1 can be considered advantageous to the recovering host.

However, this initial release of proinflammatory cytokines is ultimately short lived. For example, following mild endotoxemia in human volunteers, plasma TNFα, IL-1β and IL-6 concentrations peak within 4 hours, and disappear within 8 (34–37). IL-1 activity is mitigated by the synthesis and release of IL-1ra, which interferes with IL-1 binding to its cellular receptors (11). Similarly, TNFα activity is modulated by the subsequent shedding of the extracellular portion of its two cellular receptors, which form complexes with TNF and prevent its binding to the cellular TNF receptors (35,36). Following a mild endotoxemia, sTNFR I and II concentrations peak 1 to 2 hours after TNFα and remain elevated for longer periods (37,38). The loss of cellular TNFα receptors from target tissues serves two purposes: the transient desensitization of cells to repeated exposure of TNFα (39) and the formation of receptor-ligand complexes that attenuate peak free TNFα concentrations and may act as a reservoir to deliver low levels of cytokine over extended periods (40).

A second mechanism by which the host regulates proinflammatory cytokine production and activity is the subsequent release of mediators that suppress IL-1 and TNFα production and increase IL-1ra release. For example, increased production of prostanoids and the counterregulatory endocrine response, e.g., cortisol, CRF, and α-melanocyte stimulating hormone (αMSH), all down-regulate IL-1 and TNFα production and activity (11,41–43).

The net response to an acute nonlethal inflammatory stimulus, when viewed in this integrated manner, is an initial release of proinflammatory cytokines (TNFα, IL-1, IL-6, IL-8) that are meant to initiate and integrate the early inflammatory response. This is followed by the release of cytokine inhibitors (IL-1ra and sTNFR) and antiinflammatory mediators (glucocorticoids, prostanoids, αMSH, IL-4, and IL-10) that restrict the magnitude and duration of the inflammatory response.

We believe that catastrophic host responses to overwhelming bacterial infections, and propagation of the systemic inflammatory response syndrome with multisystem organ dysfunction in ongoing inflammatory processes represent *dysregulation* of this normal homeostatic process. For example, in acute septic shock due to gram-negative bacteremia or endotoxemia the magnitude of proinflammatory cytokine response (TNFα and IL-1) is excessive. The quantities of TNFα and IL-1 produced are greater than can be mitigated by the release of IL-1ra- and TNF-soluble receptors. Furthermore, the timing of the release of these cytokine inhibitors is sufficiently delayed in septic shock such that excess proinflammatory cytokines are produced in the reticuloendothelial system. They are also produced in the blood by circulating monocytes and vascular endothelial cells where their effects on endothelial cells lead to hemodynamic collapse (44).

Similarly, in ongoing inflammatory processes, such as those that occur in hospitalized patients with systemic inflammatory response syndrome (SIRS) or sepsis syndrome, the mechanisms that ultimately down-regulate proinflammatory cytokine release are ineffective. This is due in part to the continued external stimuli that ongoing infectious or inflammatory processes invoke. In such cases, repeated or persistent proinflammatory cytokine synthesis (TNFα, IL-1) contributes to the hemodynamic instability, coagulopathy, and multiorgan dysfunction that occurs. In both septic shock and SIRS, the beneficial aspects of proinflammatory cytokine production (including stimulation of nonspecific host immunity, increased antigen specific T-cell proliferation, macrophage and NK-cell bactericidal capacity) are offset by the adverse consequences of continued exposure to elevated TNFα and IL-1 concentrations.

CYTOKINE NETWORK

Over the past 5 years, we have developed a greater appreciation for the complexity and subtlety of the cytokine network. Earlier efforts (discussed next) attempted to equate the structure of the cytokine network in terms of the classic macroendocrine system. We now recognize that the regulation of cytokine biosynthesis differs in several regards from the macroendocrine system. Unlike the macroendocrine system, wherein hormone production is generally limited to a single tissue, individual cytokine production is scattered throughout organs and tissue systems. Tissues capable of producing IL-1, TNFα, and IL-6 include blood monocytes, tissue macrophages, endothelial cells, fibroblasts, dendritic cells, and even some cells of lymphoid lineage. Tissue macrophages and dendritic cells, for example, are widely distributed throughout organs and tissues and represent one mechanism by which local inflammatory cells communicate with adjacent tissues. Because of their direct proximity, cytokines act primarily in a paracrine or autocrine fashion, unlike the macroendocrine system.

An understanding of the importance of cytokine's paracrine actions has been late in coming and was delayed by early investigations on rodents and primates expiring from lethal endotoxemia and gram-negative septic shock. Following administration of either endotoxin or live gram-negative bacteria, there is a rapid appearance of TNFα, IL-1β, and IL-6 in the circulation, and the appearance of these cytokines precedes temporally the catastrophic host responses (Fig. 1). Since blocking the actions of either TNFα or IL-1β will prevent the pathologic consequences of lethal endotoxemia and gram-negative septic shock, several groups concluded that the systemic release of TNFα and IL-1β was a principal component of the pathology of

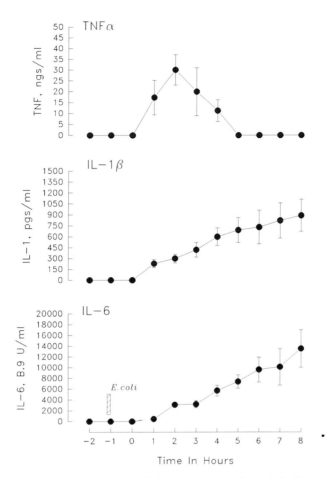

FIG. 1. Proinflammatory cytokine responses in baboons expiring from a lethal bacteremia. Following exposure to live bacteria, there is an initial appearance of TNFα, followed by a sustained production of the proinflammatory cytokines IL-1β and IL-6.

septic shock. However, efforts to document a systemic TNFα response in patients with critical illness have been less than successful. As recently as 1990, there was a general consensus that exaggerated TNFα production and appearance in the peripheral circulation was antecedent to shock and tissue injury. This was based to a large extent on earlier animal studies (45,46) that demonstrated that TNFα administration could produce tissue damage and cause mortality comparable to that seen following lethal endotoxemia or bacteremia. Based on these experimental studies and the then-recent observations of Waage and colleagues in meningococcal sepsis (47), many concluded that these cytokines acted in a classical endocrine fashion and that these circulating TNFα levels could provide predictive estimates of the degree of inflammation. Although Waage et al. reported an overall prevalence of detecting TNFα in

23% of patients with meningococcal infections, 91% of the patients who expired had detectable TNFα levels, and in subsequent studies, 100% of patients with meningococcal shock had detectable TNFα (48,49).

We investigated the appearance of plasma TNFα in 43 critically ill patients with thermal injuries (50), and in 12 postsurgical critically ill patients (51). In both cases, samples were obtained as promptly as possible after admission to the burn unit or surgical intensive care unit (SICU), respectively, and were then sampled at 3- to 4-day intervals thereafter. In patients with thermal injuries, overall frequency of detecting TNFα was only 46% (n = 250), despite the fact that the average burn size was 33%. In addition, only 49% of the patients who were septic secondary to the burn injury, and only 33% of the patients who expired from their burn wounds, had detectable TNFα. In critically ill SICU patients, the numbers were even less impressive for detecting TNFα. In a group of 12 critically ill patients with an overall mortality of 33%, TNFα could be detected in only 36% of the samples from these patients, and there was no correlation between the frequency of detecting TNFα and outcome.

These frequencies are in general agreement with the published literature of patients with sepsis syndrome (52–57), where the occurrence of detecting TNFα in the circulation has varied from 16% in the deGroot study (52) to 86% in the work of Munoz et al. (57). We now recognize that the invariable detection of TNFα in the circulation of critically ill patients is not consistent with its known biology. Rather, the data obtained from our laboratory, as well as others, confirm a principal paracrine role for TNFα in most inflammatory models, with cell-associated forms of TNFα contributing significantly to local bioactivity.

There has also been considerable controversy regarding the ability to detect IL-1 in the circulation of patients or experimental animals with inflammation. Not only are there two immunologically distinct forms of IL-1 (α and β), but each protein is first synthesized as a high molecular weight, cell–associated form, one having biological activity (preIL-1α) and the other being inactive (preIL-1β). Utilizing sensitive immunoassays, detection of IL-1β from human volunteers following endotoxin administration has generally been infrequent. Our own studies have failed to detect either IL-1α or IL-1β in plasma from human volunteers receiving endotoxin (58), an observation confirmed by others (37). Only Cannon et al. have been able to detect IL-1β reproducibly in the plasma of volunteers after an endotoxin challenge, although these authors have used an RIA based on rabbit polyclonal antisera and prior chloroform extraction of the samples (36).

We have also been unable to detect IL-1β routinely in the circulation of critically ill patients with sepsis syndrome (59). In 50 samples from 12 critically ill patients (with an overall mortality 33%), IL-1α was not detected in any samples, and IL-1β was detected in only three samples (6% frequency). Others, however, have detected IL-1β with higher frequency than we have, although the overall frequency of detection is generally less than that for TNFα (52,55,60). For example, Girardin et al. found detectable levels of IL-1β in plasma from 21% of children with gram-negative sepsis and *Purpura fulminans* (60). Of six published articles of circulating IL-1β in septic patients (36,48,55,56,60), there was a positive correlation between IL-1 detection and mortality in three. In the other three, there was either no correlation (two studies) or an inverse one (one study). For example Waage et al. described the detection of IL-1 bioactivity only in those patients with a rapid fatal outcome (48), whereas Cannon et al. reported the detection of low levels of IL-1β (<200 pg/ml) in the plasma of patients with septic shock, with higher levels occurring in surviving patients (36).

An inability to detect IL-1β (or IL-1α) in the circulation of *Papio* after experimental inflammation is consistent with the inability to detect IL-1β in critically ill patients (59). Only in animals expiring from lethal gram-negative septic shock has IL-1β (but not IL-1α) been detected with regularity (51,59,61). We have been unable to detect IL-1β or IL-1α in animals following sublethal endotoxemia (62), IL-1α administration (62), IL-8 administration (61), or sublethal TNFα administration (unpublished observation).

Despite an inability to detect TNFα and IL-1 routinely in the circulation of critically ill patients, considerable evidence has accumulated that tissue cytokine production is increased in a variety of rodent inflammatory models. Our first suggestion that TNFα synthesis and bioactivity may be principally limited to the tissue microenvironment came from observations of TNFα appearance in rodents expiring from a lethal burn coupled with *Pseudomonas* infection. In the animals that become bacteremic within 4 days, and reproducibly expire from multisystem organ failure between days 9 and 11, TNFα could only be detected in 18% of the plasma samples, despite the fact that blood was sampled daily until the animals expired (63). However, TNFα gene transcription in the liver and spleen was clearly up-regulated, as confirmed by Northern analysis. In later studies with the same model, we were able to detect immune and bioactive TNFα in the livers, in the absence of circulating protein (64). The cell-associated TNFα from the livers of burned and infected rats could be detected at both 4 and 7 days following the burn infection, suggesting that local production was continuous in this model.

Since these original findings, we have attempted to characterize the local tissue production of TNFα, IL-1, and IL-6 in other models of inflammation. Rather than rely on Northern analyses for detecting the presence of cytokine mRNA, we have used the reverse-transcriptase-PCR method. Using this technique to detect TNFα mRNA, as well as the WEHI clone 13 bioassay to quantitate TNFα bioactivity, we assessed tissue and plasma TNFα appearance in mice with a variety of infections or inflammation. In mice suffering hemorrhagic pneumonia (65) and mice infected with *Listeria* (66), as well as in mice with a cecal ligation and puncture (CLP) or a thermal injury, we were able to confirm that local production of TNFα and IL-1 occurs in the infected organs (lungs of adenovirus-induced hemorrhagic pneumonia; liver and spleen of *Listeria* infected mice), while plasma TNFα and IL-1 bioactivity could not be detected. In the hemorrhagic pneumonia and the *Listeria* models, appearance of organ TNFα bioactivity correlated temporally with evidence of tissue damage (66).

In addition, the recent description of specific inhibitors of TNFα and IL-1 bioactivity that circulate in the blood of healthy humans, which are elevated in infected patients, may be one means by which the host prevents the systemic appearance of excessive locally produced TNFα. These latter two phenomena, coupled with the tight regulatory control of TNFα biosynthesis, makes it unlikely that free TNFα appearance in the circulation is a common phenomenon after most forms of surgical injury and bacterial infection.

Studies on the local production of cytokines revealed a structural polymorphism that appears to be a common finding in the cytokine cascade, but relatively uncommon with hormones. Initial studies by Krieger and colleagues reported that TNFα existed as both a cell-associated, higher molecular weight form and a secreted low molecular weight form (67). More importantly, these investigators noted that the cell-associated form of TNFα was bioactive, implying that TNFα actions could be mediated by cell-to-cell contact in the tissue microenvironment. We subsequently confirmed the presence of cell-associated TNFα in the livers of burned and infected rats of approximately 26 to 29 kd (64). The cell-associated TNFα from the livers of burned and infected rats could be detected at both 4 and 7 days following the burn infection, suggesting that local production was continuous in this model. Jue et al. have further clarified that this high molecular weight TNFα is an intermediate in the biosynthesis of the mature 17-kd secreted form (68).

Structural polymorphism of both IL-1α and IL-1β has been known for several years. Recent studies have shown that the precursor IL-1α molecule is a 33-kd protein that, like cell-associated TNFα, is membrane-bound and functional. In fact, very little secreted IL-1α is at all detectable (11). In contrast to IL-1α, the high molecular weight form of IL-1β is neither cell-associated nor functional. Rather, preIL-1β accumulates in intracellular pools and is converted into the active form by a specific cellular protease. This accumulation of inactive cellular protein and subsequent enzymatic degradation to an active form has led Dinarello to speculate that IL-1β may play an important role in the wound and tissue microenvironments where inflammatory cell lysis is likely to occur (11). Unlike IL-1α, IL-1β appears to be more freely released into the tissue microenvironment and can be detected occasionally in the systemic circulation. Thus, IL-1α appears to be principally involved in IL-1–mediated functions that require cell-to-cell contact and functioning macrophage or dendritic cell, such as during antigen presentation, whereas IL-1β appears to be released and activated during conditions of tissue injury and cellular death.

The third hallmark of the cytokine cascade is the redundancy of cytokine actions. The actions of IL-1, TNF, and to a lesser extent IL-6 overlap and exhibit considerable synergy. This is most evident when examining TNF and IL-1 actions in producing hypotension and shock, and the capacity of IL-1, TNF and IL-6 to induce an hepatic acute-phase response. That IL-1 potentiates the toxicity of TNFα and vice versa is thought to be through the synergistic actions of these two cytokines on the production of prostanoids, as well as on the expression of endothelial adhesion molecules. Waage and Espevik have demonstrated that doses of IL-1 and TNFα in themselves are not lethal, and are uniformly so when administered together (69). Similarly, several groups have shown that each of these three proinflammatory cytokines regulate different aspects of the hepatic acute-phase protein response and that full expression of hepatic acute phase protein regulation is dependent on the production of at least two and likely all three cytokine mediators (70–72).

INTERACTIONS AMONG CYTOKINES AND THE MACROENDOCRINE SYSTEM

There is now accumulating evidence that many of the actions of these proinflammatory cytokines are modulated in part by the subsequent release of several hormones, and that the release of these macroendocrine mediators in turn regulates the continued production of cytokines. This feedback regulation has been primarily demonstrated for the proinflammatory cytokine IL-1 and the glucocorticoid response. In addition, the ultimate response by end tissues is dependent on the status of both cytokines and glucocorticoids.

Although IL-1 and TNFα are known to regulate the release of a variety of hormones, including insulin, glucagon, growth hormone, catecholamines, the mineral corticoids, αMSH, and sex hormones, this review concentrates on the interactions between proinflammatory cytokines and the release of glucocorticoids. This interaction can serve as a paradigm for the interrelationships between proinflammatory cytokines and the macroendocrine system because cytokine and glucocorticoid production and actions on end tissues are tightly interrelated.

Initial evidence for an interaction between proinflammatory cytokines and the glucocorticoid responses came from studies in which recombinant cytokine had been employed. Such studies demonstrated that coincubation of pituitary and hypothalamic cells in culture with recombinant human TNFα or IL-1 resulted in marked increases in CRF and ACTH release (73–75). These studies were confirmed in vivo when we demonstrated that administration of recombinant human IL-1α to healthy baboons produced an acute ACTH response (62). In those studies, administration of IL-1α at doses as low as 10 μg/kg BW resulted in a tenfold increase in ACTH concentrations (Table 1). It is interesting that this dose of IL-1α produced a markedly higher ACTH response than was seen in baboons given sublethal quantities of endotoxin, despite the fact that these animals responded with comparable hemodynamic and metabolic changes. We have also observed that administration of similar quan-

TABLE 1. *ACTH concentrations (pg/ml) in baboons treated with endotoxin or recombinant cytokines.*

Time (h)	Placebo	IL-1α (10 μg/kg)	TNFα (100 μg/kg)	LPS 500 μg/kg
0	135 ± 24	174 ± 43	156 ± 25	149 ± 30
1	155 ± 9	652 ± 100*	287 ± 101	160 ± 40
2	140 ± 14	1096 ± 311*	951 ± 67*	299 ± 33*
4	129 ± 17	>1200*	1076 ± 235*	251 ± 52
8	133 ± 25	154 ± 35	312 ± 75	189 ± 35

* p <0.05 versus time zero.

tities of human TNFα to the healthy baboon also results in a marked increase in ACTH responses, of similar magnitude to that seen with IL-1. Although TNFα infusions have been proposed to act in part through the endogenous production of IL-1, we were unable to demonstrate any endogenous IL-1 response in these animals (62), despite a comparable ACTH response. Such findings are consistent with the in vitro studies that suggest that both IL-1 and TNFα can induce ACTH production directly.

An observation by Roh and colleagues (76) suggests that IL-1 and TNFα induce a glucocorticoid response not only through the pituitary-hypothalamic axis, but by direct stimulation of the adrenal cortex. These investigators demonstrated that perfusion of the adrenal gland with recombinant IL-1α resulted in a direct and sustained glucocorticoid production. Thus the authors concluded that IL-1α's ability to induce a glucocorticoid response during inflammation is mediated through ACTH as well as direct adrenal stimulation.

Evidence that IL-1 can act directly on the adrenal is also supported by the rather common finding that very low dose IL-1 and TNFα administration results in multifocal adrenal cortical hemorrhage, vacuolization of adrenal cortical cells, and neutrophilic infiltration (62). The nature of these pathologic changes, however, has not been explained fully.

Van der Poll et al. confirmed these findings with TNFα administration in healthy, human volunteers (77). These investigators demonstrated that following administration of TNFα, volunteers exhibited a reproducible increase in ACTH and cortisol concentrations.

While the experimental administration of IL-1 induces several aspects of the inflammatory response, including glucocorticoid production, the contribution that individual cytokines such as IL-1 or TNFα makes to the human responses to injury or infection remains unclear. To evaluate the role that endogenously produced cytokines play in the induction of the glucocorticoid response, we have employed natural inhibitors of these individual cytokines. This approach has recently become a popular technique to isolate those endogenous responses to inflammation that are dependent on the production of individual cytokines.

Although earlier studies demonstrated that IL-1 and TNFα had the capacity to induce a glucocorticoid response, through both a direct adrenal and indirect pituitary-hypothalamic mechanism, initial rodent studies demonstrate that neither endogenously produced IL-1 nor TNFα was responsible for the corticosterone response in a mild inflammatory stress (78). In these studies, mice were passively immunized with either a monoclonal antibody against the IL-1 type I receptor or a polyclonal anti-TNFα antisera prior to the induction of a sterile turpentine abscess. This model of acute myositis produces a prompt and transient corticosteronemia as well as anorexia, cachexia, and an hepatic acute-phase protein response (Fig. 2). In preliminary studies, passive immunization against the IL-1 type I receptor and TNFα blocked the corticosterone responses to recombinant IL-1α and TNFα, respectively. However, neither IL-1 type I receptor nor TNFα blockade had any effect on the corticosteronemia seen in this mild model of inflammation. The failure to alter the corticos-

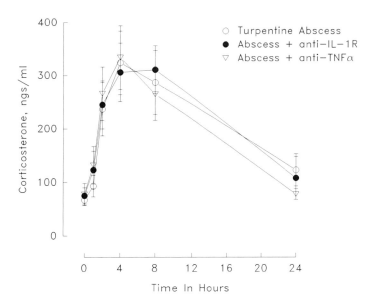

FIG. 2. Plasma corticosteronemia in mice following a sterile turpentine abscess. After induction of a turpentine abscess, plasma corticosterone concentrations increased and fell subsequently. Passive immunization with antibodies against the type I IL-1 receptor or against TNFα had no effect on this response. (From unpublished data and ref. 78).

terone response by IL-1 receptor or TNFα blockade could not be due to a failure to block endogenously produced cytokine because these therapies were effective in blocking other components of the inflammatory response. For example, IL-1 type I receptor blockade markedly attenuated the hepatic acute-phase response and the anorexia, but had no effect on either the corticosteronemia and hypoalbuminemia that developed. Thus, it is likely that in this model of mild inflammation, an endogenous corticosterone response is not dependent on the release of either IL-1 or TNFα alone.

Similar results have been obtained from human volunteers administered a mild endotoxemia. In these studies, Van Zee et al. infused recombinant human IL-1ra into healthy human volunteers during a mild endotoxemia and evaluated the macro-hormonal, physiologic, and metabolic responses (79).

IL-1ra is a member of the IL-1 superfamily and shares approximately 25% homology with IL-1β. IL-1ra has similar affinity for the IL-1 type I receptor as does IL-1β, but unlike IL-1α and IL-1β, does not have any agonist properties (11). IL-1ra is a unique cytokine whose only known function is to block the actions of another cytokine, IL-1. Site-directed mutagenesis has revealed that a single amino acid substitution in the IL-1ra molecule is responsible for its failure to have agonist properties (80).

We now believe that IL-1ra represents an endogenous mechanism by which the inflamed host acts to modulate the systemic actions of IL-1. Studies by our laboratory have revealed that IL-1ra is produced systemically under many mild inflammatory processes and circulates in the ng/ml concentrations (59). These endogenous levels are unlikely to be effective in blocking the actions of IL-1 at the local sites of IL-1 production, such as in tissue microenvironments, but are adequate to reduce the systemic responses to local IL-1 production where concentrations are much lower.

Based on this hypothesis, we and others have proposed that administration of recombinant human IL-1ra to induce levels two to three logs higher may be successful in blocking not only the systemic but the local tissue effects of endogenous IL-1 production (81). Since Eisenberg et al. cloned the protein (82), recombinant IL-1ra has been available for in vivo studies. We infused IL-1ra into septic shock baboons and demonstrated that sustained plasma concentrations of 10 μg/ml were effective in blocking the pathologic sequelae to gram-negative septic shock.

Similar quantities were administered to healthy volunteers during a mild endotoxemia and IL-1ra concentrations achieved were on the range of 10 to 20 μg/ml (79). Following administration of endotoxin, ACTH levels increased from 18 ± 3 pg/ml to 88 ± 12 pg/ml at 2 hours, and cortisol levels increased correspondingly from 152 ± 11 ng/ml to 435 ± 76 ng/ml. Infusions of IL-1ra, in themselves, had no effect on the glucocorticoid response and did not alter the steroid responses to endotoxin. Similar to the rodent studies, these findings suggest that an endogenous IL-1 response does not contribute to the glucocorticoid responses seen in a mild inflammation. Although IL-1 is one such mediator that can induce glucocorticoids, these studies emphasize that because of either redundancy or cytokine-independent mechanisms, the glucocorticoid response to mild inflammation is not dependent on an endogenous IL-1 (and probably TNFα) response.

This conclusion, though, is likely dependent on the nature and magnitude of the exogenous inflammatory stimulus. We are now recognizing that the pattern of cytokine induction is dependent not only on the magnitude of the inflammatory response but also the nature of the exogenous stimulus. This has complicated efforts to dissect the contribution of individual cytokines to host responses because such results will depend to a large extent on the stimulus.

This latter point is highlighted from our ongoing studies in baboons. Whereas IL-1 receptor blockade was ineffective at blocking any of the metabolic responses to a mild endotoxemia, identical blockade improved survival, reduced hemodynamic collapse, and attenuated the metabolic responses to lethal gram-negative bacteremia (81). In lethal gram-negative bacteremia, we have shown that there is a massive systemic release of both TNFα and IL-1β, a finding that is not seen in nonlethal endotoxemia. We have shown that both IL-1 receptor and TNFα blockade attenuated the ACTH, as well as the catecholamine, responses to a lethal bacteremia (51,81). Thus, under these experimental conditions, both an endogenous IL-1 and TNFα response contributed to the glucocorticoid and catecholamine responses.

There are several lines of evidence to suggest that the glucocorticoid responses induced by cytokines serve as a feedback mechanism by which continued cytokine production is regulated. In vitro studies revealed that glucocorticoids regulate IL-1 and TNFα biosynthesis in macrophages at two levels, transcription and translation. Remick et al. demonstrated that dexamethasone, when injected 2 to 4 hours before endotoxin, inhibited transcription of TNF mRNA, although it had no effect when given simultaneously with endotoxin (83). This regulation of TNFα production by glucocorticoids is modulated in part by another cytokine, interferon. Luedke and Cerami revealed that treatment of macrophages with interferon reversed glucocorticoid-induced suppression of TNFα production (43).

Under in vivo conditions, these interactions are complex and often yield unexpected results. For example, Barber et al. infused human volunteers with sufficient cortisol to sustain plasma concentrations approximately fivefold higher than basal and comparable to levels seen in critically ill patients and in volunteers following endotoxemia (84). When cortisol was administered for six hours prior to and six hours after a mild endotoxemia, the serum TNFα response to endotoxin was completely ablated. However, levels of the cytokine inhibitors IL-1ra and the soluble TNF receptors were unaffected. Whereas normally the response to a mild inflammation is the initial release of proinflammatory cytokines followed by the release of cytokine inhibitors, pretreatment with cortisol attenuated only the proinflammatory cytokine response. Thus corticosteroid treatment shifted the net balance between pro- and antiinflammatory cytokine responses toward antiinflammatory responses. Thus corticosteroid treatment shifted the net balance between pro- and antiinflammatory cytokine responses toward antiinflammatory responses. Thus, it was not unexpected that the volunteers showed a markedly attenuated febrile and tachycardic response, as well as diminished hepatic acute-phase protein responses with cortisol administration. Surprisingly, the plasma IL-6 response to endotoxin was unaffected by concomitant cortisol treatment. Thus, cortisol, at levels comparable to those seen in critical illness, does not uniformly suppress inflammatory cell production of proinflammatory cytokines, but rather appears to preferentially suppress TNFα production. Abrogation of the TNFα response appears adequate to attenuate many of the constitutional responses to endotoxemia.

These studies, however, reveal that the timing of exposure to increased steroids is critical. When human volunteers were exposed to hypercortisolemia 12 to 144 hours prior to endotoxin, the subsequent TNFα response was not suppressed, but surprisingly, was actually enhanced. However, despite this marked increase in the proinflammatory cytokine response, the constitutional, hemodynamic, and acute-phase protein responses were unaffected. These studies provide in vivo human correlates to previous in vitro studies. They demonstrate the intimate relationship of neuroendocrine and cytokine responses to endotoxemia via manipulation of glucocorticoid background with subsequent increases in magnitude of proinflammatory cytokine responses without toxicity to the host. It is evident from all of these studies that such responses, even if attributable in part to cytokines, are influenced by antecedent events that alter the hormonal milieu. This is likely to be of particular importance in critically ill patients in which associated hypercortisolemia exists or in whom efforts directed at modulating cytokine responses are considered.

This latter point is extremely important because it suggests that the macrohormonal milieu will affect not only the subsequent proinflammatory cytokine response but also tissue responses to the cytokine production.

This point has been highlighted repeatedly from studies evaluating the host response to cytokine administration in adrenalectomized rodents. Bertini et al. first demonstrated that adrenalectomized animals are exceedingly sensitive to the shock-producing capacity of TNFα and IL-1 (85). Replacement therapies with dexamethasone eliminate this sensitivity in adrenalectomized animals. Gelin et al. have further shown that adrenalectomized animals expiring from otherwise nonlethal administrations of IL-1 do so with pronounced hypoglycemia (86). These investigators suggest that a normal glucocorticoid response is essential for maintaining glucose homeostasis and to antagonize the hypoglycemic effects of IL-1–mediated insulin release. For example, we have shown in healthy baboons that IL-1α administration results in a rapid (<1 h) release of insulin and transient hypoglycemia that can be explained by a significant uptake of glucose by skeletal muscle without an adequate compensatory hepatic gluconeogenesis. (62). This insulin response is proposed to result from a rapid release of preformed insulin and subsequent destruction of islet β cells. Adrenalectomy prevents a compensatory increase in glucocorticoid release that serves to promote glycogenolysis and the release of glucogenic precursors from nonvisceral tissues. In addition, Warren and colleagues have demonstrated that glucocorticoids play a passive but essential role in modulating cytokine-mediated uptake of glycogenic precursors by the liver (87). Thus, in the case of glucose homeostasis in response to cytokine administration, a functioning glucocorticoid response appears essential to survival, in part to maintain adequate glucose production in the face of increased insulin-mediated demand.

Similarly, cytokine-mediated glucocorticoid responses regulate the hepatic acute-phase response. Although Gelin et al. have shown that adrenalectomy does not alter the hepatic amyloid P and albumin responses to IL-1 administration (86), there is clear evidence that corticosteroids play a passive role in modulating IL-6–mediated hepatic acute-phase protein synthesis. For example, Gauldie and colleagues have shown that IL-6, moreso than IL-1 and TNFα, is a direct regulator of the hepatic acute-phase protein response (22). However, IL-6's modulation of acute-phase protein synthesis in vitro is dependent on coincubation of hepatocytes with glucocorticoids. In the absence of glucocorticoids, IL-6 induces only a modest acute-phase response. This observation may explain the in vivo findings that IL-6 is a weak inducer of hepatic acute-phase proteins when given to healthy animals alone. IL-6, unlike IL-1 and TNFα, does not induce a glucocorticoid response in vivo (data not shown). In contrast to IL-6, IL-1 and TNFα are relatively potent in vivo inducers of hepatic acute-phase protein synthesis, but not necessarily because they act directly on hepatocytes. Rather, the in vivo capacity of IL-1 and TNF to modulate the acute-phase protein synthesis response is a result of their ability to simultaneously induce IL-6 and a glucocorticoid response, which in turn are the direct mediators of hepatic acute-phase protein synthesis.

The cytokine network represents a proximal mechanism by which inflammatory cells signal to somatic tissues the presence of infection. Unlike the classical macrohormonal system, inflammatory cells capable of producing cytokines are widely distributed in the body, cytokines act principally in a paracrine fashion signalling to adjacent tissues, and there is considerable overlap and synergy in cytokine actions. However, cytokines do not act on end tissues in a vacuum, but rather, their responses are mediated in part through, and modulated by, the classical macrohormonal system. Although cytokines are known to act directly on a variety of macroendocrine systems, including insulin, glucagon, growth hormone and the IGFs, and thyroid hormones, the complexity of the interactions has been most fully described for the glucocorticoids. Although both IL-1 and TNFα can stimulate a glucocorticoid response, both through the pituitary-hypothalamic axis and directly in the adrenal, an endogenous glucocorticoid response to mild inflammation is not dependent on either an endogenous IL-1 or TNFα response. Rather the evidence accumulated thus far suggests that sufficient redundancy in the cytokine network exists that blockade of any single cytokine is insufficient to attenuate the glucocorticoid response. This conclusion, however, is dependent on the nature of the exogenous stimulus because in lethal gram-negative infections, exaggerated TNFα and IL-1 responses contribute to the glucocorticoid and catecholamine responses.

In addition, exposure of inflammatory cells to glucocorticoids will subsequently alter the cytokine responses. Although a hypercortisolemia seen in critical illness may acutely down-regulate subsequent proinflammatory cytokine production, such exposures may also result in a delayed and heightened proinflammatory response. Finally, interactions among cytokines and glucocorticoids will ultimately determine tissue responses. This has been best demonstrated in the lethality of rodents to nonlethal quantities of IL-1 and TNFα following adrenalectomy. An endogenous glucocorticoid response is essential to maintain glucose homeostasis following cytokine administration. Thus, the cytokine network and the classical macrohormonal responses are tightly regulated to modulate the host response to inflammation.

ACKNOWLEDGMENT

Supported in part by GM-40591, GM-34695, and CA-52108, awarded by the National Institutes of Health, USPHS.

REFERENCES

1. Tracey KJ, Fong Y, Hesse DG, et al. Anti-cachectin/TNF monoclonal antibodies prevent septic shock during lethal bacteremia. *Nature* 1987;330:662–664.
2. Hinshaw LB, Tekamp-Olson P, Chang AC, et al. Survival of primates in LD100 septic shock following therapy with antibody to tumor necrosis factor (TNF alpha). *Circ Shock* 1990;30:279–292.
3. Ashkenazi A, Marsters SA, Capon DJ, et al. Protection against endotoxic shock by a tumor necrosis factor receptor immunoadhesin. *Proc Natl Acad Sci* 1991;88:10535–10539.
4. Lesslauer W, Tabuchi H, Gentz R, et al. Recombinant soluble tumor necrosis factor receptor proteins protect mice from lipopolysaccharide-induced lethality. *Eur J Immunol* 1991;21:2883–2886.
5. Ohlsson K, Bjork P, Bergenfeldt M, et al. An interleukin-1 receptor antagonist reduces mortality in endotoxin shock. *Nature* 1990;348:550–552.
6. Wakabayashi G, Gelfand JA, Burke JF, Dinarello CA. A specific receptor antagonist for interleukin-1 prevents *E. coli* induced septic shock in rabbits. *FASEB J* 1991;5:338–343.
7. Fischer E, Marano MA, Van Zee KJ, et al. Interleukin-1 receptor blockade improves survival and

hemodynamic performance in *E. coli* septic shock, but fails to alter host responses to sublethal endotoxemia. *J Clin Invest* 1992;89:1551–1557.

8. Billiau A, Matthys P. Interferon-γ, more of a cachectin than tumor necrosis factor. *Cytokine* 1992; 4:259–263.

9. Grunfeld C, Feingold KR. The role of the cytokines, interferon alpha and tumor necrosis factor in the hypertriglyceridemia and wasting of AIDS. *J Nutr* 1992;122(Suppl.):749–753.

10. Moldawer LL, Georgieff M, Lundholm KG. Interleukin 1, tumour necrosis factor-alpha and the pathogenesis of cancer cachexia. *Clin Physiol* 1987;7:263–274.

11. Dinarello CA. Interleukin-1 and interleukin-1 antagonism. *Blood* 1991;77:1627–1652.

12. Fong Y, Moldawer LL, Shires GT, Lowry SF. The biology of cytokines: implications in surgical injury. *Surg Gynecol Obstet* 1990;170:363–378.

13. Echtenacher B, Falk W, Mannel DN, Krammer PH. Requirement of endogenous tumor necrosis factor/cachectin for recovery from experimental peritonitis. *J Immunol* 1990;145:3762–3766.

14. Havell EA. Evidence that tumor necrosis factor has an important role in antibacterial resistance. *J Immunol* 1989;143:2984–2989.

15. Grau GE, Kindler V, Piquet PF, et al. Prevention of experimental cerebral malaria by anticytokine antibodies. *J Exp Med* 1988;168:1499–1504.

16. Theodos CM, Provinelli L, Molina R, et al. Role of tumor necrosis factor in macrophage leishmanicidal activity in vitro and resistance to cutaneous leishmaniasis in vivo. *Infect Immunol* 1991;59:2839–2842.

17. Nelsen S, Bagby GJ, Bainton BG, et al. Compartmentalization of intraalveolar and systemic lipopolysaccharide-induced TNF and the pulmonary inflammatory response. *J Infect Dis* 1989;159:189–194.

18. Ginsberg H, Moldawer LL, Sehgal PB, et al. A unique mouse model to investigate the molecular pathogenesis of adenovirus pneumonia. *Proc Natl Acad Sci* 1991;88:1651–1655.

19. Nijsten MWN, DeGroot ER, TenDuis HJ, et al. Serum levels of interleukin-6 and acute phase responses. *Lancet* 1987;2:921–923.

20. Tovey MG, Content J, Gresser I, et al. Genes for IL-6, TNF and IL-1 are expressed in high levels in the organs of normal individuals. *J Immunol* 1988;9:3106–3113.

21. Warren RS, Donner DB, Starnes HF Jr, Brennan MF. Modulation or endogenous hormone action by recombinant human tumor necrosis factor. *Proc Natl Acad Sci* 1987;84:8619–8622.

22. Gauldie J, Northemann W, Fey GH. IL-6 functions as an exocrine hormone in inflammation. *J Immunol* 1990;144:3804–3808.

23. Heinrich PC, Castell JV, Andus T. Interleukin-6 and the acute phase response. *Biochem J* 1990;265: 621–636.

24. Dejana E, Breviario F, Erroi A, et al. Modulation of endothelial cell functions by different molecular species of interleukin-1. *Blood* 1987;69:695–701.

25. Kohase M, May LT, Tamm I, et al. A cytokine network in human diploid fibroblasts. *Mol Cell Biol* 1987;7:273–284.

26. Van der Meer JWM, Helle M, Aarden L. Comparison of the effects of recombinant interleukin 6 and recombinant interleukin 1 on nonspecific resistance to infection. *Eur J Immunol* 1989;19:413–416.

27. Rosenwasser LM, Dinarello CA, Rosenthal AS. Adherent cell function in murine T-lymphocyte antigen recognition. *J Exp Med* 1979;150:709–715.

28. Merriman CR, Pulliam LA, Kampschmidt RF. Comparison of leukocytic pyrogen and leukocytic endogenous mediator. *Proc Soc Exp Biol Med* 1977;154:224–233.

29. Czuprynski CJ, Brown JF, Yound KM, et al. Effects of murine recombinant interleukin 1 alpha on the host response to bacterial infection. *J Immunol* 1988;140:962–968.

30. Johnson CS, Keckler DJ, Topper MI, et al. In vivo hematopoietic effects of recombinant interleukin-1α in mice. *Blood* 1989;73:678–683.

31. Bagby GC Jr. Interleukin-1 and hematopoiesis. *Blood Rev* 1989;3:152.

32. Mochizuki DY, Eisenman JR, Conlon PJ, et al. Interleukin 1 regulates hematopoietic activity, a role previously ascribed to hematopoietin 1. *Proc Natl Acad Sci* 1987;84:5267–5271.

33. Moldawer LL, Marano M, Wei H, et al. Cachectin/tumor necrosis factor-alpha alters red blood cell kinetics and induces anemia in vivo. *FASEB J* 1989;3:1637–1643.

34. Fong Y, Marano MA, Moldawer LL, et al. The acute splanchnic and peripheral tissue metabolic response to endotoxin in man. *J Clin Invest* 1990;85:1896–1904.

35. van Deventer SJH, Buller HR, ten Cate, JW, et al. Experimental endotoxemia in humans: analysis of cytokine release and coagulation, fibrinolytic and complement pathways. *Blood* 1990;76:2520–2526.

36. Cannon JG, Tompkins RG, Gelfand JA, et al. Circulating interleukin-1 and tumor necrosis factor in septic shock and experimental endotoxin fever. *J Infect Dis* 1990;161:79–84.

37. Michie HR, Manogue KR, Spriggs DR, et al. Detection of circulating tumor necrosis factor after endotoxin administration. *N Engl J Med* 1988;318:1481–1486.
38. Van Zee KJ, Kohno T, Fischer E, et al. TNF soluble receptors protect against excessive TNFα during infection and injury. *Proc Natl Acad Sci* 1992;89:4845–4849.
39. Spinas GA, Keller U, Brockhaus M. Release of soluble receptors for tumor necrosis factor in relation to circulating TNF during experimental endotoxemia. *J Clin Invest* 1992;90:533–536.
40. Porteau F, Nathan CF. Mobilizable intracellular pool of p55 (type 1) tumor necrosis factor receptors in human neutrophils. *J Leuk Biol* 1992;52:122–125.
41. Hiltz ME, Lipton JM. Anti-inflammatory activity of a COOH-terminal fragment of the neuropeptide alpha-MSH. *FASEB J* 1989;3:2282–2287.
42. Marcinkiewics J. In vitro cytokine release by activated murine peritoneal macrophages. *Cytokine* 1991;3:327–332.
43. Luedke CE, Cerami A. Interferon gamma overcomes glucocorticoid suppression of cachectin/tumor necrosis factor biosynthesis by murine macrophages. *J Clin Invest* 1990;86:1234–1240.
44. Vane JR, Anggard EE, Botting RM. Regulatory functions of the vascular endothelium. *N Engl J Med* 1990;323:27–36.
45. Tracey KJ, Beutler B, Lowry SF, et al. Shock and tissue injury induced by human cachectin. *Science* 1986;234:470–474.
46. Tracey KJ, Lowry SF, Fahey TJ III, et al. Cachectin/tumor necrosis factor induces lethal shock and stress hormone responses in the dog. *Surg Gynecol Obstet* 1987;164:415–422.
47. Waage A, Espevik T, Lamvik J. Detection of TNF cytotoxicity in serum from patients with septicemia, but not from untreated cancer patients. *Scand J Immunol* 1987;24:739–744.
48. Waage A, Brandtzaeg P, Haltensen A, et al. The complex pattern of cytokines in serum from patients with meningococcal shock: association between IL-6, IL-1 and fatal outcome. *J Exp Med* 1989;169: 333–338.
49. Waage A, Halstensen A, Espevik T. Association between tumor necrosis factor in serum and fatal outcome in patients with meningococcal disease. *Lancet* 1987;1:355–357.
50. Marano M, Moldawer LL, Fong Y, et al. Cachectin/TNF production in experimental burns and Pseudomonas infection. *Arch Surg* 1988;123:1383–1388.
51. Van Zee KJ, Kohno T, Fischer E, et al. TNF soluble receptors protect against excessive TNFα during infection and injury. *Proc Natl Acad Sci* 1992;89:4845–4849.
52. de Groote MA, Martin MA, Densen P, et al. Plasma tumor necrosis factor levels in patients with presumed sepsis: results in those treated with antilipid A antibody versus placebo. *JAMA* 1989;262: 249–251.
53. Debets JMH, Kampmeijer R, van der Linden MPMH, et al. Plasma tumor necrosis factor and mortality in critically ill septic patients. *Crit Care Med* 1989;17:489–494.
54. Damas P, Reuter A, Gysen P, et al. Tumor necrosis factor and interleukin-1 serum levels during severe sepsis in humans. *Crit Care Med* 1989;17:975–978.
55. Marks JD, Marks CB, Luce JM, et al. Plasma tumor necrosis factor in patients with septic shock: mortality rate, incidence of ARDS and effects of methylprednisolone administration. *Annu Rev Resp Dis* 1990;141:94–97.
56. Calandra T, Baumgartner JD, Grau GE, et al. Prognostic value of tumor necrosis factor, interleukin-1, interferonα, and interferonγ in the serum of patients with septic shock. *J Infect Dis* 1990;161: 982–987.
57. Munoz C, Misset B, Fitting C, et al. Dissociation between plasma and monocyte-associated cytokines during sepsis. *Eur J Immunol* 1991;21:2177–2184.
58. Fong Y, Marano MA, Moldawer LL, et al. The acute splanchnic and peripheral tissue metabolic response to endotoxin in man. *J Clin Invest* 1990;85:1896–1904.
59. Fischer E, Poutsiaka DD, Van Zee KJ, et al. Interleukin-1 receptor antagonist circulates in experimental inflammation and in human disease. *Blood* 1992;79:2196–2200.
60. Girardin E, Grau GW, Dayer JM. Tumor necrosis factor and interleukin-1 in severe infectious purpura. *N Engl J Med* 1988;319:397–400.
61. Van Zee K, DeForge L, Fischer E, et al. IL-8 in septic shock, endotoxemia and following IL-1 administration. *J Immunol* 1991;146:3478–3482.
62. Fischer E, Marano MA, Barber A, et al. A comparison between the effects of interleukin-1α administration and sublethal endotoxemia in primates. *Am J Physiol* 1991;261:R442–R452.
63. Marano MA, Fong Y, Moldawer LL, et al. Serum cachectin/TNF in critically-ill patients correlates with infection and mortality. *Surg Gynecol Obstet* 1990;170:32–38.

64. Keogh C, Fong Y, Marano MA, et al. Identification of a novel tumor necrosis factor/cachectin from the livers of burned and infected rats. *Arch Surg* 1990;125:79–85.
65. Ginsberg H, Moldawer LL, Sehgal PB, et al. A unique mouse model to investigate the molecular pathogenesis of adenovirus pneumonia. *Proc Natl Acad Sci* 1991;88:1651–1655.
66. Havell EA, Moldawer LL, Helfgott D, et al. Type I IL-1 receptor blockade exacerbates murine listeriosis. *J Immunol* 1992;148:1486–1493.
67. Kriegler M, Perez C, DeFay K, Albert I, Lu SD. A novel form of TNF/cachectin is a cell-surface cytotoxic transmembrane protein: ramifications for the complex physiology of TNF. *Cell* 1988;53: 45–53.
68. Jue DM, Sherry B, Luedke C, et al. Processing of newly synthesized cachectin/tumor necrosis factor in endotoxin-stimulated macrophages. *Biochemistry* 1990;29:8371–8377.
69. Waage A, Espevik T. Interleukin-1 potentiates the lethal effect of tumor necrosis factorα/cachectin in mice. *J Exp Med* 1988;167:1987–1992.
70. Marinkovic S, Jahreis GP, Wong GG, Baumann H. *J Immunol* 1989;142:808.
71. Ganapathi MK, Rzewnicki D, Samols D, Jiang SL, Kushner I. Effect of combination of cytokines and hormones on synthesis of serum amyloid A and C-reactive protein in HEP 3B cells. *J Immunol* 1991;147:1261–1265.
72. Kushner I. The acute phase response: an overview. *Meth Enzymol* 1988;163:373–383.
73. Bernton EW, Beachm JE, Holaday JW, et al. Release of multiple hormones by a direct action of interleukin-1 on pituitary cells. *Science* 1987;238:519–521.
74. Sapolsky R, Rivier C, Yamamato G, et al. Interleukin-1 stimulates the secretion of hypothalamic corticotropin-releasing factor. *Science* 1987;238:522–524.
75. Lumpkin MD. The regulation of ACTH secretion by IL-1. *Science* 1987;238:452–454.
76. Roh MS, Drazenovich KA, Barbose JJ, et al. Direct stimulation of the adrenal cortex by interleukin-1. *Surgery* 1987;102:140–146.
77. Van der Poll T, van Deventer SJ, Buller HR, et al. Tumor necrosis factor mimics the metabolic response to acute infection in healthy humans. *Am J Physiol* 1991;261:E457–E465.
78. Gershenwald JE, Fong Y, Fahey TJ III, et al. Interleukin-1 receptor blockade attenuates the host inflammatory response. *Proc Natl Acad Sci* 1990;87:4966–4970.
79. Van Zee KJ, Coyle SM, Calvano SE, et al. Influence of interleukin-1 receptor blockade on the human response to endotoxemia. *J Immunol (in review)*, 1994.
80. Ju G, Labriola-Tompkins E, Campen CA, et al. Conversion of interleukin-1 receptor antagonist into an agonist by site-specific mutagenesis. *Proc Natl Acad Sci* 1991;88:2658–2662.
81. Fischer E, Marano MA, Van Zee KJ, et al. Interleukin-1 receptor blockade improves survival and hemodynamic performance in *E. coli* septic shock, but fails to alter host responses to sublethal endotoxemia. *J Clin Invest* 1992;89:1551–1557.
82. Eisenberg SP, Evans RJ, Arend WP, et al. Primary structure and functional expression from complementary DNA of a human interleukin-1 receptor antagonist. *Nature* 1990;343:341–346.
83. Remick DG, Streiter RM, Lynch JP, et al. In vivo dynamics of murine tumor necrosis factor alpha gene expression. *Lab Invest* 1989;60:766–772.
84. Barber AE, Coyle SM, Marano MA, et al. Glucocorticoid therapy alters hormonal and cytokine responses to endotoxin in man. *J Immunol* 1993;150:1999–2006.
85. Bertini R, Bianchi M, Ghezzi P. Adrenalectomy sensitizes mice to the lethal effects of interleukin-1 and tumor necrosis factor. *J Exp Med* 1988;167:1708–1712.
86. Gelin J, Moldawer LL, Iresjo B-M, Lundholm KG. The role of the adrenals in the acute phase response to interleukin-1 and tumor necrosis factor. *J Surg Res* 1993;54:70–78.
87. Warren RS, Donner DB, Starnes HF Jr, Brennan MF. Modulation of endogenous hormone action by recombinant tumor necrosis factor. *Proc Natl Acad Sci* 1987;84:8619–8622.

Organ Metabolism and Nutrition:
Ideas for Future Critical Care, edited by
J. M. Kinney and H. N. Tucker.
Raven Press, Ltd., New York © 1994.

7

Molecular and Cellular Control of the Tissue-Specific Inflammatory Response

Harvey R. Colten

Department of Pediatrics, Washington University School of Medicine, St. Louis Children's Hospital, St. Louis, Missouri 63110

Inflammation is comprised of a set of programmed responses to tissue injury, toxins, and microbial agents. Even rather primitive multicellular organisms are capable of mounting an inflammatory response. That is, even in these organisms, humoral and cellular constituents of host defenses are focused by the presence of a foreign body or at a site of tissue injury. The evolution in higher organisms of a discrete circulatory system introduced an additional complexity of the interaction between the cellular and humoral constituents of the inflammatory response. This compartmentalization of host defenses imposed a need for mechanisms regulating changes in permeability of the circulatory system and for margination/directed migration of circulating cellular elements. For instance, an elaborate array of highly regulated genes expressed in endothelium, blood leukocytes, and in extravascular cells are responsible for accumulation of white cells at sites of inflammation. A set of proteins within the selectin family (1) displayed on the majority of lymphocytes, neutrophils and monocytes, and corresponding cytokine-regulated selectins on endothelium are critical for recruitment of white cells to an inflammatory site. Similar general functions are served by adhesion molecules of the integrin and immunoglobulin families (2,3). In addition, other moieties such as nitric oxide (4), arachadonic acid metabolites (5), and reactive oxygen radicals (6) generated at inflammatory sites play modulating and direct roles in leukocyte adherence, migration, and activation. This process is characterized by elaborate control mechanisms and is highly redundant even when considering only the intravascular elements. In addition, separate vascular and peripheral tissue sources of soluble components of the system evolved. This has resulted in separate regulatory mechanisms that govern availability of the intravascular and extravascular constituents.

The classically recognized features of inflammation, calor (heat), tumor (swelling), rubor (redness), and dolor (pain), are for the most part manifestations of the vascular response (dilatation and increased permeability) to the inflammatory stimulus. Historically, studies of the constituents of blood have provided convenient, relatively noninvasive access to the elements of the immune system. Less interest was generated in the local extravascular events because they were more difficult to study and were thought to be quantitatively and qualitatively of lesser importance. It is the purpose of this chapter to suggest that these extravascular local events are critical for an effective host-defense mechanism and that studies of these phenomena suggest rather elegant control mechanisms, which must be taken into account in attempts to modify inflammation for clinical purposes.

THE ACUTE-PHASE RESPONSE

Interest in the specificity of the host response to microbes was the basis for the development of immunology as a distinct discipline in the late nineteenth century. It was the recognition of primitive host-defense mechanisms that prompted Metchnikoff (7) to develop his theory of phagocytosis, one of the fundamental principles of modern immunology. The elucidation of the mechanisms generating diversity of specific antibody and the cellular responses to antigen have, in fact, been central goals of immunologists from the beginning. Nevertheless, it is clear that an effective inflammatory response can dispose of toxins, microbes, and tissue debris even in the absence of specific immunity.

Following the discovery of C reactive protein (CRP) by Tillett and Francis (8), the concept of the acute-phase response was developed (summarized in Kushner, 9). They and others observed remarkable changes in plasma protein concentrations (100- to 1,000-fold for CRP and serum amyloid A) within hours following tissue injury or infection. Moreover, this rapid change in hepatic synthesis of plasma proteins was accompanied by many other systemic changes. For example, fever, leukocytosis, changes in nitrogen balance, and fat, carbohydrate, and heavy trace metal metabolism are also features of the acute-phase response. None of these are dependent on specific immune mechanisms. It is clear, however, that the acute-phase reaction not only provides a rapid response to noxious stimuli, but also facilitates the acquisition of specific immunity.

Among the acute-phase proteins that are important in both nonspecific and specific host defenses are members of the complement system. The increase in complement proteins is neither quantitatively nor kinetically the most impressive among the acute-phase plasma proteins. For example, serum concentrations of C3 protein rise only about twofold over baseline within a week following an acute-phase stimulus (tissue injury or infection). The serum complement proteins are almost entirely of hepatic origin (10). The precise kinetics of extrahepatic induction of complement genes in vivo is not known, but data from Katz et al. (11) show that these acute-phase–induced changes in complement gene expression in extrahepatic fibroblasts and other cell types are quantitatively much greater than in hepatocytes. Several studies suggest that this is true in vivo as well. For example, the increase in extrahepatic complement expression exceeds by severalfold the increase in liver during evolution of systemic lupus erythematosus. (12–15).

COMPLEMENT

Several of the complement genes are responsive to a broad array of acute-phase stimuli, the mechanisms regulating their expression are similar to those involved in control of other acute phase response genes, and the complement gene products play an important role in host defense and other features of the acute-phase response. For example, components of the alternative pathway of complement activation (see next section) are synthesized in fat cells (16). Differentiation of pre-fat to fat cells, obesity, and starvation have a marked effect on expression of these genes (17,18). Finally, complement proteins are directly involved in facilitating specific immune recognition and antibody responses. Melchers and colleagues (reviewed in Lernhardt and Melchers, 19) have provided evidence that fragments of the third component of complement promote entry of B lymphocytes into S phase of the cell cycle (proliferation) and are important in B cell differentiation. The latter conclusion is supported by studies of immune responses in complement deficient guinea pigs (20,21), which show a dependence on complement of isotype switching especially at low antigen doses (in conditions most typical of natural infection). The balance of this chapter focuses on the acute-phase complement genes and the tissue specificity of regulated expression. Nevertheless, it must be understood that specific mechanisms governing expression of other acute-phase proteins vary, are species specific, and are developmentally determined.

COMPLEMENT ACTIVATION PATHWAYS

The complement system consists of a set of nearly 30 effector and regulatory proteins (reviewed in Muller-Eberhard, 22). The complement cascade is activated by limited proteolysis of the classical (antibody-dependent) pathway and alternative (antibody-independent) pathway proteins. Interaction of antigens with antibodies of immunoglobulin class IgM and several IgG subclasses initiates binding and activation of the classical complement pathway. The specificity of this reaction is imposed by antibody. Under some conditions, however, viral agents (23–25), DNA, CRP (26), and mitochondrial membranes (27) can activate the classical pathway in the absence of antibody. Activation of the alternative complement pathway always involves antibody-independent recognition of structures (e.g., polysaccharides) that are highly represented among pathogens. This activation is initiated by nonspecific binding of alternative pathway proteins. Localization of the alternative pathway reaction is accomplished by permissive propagation of the cascade, i.e., conditions that limit control protein inactivation of the effector proteins. Amplification is an important feature of both pathways because deposition of a few molecules results in cleavage of thousands of later components in the cascade and the appearance of complement-dependent biological activities. Further amplification results from the positive activation loop involving the proteins of the alternative pathway. The proteins of the classical pathway include C1 (a macromolecular complex comprised of the products of five genes and the fourth (C4) and second (C2) components). The latter two are encoded by genes within the major histocompatibility complex along with one of the alternative pathway proteins, factor B (28–30). The other alternative pathway constituents include factor D and C3. Two distinct unstable enzymes capable of cleaving the third component of complement (C3) are generated by complexing of active fragments of proteins of the two pathways.

The C3 protein is a principle source of biologically active cleavage products that mediate inflammation, solubilize and clear immune complexes, and further propagate the complement cascade resulting in assembly of the terminal complement protein complex (the membrane attack complex [MAC]) and cytolysis via the generation of discrete membrane channels. The complement effector proteins are controlled by a network of regulatory proteins, some of which, such as the C3b receptor (CR1), also serve as cell-surface receptors for complement activation products.

The effector and regulatory proteins of the complement cascade are synthesized in liver and in many extrahepatic tissues (31). Liver (hepatocytes and Kupffer cells) is the source of most of the complement proteins circulating in plasma (10,32). This has been known since the turn of the century when Ehrlich and Morgenroth (33) demonstrated that complement was depressed in sera of animals following experimental liver injury. Liver perfusion studies further supported the concept that the liver was a site of complement synthesis (34). Much later, Alper and coworkers (35) confirmed that the liver is a major site of serum complement synthesis in studies of patients following liver transplantation. They demonstrated a shift from the recipient allotype to the donor allotype of several complement proteins that exhibit genetic polymorphism. Based on current data, except for C1q, factor D, and properdin, liver is an important source of circulating complement effector proteins. However, Thorbecke and colleagues (36) suggested that cell types of endodermal, mesodermal, and ectodermal origin in several organs were also capable of producing proteins of the complement system. This concept has been confirmed and extended with the use of modern molecular, biological methods. Studies of complement metabolism and mRNA expression in vivo (12,13,37) and biosynthetic studies in tissue culture indicate an important role for complement produced at extrahepatic sites.

Activation of the complement cascade through C5 can be accomplished by proteins synthesized at the extrahepatic sites without a requirement for serum protein. The widespread synthesis of the prominent acute-phase complement proteins C3 and factor B, which have been identified in fibroblasts, mononuclear phagocytes, epithelial cells, and others, suggests that this extrahepatic synthesis provides a source of alternative complement proteins for local host defense that precedes and may facilitate influx of serum proteins. The synthesis of two other alternative complement proteins, factor D and properdin, at extrahepatic sites is consistent with this concept. The functional importance of this extrahepatic complement production is supported by the presence of elaborate tissue-specific and developmentally regulated controls of complement gene expression.

ACUTE-PHASE COMPLEMENT GENES

Factors B, C3, and C4 are quantitatively the most prominent of the acute-phase complement proteins in plasma. These changes result from an increase in hepatic complement gene expression. Inflammation and tissue injury also modulates complement gene expression at extrahepatic sites. As suggested, the magnitude of acute-phase induced changes in extrahepatic complement expression often exceeds the effects in liver. For example, expression of the classical activation pathway protein C2 (not an acute-phase *plasma* protein) is highly regulated at extrahepatic sites of inflammation (12,13). The acute-phase complement gene response is also affected by genetic background and development. In the past few years, the molecular bases of this phenomenon have been partially elucidated. The soluble mediators of this response and their respective receptors, the cell biological events, and the cis and transacting elements that regulate complement gene expression have been revealed.

COMPLEMENT GENES AND GENE PRODUCTS

The constituents of the classical pathway C3-cleaving enzyme (C4 and C2) are synthesized in similar cell types but the co- and postsynthetic processing of each differs considerably. C4 is a heterotrimeric glycoprotein of approximately 200 kd (38). The protein is synthesized as a single-chain precursor (pre-pro-C4) (39) programmed by a 5.5-kb mature mRNA (40). Processing of pre-pro-C4 requires proteolytic cleavage by a signal peptidase, excision of two interchain linking peptides, generation of a thiolester bridge, glycosylation of α and β chain residues via a dolichol phosphate intermediate, sulfation, and cleavage of a carboxyterminal fragment of α chain by an extracellular metalloproteinase (41–43). Processing and secretion of C4 occurs with a half-time of about 60 to 90 minutes (44). The mature C4 protein is activated by cleavage of C4a (a weak anaphylotoxin), a 9-kd NH_2 terminal fragment from alpha chain, leaving the remainder, C4b. The latter serves as a subunit of the C3-cleaving enzyme of the classical pathway.

Constitutive expression of C4 is under genetic control and is tissue specific. For example, there is a 20-fold difference in plasma C4 concentration among inbred mouse strains of different H-2 haplotypes (45). The tissue specificity of this phenomenon is evidenced by the finding of equal C4 expression in extrahepatic macrophages from C4-high and C4-low strains (46,47).

C2 is a single-chain glycoprotein (Mr $\sim$ 100,000) that binds to C4b in the presence of Mg^{2+} and is cleaved into an aminoterminal, 223 amino acid polypeptide C2b and carboxyterminal C2a (509 amino acid) fragment. The latter bears the active enzymatic site for C3 cleavage (48). The C3-cleaving enzyme C4b2a is unstable, i.e., provides an intrinsic control mechanism, but its decay is accelerated by cell-surface regulatory proteins. C2 is encoded by a gene (15 kb) that is located $\sim$400 basepairs 5′ to the factor B gene (28). Several primary translation products have been recognized, though only one is secreted (one-half time $\sim$ 45 minutes) (49). Translational control of C2 protein expression is due to differences in transcriptional initiation. These generate differences in the 5' untranslated region, the sequence of which governs the rate of C2 translation (50). A similar mechanism provides translational control of factor B production (51).

Factor B (Bf) is synthesized as an ~80-kd propolypeptide that undergoes signal peptide cleavage, glycosylation, and secretion in about 60 minutes. Two factor B transcripts generated from alternative transcriptional initiation sites have been recognized in studies of murine Bf expression in kidney and intestine (52). The larger of the two is expressed in amounts equal to the shorter message only in those two tissues; in liver, the long transcript represents <5% of Bf mRNA (53). It is this Bf long transcript that is responsible for the translational control of the Bf production previously described.

Constitutive and regulated expression of C2 and Bf has been studied extensively in mice. Conservation of overall gene structure and primary sequences between humans and mice for C2 and Bf (53,54) suggests that these studies will be relevant to humans as well. Among inbred mouse strains, marked differences in C2 and B serum concentrations are paralleled by differences in hepatic mRNA content for each (37). Expression of C2 and Bf in these strains varies independently. As was cited for expression of C4, constitutive control is tissue specific; i.e., the content of specific C2 or B mRNA in macrophages is independent of the relative hepatic expression of each among the murine strains examined. Analysis of this phenomenon in mice of different H-2 haplotypes revealed both cis and trans elements important for strain and tissue specificity of Bf expression (51).

Pre-pro C3 is programmed by an ~5.2-kb mature mRNA derived from a >40-kb gene on chromosome 19 (55) in humans and 17 in mice (56). Co- and postsynthetic modification involves cleavage of a signal peptide, excision of a single interchain linking peptide, generation of a thiolester bridge (57), and glycosylation to the native C3 protein. The native C3 protein is a disulfide-linked heterodimer of α (~110 kd) and β (75 kd) chains (58). Cleavage of C3 α chain liberates the C3a fragment, a potent anaphylatoxin that elicits histamine release, smooth muscle contraction, and noncytotoxic liberation of arachadonate metabolites (59). Covalent binding of C3b to a carboxyl or amino acceptor site is via its labile thiolester (60). Deposition of C3 on a cell is relatively inefficient (61) so that much of the metastable C3b reacts with water and cannot bind to target cells. Nevertheless, C3b, whether surface bound or hydrolyzed, can bind C5, factors B, H, properdin, and the C3b receptor CR1.

Binding and activation of factor B to C3b generates the alternative pathway amplification loop, the flux of which is controlled by intrinsic decay of the enzyme C3bBb, control/cofactor protein dissociation of the complex and cleavage of the C3b (62). Fluid-phase and cell-surface proteins participate in the regulation of the complement cascade at this point in the sequence. A second C3b bound to the C3bBb complex results in generation of a C5-cleaving enzyme and assembly of the membrane attack complex (63). Cleavage of C3b by one of the natural control proteins, factor I, is facilitated by the fluid-phase component factor H and on erythrocytes, lymphocytes, granulocytes, mononuclear phagocytes, and other cells by the C3b receptor CR1.

C3b α chain is cleaved by factor I at two sites to generate C3bi. An integrin found on phagocytes, CR3 is a specific receptor for C3bi. The C3bi undergoes further cleavage by factor I to generate C3dg, a 40-kd C3 product that remains covalently bound to the target of complement activation. A specific receptor, CR2, is found on B lymphocytes and recognizes C3dg and C3d, a further cleavage product.

The hepatic biosynthetic rate estimated in vivo from fractional catabolic rates of ^{125}I-labelled C3 is 0.45 to 2.7 mg/kg/h (64); extrahepatic rates of synthesis are not well defined. Constitutive expression of C3 (65) varies among inbred mouse strains but effects of age and sex (56) complicate the analysis. A detailed structural and functional study of the sequences 5′ to the murine and human C3 genes (66,67) has been undertaken. Sequence analysis of the 5′ flanking region of murine and human C3 revealed 51% identity overall with two segments (-36 to -1 and -146 to -68) 80% identical (66). Of the four TATA boxes upstream of the murine gene, only the most 3′ (-30) is active in hepatic-derived cells as determined by deletional analysis. Positive and negative elements for constitutive C3 expression have been identified and sequences providing enhancer and IL-1/IL-6 regulation are found between positions -90 and -41. Site-directed mutagenesis and functional studies in HepG2 showed that the IL-1 and IL-6 response elements could be partially separated and that proteins of the C/EBP and NFκB families are implicated in C3 expression.

REGULATED EXPRESSION

Endotoxin, a constituent of the cell wall of gram-negative bacteria, has a potent effect on regulation of complement gene expression. The analysis of this effect is complicated by the many genes induced by endotoxin, products of which also regulate complement gene expression. In addition, the mechanisms for recognition of endotoxin on cell surfaces and the signal transduction pathways mediating its effects, are poorly characterized. Lipopolysaccharide (LPS) administration in vivo or to mast cells in culture results in a brisk increase in net synthesis of several of the complement proteins up to >20-fold over constitutive synthesis rates (68,69). Certain cells that express complement genes such as monocytes, type II lung cells, and fibroblasts are highly LPS responsive, whereas others, the hepatocyte and intestinal epithelium, are not.

The LPS effect on C3 and factor B expression serves as a useful model to evaluate this phenomenon because the quantitative effect on these two genes is substantial and both gene products are of importance in host defenses against gram-negative bacteria. In human peripheral blood monocytes and macrophages and in murine macrophages, LPS at nanogram concentrations induces a five- to 30-fold increase in C3 and Bf synthesis and secretion (11,68,70). Most of this effect is transcriptional, but two lines of evidence suggest an important translational regulatory effect as well. In adult human fibroblasts, the increased Bf protein synthesis rates following LPS stimulation exceeds the increase in Bf mRNA. LPS does not up-regulate C3 and Bf synthesis in newborn (umbilical cord) blood monocytes, although corresponding mRNA levels are increased (70). Specific C3 and Bf mRNA is also induced in newborn fibroblasts, but there is no increase in C3 or Bf protein synthesis; in fetal cells, LPS does not induce C3 or Bf mRNA. Thus, the response to LPS involves a sequential maturation of transcriptional, then translational competence from fetal to newborn and adult. It should be noted that LPS also has counterregulatory effects on complement expression as in the case of C4 (see the following description).

Each of the cytokines associated with up-regulation of other acute-phase genes has been recognized to modulate expression of several of the complement genes as well. For instance, in the case of factor B, the complement gene most broadly responsive to cytokine control, IL-1α, IL-1β, TNF-α, IL-6, and IFN-γ are able, separately and together, to increase transcription of the Bf gene (reviewed in Colten, 71). The C3 gene is also regulated by these cytokines, though its response to IFN-γ is species specific and even within a species such as mice, strain specific. The effect of these cytokines is manifest in many different tissues and cell types, including hepatocytes, fibroblasts, macrophages, enterocytes, neuroglia, endothelial cells, and other cell types that have been less well studied. Other complement genes, such as C2 and C4, display a much more restricted cytokine responsiveness; i.e., they only up-regulate in response to IFN-γ (72).

During the course of studies of hepatic complement gene regulation (73), a variant of HepG2 permitted dissection of transacting nucleoproteins interacting with the IL-1 and IL-6 response regions of the Bf gene and distinguished them from similar proteins interacting with the corresponding C3 cis elements (66). Gel shift analysis showed at least four bands, the binding of which was dependent on cytokine (IL-1 and IL-6) stimulation of HepG2 and sequences -88 to -83 upstream of the C3 transcriptional initiation site. Functionally another region (-77 to -72) was required for IL-1 response, but not IL-6 responsiveness. However, with this method no specific proteins binding to this region could be identified. By contrast to the parent cell, IL-1 does not up-regulate Bf expression in the HepG2 mutant line, even though the mutant HepG2 responds to IL-6 and TNF stimulation. This aberrant response is selective but not exclusive (C3 is responsive to IL-1). Albumin, a negative acute-phase reactant, is also regulated by IL-6 and TNF but not IL-1 in the mutant HepG2. Equilibrium binding using ^{125}I-labelled IL-1 showed similar numbers and affinity of IL-1 receptors on the two cell lines. Gel shift patterns using a Bf probe and lysate from each of the HepG2 lines show differences in binding of C/EBP-like proteins, NFκB binding, and competition by NF-IL-6 and NFκB binding sequences. The pattern of nucleoprotein binding and response of the Bf gene in the two cell lines is qualitatively and quantitatively different following IL-1 stimulation, identifying one level at which these cells differ and a probe of mechanisms for cytokine regulation of Bf expression.

Counterregulation of the effects of these cytokines by the growth factors IL-4, FGF, PDGF, and EGF (74) has prompted questions regarding the mechanisms by which the acute-phase response is terminated. In other words, is the return to constitutive expression of these genes simply a result of less stimulation or is it an active extinction (down-regulation) of gene expression? In any case, the effects on complement genes of the growth factors are cytokine specific, gene specific, and are independent of (precede) their effect on the proliferative response. That is, pretranslational Bf up-regulation by IL-1 and TNF is counterregulated by the growth factors, but there is no effect on C3 and factor H induction, thus ruling out an effect mediated by changes in cytokine receptor or postreceptor transduction mechanisms common to C3 and Bf. The effect on Bf is manifest within 4 to 8 hours and persists for up to 4 hours after removal of the growth factor. Counterregulation is blocked by inhibition of protein synthesis. Not only growth factors have the capacity to counterregulate cytokine-mediated induction of complement. For instance, LPS completely counters the up-regulation of C4 by IFN-γ, though it augments the effect of IFN-γ on Bf expression (72). These differences offer an advantage in working out the mechanisms responsible for this interesting set of phenomena. In contrast to inhibitory effects of these growth factors on Bf, there is a marked enhancement (25-fold) of PDGF on IL-1 stimulation of metalloproteinase/antiproteinases in skin fibroblasts (75).

In at least two experimental models, abundant evidence supports the hypothesis that local tissue-specific regulation of complement gene expression has an important effect on the pathogenesis of tissue injury associated with systemic lupus erythematosus (SLE) (12,13). These data support clinical studies that suggest similar conclusions (14,15,76); i.e., in target organs (kidney, heart, lung, etc.) a marked increase in C3, C4, C2, and Bf expression is observed with advancing age in mice (MRL and NZB xNZW) that spontaneously develops SLE. At a whole-organ level, this complement gene response is qualitatively similar in mice injected with endotoxin and in the two strains developing SLE. In none of the earlier work was the complement-producing cell identified either under constitutive or stimulated conditions. Current studies addressing this question suggest that this line of investigation will provide new insights into the role of complement in local and systemic inflammation. For example, utilizing an in situ hybridization procedure, we found distinctly different patterns of complement gene induction in the kidney from LPS-injected mice as compared to SLE nephritic samples. A cortical pattern of C3 expression is seen on cut section of kidney from LPS-injected mice. In contrast, lupus nephritis yields a punctate pattern throughout. These differing patterns are due to differences in the cell type responsive to the different stimuli; i.e., in the LPS-stimulated mice there is a marked increase in epithelial C3 and Bf expression whereas in SLE the increase is in perivascular inflammatory cells. The functional importance of these observations remains to be elucidated.

The data presented in this brief review suggest that the diversity of cellular sites of complement gene expression and the tissue specificity of complement gene regulation has the potential for uncovering novel strategies for the selective control of inflammation. Complement represents only a model system so that these principles have wide application to the many other components of the inflammatory response. It may be possible to modify events associated with the acute-phase response that are elicited during immunopathologic events. Hence, a study of the molecular control of tissue-specific inflammation could have practical as well as basic consequences.

REFERENCES

1. McEver RP. Leukocyte interactions mediated by selectins. *Thromb Haemost* 1991;66:80–87.
2. Springer TA. Adhesion receptors of the immune system. *Nature* 1990;346:425–434.
3. Kishimoto TK, Larson RS, Carbi AL, Dustin ML, et al. The leukocyte integrins. In: Dixon FJ, ed. *Advances in Immunology*. New York: Academic Press, 1989;46:149–182.
4. Kubes P, Suzuki M, Granger DN. Nitric oxide: an endogenous modulator of leukocyte adhesion. *Proc Natl Acad Sci USA* 1991;88:4651–4655.
5. Smith MJH, Ford-Hutchinson AW, Bray MA. Leukotriene B: a potential mediator of inflammation. *J Pharm Pharmacol* 1980;32:517–518.
6. Patel KD, Zimmerman GA, Prescott SM, et al. Oxygen radicals induce human endothelial cells to express GMP-140 and bind neutrophils. *J Cell Biol* 1991;112:749–759.
7. Metchnikoff E. *Immunity in Infective Disease*. London: Cambridge University Press, 1905;591.
8. Tillett WS, Francis T, Jr. Serological reactions in pneumonia with non-protein somatic fraction of *Pneumococcus*. *J Exp Med* 1930;52:561–571.
9. Kushner I. The phenomenon of the acute phase response. *Ann NY Acad Sci* 1982;389:39–48.
10. Alper CA, Raum D, Awdeh Z, et al. Studies of hepatic synthesis in vivo of plasma proteins including orosomucoid, transferrin, alpha-1-antitrypsin, C8 and factor B. *Clin Immunol Immunopathol* 1980;16:84–89.
11. Katz Y, Cole FS, Strunk RC. Synergism between interferon-gamma and lipopolysaccharide for synthesis of factor B, but not C2, in human fibroblasts. *J Exp Med* 1988;167:1–14.
12. Passwell J, Schreiner GF, Nonaka M, et al. Local extrahepatic expression of complement genes C3, factor B, C2 and C4 is increased in murine lupus nephritis. *J Clin Invest* 1988;82:1676–1684.
13. Passwell JH, Schreiner GF, Wetsel RA, Colten HR. Complement gene expression in hepatic and extrahepatic tissues of NZB and NZBxW (F1) mouse strains. *Immunology* 1990;71:290–294.
14. Ahrenstedt O, Knutson L, Nilsson B, et al. Enhanced local production of complement components in the small intestines of patients with Crohn's disease. *N Engl J Med* 1990;322:1345–1349.
15. Welch TR, Witte DP, Beischel LS. Differential expression and cellular localization of messenger RNA for C3 and C4 in the human kidney. *Complement Inflamm* 1991;8:141.
16. White RT, Damm D, Hancock N, et al. Human adipsin is identical to complement factor D and is expressed at high levels in adipose tissue. *J Biol Chem* 1992;267:9210–9213.
17. Wilkison WO, Min HY, Claffey KP, et al. Identification of distinct nuclear factors binding to single- and double-stranded DNA. *J Biol Chem* 1990;265:477–482.
18. Rosen BS, Cook KS, Yaglom J, et al. Adipsin and complement factor D activity: an immune-related defect in obesity. *Science* 1989;244:1483–1487.
19. Lernhardt W, Melchers F. The role of C3 and its fragments in the control of S phase entry of activated mouse B lymphocytes via the complement receptor type 2. *Exp Clin Immunogenet* 1988;5:115–122.
20. Berger R, Gordon J, Stevenson G, et al. An inherited deficiency of the third component of complement, C3, in guinea pigs. *Eur J Immunol* 1986;16:7–11.
21. Bottger EC, Hoffman T, Hadding U, Bitter-Suermann D. Guinea pigs with inherited deficiencies of complement components C2 or C4 have characteristics of immune complex disease. *J Clin Invest* 1986;78:689–695.
22. Muller-Eberhard HJ. Complement: chemistry and pathways. In: Gallin JI, Goldstein IM, Snyderman R, eds. *Inflammation: Basic Principles and Clinical Correlates, 2nd Ed.* New York: Raven Press, 1992;33–61.
23. Welsh RM, Cooper NR, Jensen FC, Oldstone MBA. Human serum lyses RNA tumor viruses. *Nature* 1975;257:612–614.
24. Cooper NR, Jensen FC, Welsh RM, Oldstone MBA. Lysis of RNA tumor viruses by human serum: direct antibody-independent triggering of the classical complement pathway. *J Exp Med* 1976;144:970–984.
25. Bartholomew RM, Esser AF. Mechanism of antibody-independent activation of the first component of complement (C1) on retrovirus membranes. *Biochemistry* 1980;19:2847–2853.
26. Kaplan MH, Volanakis JE. Interaction of C-reactive protein complexes with the complement system. I. Consumption of human complement associated with the reaction of C-reactive protein with pneumococcal C-polysaccharide and with choline phosphatides, lecithin and sphingomyelin. *J Immunol* 1974;112:2135–2147.
27. Storrs SB, Kolb WP, Pinckard RN, Olson MS. Characterization of the binding of purified human C1q to heart mitochondrial membranes. *J Biol Chem* 1981;256:10924–10929.

28. Carroll MC, Campbell RD, Bentley DR, Porter RR. A molecular map of the human major histocompatibility complex class III region linking complement genes C4, C2 and factor B. *Nature* 1984;307: 237–241.
29. Chaplin DD, Sackstein R, Perlmutter DH, et al. Expression of hemolytically active murine fourth component of complement in transfected L-cells. *Cell* 1984;37:569–576.
30. Chaplin DD, Woods DE, Whitehead AS, et al. Molecular map of the murine S region. *Proc Natl Acad Sci USA* 1985;80:6947–6951.
31. Colten HR. The biosynthesis of complement components. In: Harrison RA, ed. *New Comprehensive Biochemistry*. Amsterdam: Elsevier (in press).
32. Perlmutter DH, Colten HR. Complement: molecular genetics. In: Gallin JI, Goldstein IM, Snyderman R, eds. *Inflammation,* 2nd Ed. New York: Raven Press, 1992;81:102.
33. Ehrlich P, Morgenroth J. Ueber Haemolysine. *Berlin Klin Wochenschr* 1900;37:453–458.
34. Muller I. *Zentralbl Bacteriol Parasiter Infectionshr* 1911;57:577.
35. Alper CA, Johnson AM, Birtch AG, Moore RD. Human C3: evidence for the liver as the primary site of synthesis. *Science* 1969;163:286–288.
36. Thorbecke GJ, Hochwald GM, Van Furth LR, et al. Problems in determining the sites of synthesis of complement components. In: Wolstenholme GEW, Knight J, eds. *CIBA Symposium: Complement*. London: Churchill, 1965;99–119.
37. Falus A, Beuscher HU, Auerbach HS, Colten HR. Constitutive and IL-1 regulated murine complement gene expression is strain and tissue specific. *J Immunol* 1987;138:856–860.
38. Schreiber RD, Muller-Eberhard HJ. Fourth component of human complement: description of a three polypeptide chain structure. *J Exp Med* 1974;140:1324–1335.
39. Hall RE, Colten HR. Cell-free synthesis of the fourth component of guinea pig complement (C4): identification of a precursor of serum C4 (pro-C4). *Proc Natl Acad Sci USA* 1977;75:1707–1710.
40. Whitehead AS, Goldberger G, Woods DE, et al. Use of a cDNA clone for the fourth component of human complement for analysis of a genetic deficiency of C4 in guinea pig. *Proc Natl Acad Sci USA* 1983;80:5387–5391.
41. Goldberger G, Colten HR. Precursor complement protein (pro-C4) is converted in vitro to native C4 by plasmin. *Nature* 1980;286:514–516.
42. Karp DR. Post-translational modification of the fourth component of complement. Sulfation of the alpha chain. *J Biol Chem* 1983;258:12745–12748.
43. Karp DR. Post-translational modification of the fourth component of complement: Effect of tunicamycin and amino acid analogs on the formation of the internal thiol ester and disulfide bonds. *J Biol Chem* 1983;258:14490–14495.
44. Roos MH, Kornfeld S, Shreffler DC. Characterization of the oligosaccharide units of the fourth component of complement (Ss protein) synthesized by murine macrophages. *J Immunol* 1980;124: 2860–2861.
45. Shreffler DC. The S region of the mouse major histocompatibility complex (H-2): genetic variation and functional role in complement system. *Transplant Rev* 1976;32:140–167.
46. Sackstein R, Colten HR. Molecular regulation of MHC class III (C4 and factor B) gene expression in mouse peritoneal macrophages. *J Immunol* 1984;133:1618–1626.
47. Cox BJ, Robins DM. Tissue-specific variation in C4 and Slp gene regulation. *Nucleic Acids Res* 1988; 16:6857–6870.
48. Cooper NR. Enzymatic activity of the second component of complement. *Biochemistry* 1975;14: 4245–4251.
49. Perlmutter DH, Cole FS, Goldberger G, Colten HR. Distinct primary translation products from human liver mRNA give rise to secreted and cell-associated forms of complement protein C2. *J Biol Chem* 1984;259:10380–10385.
50. Horiuchi T, Macon KJ, Kidd VJ, Volanakis JE. Translational regulation of complement protein C2 expression by differential utilization of the 5'-untranslated region of mRNA. *J Biol Chem* 1990;265: 6521–6524.
51. Garnier G, Ault B, Kramer M, Colten HR. Cis and trans elements differ among mouse strains with high and low extrahepatic complement factor B gene expression. *J Exp Med* 1992;175:471–479.
52. Nonaka M, Ishikawa N, Passwell J, et al. Tissue specific initiation of murine complement factor B mRNA transcription. *J Immunol* 1989;142:1377–1382.
53. Ishikawa N, Nonaka M, Wetsel RA, Colten HR. Murine complement C2 and factor B genomic and cDNA cloning reveals different mechanisms for multiple transcripts of C2 and B. *J Biol Chem* 1990; 265:19040–19046.

54. Bentley DR. Primary structure of human complement component C2: homology of two unrelated protein families. *Biochem J* 1986;239:339–345.
55. Whitehead AS, Solomon E, Chambers S, et al. Assignment of the structural gene for the third component of human complement of chromosome 19. *Proc Natl Acad Sci USA* 1982;79:5021–5025.
56. DaSilva FP, Hoecker GE, Day NK, et al. Murine complement component 3: genetic variation and linkage to H-2. *Proc Natl Acad Sci USA* 1978;75:963–965.
57. Khan SA, Erickson BW. An equilibrium model of the metastable binding sites of alpha 2 macroglobulin and complement proteins C3 and C4. *J Biol Chem* 1982;257:11864–11867.
58. Tack BF, Janatova J, Thomas ML. The third, fourth, and fifth components of human complement: isolation and biochemical properties. *Methods Enzymol* 1981;80:64–101.
59. Hugli TE. Biochemistry and biology of anaphylotoxins. *Complement* 1986;3:111–127.
60. Wetsel RA, Barnum SR. Molecular biology and biochemistry of the third (C3) and fifth (C5) complement components. In: Sim RB, ed. *Biochemistry and Molecular Biology of Complement.* Lancaster: MTP Press Ltd. (in press).
61. Colten HR, Alper CA. Hemolytic efficiencies of genetic variants of human C3. *J Immunol* 1972;108: 1184–1187.
62. Pangburn MK. The alternative pathway. In: Ross GD, ed., *Immunobiology of the Complement System.* New York: Academic Press, 1986;45–62.
63. Muller-Eberhard HJ. Molecular organization and function of the complement system. *Annu Rev Biochem* 1988;57:321–347.
64. Alper CA, Abramson N, Johnston RB, et al. Increased susceptibility to infection associated with abnormalities of complement-mediated functions and of the third component of complement (C3). *N Engl J Med* 1970;282:349–354.
65. Dieli F, Lio D, Sereci G, Salerno A. Genetic control of C3 production by the S region of the mouse MHC. *J Immunogenet* 1988;15:339–343.
66. Kawamura N, Singer L, Wetsel RA, Colten HR. Cis- and transacting elements required for constitutive and cytokine (IL-1/IL-6) regulated expression of the murine complement C3 gene. *Biochem J* 1992;283:705–712.
67. Wilson DR, Juan TSC, Wilde MD, et al. A 58-base pair region of the human C3 gene confers synergistic inducibility by interleukin-1 and interleukin-6. *Mol Cell Biol* 1990;10:6181–6191.
68. Strunk RC, Whitehead AS, Cole FS. Pretranslational regulation of the synthesis of the third component of complement in human mononuclear phagocytes by the lipid A portion of lipopolysaccharide. *J Clin Invest* 1985;76:985–990.
69. Beutler B, Cerami A. The biology of cachectin/tumor necrosis factor—a primary mediatory of the host response. *Ann Rev Immunol* 1989;7:625–656.
70. St. John Sutton MB, Strunk RC, Cole FS. Regulation of the synthesis of the third component of complement and factor B in cord blood monocytes by lipopolysaccharide. *J Immunol* 1986;136: 1366–1372.
71. Colten HR. Tissue specific regulation of inflammation. *J Appl Physiol* 1992;72:1–7.
72. Kulics J, Colten HR, Perlmutter DH. Counter-regulatory effects of interferon-γ and endotoxin on expression of the human C4 genes. *J Clin Invest* 1990;85:943–949.
73. Perlmutter DH, Colten HR. Molecular basis of complement deficiencies. *Immunodeficiency Rev* 1989;1:105–134.
74. Circolo A, Pierce GF, Katz Y, Strunk RC. Antiinflammatory effects of polypeptide growth factors. Platelet-derived growth factor, epidermal growth factor, and fibroblast growth factor inhibit the cytokine-induced expression of the alternative complement pathway activator factor B in human fibroblasts. *J Biol Chem* 1990;265:5066–5071.
75. Circolo A, Welgus HG, Pierce GF, et al. Differential regulation of the expression of proteinases/ antiproteinases in fibroblasts. Effects of interleukin-1 and platelet-derived growth factor. *J Biol Chem* 1991;266:12283–12288.
76. Ruddy S, Colten HR. Rheumatoid arthritis: biosynthesis of complement proteins by synovial tissues. *N Engl J Med* 1974;290:1284–1288.

Organ Metabolism and Nutrition:
Ideas for Future Critical Care, edited by
J. M. Kinney and H. N. Tucker.
Raven Press, Ltd., New York © 1994.

8

Tolerance and Susceptibility to Bacterial Endotoxins

Sander J. H. van Deventer

Center for Thrombosis, Hemostasis, Atherosclerosis, and Inflammation Research, Academic Medical Center, 1105 AZ, Amsterdam, The Netherlands

Serious bacterial infections cause profound immunologic and metabolic changes that are thought to enable a normal host-defense response. In this process, the coagulation, fibrinolytic, and complement pathways also become activated, and leukocytes are induced to release eicosanoids, oxygen radical species, and proinflammatory proteins. These host-defense responses constitute a fine-tuned immune defense network that is necessary for successful clearance of bacterial infections. Uncontrolled release of inflammatory mediators, however, may cause profound tissue damage and organ failure and, finally, even may result in the demise of the host. Overwhelming gram-negative and gram-positive bacterial infections cause very similar clinical syndromes, generally referred to as "sepsis syndrome," or, more recently, as "systemic immune response syndrome" (SIRS). The mortality of these syndromes is at least 30%, and, when complicated by shock or the adult respiratory distress syndrome (ARDS), may approach 80%. For many years, gram-negative bacterial lipopolysaccharides, endotoxins, have been recognized as important toxic molecules that are intimately involved in the pathogenesis of sepsis. The biological effects of endotoxin (referred to as "endotoxicity") are almost completely caused by induction of the biosynthesis and release of endogenous inflammatory and immunomodulating proteins (cytokines), in particular, tumor necrosis factor, interleukin-1, and interferon γ. Hence, the sepsis syndrome can be considered a disregulated host immune reaction, that, in the case of gram-negative infection, is incited by endotoxin and mediated by uncontrolled cytokine release. It should be appreciated that, with the exception of fulminant meningococcemia, no clear relationship exists between the amount of circulating endotoxin and clinical outcome. Patients may succumb with circulating endotoxin levels that in healthy volunteers cause only minor discomfort, whereas others may survive significant endotoxemia. These observations indicate that individual patients differ in their susceptibility to endotoxin, and that these differences are important for outcome. In fact, results from experimental sepsis studies have indicated that even within one individual the effects of endotoxin may dramatically change in the course of bacterial infection. This chapter discusses genetic and phenotypic bases for differences in sensitivity to endotoxin that have been observed in experimental animals and in humans. Evidence is presented that high and low endotoxin responder phenotypes are in linkage disequilibrium with certain HLA-haplotypes as well as specific restriction fragment polymorphisms within the HLA class III region. Specific responder types may also be related to an increased susceptibility to (autoimmune) inflammatory diseases. Furthermore, studies are reviewed that provide data that the genetically determined individual susceptibility to endotoxin in large part, but not exclusively, results from differences in the endogenous production of cytokines, in particular, interferon-γ (IFNγ) and tumor necrosis factor-α (TNF). Several other proteins importantly modulate endotoxin sensitivity by enhancing or preventing the binding of endotoxin to membrane proteins on immunocompetent cells or by neutralization of endotoxin. Because the serum concentrations of these proteins are influenced by bacterial infections, they may become additional factors that determine endotoxin sensitivity in the course of infectious disease.

ENDOTOXIN

Endotoxins constitute a family of lipopolysaccharides that are present in the gram-negative bacterial outer-cell membrane. Although extensive structural heterogeneity exists between endotoxins that are derived from different bacteria, some general principles exist. Endotoxins consist of a polysaccharide chain (extending in the environment) and a lipid moiety, named lipid A, that in its natural conformation serves to anchor the endotoxin molecule within the bacterial membrane (1). The polysaccharide chain is antigenically the most diverse structure but contributes little if anything to endotoxicity. On the other hand, in pathogenic gram-negative bacteria, lipid A is relatively well conserved and is responsible for nearly all endotoxin effects. Lipid A's from enterobacteria consist of a β-1'6-linked biphosphorylated D-diglucosamine backbone to which, in general, four hydroxy fatty acids are attached. The number, position, and conformation of these fatty acids has been shown to be a major determinant of endotoxicity (2). Although all enterobacterial lipid A's tested thus far are active in standard endotoxin assays, such as Limulus activation, rabbit pyrogenicity, Shwartzman reaction, and tolerance induction, their relative biological potency may vary. The only biological assay with sufficient sensitivity to detect endotoxin in blood is the Limulus assay, which is based on activation of certain coagulation factors present in a lysate of hemolymph of the horseshoe crab *(Limulus polyphemus)*. In the original assay, the presence of endotoxin was detected by the formation of a gel from a lysate of Limulus amebocyte lysate. The introduction of chromogenic substrates has improved the sensitivity of the assay and enabled quantitative assessment (3). When interpreting endotoxin test results from clinical trials, it should be kept in mind that over- or underestimation of the amount of endotoxin measured is a result of comparison of Limulus activation by the various enterobacterial endotoxins present in the test sample with a standard curve produced with *Escherichia coli* endotoxin.

Furthermore, it is important to consider the complex relationship between gram-negative bacteremia and endotoxemia. In its natural conformation, completely embedded within the outer membrane, it is not likely that lipid A can have biological effects. In order to cause toxicity, endotoxin therefore needs to be released from bacteria. Endotoxin release can follow death of bacteria and in this process can be enhanced by complement factors, phagocytic cells, and antibiotic treatment. When quantitatively cultured, the number of viable circulating bacteria in gram-negative sepsis frequently is less than 10^2/ml, which, even in case of complete lysis and endotoxin liberation, is not enough to generate a sufficient amount of endotoxin to result in a positive Limulus assay, indicating that most endotoxin detected in these cases is derived from dead bacteria that have either disintegrated within the circulation or at local tissue sites. Likewise, in experimental gram-negative bacteremia a rise in endotoxin levels can be detected following antibiotic treatment, coinciding with a rapid decline in bacterial counts (4). In this model the animals may ultimately succumb with low bacterial counts but high endotoxin levels. Finally, in nonselected febrile patients, gram-negative bacteremia may often be present in the absence of measurable endotoxemia, and these patients are not likely to develop clinical criteria for the sepsis syndrome (5). In patients who are both bacteremic and endotoxemic, however, a high risk for the subsequent development of clinical symptoms of sepsis, such as hypotension, oliguria, and coagulation activation, was demonstrated (5).

TUMOR NECROSIS FACTOR

History and Biological Effects

Circulating bioactive human TNF is a 51-kd nonglycosylated protein that consists of three identical noncovalently linked subunits. TNF was originally isolated as a serum factor that transferred necrosis of certain tumors in BCG-treated mice (6). Although TNF is toxic for certain tumor cells, the observed hemorrhagic necrosis of transplantable mouse tumors more likely results from its procoagulant effects, which cause thrombosis of the vessels feeding the tumor (7), than from cytotoxicity. A few years after its initial discovery, TNF was shown to be identical to cachectin, a protein that caused down-regulation of lipoprotein lipase on 3T3 adipocytes, and was held responsible for the hypertriglyceridemia and cachexia that complicates canine trypanosomiasis (8). The metabolic effects of TNF, as well as its relationship to cachexia, are complex, however, and are presently subject to controversy. Soon after the disclosure of the identity of TNF and cachectin, TNF's pivotal role in the pathogenesis of sepsis was demonstrated. Injection of purified murine TNF in mice caused hypotension and organ damage (9), and pretreatment with fab_2 anti-TNF antibody fragments prevented death in baboons that were challenged with *Escherichia coli* (10). These findings, as well as clinical studies that demonstrated a correlation between serum TNF levels and mortality in sepsis (11), led to the identification of TNF as a target for intervention immunotherapy in sepsis. Subsequent studies using various anti-TNF antibodies in various experimental sepsis models have yielded miscellaneous results, however. In general, protection of anti-TNF strategies was shown in most models that were characterized by acute overwhelming intravascular infection. In contrast, in an increasing number of experimental models of more chronic local infection caused by either bacteria or parasites, neutralization of TNF has been reported to increase morbidity or mortality (12). These studies indicate that TNF is a necessary host-defense factor, but that either overproduction or increased sensitivity to its biological effects can be detrimental. It therefore became important to identify factors that regulate TNF biosynthesis and to correlate TNF "responsiveness" to human disease.

Regulation of TNF Gene Transcription

Because TNF was found to be such an important inflammatory mediator, considerable attention has focused on the regulation of TNF gene transcription. Early studies focused on the mouse TNF gene, but the elements that have been found to be important for regulation of the murine TNF gene have been found to be relatively well conserved among mammalian species. Nevertheless, the interspecies homology of the TNF genes is strongest in the coding regions. The murine as well as the human TNF genes are located in tandem with the lymphotoxin gene, and the two genes are separated by a mere 1,000 base pairs. Such diverse stimuli as ionizing radiation, cell adherence, and various bacterial products may increase TNF synthesis, but the most potent TNF inducer known is endotoxin. Because in many cells endotoxin importantly induces TNF, but not lymphotoxin, it was hypothesized that most TNF gene regulatory elements would be located in the 5', 1,000 base pair untranslated region that separates the two genes. These *cis*-acting regulatory elements in the mouse TNF gene have been studied using 5' deletion analysis as well as electrophoretic mobility shift assays that detect DNA/transcription factor binding interactions (13,14). More recently, constructs have been engineered in which TNF gene promoter sequences were coupled to reporter genes (15). In summary, these experiments disclosed the importance of nuclear factor kappa B (NFκB) as a major regulator of TNF gene transcription. Kappa B is defined as a DNA sequence that forms a potential binding site for NFκB, an endotoxin-inducible transcription factor that consists of a 50- to 67-kd protein heterodimer (16). Assessment of the functional importance of these binding sites in the murine TNF promoter revealed that at least two of the five κB sites present in the murine TNF promoter can bind NFκB (15). In addition, the κB sites may also bind another transcription factor, nuclear factor granulocyte-monocyte-a (NFGMa) (17,18). NFGMa has been shown to be able to bind to at least two of the NFκB sites in the murine TNF promoter, but at present it remains unknown whether binding results in increased TNF gene transcription. It is even possible that NFGMa competes with NFκB and therefore negatively influences TNF gene transcription. Although NFκB has been identified as a major regulator of TNF gene transcription, other transcription factor binding sites, including NF-Y are located in the TNF promoter region (15), and potentially are involved in TNF synthesis regulation.

Other regulatory mechanisms contribute to the rate of TNF production, and probably serve to safeguard against the potentially lethal consequences of its uncontrolled release. TNF mRNA has a very short half-life, presumably because of rapid degradation. The TNF mRNA instability is related to the presence of AU-rich motifs (UUAU-UUAU) in the 3' untranslated region (19). These elements, are also known as Kamen and Shaw regions (20), are present in many cytokine and oncogene mRNAs and may represent a ribonuclease (RNA-se) attack site (21). In addition, these AU motifs have been demonstrated to interfere with translation of TNF mRNA (22,23) and therefore are important for the regulation of TNF synthesis at multiple levels. Recently, the importance of the 3'-untranslated region for expression of the TNF gene was demonstrated using constructs of a chloramphenicol reporter gene with 5'- and 3'-untranslated TNF sequences (24). These experiments, which were performed in nonhematopoietic cells (that do not normally synthesize TNF), indicated that (constitutive) expression of TNF in these cells is silenced by the presence of the 3'-untranslated region. In constructs that lacked the 3'-untranslated region, CAT expression was demonstrated even when NFκB sites were lacking.

Other experiments have demonstrated an important additional synthesis regulatory function of the TNF translation process. Endotoxin, for example, does not only increase TNF transcription, but also importantly enhances the translation rate (25), and the well-known inhibitory effect of corticosteroids on TNF synthesis in part results from interference with endotoxin-induced translation derepression (26). Similarly, cyclosporin inhibits TNF transcription as well as translation, although the mechanism of action remains to be determined (27).

In conclusion, TNF transcription is tightly regulated at both the transcriptional and translational levels. NFκB is a major regulator of TNF gene transcription, whereas the function of NFGMa remains to be determined. AU-rich motifs in the 3'-untranslated region render TNF mRNA short-lived and interfere with its translation. Finally, other yet to be identified factors tightly regulate the TNF mRNA translation rate, possibly by constitutive repression.

TNF Gene Polymorphisms, TNF Responsiveness, and (Autoimmune) Disease

The TNF and lymphotoxin genes are located in tandem within the major histocompatibility complex (MHC) between the HLA-B and the HLA class III genes (28,29). Because multiple associations between certain HLA haplotypes and autoimmune diseases are known, it has been hypothesized that differences in TNF synthesis rate (or bioactivity) might explain this relationship. Presumptive evidence for this hypothesis was provided by experiments in a mouse model for lupus nephritis (30). (NZBxNZW)F1 mice develop lupuslike nephritis and have a *decreased* capability to synthesize TNF that correlates to a certain restriction fragment length polymorphism (RFLP). Moreover, TNF administration in this model prevents the development of lupus nephritis (30). DR2- and DQW1-positive patients with systemic lupus erythematosus have an increased risk for nephritis, and both HLA-haplotypes are also correlated to a decreased capability to synthesize TNF after stimulation of peripheral blood lymphocytes (31). Encouraged by these findings, several groups have searched for individual differences in TNF synthesis rates ("TNF responder types") (32,33) and for markers within the TNF gene that would facilitate linkage of HLA-haplotypes or TNF responder types with (auto)immune disease. Indeed, large interindividual differences were demonstrated in the amount of TNF produced in whole blood, by peripheral blood mononuclear cells, or by enriched monocytes after stimulation with either PMA or endotoxin. Experiments in endotoxin-challenged volunteers also revealed large differences in the individual endotoxin responsiveness. After injection of endotoxin (lot EC-5, 2 ng/kg), a short-lived (45 minutes) low-level (peak level 12 to 15 ng/l) endotoxemia was detected using a chromogenic Limulus assay, and the endotoxin levels in all volunteers were very similar. Nearly tenfold differences in TNF response were demonstrated, however (34), and the TNF level closely correlated with the levels of IL-6, granulocytopenia, fever, and with parameters for activation of the coagulation and fibrinolytic systems (35). Clearly, the interindividual differences in TNF responder type are not in vitro artifacts. The quest for detectable polymorphisms in the TNF gene that could be used to rapidly demonstrate differences in TNF-responder types has been less successful, however. In contrast to the HLA-class I (A genes), class II (DR genes) regions, and the class III complement genes, the human TNF gene displays no diversity when analyzed with pulsed-field megabase scale electrophoresis of restriction fragments (36). A more detailed restriction fragment analysis of the TNF gene, using multiple restriction enzymes, revealed only a single Nco1 polymorphism, characterized by a 10.5-kb allele and a less frequent 5.3-kb allele (37). Nevertheless, this restriction fragment polymorphism has been linked to primary biliary cirrhosis, which is negatively associated with the 10.5-kb allele (38), and to diabetes mellitus, in which disease group 5.3- to 10.5-kb allele heterozygotes are overrepresented (39). It has been subsequently reported, however, that the Nco1 polymorphism is in fact located within the first intron of the lymphotoxin gene rather than in the TNF gene, and that the Nco1 polymorphism corresponds to a decreased level of lymphotoxin (rather than TNF) production (40), although these latter results have not been confirmed by others (41). Hence, the Nco1 polymorphism, previously thought to indicate a TNF gene polymorphism, has been shown to have no direct relationship with TNF responsiveness. These results notwithstanding, the case for differences in TNF production rate as a pathogenic factor in autoimmune disease is not closed. In recent years, "microsatellites" have proven their usefulness as markers for polymorphism. Microsatellites are short $(CA)_n$ or $(CT)_n$ repeats within the genome that differ in the number of dinucleotide repeats. The length of a certain microsatellite after polymerase chain reaction (PCR) amplification can therefore be used as an allelic marker. The discovery of a unique microsatellite polymorphism within the ("autoimmune") NZW mouse strain TNF gene promoter region, closely linked to the Y-box (42), led to speculations on the possible role of this CA repeat in TNF gene regulation and prompted a renewed search for TNF polymorphisms in (autoimmune) diseases. Using PCR-based microsatellite mapping techniques, three polymorphic microsatellites (named TNFa, TNFb, and TNFc) have been identified within a 12-kb region of the human histocompatibility complex that includes the TNF gene (43). The TNFc microsatellite is located within the first intron of the lymphotoxin gene, whereas TNFa and TNFb, which display extensive polymorphism (13 and 7 alleles, respectively), are located about 3.5 kb upstream of the lymphotoxin gene. Hence, in the human genome (in contrast to mice), no microsatellites are located within the TNF promoter region, which makes a direct regulatory function unlikely. These polymorphisms are useful, however, to study the relationship between TNF gene-related polymorphisms in more detail, in particular in view of their linkage disequilibrium with alleles located in the HLA class I, class II, and class III loci and their association with some extended HLA haplotypes. The association of certain TNF microsatellite alleles with TNF responder types has not yet been reported, however.

In conclusion, their is ample evidence that individuals differ in the amount of TNF produced by mononuclear cells in response to various stimuli, including endotoxin. These differences are linked to certain HLA haplotypes and polymorphisms in the TNF gene locus. Microsatellite mapping now provides an important tool for investigating these relationships in more detail.

SERUM PROTEINS THAT BIND ENDOTOXIN

Many proteins present in normal human serum bind endotoxin, and most of these interactions are nonspecific. Using a radioiodinated photoactivatible endotoxin derivative that transfers the radiolabeled to the proteins that it binds, labeling of albumin, immunoglobulin G, complement component 3, apolipoproteins, and several unidentified proteins has been reported (44). Results from recent studies indicate that two related proteins are of particular importance for the regulation of endotoxicity. First identified as a factor that interfered with binding of endotoxin to lipoproteins, lipopolysaccharide-binding protein (LBP) is now known to importantly regulate the effects of endotoxin on target cells. LBP is an acute-phase protein with an apparent molecular weight of 55 kd that binds to lipid A (45). The endotoxin-LBP complex can subsequently bind to CD14, a phosphatidyl inositol-linked membrane protein present on monocytes and macrophages (46), and this results in a ten- to 100-fold upregulation of the amount of TNF that is produced by monocytes in response to endotoxin stimulation. It should be noted that in the complete absence of LBP (or CD14), monocytes can be activated by endotoxin, although the amount of TNF produced is less than in the presence of an intact CD14/LBP pathway. Although none of the candidate proteins has yet been cloned, these results are compatible with the existence of specific endotoxin receptors (see discussion that follows). Activation of CD14 presumably causes an additional signal that up-regulates the responsiveness to endotoxin stimulation. Because LBP is an acute-phase protein, its levels are expected to increase during the course of infection, thereby potentially enhancing the susceptibility of the host. A second protein, related to LBP, that is involved in modulation of the biological effects of endotoxin in vivo is bactericidal permeability-increasing protein (BPI). This protein was first identified as one of several neutrophil-derived bactericidal proteins (47), and subsequently it was demonstrated that BPI binds endotoxin (48), resulting in a neutralization of several of its biological effects. After stimulation with endotoxin, TNF, or f-methionyl-leucyl-phenylaline (fMPL), most BPI remains bound to the neutrophil membrane, and it is possible that, in that position, it scavenges endotoxin. Free circulating BPI (in levels up to 100 ng/l) can be detected in patients with gram-negative sepsis, however, (von der Möhlen and Marra, manuscript in preparation), and it is tempting to speculate about its role as a circulating endotoxin-neutralizing protein. Finally, most healthy humans have substantial levels of antibodies that recognize endotoxin. Antibodies that are generated against epitopes on the outer polysaccharide endotoxin chain may neutralize endotoxin and are responsible for the phenomena of "late tolerance" (see next section). In addition some of the "naturally" occurring antibodies are crossreactive (in particular when the epitopes recognized are on conserved parts of the molecule, such as the core region or lipid A) and may in part determine outcome in septic shock.

ENDOTOXIN RESISTANCE AND HYPERRESPONSIVENESS

C3H/HeJ Mice

In 1965 a mouse strain (C3H/HeJ) was reported to be highly resistant to Salmonella endotoxin (49; for comprehensive review see ref. 50). The greatly reduced sensitivity of C3H/HeJ mice to endotoxin-induced lethality was subsequently mapped to a locus (named *Lps*) on chromosome 4, in close proximity to the interferon α genes (51). The cause of the reduced responsiveness of C3H/HeJ mice to endotoxin has not been completely unraveled. Fusion of cells from C3H/HeJ mice with endotoxin-responsive cells confers endotoxin responsiveness (52). Because Sendai virus-induced insertion of fragments of normal cell membrane in C3H/HeJ cells also restored endotoxin responsiveness (53), it is probable that the C3H/HeJ defect is associated with alterations of the cell membrane. Differences in accessibility of gangliosides between normal and C3H/HeJ membranes have been described (54), and because certain gangliosides can bind endotoxin (55), these differences may be involved in altered recognition of endotoxin by C3H/HeJ cells. Interestingly, an 80-kd endotoxin-binding protein (that possibly represents an endotoxin receptor) is normally expressed on C3H/HeJ cells (56), but activation of the receptor by agonistic monoclonal antibodies on C3H/HeJ macrophages did not cause the increased tumoricidal effects that were observed in normal cells (57). In vivo endotoxin sensitivity in large part is a result of macrophage responsiveness. C3H/HeJ macrophages are poor producers of many endotoxin-inducible inflammatory factors, including TNF, IL-1, IL-6, interferons, and prostaglandins, and transplantation of normal bone marrow to irradiated C3H/HeJ mice rendered normal endotoxin sensitivity to the recipients (58). More specifically, a defect of C3H/HeJ macrophages to synthesize interferon α/β may explain the increased sensitivity of C3H/HeJ mice to bacterial infections (see sections that follow). Furthermore, in recent years it has become apparent that many cytokines play an important role in the host-defense system, and subnormal production or therapeutic neutralization of TNF and IL-1 may result in an inability to clear bacterial infections (59). This in part may explain why C3H/HeJ mice have an increased susceptibility to infection.

Galactosamine

Like most other experimental animals, mice are relatively resistant to the effects of endotoxin in comparison with humans. Mice can be rendered more than 100,000 times more sensitive to endotoxin, however, by pretreatment with D-galactosamine. The endotoxin-sensitizing effect of D-galactosamine is related to its effect on hepatocytes, but it is unrelated to the well-known D-galactosamine hepatoxicity. Liver injury occurs only after prolonged D-galactosamine administration, whereas the endotoxin-sensitizing effect is apparent almost immediately and extends for only a few hours. Although endotoxin sensitization by D-galactosamine has been shown to be correlated in time with depletion of uridine triphosphate (UTP) from the liver (60), and uridine administration prevents this effect, the exact biochemical basis for its effect has not been defined exactly (for review, see 61). D-galactosamine–induced hepatocyte UTP depletion occurs in endotoxin-resistant as well as endotoxin-sensitive mice, but sensitization occurs only in LPS-sensitive mice. D-galactosamine also potently sensitizes mice to TNF, and in this respect the endotoxin-sensitive and -resistant mice respond equally (61). In summary, D-galactosamine, through a yet unknown effect on hepatocytes that is related to depletion of UTP, causes potent sensitization to the effects of TNF in both endotoxin-resistant and endotoxin-sensitive mice, but sensitization to endotoxin in endotoxin-sensitive mice only. These data indicate that C3H/HeJ mice completely lack the capacity to respond to (purified) endotoxin, but their more peripheral inflammatory responses seem to be normal.

Bacterial Infections and Interferon Gamma

In the course of bacterial infections, the sensitivity to endotoxin may dramatically increase. One of the well-known models of sensitization of mice to the effects of endotoxin, for example, is infection with live bacille Calmette-Guérin (BCG) (62). Interestingly, even C3H/HeJ mice can be rendered endotoxin-sensitive by mycobacterial infection, even though they remain endotoxin resistant after D-galactosamine pretreatment (63). Normal and endotoxin-resistant mice can also be sensitized to endotoxin by gram-negative bacteria, for example by *Salmonella typhimurium* (64). In this experimental model, the amount of circulating TNF following injection of endotoxin dramatically and progressively increases 3 days after the onset of infection. Not only does bacterial infection increase the sensitivity to endotoxin, infected animals also become more sensitive to the biological effects of TNF. In the *S. typhimurium* model, for example, the LD_{50} of TNF increased tenfold (61). Endotoxin-sensitization by gram-negative bacterial infection presumably does not (entirely) depend on the endotoxin because it also occurs during gram-positive infections and in animals that bear growing malignant tumors (65), and it can be induced in C3H/HeJ mice.

Endotoxin is a relatively poor inducer of IFN-γ in mice (66), but substantial serum levels can be detected in lethal gram-negative bacteremia in baboons and in patients with fulminant meningococcemia (11). In mice, the ability to produce IFN subsides several days after splenectomy (67) and can be restored either by transfer of rat or (glass adherent) mouse splenocytes or by transfer of splenocyte culture supernatants (for review, see ref. 68). The ability of C3H/HeJ mice to synthesize IFN in response to endotoxin was also restored by transplantation of bone marrow from syngeic endotoxin-sensitive (C3H/HeN) mice (58). It therefore seems that bone marrow–derived cells (or a soluble factor derived from these cells) are necessary for endotoxin-induced IFN production, and indeed, macrophages may be stimulated in vitro by endotoxin to secrete IFN (69). It should be noted, however, that different macrophages have a different capacity to produce IFN, that some macrophages need to be "primed" in order to produce significant amounts of IFN (70), and that most IFN produced in these experiments has been characterized as IFN-α and IFN-β (71). In animals that have been rendered hypersensitive for endotoxin by bacterial infections, large amounts of immunoreactive IFN-γ can be detected in the circulation, however (72). The cellular source of the IFN-γ that is released in endotoxin hypersensitivity states is not precisely known, but it appears that both macrophages and T cells are necessary for its induction (63). One study reported that after stimulation by gram-positive bacteria and endotoxin, macrophages synthesized soluble factors that stimulated IFN-γ production by IL-2 pretreated NK cells (63), and TNF was necessary, but not sufficient for this effect. Results from several recent studies in mice are in accordance with the concept that IFN-γ is intimately involved in the endotoxin hypersensitivity that arises in the course of bacterial infection. Administration of IFN-γ antibodies importantly reduced the amount of TNF that was induced in mice rendered endotoxin hypersensitive by *Proprionibacterium acnes* injection (61). Neutralization of IFN-γ in this model in fact prevented the sensitization to endotoxin, and the LD_{50} for endotoxin in antibody-treated mice was 1,000-fold higher than in control (endotoxin-sensitized) animals. Another important finding in this study was that administration of IFN-γ antibodies still decreased mortality when administered as late as 7 days after the onset of infection, albeit that early treatment yielded better results. In another study, neutralization of IFN-γ also prevented the endotoxin-induced local and generalized Shwartzman reaction (73), and a similar intervention recently has been reported to reduce the mortality of *E. coli* sepsis in mice (74). The latter experiment importantly differs from the *Corynebacterium parvium* or BCG models of endotoxin hypersensitivity. In the endotoxin-sensitization experiments, hypersensitivity is first induced by low-grade bacterial infection and later tested by injection of endotoxin or TNF, whereas in the *E. coli* sepsis model, the infecting bacteria directly are responsible for the observed mortality. In addition, in contrast to endotoxin-sensitization models, no decrease of the amount of endotoxin-induced TNF release was observed following IFN-γ antibody treatment of *E. coli* sepsis. Nevertheless, the beneficial results of IFN-γ antibody treatment of gram-negative sepsis in mice are compatible with the hypothesis that, even in acute and fulminant sepsis, an endotoxin hypersensitivity state exists, and that in this situation, the responsiveness to TNF may be increased.

Endotoxin Tolerance

Not only can sensitivity to endotoxin be increased, in certain circumstances substantial tolerance to its biological activities can be achieved. The first observations on endotoxin tolerance stem from clinical experiences with continuous infusion of (pyrogenic) gram-negative "therapeutic" vaccines (for review, see ref. 75). It was noted that although a pyrogenic response invariably was detected early after the start of the infusion of such vaccines, several hours later the body temperature returned to normal, despite continuous infusion, indicating that tolerance to the pyrogenic effects of the vaccine had occurred. In healthy volunteers, tolerance can also be induced by continuous infusion of endotoxin (76), but does not occur when the endotoxin infusion is interrupted and resumed on the next day (75). In fact, interrupted endotoxin infusion causes an exaggerated febrile response upon reinfusion on the second day, which only blunts after several days of interrupted endotoxin challenges. These experiments therefore revealed two types of endotoxin tolerance: "early" and "late" tolerance. It is now known that the biological mechanisms responsible for early and late tolerance differ importantly. Late tolerance can be transferred by infusion of plasma or serum (77) and is endotoxin specific. In other words, serum obtained in animals that are in a state of late tolerance against a specific endotoxin molecule does not confer tolerance against that particular endotoxin molecule but not against antigenically different endotoxin molecules. These observations therefore led to the now well-accepted notion that late tolerance resulted from the generation of antiendotoxin antibodies (particularly against the O-chain), which formed the basis for clinical trials in septic patients using crossreactive hyperimmune antiendotoxin antisera (78).

Early tolerance importantly differs from late tolerance because it cannot be transferred by plasma or serum and crossprotects against antigenically different endotoxins. Akin to endotoxin sensitization, early endotoxin tolerance results from modulation of the endotoxin responsiveness of mononuclear cells and can be demonstrated in vitro (79). Importantly, in this latter experiment the (minute) endotoxin dose that was used to produce tolerance did not induce detectable TNF mRNA induction, but it prevented TNF induction by a subsequent challenge using a high endotoxin dose. D-galactosamine pretreated mice can also be rendered endotoxin tolerant by low-dose endotoxin, and in this model the amount of TNF that is generated in response to the second endotoxin challenge is importantly reduced (61). Of potential clinical importance was the observation that tolerance could be induced in mice that were rendered endotoxin hypersensitive by bacterial infections (61). The tolerance that was achieved in this model, however, was shorter-lived (5 to 24 hours as opposed to several days) and less absolute when compared with the tolerance induced in D-galactosamine–sensitized mice. Although at present clinical experience is limited, it appears that lipid A analogs that have reduced endotoxicity may induce endotoxin tolerance in humans. One of these analogs is monophosphoryl lipid A (MLA), which is derived from endotoxin by acid hydrolysis (for review, see ref. 80), and recently a lipid A precursor has also been shown to block endotoxin-induced TNF synthesis in whole human blood (81).

Endotoxin interacts in a complicated manner with the human host. Endotoxin-induced release of cytokines is necessary for a normal host-defense response, and complete inhibition of this response may cause immunologic paralysis. On the other hand, endotoxin has been implicated as one of the main causal factors in the pathogenesis of gram-negative shock. In nonmeningococcal septic shock, however, no clear dose-effect relationship seems to exist between the amount of circulating endotoxin and clinical outcome, and septic patients may die with rather low endotoxin levels. Large interindividual differences exist in the susceptibility to endotoxin, which is in part genetically determined. Apart from a genotypic "endotoxin responder type," bacterial infections, as well as endotoxin itself, can alter importantly the reactivity to endotoxin, resulting in either hyperresponsiveness or tolerance. Based on these observations, it is likely that septic shock in patients with low-level endotoxemia results from endotoxin hyperresponsiveness. In addition to IFN-γ and TNF, it may be that BPI and LBP are involved in endotoxin responsiveness and may open new opportunities for the treatment of sepsis.

REFERENCES

1. Rietschel E, Brade L, Lindner B, Zähringer U. Molecular biochemistry of lipopolysaccharides. In: Ryan JL, Morrison DC, eds. *Bacterial Endotoxic Lipopolysaccharides*, vol. 1. Boca Raton: CRC Press, 1992:3–42.
2. Takada H, Kotani S. Structure-function relationships of lipid A. In: Ryan JL, Morrison DC, eds. *Bacterial Endotoxic Lipopolysaccharides*, vol. 1. Boca Raton: CRC Press, 1992;107–134.
3. Van Deventer SJH, Pauw W, ten Cate JW, et al. Clinical evaluation of febrile patients of an optimized endotoxin assay in blood. *Prog Clin Biol Res* 1987;231:489–499.
4. Shenep JL, Flynn PM, Barrett FF, Stidham GL, et al. Serial quantitation of endotoxemia and bacteremia during therapy for gram-negative bacterial sepsis. *J Infect Dis* 1988;157:565–568.
5. Van Deventer SJH, Büller HR, ten Cate JW, et al. Endotoxaemia: an early predictor of septicaemia in febrile patients. *Lancet* 1988;I:605–609.
6. Carswell EA, Old LJ, Kassel RJ, et al. An endotoxin-induced serum factor that causes necrosis of tumors. *Proc Natl Acad Sci USA* 1975;72:3666–3670.
7. Clauss M, Ryan J, Stern D. Modulation of endothelial cell hemostatic properties by TNF: insights into the role of endothelium in the host response to inflammatory stimuli. In: Beutler B, ed. *Tumor Necrosis Factors. The Molecules and Their Emerging Role in Medicine*. New York: Raven Press, 1922;49–63.
8. Beutler B, Greenwald D, Hulmes JD, et al. Identity of tumour necrosis factor and the macrophage-secreted factor cachectin. *Nature* 1985;316:552–554.
9. Beutler B, Milsark IW, Cerami A. Passive immunization against cachectin/tumor necrosis factor (TNF) protects mice from the lethal effect of endotoxin. *Science* 1985;229:869–871.
10. Tracey KJ, Fong Y, Hesse DG, et al. Anti-cachectin/TNF monoclonal antibodies prevent septic shock during lethal bacteraemia. *Nature* 1987;330:662–664.
11. Girardin E, Grau GE, Dayer JM, et al. Tumor necrosis factor and interleukin-1 in the serum of children with severe infectious purpura. *N Engl J Med* 1988;319:397–400.

12. Bagby GJ, Plessala KJ, Wilson LA, et al. Divergent efficacy of antibody to tumor necrosis factor-alpha in intravascular and peritonitis models of sepsis. *J Infect Dis* 1991;163:83–88.
13. Collart MA, Bäuerle P, Vassali P. Regulation of tumor necrosis factor-α transcription in macrophages: involvement of four κB-like motifs and of constitutive and inducible forms of NF-κB. *Mol Cell Biol* 1990;10:1498–1506.
14. Shakhov AN, Collart MA, Vassalli P, et al. κB-type enhancers are involved in lipopolysaccharide-mediated transcriptional activation of the tumor necrosis factor-α gene in primary macrophages. *J Exp Med* 1990;171:35–47.
15. Jongeneel CV. The TNF and lymphotoxin promoters. In Beutler B, ed. Tumor necrosis factors, the molecules and their emerging role in medicine. New York: Raven Press, 1992;539–559.
16. Sen R, Baltimore D. Multiple nuclear factors interact with the immunoglobulin enhancer sequences. *Cell* 1986;46:705–716.
17. Schreck R, Bäuerle PA. NF-κB as inducible transcriptional activator of the granulocyte-macrophage colony-stimulating factor gene. *Mol Cell Biol* 1990;10:1281–1286.
18. Shannon MF, Gamble JR, Vadas MA. Nuclear proteins interacting with the promoter region of the human granulocyte/monocyte colony-stimulating factor gene. *Proc Natl Acad Sci USA* 1988;85:674–678.
19. Caput D, Beutler B, Hartog K, et al. Identification of a common nucleotide sequence in the 3'-untranslated region of mRNA molecules specifying inflammatory mediators. *Proc Natl Acad Sci USA* 1986;83:1670–1674.
20. Shaw G, Kamen R. A conserved AU-rich sequence from the 3' untranslated region of GM-CSF mRNA mediates selective mRNA degradation. *Cell* 1986;46:659–667.
21. Wilson T, Treisman R. Removal of poly(A) and consequent degradation of c-fos mRNA facilitated by 3' AU-rich sequences. *Nature* 1988;336:396–399.
22. Kruys VI, Wathelet MG, Huez GA. Identification of a translation inhibitory element (TIE) in the 3' untranslated region of the human interferon-β mRNA. *Gene* 1988;72:191–200.
23. Kruys V, Marinx O, Shaw G, et al. Translational blockade imposed by cytokine-derived AU-rich sequences. *Science* 1989;245:852–855.
24. Kruys V, Kemmer K, Shakhov A, et al. Constitive activity of the tumor necrosis factor promoter is canceled by the 3' untranslated region in nonmacrophage cell lines; a transdominant factor overcomes this suppressive effect. *Proc Natl Acad Sci USA* 1992;89:673–677.
25. Han J, Brown T, Beutler B. Endotoxin-responsive sequences control cachectin/tumor necrosis factor biosynthesis at the translational level. *J Exp Med* 1990;171:465–475.
26. Han J, Thompson P, Beutler B. Dexamethasone and pentoxitylline inhibit endotoxin-induced cachectin/tumor necrosis factor synthesis at separate points in the signaling pathway. *J Exp Med* 1990;172:391–394.
27. Remick D, Nguyen DT, Eskandari MK, et al. *Biochem Biophys Res Commun* 1989;161:551–555.
28. Dunham I, Sargent CA, Trowsdale J, Campbell RD. Molecular mapping of the human major histocompatibility complex by pulsed-field gel electrophoresis. *Proc Natl Acad Sci USA* 1987;84:7237.
29. Carroll MC, Katzman P, Alicott EM, et al. Linkage map of the human major histocompatibility complex including the tumor necrosis factor genes. *Proc Natl Acad Sci USA* 1987;84:8535.
30. Jacob CO, McDevitt HO. Tumor necrosis factor α in murine autoimmune 'lupus' nephritis. *Nature* 1988;331:356.
31. Jacob CO, Fronel Z, Lewis GD, et al. Heritable major histocompatibility complex class II-associated differences in production of tumor necrosis factor α: relevance to genetic predisposition to systemic lupus erythematosus. *Proc Natl Acad Sci USA* 1990;87:1233–1237.
32. Bendtzen K, Morling A, Fomsgaard A, et al. Association between HLA-DR2 and production of tumour necrosis factor α and interleukin 1 by mononuclear cells activated by lipopolysaccharide. *Scand J Immunol* 1988;28:599–606.
33. Santamaria P, Gehrz RC, Bryan MK, Barbosa JJ. Involvement of class II MHC molecules in the LPS-induction of IL1/TNF secretion by human monocytes. *J Immunol* 1989;143:913–922.
34. Derkx HHF, Bruin KF, Jongeneel CV, van Deventer SJH. LPS reactivity of monocytes and TNF gene polymorphism. In: R van Furth, ed. *Mononuclear Phagocytes. Biology of Monocytes and Macrophages.* Boston: Kluwer Dordrecht, 1992;355–358.
35. Van Deventer SJH, Buller HR, ten Cate JW, et al. Experimental endotoxemia in humans: analysis of cytokine release and coagulation, fibrinolytic and complement pathways. *Blood* 1990;76:2520–2526.
36. Lawrence SK, Smith CL. Megabase scale restriction fragment length polymorphism in the human major histocompatibility complex. *Genomics* 1990;8:394–399.

37. Dawkins RL, Leaver A, Cameron PU, et al. Some disease-associated ancestral haplotypes carry a polymorphism of TNF. *Hum Immunol* 1989;26:91.29.
38. Fugger L, Morling N, Ryder LP, et al. Nco1 restriction length polymorphism (RFLP) of the tumor necrosis factor (TNF-α) region in primary biliary cirrhosis and in healthy Danes. *Scand J Immunol* 1989;30:185.
39. Badenhoop K, Schwartz G, Trowsdale J, et al. TNF-α gene polymorphism in type 1 (insulin-dependent) diabetes mellitus. *Diabetologica* 1989;32:445.
40. Messer G, Spengler U, Jung MC, et al. Polymorphic structure of the tumor necrosis factor (TNF) locus: an Nco1 polymorphism in the first intron of the human TNF-β gene correlates with a variant amino acid in position 26 and a reduced level of TNF-β production. *J Exp Med* 1991;173:209–219.
41. Sachs JA, Whichelow CE, Hitman GA, et al. The effect of HLA and insulin dependent diabetes mellitus on the secretion levels of tumor necrosis factor alpha and beta and gamma interferon. *Scand J Immunol* 1990;32:703–708.
42. Jongeneel CV, Acha-Orbea H, Blankenstein T. A polymorphic microsatellite in the tumor necrosis factor α promoter identifies an allele unique to the NZW mouse strain. *J Exp Med* 1990;171:2141–2146.
43. Jongeneel CV, Briant L, Udalova IA, et al. Extensive genetic polymorphism in the human tumor necrosis factor region and relation to extended HLA haplotypes. *Proc Natl Acad Sci USA* 1991;88: 9717–9721.
44. Tesh VL, Vukajlovitch SW, Morrison DC. Endotoxin interactions with serum proteins. Relationship to biological activity. *Prog Clin Biol Res* 1988;272:47–62.
45. Tobias PS, Soldau K, Ulevitch RJ. Identification of a lipid A binding site in the acute phase reactant lipopolysaccharide binding protein. *J Biol Chem* 1989;264:10867–10871.
46. Wright SD, Ramos RA, Tobias PS, et al. CD14, a receptor for complexes of lipopolysaccharide (LPS) and LPS binding protein. *Science* 1990;249:1431–1433.
47. Weiss J, Elsbach P, Olsson I, Odeberg H. Purification and characterization of a potent bactericidal and membrane active protein from the granules of human polymorphonuclear proteins. *J Biol Chem* 1978;253:2664.
48. Marra M, Wilde CG, Collins MS, et al. The role of bactericidal/permeability-increasing protein as a natural inhibitor of bacterial endotoxin. *J Immunol* 1992;148:532–537.
49. Heppner G, Weis DW. High susceptibility of strain A mice to endotoxin and endotoxin-red blood cell mixtures. *J Bacteriol* 1965;90:696–703.
50. Vogel SN. The LPS gene. In: Beutler B, ed. *Tumor Necrosis Factors. The Molecules and Their Emerging Role in Medicine.* New York: Raven Press, 1992;485–513.
51. Fultz MJ, Vogel SN. The physical separation of LPS and Ia loci in BXH recombinant inbred mice. *J Immunol* 1989;143:3001–3006.
52. Watanabe T, Ohara J. Functional nuclei of LPS-non-responder C3H/HeJ mice after transfer into LPS-responder C3H/HeN cells by cell fusion. *Nature* 1981;290:58–59.
53. Jacobavits A, Sharon N, Zan-Bar I. Acquisition of mitogenic responsiveness by nonresponding lymphocytes upon insertion of appropriate membrane components. *J Exp Med* 1982;156:1274–1279.
54. Yohe HC, Berenson CS, Cuny CL, et al. Altered B-lymphocyte membrane architecture indicated by ganglioside accessibility in C3H/HeJ mice. *Infect Immun* 1990;58:2888–2894.
55. Ryan JL, Gobran L, Morrison DC. Modulation of murine macrophage metabolism by glycolipids: inhibition of LPS-induced metabolism by specific gangliosides. *J Leukocyte Biol* 1989;40:367–379.
56. Bright SW, Chen T-Y, Flebbe LM, et al. Generation and characterization of hamster/mouse hybridomas secreting monoclonal antibodies with specificity for lipopolysaccharide receptor. *J Immunol* 1990;145:1–7.
57. Chen T-Y, Bright SW, Pace JL, et al. Induction of macrophage-mediated tumor cytotoxicity by a hamster monoclonal antibody with specificity for lipopolysaccharide receptor. *J Immunol* 1990;145: 8–12.
58. Michalek SM, Moore RN, McGhee, et al. The primary role of lymphoreticular cells in the mediation of host responses to bacterial endotoxin. *J Infect Dis* 1980;141:55–63.
59. Echtenacher B, Falk W, Mannel DN, Krammer PH. Requirement of endogenous tumor necrosis factor/cachectin for recovery from experimental peritonitis. *J Immunol* 1990;145:3762–3766.
60. Galanos C, Freudenberg MA, Reutter W. Galactosamine-induced sensitization to the lethal effects of endotoxin. *Proc Natl Acad Sci USA* 1979;76:5939.
61. Galanos C, Freudenberg MA, Katschinski T, et al. Tumor necrosis factor and host response to endotoxin. In: Ryan JL, Morrison DC, eds. *Bacterial Endotoxic Lipopolysaccharides*, vol. 2. Boca Raton: CRC Press, 1992;75–104.

62. Suter E, Ullman GE, Hoffmann RG. Sensitivity of mice to endotoxin after vaccination with BCG (Bacillus Calmette Guerin). *Proc Soc Exp Biol Med* 1958;99:167.
63. Vogel SN, Moore RN, Sipe JD, Rosenstreich DL. BCG-induced enhancement of endotoxin sensitivity in C3H HeJ mice. I. In vivo studies. *J Immunol* 1980;124:2004.
64. Matsuura M, Galanos C. Induction of hypersensitivity to endotoxin and tumor necrosis factor by sublethal infection with *Salmonella typhymurium*. *Infect Immun* 1990;58:935.
65. Bartoleyns J, Freudenberg MA, Galanos C. Growing tumors induce hypersensitivity to endotoxin and tumor necrosis factor. *Infect Immun* 1987;55:2230.
66. Heinzel FP. The role of IFN-γ in the pathology of experimental endotoxemia. *J Immunol* 1990;145: 2920.
67. Ito Y, Kunii A, Mori N, Nagata I. Effects of splenectomy on production of endotoxin type interferon in mice. *Virology* 1971;44:638.
68. Vogel SN. Lipopolysaccharide-induced interferon. In: Ryan JL, Morrison DC, eds. *Bacterial Endotoxic Lipopolysaccharides*, vol. 2. Boca Raton: CRC Press, 1992;165–196.
69. Fleit HB, Rabinovitch M. Production of interferon by in vitro derived bone marrow macrophages. *Cell Immunol* 1981;51:495.
70. Havell EA, Spitalny GL. Endotoxin-induced interferon synthesis in macrophages cultures. *J Reticuloendothel Soc* 1983;33:369.
71. Belardelli F, Gessani S, Proietti E, et al. Studies on the expression of spontaneous and induced interferons in mouse peritoneal macrophages by means of monoclonal antibodies to mouse interferons. *J Gen Virol* 1987;68:2203.
72. Kiener PA, Marek F, Rodgers G, et al. Induction of tumor necrosis factor, IFN-γ, and acute lethality in mice by toxic and non-toxic forms of lipid A. *J Immunol* 1988;141:870.
73. Heremans H, van Damme J, Dillen C, et al. Interferon gamma, a mediator of lethal lipopolysaccharide-induced Shwartzman-like shock reactions in mice. *J Exp Med* 1990;171:1853–1869.
74. Silva AT, Cohen J. Role of interferon-γ in experimental gram-negative sepsis. *J Infect Dis* 1992;166: 331–335.
75. Johnston CA, Greisman SE. Mechanisms of endotoxin tolerance. In: Hinshaw LB, ed. *Handbook of Endotoxin*, vol II. Amsterdam: Elsevier, 1985;359–401.
76. Greisman SE, Woodward WE. Mechanisms of endotoxin tolerance. III. The refractory state during continuous intravenous infusions of endotoxin. *J Exp Med* 1965;121:911–933.
77. Greisman SE, Young EJ, DuBuy B. Mechanisms of endotoxin tolerance. VIII. Specificity of serum transfer. *J Immunol* 1973;111:1349–1360.
78. Ziegler EJ, McCutchan JA, Fierer J, et al. Treatment of gram-negative bacteremia and shock with human antiserum to a mutant *Escherichia coli*. *N Engl J Med* 1982;307:1225–1230.
79. Mathison JC, Virca GD, Wolfson E, et al. Adaptation to bacterial lipopolysaccharide controls lipopolysaccharide-induced tumor necrosis factor production in rabbit macrophages. *J Clin Invest* 1990;85: 1108.
80. Von Eschen K. Monophosphoryl lipid A and immunotherapy. In: Ryan JL, Morrison DC, eds. *Bacterial Endotoxic Lipopolysaccharides*, vol II. Boca Raton: CRC Press, 1992;411–428.
81. Kovak NL, Yee E, Munford RS, et al. Lipid IV_A inhibits synthesis and release of tumor necrosis factor induced by lipopolysaccharide in human whole blood *ex vivo*. *J Exp Med* 1990;172:77.

Organ Metabolism and Nutrition:
Ideas for Future Critical Care, edited by
J. M. Kinney and H. N. Tucker.
Raven Press, Ltd., New York © 1994.

9

Cytokine Interaction and Clinical Response

Terje Espevik, Anders Sundan, Nina B. Liabakk, and
Anders Waage

The Institute of Cancer Research, University Medical Center, Trondheim N-7005, Norway

Cytokines are protein hormones that transmit signals from one cell to another. This family of proteins has potent effects on different cell types, and the activity of one particular cytokine can often be enhanced or inhibited by other cytokines. Thus, cytokines interact with each other and constitute a complex network of overlapping signals. These proteins mediate their effects by first binding to specific receptors on the cell membrane. The main function of cytokines is to regulate cell responses associated with inflammation and immunity. Several cytokines such as tumor necrosis factor (TNF), interleukin-1 (IL-1), IL-6, and interferon-γ (IFN-γ) have been implicated as mediators of gram-negative sepsis. In this chapter we focus on our work on mechanisms of cytokine induction by lipopolysaccharide (LPS). In relevance to this we also review some of our data on the involvement of cytokines and cytokine interaction during gram-negative sepsis.

MECHANISMS OF LIPOPOLYSACCHARIDE EFFECTS

Lipopolysaccharide from gram-negative bacteria consists of a lipid A and a polysaccharide part of various size and complexity (1). Monocytes produce large quantities of TNF in response to LPS, which stimulates both translation and transcription of TNF mRNA (2). Addition of LPS to monocytes results in a rapid and transient accumulation of TNF in perinuclear vesicles, which can be detected by immunofluorescence microscopy after 20 minutes (3). Production of TNF from monocytes follows the pathway typical for secretory proteins as it involves passage through the secretory apparatus (3). The release of LPS during gram-negative infections may result in high levels of TNF, which has been shown to be one of the effector molecules in septic shock (4,5).

Many of the toxic and immunomodulating activities of LPS are reported to be mediated by the lipid A part (6,7). However, synthetic lipid A has weak or no cytokine stimulatory activity on monocytes (8), suggesting that the lipid A and the polysaccharide part of LPS are cooperatively involved for maximal cytokine stimulation. Recent studies have shown that LPS may interact with monocytes by first forming a complex with LPS-binding protein (LBP) (9,10). The binding of LPS-LBP complex to membrane-bound CD14, a glycosylphosphatidyl inositol (GPI)–anchored protein, results in TNF production from monocytes, indicating that CD14 is one of the functional receptors for LPS (10). We have found that defined polysaccharides such as β1-4 linked poly uronic acids also induce TNF production through mechanisms which involve CD14 (11). The implication of this finding is that the involvement of CD14 in the stimulation of TNF production is not restricted to LPS.

Recent studies have indicated that serum also contains an activity distinct from LBP, termed "septin," which enables LPS to bind to CD14 (12). This novel LPS opsonic activity in plasma is blocked by addition of protease inhibitors, and the properties of septin are suggestive of the action of a protease cascade distinctly different from the complement system (12).

Lipopolysaccharide can also stimulate cells that do not express membrane CD14, which indicates that a wide variety of different cell types are affected by LPS. For example, human umbilical vein endothelial cells respond to LPS with increased expression of tissue factor (13), endothelial-leukocyte adhesion molecule 1 (ELAM-1) (14), and IL-6 (15). Lipopolysaccharide may also have toxic effects on endothelial cells. Of particular importance is that LPS toxicity on endothelial cells is enhanced by cytokines such as TNF and IL-1 (16). The astrocytoma cell line U373 responds to LPS with strong synthesis of IL-6 (11). CD14 has not been reported to be present on the surface of U373 cells or endothelial cells. We found that CD14 is essential for response of each of these cell types to LPS, but that the CD14 is derived from the soluble CD14 present in serum, not from the surface of the responding cell (16). This phenomenon is illustrated for U373 cells in Fig. 1. U373 cells respond to LPS in a serum-dependent manner by secretion of IL-6. Addition of LBP will not enhance the LPS response in these cells, which do not express CD14 on their surface. This result confirms that binding of LPS-LBP complexes to membrane CD14 does not account for the observed IL-6 production in U373 cells and indicates that serum contains factors in addition to LBP that are required for cell stimulation. Addition of soluble CD14 enables a strong LPS-dependent stimulation of IL-6 production (Fig. 1; ref. 17). These data suggest that soluble CD14 in plasma may play a significant role in response of animals to LPS, and that CD14 may play a role in the responses of many cell types lacking membrane CD14 (Table 1). How soluble CD14, without a GPI anchor, mediates signal transduction is unclear. One possibility is that soluble CD14 interacts with an additional receptor subunit on U373 cells and endothelial cells after binding of CD14 to LPS-LBP or LPS-septin complexes. This hypothesis is similar to the IL-6 receptor where the ligand-binding 80-kd subunit of the IL-6 receptor interacts with a signal-transducing 130-kd subunit only after binding to IL-6 (18). In addition, both soluble as well as membrane-bound 80-kd proteins may bind IL-6, associate with the 130-kd subunit, and transduce a signal (18). A lot more work is still required to understand the LPS recognition mechanisms and the subsequent intracellular events involved in LPS responses.

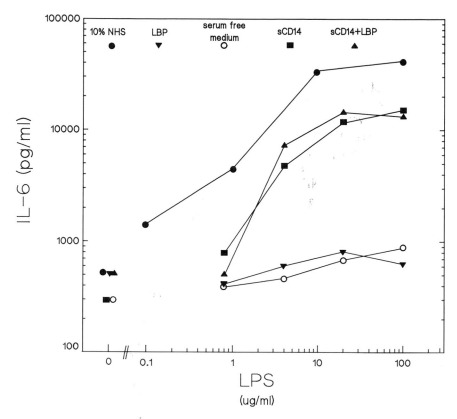

FIG. 1. Soluble CD14 is required for induction of IL-6 in U373 cells by LPS. Different concentrations of LPS were added to U373 cells in AIM serum-free medium (Gibco) (o) with 100 ng/ml LPS-binding protein (LBP) (▼), 10 ng/ml soluble CD14 (■), or 100 ng/ml LPB + 10 ng/ml soluble CD14 (▲). The LPS response in 10% normal human serum (NHS) (●) was included for comparison. Supernatants were harvested after 24 hours and assayed for IL-6 levels. Reproduced from Frey et al. (17), with permission.

TABLE 1. *Summary of effects of LPS on monocytes and U373 cells.*

	Monocytes	U373
Expression of membrane CD14	Yes	No
Effects induced by LPS	Cytokine production	IL-6 production
Serum-dependent LPS response	Yes	Yes
LPS response increased by LBP	Yes	No
Inhibition of LPS response by antiCD14	Yes	Yes
LPS response increased by sCD14*	No	Yes

* sCD14; soluble CD14 isolated from urine of nephrotic patients.

CYTOKINES IN SEPTIC SHOCK

The Role of Tumor Necrosis Factor

Release of LPS from gram-negative bacteria may result in sepsis, which is characterized by hypotension, tachycardia, hyperglycemia, electrolyte abnormalities, fluid retention, and fever. The manifestation of the sepsis is apparently induced by host-derived mediators such as cytokines. The evidence that TNF is involved in septic shock was originally provided by Beutler et al. who treated mice with antiserum against TNF and observed a significant reduction in LPS lethality (4). Further support for the involvement of TNF in septic shock comes from histopathologic and pathophysiologic studies showing similarities between LPS and TNF effects in dogs and rats (19,20). Histopathologic studies of TNF-treated mice show pronounced accumulation of granulocytes in small vessels in intestine, lungs, kidney, liver, and uterus, apparently adherent to the endothelial lining (21). Injection of TNF induces parenchymal cell damage in the kidney, with necrosis of single cells of the distal tubular epithelium (21). Similar histopathologic changes can also be observed in the liver and lung after TNF administration. The fact that the kidney, lungs, and liver were the organs most affected is consistent with biodistribution studies demonstrating that these organs contained the highest levels of administered TNF per milligram of tissue in mice (22). The detailed mechanism behind TNF lethality is not known. However, the severe vessel congestion that occurs in the lung after TNF administration may result in respiratory failure. In addition, the procoagulant activity of TNF appears to be important (23) and may contribute to the disseminated intravascular coagulation seen in most patients with septic shock.

Further support for the view that TNF is a mediator of septic shock comes from patients with meningococcal disease (5). In a study of 79 patients we found that 10 of 11 patients who died had TNF in serum, whereas only 8 of 68 patients who survived had TNF in serum. In addition, there appeared to be a critical serum TNF concentration above which all patients died. This study demonstrated that TNF in serum is strongly associated with septic shock and fatal outcome.

The Role of IL-1

TNF and IL-1 share many biological activities, and IL-1 is likely to be an important mediator in septic shock. In rabbits, IL-1 induces hypotension and histopathologic changes similar to TNF (24,25). IL-1 is lethal for actinomycin-D–treated mice, although with a less potency than TNF (21). When IL-1 is given together with TNF to mice, it markedly potentiates the lethal effects of TNF (26). Figure 2 shows results from experiments with combinations of TNF and IL-1 administered to mice. In the group of mice receiving recombinant IL-1α, all mice survived, whereas 14 of 15 survived in the group receiving 0.5 μg of recombinant murine TNF. However, when IL-1 and TNF were given together, all mice died. This result demonstrates that IL-1 potentiates the lethal effects of TNF and illustrates very clearly how cytokines may interact to increase biological effects.

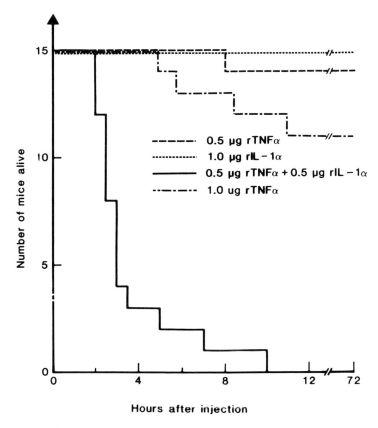

FIG. 2. Effects of TNF and/or IL-1 on lethality in mice. Reproduced from Waage and Espevik (26), with permission.

IL-1 activity can also be detected in serum from patients with meningococcal disease (27). Of patients studied who had TNF in serum, the patients with IL-1 activity in serum had the shortest life expectancy. This observation is consistent with the IL-1 potentiating effect of TNF in mice. The involvement of IL-1 in septic shock has been elegantly shown by Ohlsson et al. (28) who demonstrated protection of LPS lethality in rabbits by administrating IL-1 receptor antagonist (IL-1ra) to the animals. Injection of IL-1ra reduces the severity of diseases in several animal models, which illustrates the importance of IL-1 as an effector molecule in many pathologic conditions (for review, see ref. 29).

The Role of IFN-γ, IL-6, and IL-8

Similar to TNF, high levels of IFN-γ are associated with severe shock and fatal outcome in patients with meningococcal disease (30). IFN-γ is a T-cell–derived cytokine that can be detected in serum during bacteraemia (31). Injection of IFN-γ in actinomycin-D–sensitized mice indicates that this cytokine alone is well tolerated (21); however, IFN-γ potentiates the lethal effect of TNF (32). Recently, Doherty et al. (33) showed that antibodies against IFN-γ markedly reduced the toxic and lethal effects of both LPS and TNF, suggesting that IFN-γ activity is required for the lethal effects of TNF.

Another cytokine, IL-6, has also been thought to play a role in acute infection. IL-6 was detected in almost all serum samples from patients with meningococcal meningitis, bacteremia, septic shock, or a combination of these (27). However, patients with septic shock had about 1,000 times higher concentrations compared to patients with other manifestations. In experimental models IL-6 does not mediate any lethal effects (21) and does not seem to potentiate the lethal effects of TNF (Waage, unpublished data). IL-6 induces the production of acute-phase proteins (34) and induces fever (35). The involvement of IL-6 in septic shock is not clear. Starnes et al. (36) have provided data indicating that antibodies against IL-6 protect mice against lethal *Escherichia coli* infection. It has also been proposed that IL-6 may play a protective role in this syndrome, as IL-6 inhibits both IL-1 and TNF production (37). Altogether, the exact role of IL-6 in septic shock is not clear.

Lipopolysaccharide can stimulate monocytes to produce several cytokines in addition to IL-1, TNF, and IL-6. Neutrophil-activating protein–IL-8 is a recently characterized cytokine that functions as a chemoattractant and activator for neutrophils and also as a chemoattractant for lymphocytes. IL-8 is produced in response to LPS and zymosan as well as the cytokines TNF and IL-1. Circulating levels of IL-8 have been detected in patients with septic shock (38). Furthermore, elevated levels of IL-8 in serum are associated with lethality in meningococcal disease (39). Despite these indications of possible involvement of IL-8 in septic shock, IL-8 is not lethal when injected into actinomycin-treated mice (21). However, despite lack of evidence that IL-8 has acute toxicity, IL-8 may interact with TNF and IL-1 to attract neutrophils to the tissue sites of inflammation. Thus, the chemotactic activity of IL-8 could result in complications at later time points in septic infections.

The detection of granulocyte colony–stimulating factor in a patient with bacterial infection has been reported (40), but the role of this cytokine in relation to the pathogenesis of infection or shock is unclear. Serum samples from patients with meningococcal disease have also been examined for the presence of IL-2 and lymphotoxin, but all samples were negative (27).

KINETICS OF PRODUCTION AND ELIMINATION OF CYTOKINES

Lipopolysaccharide is the principal inducer of TNF production, and the main source of systemically released TNF is likely to be the monocytes and macrophages. When LPS is injected into human volunteers, the TNF levels markedly rise within 2 hours and thereafter decline to background levels after 4 hours (41). The same release pattern has been demonstrated in all species investigated and seems to be universal (42–44). The burst release of TNF is thus an early event in endotoxinemia.

In patients with meningococcal septic shock we analyzed consecutively collected serum samples for the presence of TNF (27). The first samples were taken at admission time, which appeared to be later than the peak concentration. Tumor necrosis factor was eliminated at a constant rate in half of the patients, and the half-life of TNF was calculated to be 72 minutes in these patients. In the other half of the patients there was a constant elimination rate of TNF after admission, but additional release occurred at a later time. In all patients TNF activity was completely eliminated within 18 hours. The release and elimination pattern in meningococcal patients is thus similar to that in experimental animals, although there may be other release mechanisms responsible for the late release of TNF observed in some patients.

IL-1 is difficult to measure in serum by bioassays due to the presence of inhibitory activity (45). During experimental endotoxemia in humans, the IL-1β levels rarely exceed 500 pg/ml, and production of a small amount of IL-1 and a large amount of the IL-1ra appears to be a natural response in serum to bacterial infections (46). In other compartments of the organism, such as the subarachnoid space, the LPS-induced IL-1 release occurs later than TNF but prior to IL-6 (47). It is reasonable to believe that the same situation takes place in the systemic circulation as well. The peak of IL-6 occurs about 2 hours after injection of LPS in mice (48), and the same kinetics of release are also found in human volunteers (49). Thus, IL-6 is released after TNF under experimental conditions. The release of IL-6 after TNF can also be observed in serum samples consecutively drawn from meningococcal septic shock patients (27). Tumor necrosis factor and IL-1 are potent inducers of IL-6, especially in endothelial cells (15). Peak concentrations of IL-6 in serum from mice can be detected 1 hour after injection of TNF, IL-1, or LPS (48). Thus, TNF and IL-1 may be involved in LPS-induced IL-6 production in vivo. Injection of mice with antibodies against TNF concomitantly with LPS results in a significant reduction in IL-6 peak levels (48), suggesting that TNF may act as an intermediate mediator in LPS-induced IL-6 production.

In summary, the following initial reactions are likely to occur in septic shock. Gram-negative bacteria invade the organism and multiply in the circulation, resulting in increasing serum levels of LPS. When a certain LPS level is attained, a burst of TNF is released from the monocytes within 1 to 2 hours. Thirty to 60 minutes after the TNF burst, IL-6 is released into the circulation in a similar manner, partly because of TNF–IL-1 stimulation of monocytes and endothelial cells. The release of IL-1 in serum probably occurs inbetween that of TNF and IL-6.

TOLERANCE TO LIPOPOLYSACCHARIDE AND THE PROTECTIVE ROLE OF TUMOR NECROSIS FACTOR–IL-1 IN BACTERIAL INFECTIONS

After the initial burst of TNF release, the monocytes become resistant to the TNF-inducing effect of LPS. This can, for example, be demonstrated in rats. By giving two consecutive bolus injections of LPS, it can be shown that the peak concentration of TNF after the second injection is only 15% of the peak concentration after the first injection (44). This LPS tolerance in rats lasts for at least 3 days (44). In addition, macrophages isolated from patients with sepsis do not produce TNF upon LPS stimulation (50). This may be explained by exposure of LPS during the early phase of the disease, resulting in resistance of the macrophages to LPS.

The release of a burst of high amounts of TNF and other cytokines during septic shock clearly mediates harmful effects to the organism. However, there are several studies indicating that the physiologic effects of TNF and IL-1 is to protect the organism against bacterial infections. The dual role of TNF was first proposed for infections with malaria parasites (51). Low concentrations of TNF appeared to protect against malaria disease, whereas high TNF concentrations were present concomitantly with the manifestation of severe malaria. Small doses of TNF, IL-1, or LPS given to mice before injection of a lethal dose of TNF or LPS results in marked protection against lethality. A similar protection by TNF and IL-1 can also be observed in bacterial infections (52,53). Injection of β1-4–linked polyuronic acids, which specifically stimulates CD14 positive cells (11) to produce cytokines, also protects against lethal LPS doses as well as lethal bacterial infections (Espevik, unpublished observations). The mechanism of protection by pretreatment with certain cytokines and cytokine inducers against bacterial infections or lethal LPS and TNF effects is not known in detail. TNF may cause down-regulation of the TNF receptors on the cell membrane due to internalization of the ligand-receptor complex, which, in turn, may decrease target cell interactions with TNF at later times. Tumor necrosis factor and IL-1 may also induce production of protective or repair proteins in target cells. For example, TNF and IL-1β have been shown to induce the production of manganous superoxide dismutase (54), which is a scavenger of toxic reactive oxygen species that are released in response to TNF treatment (55). The fact that protein-RNA synthesis inhibitors, such as Act-D, increase the susceptibility of mice to TNF lethality further emphasizes a role for induced proteins in the protection mechanism. Soluble TNF receptors, which are induced during sepsis, could be another protein source involved in the protection against TNF lethality.

SOLUBLE TUMOR NECROSIS FACTOR RECEPTORS

Tumor necrosis factor mediates a wide variety of biological responses that are likely to be due to the fact that TNF receptors (TFNRs) have been identified on most cell types in the organism. Two types of TNFRs with different molecular weights of 55 kd (p55) and 75 kd (p75), glycosylation pattern, and immunologic characteristics have been identified (56). The gene for both human and mouse TNFRs have been cloned and expressed (57–62). The cysteine rich extracellular domains of p55 and p75 share homology with each other and other cell-surface proteins (63,64), while the intracellular domains show no identity with each other, which indicates that p55 and p75 may use different mechanisms for intracellular signaling (65). Under physiologic conditions TNF is a trimer suggesting that aggregation of the TNFRs is necessary for transducing the signal into the cell. This is supported by data showing that divalent TNFR mabs may mimic different TNF activities (66). Data from Tartaglia and Goeddel suggest that p55 and p75 are involved in different cellular responses. For example, p55 is proposed to be involved in cytotoxicity, antiviral activity, fibroblast proliferation, and induction of NFκB, while p75 is involved in thymocyte proliferation and cytotoxic T-cell proliferation (67). On the other hand, we have found that antibodies against both p55 and p75 inhibit TNF-induced killing of U937 cells, suggesting that both types are involved in cytotoxicity (68). Heller et al. (69) have provided evidence also for the involvement of p75 in TNF-induced cytotoxicity. Human TNF binds to murine p55 but not murine p75 TNFR (65). Because human TNF is approximately 50-fold less toxic than murine TNF for mice, it has been suggested that the p75 is responsible for the systemic TNF toxicity in mice (70).

The extracellular domains of the TNFRs also exist in soluble forms in different biological fluids. Quantification of soluble TNFR fragments can be done by using mabs detecting a non-TNF binding site on the receptor and by using digoxigenin-labeled TNF as a probe for receptors immobilized to the TNFR mabs. We have developed mabs against non–TNF-binding sites of both p55 and p75 and applied them in immunoassays based on this principle (Fig. 3).

Increased levels of soluble TNFR have been observed in various conditions, such as fever (71), chronic lymphatic leukemia and various cancer types (72,73), and pregnancies (74). Increased serum levels of TNFR are also detected during meningococcal sepsis where the amounts of p75 are higher than p55 (75). Of particular interest is that the TNF-TNFR ratios are higher in patients with fatal outcome of meningococcal sepsis when compared with survivors (75). Thirty and 300 molar excesses of soluble p55 and p75, respectively, are required to inhibit TNF cytotoxicity by 50%, suggesting that p55 is more effective than p75 in neutralizing TNF activity (76). On the cell membrane, however, the affinity of p75 for TNF appears to be higher than for p55 (Fig. 4). Injection of LPS into human volunteers results in a serum TNFR peak 3 hours after injection (76). In these studies the p55 serum levels are slightly elevated compared with p75 levels. Several cell types are likely to be involved in the TNFR release during septic shock. Spinas et al. have obtained data indicating that the release in vivo of p55 and p75 fragments upon a short LPS exposure is regulated differently (77). Addition of LPS to human monocytes results in release of significant amounts of p75; however, the release of p55 was not above background (Fig. 5). In contrast to monocytes, LPS-responsive endothelial cells only release p55 fragments (Liabakk and Espevik, unpublished observations). These data suggest that monocytes and endothelial cells may contribute to the differential release of p55 and p75 TNFRs during septic shock.

Little is known about the exact mechanisms of TNFR release from cells. Lipopolysaccharide and TNF have been shown to induce TNFR release from monocytes and HL-60 cells, respectively (Fig. 5; ref. 78). In addition, IL-2, IL-7, and IL-12 stimulate NK cells to produce significant amounts of soluble p75 TNFR (79). Porteu et al. (80) have shown that the azurophilic granules of neutrophils contain a proteolytic activity that acts specifically on p75 and not on p55, resulting in shedding of p75 fragments from the cell surface. The TNFR-releasing effect was identified as an elastase-like

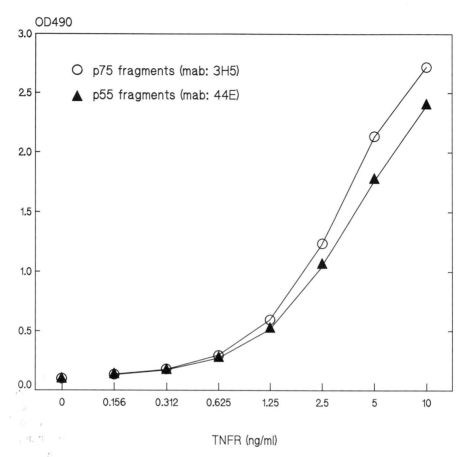

FIG. 3. Immunoassays for detection of p55 and p75 TNFR fragments. Immunowells were coated with monoclonal antibodies against p55 (44E) or against p75 (3H5). These two antibodies detect non–TNF-binding sites on the TNFRs. Different concentrations of recombinant p55 and p75 TNFR fragments were added to the wells. Bound TNFRs were quantitated by adding digoxigenin (DIG)–labeled TNF and peroxydase-conjugated anti-DIG. These TNFR assays are valuable tools for detecting TNFR fragments in various biological fluids.

activity. A proteolytic cleavage site in p55 has also been suggested (81). We have found that stimulation of monocytic leukemia cells (U937) with phorbol myristate acetate (PMA) resulted in release of p55 fragments in a biphasic manner (82). The first phase showed a rapid increase in the release of p55 fragments after PMA stimulation, while the second phase occurred at a much slower rate. Inhibitors of intracellular transport (brefeldin A and monensin) and protein synthesis (cycloheximide) inhibit the PMA-induced p55 release in the second phase but not in the first phase. In addition, increase in p55 mRNA expression can be observed only in the second phase. These data suggest that release of p55 from cells involves shedding and also requires protein synthesis (82).

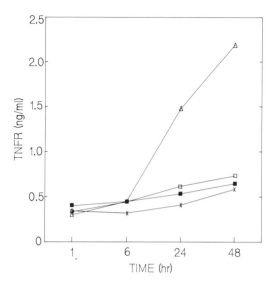

FIG. 4. Induction of soluble p75 TNFR fragments (△) in monocytes stimulated with 100-ng/ml LPS. Supernatants from monocytes were collected at the indicated times and assayed for TNFRs by the assay described in Fig. 3. LPS at 100 ng/ml did not result in increased p55 release (x) compared to unstimulated monocytes (■). The symbol (□) indicates the p75 TNFR levels in supernatants from unstimulated monocytes.

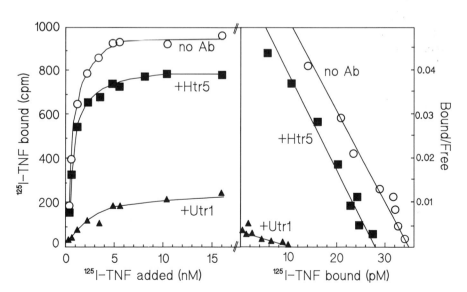

FIG. 5. Binding of ^{125}I-TNF to U937 cells in the absence or presence of either anti-p55 TNFR (Htr5) or anti-p75 TNFR (Utr1). The affinities of TNF binding in the presence of antibodies were estimated from the left panel and found to be $K_d^{TNF} = 0.5$ nM, $K_a^{p75} = 0.5$ nM, and $K_d^{p55} = 3.3$ nM. These data suggest that p75 has higher affinity for TNF than does p55.

Soluble Tumor Necrosis Factor Receptors and Protection Against Septic Shock

The physiologic significance of increased TNFR release in septic shock is not clear. TNFR release occurs during several and various conditions and is therefore not restricted to septic shock. Because TNFRs are expressed on all types of nucleated cells, TNFR release may occur easily during stress situations and may not have a particular physiologic function in vivo. On the other hand, soluble TNFR fragments may represent naturally occurring TNF inhibitors, which increase during inflammation and which may play an important role in modulating the biological activity of TNF. Neutralization of TNF may not be the sole function of soluble TNFR in vivo. Aderka et al. (83) have found that soluble TNFRs may augment TNF activities, probably by stabilizing its structure and preserving its activity. The ability of soluble TNFRs to stabilize TNF is not likely to be of any significance in the circulation where the clearance of TNF is rapid ($t_{0.5}$ ≈6 minutes) (84), unless it turns out that TNF is cleared at a much slower rate when bound to its receptor (83). In closed compartments, such as at an inflammatory site where the TNF clearance rate is much slower, soluble TNFRs may function as a buffer mechanism or "slow release reservoir" of bioactive TNF (83).

Administration of TNF inhibitors may provide a new treatment approach for sepsis. Clinical trials with TNF antibodies are now being performed both in the United States and Europe. An alternative to TNF antibodies for treatment of septic shock is the use of soluble TNFRs. Chimeric proteins containing the extracellular portion of human p55 TNFR and the hinge and Fc regions of human IgG heavy chain (p55-IgG) protect mice against lethal doses of LPS (84,85). The p55-IgG has significant higher affinity for TNF than soluble monomeric p55, which may be due to the bivalent binding to TNF. Protection against LPS lethality can be seen even when the p55-IgG is given shortly after LPS, which suggests that the time-window for treatment of septic shock may be extended by using p55-IgG. Administration of TNFR-IgG may represent a new therapeutic strategy that, hopefully, will have beneficial effects for the treatment of septic shock.

ACKNOWLEDGMENTS

This work has been supported by grants from the Norwegian Cancer Society, the Norwegian Technical Research Council, and the Norwegian Research Council for Science and Humanities.

REFERENCES

1. Raetz CRH. Biochemistry of endotoxins. *Annu Rev Biochem* 1990;59:129–170.
2. Beutler B, Krochin N, Milsark IW, et al. Control of cachectin (tumor necrosis factor) synthesis: mechanisms of endotoxin resistance. *Science* 1986;232:977–980.
3. Hofsli E, Bakke O, Nonstad U, Espevik T. A flow cytometric and immunofluorescence microscopic

study of tumor necrosis factor production and localization in human monocytes. *Cell Immunol* 1989; 122:405–415.
4. Beutler B, Milsark IW, Cerami AC. Passive immunization against cachectin/tumor necrosis factor protects mice from lethal effect of endotoxin. *Science* 1985;229:869–871.
5. Waage A, Halstensen A, Espevik T. Association between tumour necrosis factor in serum and fatal outcome in patients with meningococcal disease. *Lancet* 1987;i:355–357.
6. Feist W, Ulmer AJ, Musehold J, et al. Induction of tumor necrosis factor-alpha release by lipopolysaccharide and defined lipopolysaccharide partial structures. *Immunobiology* 1989;179:293–307.
7. Loppnow H, Brade H, Durrbaum I, et al. IL-1 induction-capacity of defined lipopolysaccharide partial structures. *J Immunol* 1989;142:3229–3238.
8. Rietschel ET, Seydel U, Zähringer U, et al. Bacterial endotoxin: molecular relationships between structure and activity. *Infect Dis Clin North Am* 1991;5:753–779.
9. Schumann RR, Leong SR, Flaggs GW, et al. Structure and function of lipopolysaccharide binding protein. *Science* 1990;249:1429–1433.
10. Wright SD, Ramos R, Tobias TS, et al. CD14, a receptor for complexes of lipopolysaccharide (LPS) and LPS binding protein. *Science* 1990;249:1431–1433.
11. Espevik T, Otterlei M, Skjåk-Bræk G, et al. The involvement of CD14 in stimulation of cytokine production by uronic acid polymers. *Eur J Immunol* 1993;23:255–261.
12. Wright SD, Ramos RA, Patel M, Miller DS. Septin: a factor in plasma that opsonizes lipopolysaccharide-bearing particles for recognition by CD14 on phagocytes. *J Exp Med* 1992;176:719–727.
13. Stern DM, Bank I, Nawroth PP, et al. Self-regulation of procoagulant events on the endothelial cell surface. *J Exp Med* 1985;162:1223–1235.
14. Bevilacqua MP, Pober JS, Mendrick DL, et al. Identification of an inducible endothelial-leukocyte adhesion molecule. *Proc Natl Acad Sci USA* 1987;84:9238–9242.
15. Shalaby MR, Waage A, Espevik T. Cytokine regulation of interleukin 6 production by human endothelial cells. *Cell Immunol* 1989;121:372–382.
16. Sharma SA, Olchowy TWJ, Yang Z, Breider MA. Tumor necrosis factor α and interleukin 1α enhance lipopolysaccharide-mediated bovine endothelial cell injury. *J Leukocyte Biol* 1992;51:579–585.
17. Frey EA, Miller DS, Gullstein Jahr T, et al. Soluble CD14 participates in the response of cell to lipopolysaccharide. *J Exp Med* 1992;176:1665–1671.
18. Taga T, Hibi M, Hirata Y, et al. Interleukin-6 triggers the association of its receptor with a possible signal transducer, gp130. *Cell* 1989;58:573–581.
19. Tracey KJ, Beutler B, Lowry SF, et al. Shock and tissue injury induced by recombinant human cachectin. *Science* 1986;234:470–474.
20. Tracey KJ, Lowry SF, Fahey TJ III, et al. Cachectin-tumor necrosis factor induces lethal shock and stress hormone responses in the dog. *Surg Gynecol Obstet* 1987;164:415–422.
21. Shalaby MR, Halgunset J, Haugen OA, et al. Cytokine-associated tissue injury and lethality in mice: a comparative study. *Clin Immunol Immunopathol* 1991;61:69–82.
22. Palladino MA, Shalaby MR, Kramer SM, et al. Characterization of the antitumor activities of human tumor necrosis factor-α and the comparison with other cytokines: induction of tumor-specific immunity. *J Immunol* 1987;138:4023–4032.
23. Bevilacqua MP, Pober JS, Majeau GR, et al. Recombinant tumor necrosis factor induces procoagulant activity in cultured human vascular endothelium: characterization and comparison with the actions of interleukin 1. *Proc Natl Acad Sci USA* 1986;83:4533–4537.
24. Okusawa S, Gelfrand JA, Ikejima T, et al. Interleukin 1 induces a shock-like state in rabbits. Synergism with tumor necrosis factor and the effect of cyclooxygenase inhibition. *J Clin Invest* 1988;81:1162–1172.
25. Weinberg JR, Wright DJM, Guz A. Interleukin-1 and tumour necrosis factor cause hypotension in the conscious rabbit. *Clin Sci* 1988;75:251–255.
26. Waage A, Espevik T. Interleukin 1 potentiates the lethal effect of tumor necrosis factor α/cachectin in mice. *J Exp Med* 1988;167:1987–1992.
27. Waage A, Brandtzaeg P, Halstensen A, et al. The complex pattern of cytokines in serum from patients with meningococcal septic shock. *J Exp Med* 1989;169:333–338.
28. Ohlsson K, Björk P, Bergenfeldt M, et al. Interleukin 1 receptor antagonist reduces mortality from endotoxin shock. *Nature* 1090;348:550–552.
29. Dinarello CA. Role of interleukin-1 and tumor necrosis factor in systemic responses to infection and inflammation. In: Gallin JI, Goldstein IM, Snyderman R, eds. *Inflammation: Basic Principles and Clinical Correlates,* 2nd ed. New York: Raven Press, 1992;211–232.

30. Girardin E, Grau GE, Dayer J-M, et al. Tumor necrosis factor and interleukin-1 in the serum of children with severe infectious purpura. *N Engl J Med* 1988;319:397–400.
31. Hesse DG, Tracey KJ, Fong Y, et al. Cytokine appearance in human endotoxemia and primate bacteremia. *Surg Gynecol Obstet* 1988;166:147–153.
32. Talmadge JE, Bowersox O, Tribble H, et al. Toxicity of tumor necrosis is synergistic with γ-interferon and can be reduced with cyclooxygenase inhibitors. *Am J Pathol* 1987;128:410–425.
33. Doherty GM, Lange JR, Langstein HN, et al. Evidence for IFN-γ as a mediator of the lethality of endotoxin and tumor necrosis factor-α. *J Immunol* 1992;149:1666–1670.
34. Gauldie J, Richards C, Harnish D, et al. Interferon β₂/B-cell stimulatory factor type 2 shares identity with monocyte-derived hepatocyte-stimulating factor and regulates the major acute phase protein response in liver cells. *Proc Natl Acad Sci USA* 1987;84:7251–7255.
35. Helle M, Brakenhoff JPJ, de Groot E, Aarden LA. Interleukin 6 is involved in interleukin 1-induced activities. *Eur J Immunol* 1988;18:957–959.
36. Starnes HF Jr, Pearce MK, Tewari A, et al. Anti-IL-6 monoclonal antibodies protect against lethal *Escherichia coli* infection and lethal tumor necrosis factor-α challenge in mice. *J Immunol* 1990;145:4185–4191.
37. Schindler R, Mancilla J, Endres S, et al. Correlations and interactions in the production of interleukin-6 (IL-6), IL-1, and tumor necrosis factor (TNF) in human blood mononuclear cells: IL-6 suppresses IL-1 and TNF. *Blood* 1990;75:40–47.
38. Hack CE, Hart M, van Schijndel JMS, et al. Interleukin-8 in sepsis: relation to shock and inflammatory mediators. *Infect Immun* 1992;60:2835–2842.
39. Halstensen A, Ceska M, Brandtzæg P, et al. Interleukin-8 in serum and cerebrospinal fluid from patients with meningococcal disease. *J Infect Dis* 1993; 167:471–475.
40. Watari K, Asano S, Shirafuji N, et al. Serum granulocyte colony-stimulating factor levels in healthy volunteers and patients with various disorders as estimated by enzyme immunoassay. *Blood* 1989;73:117–122.
41. Michie HR, Manogue KR, Spriggs DR, et al. Detection of circulating tumor necrosis factor after endotoxin administration. *N Engl J Med* 1988;318:1481–1486.
42. Beutler BA, Milsark IW, Cerami A. Cachectin/tumor necrosis factor: production, distribution and metabolic fate in vivo. *J Immunol* 1985;3972–3977.
43. Flick DA, Gifford GE. Production of tumor necrosis factor in unprimed mice: mechanism of endotoxin-mediated tumor necrosis. *Immunobiology* 1986;171:320–328.
44. Waage A. Production and clearance of tumor necrosis factor in rats exposed to endotoxin and dexamethasone. *Clin Immunol Immunopathol* 1987;45:348–355.
45. Larrick JW. Native interleukin 1 inhibitors. *Immunol Today* 1989;10:61–66.
46. Dinarello CA. Role of interleukin-1 in infectious diseases. *Immunol Rev* 1992;127:119–146.
47. Waage A, Halstensen A, Shalaby R, et al. Local production of tumor necrosis factor α, interleukin 1, and interleukin 6 in meningococcal meningitis: relation to the inflammatory response. *J Exp Med* 1989;170:1859–1867.
48. Shalaby R, Waage A, Aarden L, Espevik T. Endotoxin, tumor necrosis factor-alpha/cachectin and interleukin 1 induce interleukin 6 production in vivo. *Clin Immunol Immunopathol* 1989;53:488–498.
49. van Deventer SJH, Büller HR, Ten Cate JW, et al. Experimental endotoxemia in humans: analysis of cytokine release and coagulation, fibrinolytic, and complement pathways. *Blood* 1990;76:2520–2526.
50. Simpson SQ, Casey LC. Role of tumor necrosis factor in sepsis and acute lung injury. *Crit Care Clinics* 1989;5:27–47.
51. Clark IA. Cell-mediated immunity in protection and pathology of malaria. *Parasitol Today* 1987;3:300–305.
52. Cross AS, Sadoff JC, Kelly N, et al. Pretreatment with recombinant murine tumor necrosis factor α/cachectin and murine interleukin 1α protects mice from lethal bacterial infection. *J Exp Med* 1989;169:2021–2027.
53. van der Meer JWM, Barza M, Wolff SM, Dinarello CA. A low dose of recombinant interleukin 1 protects granulocytopenic mice from lethal gram-negative infection. *Proc Natl Acad Sci USA* 1988;85:1620–1623.
54. Wong GHW, Goeddel DV. Induction of manganous superoxide dismutase by tumor necrosis factor: possible protective mechanism. *Science* 1988;242:941–944.
55. Krosnick JA, McIntosh JK, Mule JJ, Rosenberg SA. Studies of the mechanism of toxicity of the administration of recombinant tumor necrosis factor α in normal and tumor-bearing mice. *Cancer Immunol Immunother* 1989;30:133–138.

56. Hohmann HP, Remy R, Brockhaus M, van Loon APGM. Two different cell types have different major receptors for human tumor necrosis factor (TNFα). *J Biol Chem* 1989;264:14927–14934.
57. Loetscher H, Pan Y-CE, Lahm H-W, et al. Molecular cloning and expression of the human 55 dD tumor necrosis factor receptor. *Cell* 1990;61:351–359.
58. Schall TJ, Lewis M, Koller KJ, et al. Molecular cloning and expression of a receptor for human tumor necrosis factor. *Cell* 1990;61:361–370.
59. Gray PW, Barrett K, Chantry D, et al. Cloning of human tumor necrosis (TNF) receptor cDNA and expression of recombinant soluble TNF-binding protein. *Proc Natl Acad Sci USA* 1990;87:7380–7384.
60. Smith CA, Davis T, Anderson D, et al. A receptor for tumor necrosis factor defines an unusual family of cellular and viral proteins. *Science* 1990;248:1019–1023.
61. Nophar Y, Kemper O, Brakebush C, et al. Soluble forms of tumor necrosis factor receptors (TNF-Rs). The cDNA for the type I TNF-R, cloned using amino acid sequence data of its soluble form, encodes both the cell surface and a soluble form of the receptor. *EMBO J* 1990;9:3269–3278.
62. Goodwin RG, Anderson D, Jerzy R, et al. Molecular cloning of the type 1 and type 2 murine receptors for tumor necrosis factor. *Mol Cell Biol* 1991;11:3920–3926.
63. Itoh N, Yonehara S, Ishii A, et al. The polypeptide encoded by cDNA for human cell surface antigen Fas can mediate apoptosis. *Cell* 1991;66:233–243.
64. Camerini D, Waltz G, Loenen WA, et al. The T cell activation antigen CD27 is a member of the nerve growth factor/tumor necrosis factor gene family. *J Immunol* 1991;147:3165–3169.
65. Lewis M, Tartaglia LA, Lee A, et al. Cloning and expression of cDNA for two distinct murine tumor necrosis factor receptors demonstrate one receptor is species specific. *Proc Natl Acad Sci USA* 1991; 88:2830–2834.
66. Espevik T, Brockhaus M, Loetscher H, et al. Characterization of binding and biological effects of monoclonal antibodies against a human tumor necrosis factor receptor. *J Exp Med* 1990;171:415–426.
67. Tartaglia LA, Goeddel DV. Two TNF receptors. *Immunol Today* 1992;13:151–153.
68. Shalaby MR, Sundan A, Loetscher H, et al. Binding and regulation of cellular functions by monoclonal antibodies against human tumor necrosis factor receptors. *J Exp Med* 1990;172:1517–1520.
69. Heller RA, Song K, Fan N, Chang DJ. The p70 tumor necrosis factor receptor mediates cytotoxicity. *Cell* 1992;70:47–56.
70. Van Ostade X, Vandenabeele P, Everaerdt B, et al. Human TNF mutants with selective activity on the p55 receptor. *Nature* 1993;361:266–269.
71. Liabakk N-B, Sundan A, Waage A, et al. Development of immunoassays for the detection of soluble tumour necrosis factor receptors. *J Immunol Methods* 1991;141:237–243.
72. Waage A, Liabakk N, Lien E, et al. p55 and p75 tumor necrosis factor receptors in patients with chronic lymphocytic leukemia. *Blood* 1992;80:2577–2583.
73. Aderka D, Engelmann H, Hornik V, et al. Increased serum levels of soluble receptors for tumor necrosis factor in cancer patients. *Cancer Res* 1991;51:5602.
74. Austgulen R, Liabakk N-B, Brockhaus M, Espevik T. Soluble TNF receptors in amniotic fluid and in urine from pregnant women. *J Reprod Immunol* 1992;22:105–116.
75. Girardin E, Roux-Lombard P, Grau GE, et al. Imbalance between tumour necrosis factor-alpha and soluble TNF receptor concentrations in severe meningococcaemia. *Immunology* 1992;76:20–23.
76. Van Zee KJ, Kohno T, Fischer E, et al. Tumor necrosis factor soluble receptors circulate during experimental and clinical inflammation and can protect against excessive tumor necrosis factor α in vitro and in vivo. *Proc Natl Acad Sci USA* 1992;89:4845–4849.
77. Spinas GA, Keller U, Brockhaus M. Release of soluble receptors for tumor necrosis factor (TNF) in relation to circulating TNF during experimental endotoxinemia. *J Clin Invest* 1992;90:533–536.
78. Lantz M, Gullberg U, Nilsson E, Olsson I. Characterization in vitro of a human tumor necrosis factor-binding protein. A soluble form of a tumor necrosis factor receptor. *J Clin Invest* 1990;86:1396–1402.
79. Naume B, Johnsen A-C, Espevik T, Sundan A. Gene expression and secretion of cytokines and cytokine receptors from highly purified CD56+ NK cells stimulated with IL-2, IL-7 and IL-12. *Eur J Immunol* 1993;23:1831–1838.
80. Porteu F, Brockhaus M, Wallach D, et al. Human neutrophil elastase releases a ligand-binding fragment from the 75-kDa tumor necrosis factor (TNF) receptor. *J Biol Chem* 1991;266:18846–18853.
81. Gullberg U, Lantz M, Lindvall L, et al. Proteolytic cleavage site in the p55 tumor necrosis factor receptor. *Eur Cytokine Network* 1992;3:140(no. A-14).

82. Liabakk N-B, Sundan A, Lien E, et al. The release of p55 TNF receptor from U937 cells studied by a new p55 immunoassay. *J Immunol Methods* 1993;163:145–154.
83. Aderka D, Engelmann H, Maor Y, et al. Stabilization of the bioactivity of tumor necrosis factor by its soluble receptors. *J Exp Med* 1992;1275:323–329.
84. Beutler B, Milsark IW, Cerami A. Cachectin/tumor necrosis factor: production, distribution, and metabolic fate in vivo. *J Immunol* 1985;135:3972–3977.
85. Ashkenazi A, Marsters SA, Capon DJ, et al. Protection against endotoxic shock by a tumor necrosis factor receptor immunoadhesin. *Proc Natl Acad Sci USA* 1991;88:10535–10539.
86. Lesslauer W, Tabuchi H, Gentz R, et al. Recombinant soluble tumor necrosis factor receptor proteins protect mice from lipopolysaccharide-induced lethality. *Eur J Immunol* 1991;21:2883–2886.

Organ Metabolism and Nutrition:
Ideas for Future Critical Care, edited by
J. M. Kinney and H. N. Tucker.
Raven Press, Ltd., New York © 1994.

Overview: Interleukin-1 and Tumor Necrosis Factor in Inflammatory Disease and the Effect of Dietary Fatty Acids on Their Production

Charles A. Dinarello

Department of Geographic Medicine and Infectious Diseases, New England Medical Center, Boston, Massachusetts 02111

Tumor necrosis factor (TNF) and interleukin-1 (IL-1) are the cytokines most often implicated in the pathogenesis of disease. This is because the biological properties of these cytokines closely resemble the spectrum of physiologic and biochemical (metabolic) changes observed in many inflammatory and infectious diseases. Moreover, these two cytokines act in a synergistic fashion. In terms of catabolism, these two cytokines contribute to the negative nitrogen balance of acute or chronic disease. First, there is ample evidence that injections of either IL-1 or TNF can result in anorexia. Second, there is a component of the cachexia of disease that is due to loss of mean body mass. The direct effect of IL-1 or TNF on the loss of protein from muscle plays a role in the loss of mean body mass, although the precise mechanism for the interaction of cytokines with muscle tissue remains clouded. One mechanism, however, appears to be mediated by IL-1 and TNF-induced cyclooxygenase.

Interferon-γ (IFNγ) also contributes to the spectrum of disease at many levels but its effects on hepatic protein gene expression and cytokine receptors appears to be relevant to the biological activities of TNF and IL-1. IFNγ up-regulates the responsiveness to TNF and increases the production of IL-1 and TNF in cells stimulated with endotoxin (LPS). Recent studies using knockout mice for the IFNγ receptor have revealed an essential role for IFNγ in host defense against intracellular parasites and *Mycobacteria*.

The strongest evidence that inflammatory cytokines are important players in the pathogenesis of disease can be found in recent studies using specific cytokine blockade. Blocking either IL-1 or TNF can reduce the severity of disease. Specific blockade of these cytokines has entered clinical trials and it seems certain that within the next 5 years, anticytokine therapy will be used in a variety of disease states. The basis for the role of the cytokines IL-1 and TNF in inducing inflammation is now well supported in hundreds of published papers. What is also clear is that other cytokines are playing a negative role and that the balance of pro- and antiinflammatory cytokines likely determines the outcome or progression of disease. An example of this balance is the cytokine IL-1 because its naturally occurring receptor antagonist functions to block the biological activity of IL-1 itself. The other example is TNF for which two naturally occurring soluble receptors are produced during disease that bind and block the activity of this cytokine. This overview will focus on two themes: first, the role of IL-1 and TNF in disease and second, the effect of dietary fatty acids in the control of IL-1 and TNF production in human subjects.

INTERLEUKIN

The IL-1 family consists of three structurally related polypeptides; the first two are IL-α and IL-1β and the third member is IL-1 receptor antagonist (IL-1ra) which inhibits the activities of IL-1. Among the properties of IL-1 (α and β) are the ability to induce fever, sleep, anorexia, and hypotension. IL-1 stimulates the release of pituitary hormones, increases the synthesis of collagenases, resulting in cartilage destruction, and stimulates prostaglandin production, leading to a decrease in pain threshold. IL-1 also has been implicated in destruction of beta-cells of the islets of Langerhans, growth of acute and chronic myelogenous leukemia cells, inflammation associated with arthritis and colitis, and development of atherosclerotic plaques.

The third member of the interleukin-1 family, IL-1ra, provides some protection against the disease-provoking effects of IL-1. IL-1ra is a specific inhibitor of IL-1 activity (1,2) that acts by blocking the binding of IL-1 to its cell surface receptors (2–4). The preliminary results of clinical studies with IL-1ra suggest that it may be beneficial in patients with sepsis syndrome, arthritis, and some forms of chronic myelogenous leukemia, and that it is safe.

TUMOR NECROSIS FACTOR

The TNF family consists of TNFα, primarily a product of the monocyte and macrophage, and TNFβ (also called "lymphotoxin"), a product of lymphocytes. The natural antagonists of the biological activity of TNF are the solubilized extracellular portions of its two cell-surface receptors, p55 and p75. The soluble TNF receptors (TNFRp55 and TNFRp75) block the biological activity of TNF by binding to TNF and preventing its interaction with the cell-surface TNFR (5).

In addition, IL-1 and TNF have some host-defense properties. For example, IL-1 and TNF stimulate T and B lymphocytes and, in animals, protect bone marrow stem cells from radiation-induced death (6). They can reduce the mortality from bacterial infections in animals (7). Tumor necrosis factor reduces the size and number of metastatic tumors in animals. Because of these beneficial effects, IL-1 or TNF has been given to humans. In phase I trials, IL-1 increased the numbers of bone marrow precursor cells and circulating platelets and neutrophils (8,9). However, increasing doses caused fever, gastrointestinal disturbances, myalgia, arthralgia, and hypotension (9). Similar results have been reported in humans receiving TNF (10–12).

ROLE IN NORMAL PHYSIOLOGY

Neither TNFα, IL-1α, nor β mRNA is present in monocytes from normal subjects. Plasma levels of IL-1β are elevated in women who have recently ovulated or in subjects after strenuous exercise. IL-1α is found in normal skin where it is thought to play a role in maturation of keratinocytes. Tumor necrosis factor is not found in normal skin. Various epithelial cells, neurons, and adrenal cortical cells contain IL-1β. However, an essential role for IL-1 or TNF in homeostasis has not been demonstrated.

INTERLEUKIN-1 AND TUMOR NECROSIS FACTOR AS MEDIATORS OF DISEASE

IL-1 and TNF have actions both directly on specific target tissues and as effector molecules. An example of a direct effect of IL-1 or TNF is the septic shock syndrome in which infection leads to the synthesis and release of large amounts of these cytokines that directly induce hypotension. An example of IL-1 or TNF as effector molecules is autoimmune disease in which IL-1 and TNF contribute to tissue destruction because of their ability to stimulate collagenases and prostaglandins, which induce bone resorption.

In most autoimmune diseases, T lymphocytes and not IL-1–producing phagocytic cells are the critical determinants of disease. The various treatments, such as cyclosporine, affect T-lymphocytes rather than mononuclear phagocytosis. Any reduction in IL-1 or TNF production associated with immunosuppressive therapies is likely secondary to reduced T-lymphocyte stimulation of IL-1- and TNF-producing cells. Reducing the production of TNF or IL-1 in autoimmune diseases reduces the inflammatory effects on target tissues such as the synovium, pancreatic islet cells or intestinal lining cells.

INTERLEUKIN-1 AND TUMOR NECROSIS FACTOR IN THE SEPSIS SYNDROME

The mechanism of TNF- and IL-1–induced shock appears to be its ability to increase the plasma concentrations of small mediator molecules such as platelet-activating factor, prostaglandins, and nitric oxide. These substances are potent vasodilators and induce shock in experimental animals. Blocking the action of IL-1 or TNF prevents the synthesis and release of these mediators. In animals, a single intravenous injection of TNF or IL-1 decreases mean arterial pressure, lowers systemic vascular resistance, and induces leukopenia and thrombocytopenia (13,14). In humans, intravenous administration of TNF or IL-1 also decreases blood pressure rapidly, and doses of 300 ng/kg or greater of IL-1 may cause severe hypotension (9). In experimental animals, the effects of the two cytokines are far greater than those of either cytokine alone (13). In addition, TNF can stimulate IL-1 production and hence both molecules are likely to be involved in the mediation of septic shock. In a study of patients with septic shock treated with a constant infusion of IL-1Ra (2 mg/kg/hr) for 3 days, the 28-day mortality was reduced by 22% ($p = 0.03$) compared with high-risk patients who received a placebo infusion (15). Monoclonal antibodies to TNF have similar reductions in mortality rates in humans with sepsis and shock.

Therapeutic advantage of blocking the action of IL-1 or TNF resides in preventing their deleterious biological effects without interfering with the production of intermediary molecules that have a role in homeostasis. For example, prostaglandins have a role in protecting gastric mucosa from acid. Although drugs blocking the synthesis of prostaglandins reduce hypotension in animals, these drugs lead to well-known toxicities because they also block the normal synthesis of prostaglandins in many tissues. A similar case can be made for blocking nitric oxide. The use of prostaglandin or nitric oxide synthesis inhibitors in shock will likely alter the function of these mediators in homeostasis, whereas reducing the action of IL-1 or TNF will reduce only that portion of prostaglandin and nitric oxide synthesis due to elevated IL-1 and TNF, sparing the synthesis of these intermediary molecules for homeostasis.

RHEUMATOID ARTHRITIS

IL-1 and TNF are present in the synovial lining cells and synovial fluid of patients with rheumatoid arthritis and explants of synovial tissue from those patients produce IL-1 in vitro. When injected directly into the joint space of experimental animals, IL-1 induces increased leukocyte infiltration, cartilage breakdown, and periarticular bone remodeling. In isolated cartilage and bone cells in vitro, IL-1 and TNF trigger expression of the genes for collagenases as well as phospholipases and cyclooxygenase and blocking IL-1 action reduces bacterial cell-wall–induced arthritis in rats (16).

INFLAMMATORY BOWEL DISEASE

Ulcerative colitis and Crohn's disease are characterized by infiltrative lesions of the bowel wall that contain activated neutrophils and macrophages. Two biological actions of IL-1 are particularly relevant to the pathogenesis of inflammatory bowel disease. They are its ability to stimulate the production of inflammatory eicosanoids (17), namely prostaglandin E2 and leukotriene B4. The reduction in inflammation is likely to do with a reduced production of IL-8, an inflammatory cytokine with neutrophil chemoattractant and neutrophil-stimulating properties (18), which seems to be under the control of IL-1 (19). The tissue concentrations of prostaglandin E2 and leukotriene B4 correlate with disease severity in patients with ulcerative colitis and tissue concentration of IL-8 are high in patients with inflammatory bowel disease.

The best evidence that IL-1 contributes to the pathogenesis of inflammatory bowel disease comes from studies of animals with acute, immune-complex–mediated colitis in which blocking IL-1 action with IL-1ra reduces the severity of acute inflammation and decreases eicosanoid concentrations in affected bowel (20). A likely mechanism for these is that blocking the action of IL-1 reduces the amount of IL-8 that is produced in the inflamed bowel. The intestinal tissue of patients with inflammatory bowel disease contains IL-1. The increased production of IL-1 and IL-8 in tissue specimens from patients with inflammatory bowel disease appears to come from mononuclear cells in the lamina propria of the bowel wall.

OTHER DISEASES

The pathogenesis of transplant rejection, graft-versus-host disease, atherosclerosis, psoriasis, asthma, acute myelogenous leukemia, osteoporosis, peridontal disease, autoimmune thyroiditis, and alcoholic hepatitis has been linked to IL-1 and TNF. Most studies making these linkages are based on findings of increased concentrations of circulating IL-1 or TNF or evidence of gene expression in affected tissues. Since other cytokines are also produced in these diseases, the role of IL-1 and TNF in their pathogenesis or even their manifestations is uncertain. However, since the severity of various related diseases in experimental animals is reduced when the action(s) of IL-1 or TNF are blocked, it is likely that these cytokines are important in their expression if not their causation. For example, in mice undergoing a graft-versus-host reaction to allogeneic bone marrow, administration of IL-1ra reduced mortality without impairing graft function (21). Anti-TNF antibodies accomplish the same effect.

INTERLEUKIN-1 AND TUMOR NECROSIS FACTOR ON CATABOLIC PROCESSES

The role of TNF in mediating the cachexia of disease has been reviewed (22). In short, when administered to mice, weight loss is observed that is not entirely due to anorexia. Nude mice injected with cells that are genetically engineered to produce large amounts of TNF develop a distinct wasting syndrome. Part of the wasting is the inability to metabolize fat because TNF inhibits the synthesis of lipoprotein lipase. There is less of a role for IL-1 in the inhibition of lipoprotein lipase, although IL-1 possesses this property.

Muscle Protein Degradation

Using semipurified IL-1 from human monocytes incubated with rat muscle strips, increased protein degradation was observed (23). This increased rate of muscle protein breakdown in vitro was not observed, however, when recombinant IL-1 was used. Even combinations of recombinant IL-1 and TNF added to muscle strips ex vivo were not able to reproduce the observation that was made using semipurified IL-1. Later it was shown that a small molecular weight protein(s) in the 6,000-Dalton range isolated from the plasma of humans with fever and infection or from stimulated human blood monocytes would induce protein degradation in isolated rat muscle strips (24). The structural nature of this (or these) proteins remains to be defined.

Although the in vitro model of muscle protein breakdown has not been shown using recombinant cytokines, infusions of these cytokines into rats results in metabolic changes that are consistent with a direct effect on muscle protein breakdown and fits a model of chronic cachexia. When rats were infused with TNF for 6 hours (20 μg/kg), there was increased excretion of urinary nitrogen (25). This was not observed with infusions of IL-1; however, when a combination of TNF and IL-1 (both human recombinant forms) was used, the increase in loss of mean body mass was greater than either TNF or IL-1 alone (25). In this model, the combination of TNF and IL-1 resulted in increased muscle proteolysis as measured by ^{14}C-leucine turnover. The effect was not due to changes in regional muscle blood flow induced by these cytokines but rather appeared to be due to the direct effect on the balance of muscle protein synthesis and degradation (25). These studies support the concept that inflammatory cytokines play a role in wasting, primarily through muscle protein breakdown. However, the mechanism of this action at the level of the muscle tissue remains unclear.

Effect of Interleukin-1 and Tumor Necrosis Factor on Lipid Metabolism

Hyperlipidemia is one of the hallmarks of wasting in infectious and inflammatory diseases. Although TNF and IL-1 reduce the synthesis of lipoprotein lipases in cultured cells, only TNF appears to induce lipolysis in vivo as measured by increased free fatty acids in the plasma (26). The ability of either IL-1 or TNF to induce lipolysis in cultured cells is blocked by inhibitors of cyclooxygenase (26).

However, other effects of these cytokines on lipid metabolism contribute to the hyperlipidemia. Administration of a single injection of TNF or IL-1 to rats or mice increases hepatic fatty-acid synthesis within 120 minutes and the effect lasts for 16 hours. Hepatic cholesterol synthesis is also increased (27). The mechanism for the cytokine-induced increases in fatty-acid synthesis is due to increased hepatic citrate levels, the primary activator of acetyl-Co-A carboxylase, the rate-limiting enzyme for fatty-acid synthesis (28). Interestingly, interferons, which also increase de novo fatty-acid synthesis, do not increase citrate levels, and the mechanism for IFN-mediated increased fatty-acid synthesis is unknown (28).

A single injection of IL-1 at doses that cause fever in rodents, results in elevated triglyceride levels; this elevation persists 17 hours (29). The mechanism is not via reduced lipolysis because IL-1 in these animals does not result in increased circulating levels of free fatty acids or glycerol (29). In vitro, IL-1 and TNF stimulate hepatic cell synthesis of triglyceride as measured by the incorporation of ^{3}H glycerol into triglyceride (30). The concentration of IL-1 (300 pg/ml), which induces triglyceride synthesis, is in the range of levels measured in the circulation of patients with mild-to-moderate inflammatory disease (31). Similar to other studies, the cytokine IL-4 suppresses the ability of IL-1 and TNF to stimulate fatty-acid synthesis (32).

In models of infection or inflammation, LPS induces hypertriglyceridemia, and current interpretation would suggest that this is mediated by IL-1 and TNF. However, when IL-1ra was administered to mice, there was no effect on LPS-induced hypertri-glyceridemia (33). To control this experiment, it was shown that IL-1ra was able to block the hypertriglyceridemia induced by IL-1 itself. Antibodies to TNF also did not alter the hypertriglyceridemia induced by LPS, although these antibodies blocked TNF-induced hypertriglyceridemia (33).

Role of Interleukin-1 and Tumor Necrosis Factor in the Anorectic Contribution to Wasting

There are several studies documenting the ability of IL-1 and TNF to suppress appetite (34,35). Recently, it was shown that a single intraperitoneal injection of IL-1 reduced food intake in rats but that this was mediated by prostaglandins because ibuprofen prevented the IL-1–induced effect (36). As in other studies using either IL-1 or TNF, tachyphylaxis develops and attenuates the weight loss. Besides inhibit-ing the anorectic effect of IL-1 with ibuprofen, a diet rich in fish oil (see next section) also attenuated the anorexia, and the effect of fish oil appeared due to reduced synthe-sis of PGE2 (36). Rats fed corn oil, on the other hand, did not have an attenuated anorectic response to injections of IL-1.

BLOCKING INTERLEUKIN-1 RECEPTORS

Considerable information has accumulated pertaining to the blockade of IL-1 recep-tors using the naturally occurring IL-1Ra (3,4). This IL-1 antagonist belongs to the IL-1 gene family, it is produced by the same cells, and it has the same molecular size of mature IL-1 and is structurally related to it. Similar to the findings of IL-1, IL-1Ra is not present in peripheral blood monocytes or plasma from normal subjects but is found in the keratinocytes of the skin and in neuronal cells. IL-1Ra binds to cellular IL-1 receptors but that binding does not initiate any biological response. Lacking biological activity, it can be given in doses sufficient to occupy IL-1 receptors and therefore prevent IL-1 from binding to these same receptors in contrast to soluble IL-1 receptors that achieve the same result by binding IL-1 before it can interact with the cell receptors. Since both IL-1Ra and soluble IL-1R are specific inhibitors of IL-1, any modification of disease with the use of these agents would indicate a role for IL-1 in that particular disease. In fact, administration of IL-1Ra to animals, as with administration of soluble IL-1R, reduces the severity of inflammation in some pathologic processes and improves survival.

IL-1Ra appears to be a pure receptor antagonist. In a phase I trial in normal subjects, raising the plasma IL-1Ra concentrations to 25 to 30 μg/ml caused no symptoms or changes in vital signs and did not alter white blood cell counts or routine biochemical and endocrinologic tests (37). These results are consistent with the concept that IL-1 does not play an important role in normal homeostasis. In animals, administration of antibodies to IL-1 receptors reduces inflammation and anorexia due to endotoxins and other inflammation-inducing agents (38).

TUMOR NECROSIS FACTOR ANTAGONISM

Numerous animal studies have shown that infusions of neutralizing anti-TNF antibodies prevent shock and death due to bacterial sepsis or endotoxemia. Based on these studies, humans have received either mouse antihuman monoclonal anti-TNF antibodies or "humanized" forms of these antibodies for the treatment of septic shock. Monoclonal anti-TNF antibodies are now in phase III trials in patients with sepsis. Preliminary data suggest that there is improved survival in patients with documented bacteremia. Although the use of monoclonal antibodies to TNF indicate preliminary clinical efficacy in sepsis and organ rejection, soluble TNFRs are likely to be equally efficacious. These soluble receptors bind TNF and prevent its binding to the cell-surface receptors, similar to the binding by anti-TNF antibodies. The advantage of monoclonal antibody treatment is that a single injection may afford protection, whereas soluble receptors will likely require frequent infusion. In general, affinities of soluble receptors for their ligands are greater than those of antibodies for the same ligand, making soluble receptors ideally suited for effective treatment.

Soluble Tumor Necrosis Factor Receptors

There are two soluble TNFRs that represent the extracellular domains of the two TNFR (type I and type II). The type I receptor is also termed p55 and the type II receptor, p75. The extracellular domains of both receptors were initially discovered in and purified from the urine of healthy humans (39–41). The soluble TNFRs are proteolytic cleavage products of the cell-bound TNFRs. When given to baboons to combat *Escherichia coli*–induced shock, soluble receptors to the type I TNFR reduced the severity of the shock (42).

Naturally occurring soluble TNFRs are glycosylated proteins; however, recombinant forms can be either glycosylated or nonglycosylated. In order to prolong the half-life of soluble TNFR in the circulation, chimeric molecules have been constructed consisting of two extracellular domains of the type TNFR linked covalently to the complement-binding portion of immunoglobulin. This results in a molecule with a longer half-life in the circulation and an ability to bind two TNF molecules (43). However, unlike the glycosylated monomeric soluble TNFR, the chimeric soluble TNFR molecules are not naturally occurring and may be immunogenic.

As in the case of the IL-1ra, the host response to infection includes a brisk production of TNF-soluble receptor molecules. Circulating levels of both soluble TNFR are elevated in patients during infection and autoimmune and metastatic disease (5). Circulating levels of the type II (p75) are higher than those of the type I (p55). As in the case of IL-1Ra, it is presently unclear whether the amount of soluble TNFR produced in disease reduces the activity of endogenous TNF.

Blocking Both Interleukin-1 and Tumor Necrosis Factor

Despite evidence that TNF and IL-1 produce a shocklike state and that their biological properties are consistent with the host's response to disease, only by specifically blocking either TNF or IL-1 has the critical role for these cytokines in infections as well as in other disease states been revealed. It is likely that the pathophysiologic events of infectious or inflammatory diseases is due to a synergism between IL-1 and TNF. Therefore, blocking *either* cytokine reduces the severity of the disease. In the case of septic shock, no doubt an extreme example of the lethal consequences of host responses to infection, blocking either IL-1 or TNF reduces the impact of the cytokine cascade leading to the terminal event. It has not been determined whether blocking both cytokines will improve outcomes over those of blocking both cytokines.

Blocking IL-1R is not easily accomplished because triggering of only 5% of the receptors induces a biological response and thus these nearly all IL-1R require blockade. A single injection of an antibody to the type I receptor would maintain blockade for several days, whereas a constant infusion of IL-1Ra is required for the same degree of blockade. The disadvantage of maintaining high levels of IL-1Ra opens the door for a more effective approach, and antireceptor antibodies with high affinities appear to offer several advantages. The advantage of short-lived IL-1Ra therapy is that adverse effects on host defense can be easily reversed. The same argument may be raised for soluble TNFRs. For the time being, however, these antagonists will be infused in critically ill patients with increasing frequency and presumably success in reducing acute disease.

DOES BLOCKING INTERLEUKIN-1 AND TUMOR NECROSIS FACTOR ACTION IMPAIR HOST-DEFENSE MECHANISMS?

Short-term blockade of TNF or IL-1 appears to be safe and effective. The remaining question is whether a more prolonged blockade will interfere with fundamental host-defense mechanisms. Both cytokines, particularly at low concentrations, increase natural resistance to certain infections and in some animal models, blocking IL-1 or TNF increases mortality. Antibodies to TNF have a longer half-life in the circulation than TNF-soluble receptors and therefore may result in greater effects on host defense.

Patients with sepsis have plasma concentrations of IL-1β in the range of 250 to 500 pg/ml and occasionally over 1,000 pg/ml. Raising the plasma concentrations of IL-1Ra to 20 to 30 μg/ml (representing a 10,000-fold molar excess) by intravenous infusion of IL-1Ra for 3 days in patients with septic shock is associated with improved survival and in normal subjects, the same plasma IL-1Ra concentrations had no deleterious effects on immune responses (37). These results are consistent with in vitro experiments in which blocking IL-1 action did not diminish the response of human T cells to antigens (44). Thus, blocking IL-1 action is likely to be safe, at least in the short term. Since IL-1Ra treatment of some diseases thought to be mediated by IL-1 may require prolonged use, the question arises whether sustained blockade of IL-1 action will weaken host-defense mechanisms.

There is no dearth of experimental data illustrating a role for IL-1 and TNF in boosting natural host-defense mechanisms. For example, IL-1 and TNF protect the early stem cells against radiation damage (6), IL-1 augments immune responses (45), and IL-1 and TNF improve survival of granulocytopenic mice with lethal *Pseudomonas* infection (7). How can both IL-1 or TNF administration and blocking IL-1 or TNF action have the same effect? An example of this type of duality in biology is well documented for trace elements—low levels are essential for several metabolic pathways whereas high levels are toxic (46). Thus, small amounts of IL-1 or TNF may be necessary for maintenance of host defenses, but large amounts of IL-1 and TNF are injurious. Clinical evidence supports this concept. Blocking the action of high IL-1 and TNF concentrations reduces the inflammatory and other actions of the cytokine. Whether total blockade of these cytokines is advisable, or even possible, is not known.

EFFECT OF DIETARY N-3 FATTY ACIDS ON THE PRODUCTION OF INTERLEUKIN-1 AND TUMOR NECROSIS FACTOR

The pathway for the synthesis of IL-1 and TNF includes products of arachidonic acid metabolism. Because dietary fatty acids influence the type of prostaglandin or leukotriene released from phospholipids, the type of fatty acid incorporated into the monocyte-macrophage cell membrane affects membrane fluidity, receptor function, and enzyme activity. Furthermore, changing the monocyte membrane ratio of arachidonic acid to eicosapentaenoic acid (EPA) affects the production of IL-1 and TNF. Diets rich in N-3 fatty acids have beneficial cardiovascular effects (47). In addition, dietary supplementation with fish oils (rich in N-3 fatty acids) are of benefit in ulcerative colitis (48), rheumatoid arthritis (49), hypertension (50,51), and psoriasis. Since IL-1 and TNF are thought to play a pathogenic role in each of these diseases, what is the evidence that increasing the N-3 fatty acid content in cell membranes affects the production of these two inflammatory cytokines?

In an attempt to relate the epidemiologic and clinical studies on populations that consume more fish, we initiated a series of studies to examine the effect of dietary N-3 fatty acids supplementation on the synthesis of IL-1 and TNF from blood mononuclear cells ex vivo. Animal studies have not provided a consistent pattern, as reviewed in Meydani et al. (52). The fundamental design of these studies was to first test the pre-dietary production level of these cytokines in human volunteers, initiate the intake of N-3 fatty acids, retest for the production after various time periods, and retest again after a wash-out period.

In each of our studies, peripheral blood mononuclear cells (PBMC) were taken from volunteers on two or three occasions during the pre-diet period. This method establishes the pre-diet baseline level with greater accuracy than does a single reading. The determination of cytokine production from these various time points is made using various stimuli such as LPS, mitogens, cytokines themselves, and dead bacteria. After the incubations, the cultures are frozen and each cytokine is determined in a single radioimmunoassay or ELISA test so that the pre-diet, dietary, and wash-out phases are assessed within the same assay. We believe this design eliminates or reduces the variability inherent in single-point determinations and that the wash-out time point supports the concept that the results are indeed secondary to the dietary intervention. In addition, we have established that without dietary intervention, the production of cytokines from PBMC remains constant over a 6-month period (53).

In previous studies in which neutrophil function was studied, volunteers consumed 18 grams of medhaden oil per day for 6 weeks. Medhaden oil (commonly called "fish oil") is a preparation rich in N-3 fatty acids. The volunteers for the cytokine study also consumed 18 g/d of fish oil containing 2.7 grams of EPA and 1.85 grams of docosahexaenoic acid (DHA) per day. The subjects were not restricted to change their regular consumption of calories or fats (54). Under these conditions, relatively large amounts of N-3 fatty acids are needed to change the ratio of arachidonic acid to EPA in the plasma. Using a diet in which the total calories from fat were reduced to 30%, the conversion to high levels of EPA can be accomplished with dietary fish rather than fish oil supplements (55).

Using a 6-week supplementation diet of menhaden oil in male volunteers, there was a 50% decrease in PBMC production of IL-1 and TNF (54). The effect was maximal 6 weeks after stopping the supplementation, but after an additional 20 weeks of the wash-out period, the production of these cytokines returned to the baseline levels. Associated with the suppression of IL-1 and TNF production, there was a comparable reduction in IL-2 production and proliferation of PBMC to phytohemagglutinin. These parameters also returned to baseline levels 20 weeks after stopping the fish oil (54).

A second study with a comparable design was carried out in two groups of women (56). One group was premenopausal and the second group was comprised of older, postmenopausal women. Women consumed a lower amount of EPA (1.68 g/d) and DHA (0.720 mg/d) than was used in the study with males. Again, we observed comparable decreases in cytokine production and mitogen responses. The reduction was greater in the older compared to younger women. Lymphocyte proliferative responses and IL-2 production was also decreased in the fish oil group.

The third study was conducted using food as a source of N-3 fatty acids. The basis of the study was the National Cholesterol Education Program (NCEP) Step-2 recommendation diet following a myocardial infarction. In this diet, total calories from fat are reduced to 20% and the amount of fat from saturated fats is reduced further. PBMC were taken from volunteers on three occasions to reflect the baseline cytokine production on an American diet. For the next 24 weeks, the volunteers consumed all meals prepared by a special kitchen, which contained approximately 121 to 188 grams of fish per day comprised of sole, salmon, and tuna fish (55). The total amount of EPA and DHA was 1.23 g/d and accounted for 0.54% of the total polyunsaturated fatty acids consumed. The cytokine production was assessed after 24 weeks to reflect the effect of the NCEP diet. There was a 40% reduction in IL-1β production ($p < 0.03$). There was also a fall in the production of TNF (35%; $p < 0.05$). These changes in the IL-1β and TNF production were associated with similar reductions in other cytokines (IL-2, GM-CSF, and IL-6).

Because of the dramatic effects of these dietary sources of EPA on cytokine production, we repeated the study in which volunteers consumed protein from chicken and turkey rather than from fish. In this diet, the total EPA and DHA was 0.27 g/d. Using the same methods, we found an increase in IL-1β (62%) and TNF (47%), $p = 0.003$. These studies suggest that during low-fat diets, the alterations in cytokine production is due to EPA/DHA consumption and not to decreased fats per se.

Are Fish Oil Diets Dangerous?

In each of these studies, we have documented a decrease in IL-2 production, proliferation to mitogen and in the NCEP Step-2 diet, a depressed skin test response to antigens. Although this latter study requires confirmation, the data from several studies suggest that in addition to reducing the production of inflammatory cytokines, N-3 fatty acids also decrease cellular immunity. Part of the depressed immune parameters may be due to peroxidation of cell membrane lipids. Animals consuming high amounts of EPA and DHA have increased lipid peroxidation. The oxidative pathway of N-3 fatty includes free radical formation, which may contribute to the suppression of T-lymphocytes. In addition to increased oxidative pathways for N-3 fatty acids, the reduction in antioxidants may contribute further to suppression of immune parameters. The plasma levels of Vitamin E, a major antioxidant, are reduced in persons taking N-3 fatty-acid supplements (57). In the studies cited previously, low doses (6 U/d) of Vitamin E were added to the fish oil diets and there was no change in Vitamin E levels in the plasma. However, in order to provide sufficient antioxidant protection, higher doses of Vitamin E may be required. In elderly human subjects, a high dose (800 U/d) of Vitamin E increased the responsiveness of peripheral T-cells to mitogens.

Whether the immune suppression of N-3 fatty acids is of clinical consequence remains to be shown. Certainly, epidemiologic studies in Eskimos are complicated by economic and social factors that may contribute to death from causes unrelated to immune status. Furthermore, rural Japanese and Chinese have lifelong high consumption of N-3 fatty acids associated with increased longevity. "Immunosuppression" is based on a comparison of clinical immunologic testing parameters of certain patients with those of a cohort of "normals"; however, these normals eat diets high in saturated fats, high in N-6, but low in N-3 fatty acids. Are we measuring the "high" end of the immune responses to mitogens and antigens, when, in fact, the true normal is defined by a different diet? Interestingly, the NCEP Step-2 diet study revealed an increase over the baseline immunologic parameters in a control group eating low fish, in which the major source of polyunsaturated fats were N-6 fatty acids. Is the higher incidence of autoimmune disease in developed countries due, in part, to a vigorous immunologic response to environmental or microbial antigens such that they trigger a larger repertoire of idiotypic antibodies? At present, there is no evidence that consuming N-3 fatty acids to the level of dietary fish intake (120 to 180 g/d) containing 1.25 g/d of EPA/DHA is producing immunosuppression.

In this overview, the role IL-1 and TNF play in mediating the physiologic and metabolic consequences of inflammatory disease is presented. Both cytokines depress food intake, participate in the loss of nitrogen, increase lipid synthesis, and suppress lipolysis. There are two fundamental approaches to reducing the impact of these cytokines in order to reduce the severity of disease: First, reduce their production and second, reduce their activity. This latter strategy is accomplished by preventing the binding of each cytokine to their specific cell-bound receptors. Although this approach is seeing early success in treating acute diseases such as septic shock, it is not likely to be useful in treating chronic inflammatory diseases. Reducing the synthesis of IL-1 and TNF by increasing the amount of N-3 fatty acids in the cell membrane is accomplished by increasing oral intake by either supplements or the amount of these fatty acids in the diet. The reduction in disease severity in atherosclerosis, arthritis, psoriasis, hypertension, and inflammatory bowel disease reported in humans with increased intake of N-3 fatty acids may be due to the reduction in IL-1 and TNF production.

ACKNOWLEDGMENTS

These studies are supported by NIH Grant AI 15614. The author thanks Drs. Simin Meydani and Stefan Endres for their contributions to these studies.

REFERENCES

1. Arend WP, Joslin FG, Massoni RJ. Effects of immune complexes on production by human monocytes of interleukin 1 or an interleukin 1 inhibitor. *J Immunol* 1985;134:3868–3875.
2. Seckinger P, Lowenthal JW, Williamson K, et al. A urine inhibitor of interleukin-1 activity that blocks ligand binding. *J Immunol* 1987;139:1546–1549.
3. Arend WP. Interleukin-1 receptor antagonist. *J Clin Invest* 1991;88:1445–1451.
4. Dinarello CA, Thompson RC. Blocking IL-1: effects of IL-1 receptor antagonist in vitro and in vivo. *Immunol Today* 1991;12:404–410.
5. Aderka D, Engelmann H, Hornik V, et al. Increased serum levels of soluble receptors for tumor necrosis in cancer patients. *Cancer Res* 1991;51:5602–5607.
6. Neta R, Oppenheim JJ, Douches SD. Interdependence of the radioprotective effects of human recombinant interleukin 1 alpha, tumor necrosis factor alpha, granulocyte colony-stimulating factor, and murine recombinant granulocyte-macrophage colony-stimulating factor. *J Immunol* 1988;140:108–111.
7. van der Meer JWM, Barza M, Wolff SM, Dinarello CA. A low dose of recombinant interleukin 1

protects granulocytopenic mice from lethal gram-negative infection. *Proc Natl Acad Sci USA* 1988; 85:1620–1623.

8. Tewari A, Buhles WC Jr, Starnes HF Jr. Preliminary report: effects of interleukin-1 on platelet counts. *Lancet* 1990;336:712–714.

9. Smith J, Urba W, Steis R, et al. Interleukin-1 alpha: results of a phase I toxicity and immunomodulatory trial. *Am Soc Clin Oncol* 1990;9:717.

10. van der Poll T, Bueller HR, ten Cate H, et al. Activation of coagulation after administration of tumor necrosis factor to normal subjects. *N Engl J Med* 1990;322:1622–1627.

11. van der Poll T, Romijn JA, Wiersinga WM, Sauerwein HP. Tumor necrosis factor: a putative mediator of the sick euthyroid syndrome in man. *J Clin Endocrinol Metab* 1990;71:1567.

12. van der Poll T, Sander JH, van Deventer SJH, et al. Effects of leukocytes after injection of tumor necrosis factor into healthy humans. *Blood* 1992;79:693–698.

13. Okusawa S, Gelfand JA, Ikejima T, et al. Interleukin 1 induces a shock-like state in rabbits. Synergism with tumor necrosis factor and the effect of cyclooxygenase inhibition. *J Clin Invest* 1988;81: 1162–1172.

14. Fischer E, Marano MA, Barber A, et al. A comparison between the effects of interleukin-1a and sublethal endotoxemia in primates. *Am J Physiol* 1991;261:R442–R452.

15. Fisher CJJ, Dhainaut J-F, Pribble JP, et al. A study evaluating the safety and efficacy of human recombinant interleukin-1 receptor antagonist in the treatment of patients with sepsis syndrome. Presented at 13th International Symposium on Intensive Care and Emergency Medicine, March 23, 1993, Brussels, Belgium.

16. Schwab JH, Anderle SK, Brown RR, et al. Pro- and anti-inflammatory roles of IL-1 in recurrence of bacterial cell wall-induced arthritis in rats. *Infect Immun* 1992;59:4436–4442.

17. Cominelli F, Nast CC, Dinarello CA, et al. Regulation of eicosanoid production in rabbit colon by interleukin-1. *Gastroenterology* 1989;1400–1405.

18. Baggiolini M, Walz A, Kunkel SL. Neutrophil-activating peptide-1/interleukin 8, a novel cytokine that activates neutrophils. *J Clin Invest* 1989;84:1045–1049.

19. Porat R, Poutsiaka DD, Miller LC, et al. Interleukin-1 (IL-1) receptor blockade reduces endotoxin and *Borrelia burgdorferi*-stimulated IL-8 synthesis in human mononuclear cells. *FASEB J* 1992;6: 2482–2486.

20. Cominelli F, Nast CC, Clark BD, et al. Interleukin 1 (IL-1) gene expression, synthesis, and effect of specific IL-1 receptor blockade in rabbit immune complex colitis. *J Clin Invest* 1990;86:972–980.

21. McCarthy PL, Abhyankar S, Neben S, et al. Inhibition of interleukin-1 by an interleukin-1 receptor antagonist prevents graft-versus-host disease. *Blood* 1991;78:1915–1918.

22. Beutler B, Cerami A. Cachectin: more than a tumor necrosis factor. *N Engl J Med* 1987;316:379–385.

23. Baracos V, Rodemann HP, Dinarello CA, Goldberg AL. Stimulation of muscle protein degradation and prostaglandin E2 release by leukocytic pyrogen (interleukin-1). A mechanism for the increased degradation of muscle proteins during fever. *N Engl J Med* 1983;308:553–558.

24. Dinarello CA, Clowes GHJ, Gordon AH, et al. Cleavage of human interleukin 1: isolation of a peptide fragment from plasma of febrile humans and activated monocyts. *J Immunol* 1984;133:1332–1338.

25. Flores EA, Bistrian BR, Pomposelli JJ, et al. Infusion of tumor necrosis factor/cachectin promotes muscle catabolism in the rat. A synergistic effect with interleukin 1. *J Clin Invest* 1989;83:1614–1622.

26. Feingold KR, Doerrler W, Dinarello CA, et al. Stimulation of lipolysis in cultured fat cells by tumor necrosis factor, interleukin-1, and the interferons is blocked by inhibition of prostaglandin synthesis. *Endocrinology* 1992;130:10–16.

27. Feingold KR, Soued M, Serio MK, et al. Multiple cytokines stimulate hepatic lipid synthesis *in vivo*. *Endocrinology* 1989;25:267–274.

28. Grunfeld C, Soued M, Adi S, et al. Evidence for two classes of cytokines that stimulate hepatic lipogenesis: relationships among tumor necrosis factor, interleukin-1 and interferon-α. *Endocrinology* 1990;127:46–54.

29. Feingold KR, Soued SA, Adi S, et al. Effect of interleukin-1 on lipid metabolism in the rat; similarities to and differences from tumor necrosis factor. *Arterio Thromb* 1991;11:495–500.

30. Grunfeld C, Dinarello CA, Feingold KR. Tumor necrosis factor-α, interleukin-1, and interferon alpha stimulate triglyceride synthesis in HepG2 cells. *Metabolism* 1991;40:894–898.

31. Cannon JG, Friedberg JS, Gelfand JA, et al. Circulating interleukin-1β and tumor necrosis factor-α after burn injury in humans. *Crit Care Med* 1992;20:1414–1419.

32. Grunfeld C, Soued M, Adi S, et al. Interleukin 4 inhibits stimulation of hepatic lipogenesis by tumor necrosis factor, interleukin 1, and interleukin 6 but not by interferon-α. *Cancer Res* 1991;51:2803–2807.

33. Feingold KR, Staprans I, Memon RA, et al. Endotoxin rapidly induces changes in lipid metabolism that produce hypertriglyceridemia: low doses stimulate hepatic triglyceride production while high doses inhibit clearance. *J Lipid Res* 1992;33:1765–1776.

34. McCarthy DO, Kluger MJ, Vander AJ. Suppression of food intake during infections: is interleukin-1 involved? *Am J Clin Nutr* 1985;42:1179–1182.

35. Moldawer LL, Andersen C, Gelin J, Lundholm KG. Regulation of food intake and hepatic protein synthesis by recombinant derived cytokines. *Am J Physiol* 1988;254:G450–G456.

36. Hellerstein MK, Meydani SN, Meydani M, et al. Interleukin-1-induced anorexia in the rat. Influence of prostaglandins. *J Clin Invest* 1989;84:228–235.

37. Granowitz EV, Porat R, Mier JW, et al. Pharmacokinetics, safety, and immunomodulatory effects of human recombinant interleukin-1 receptor antagonist in healthy humans. *Cytokine* 1992;4:353–360.

38. Gershenwald JE, Fong YM, Fahey TJ, et al. Interleukin 1 receptor blockade attenuates the host inflammatory response. *Proc Natl Acad Sci USA* 1990;87:4966–4970.

39. Engelmann H, Holtmann H, Brakebusch C, et al. Antibodies to a soluble form of a tumor necrosis factor (TNF) receptor have TNF-like activity. *J Biol Chem* 1990;265:14497–14504.

40. Engelmann H, Aderka D, Rubinstein M, et al. A tumor necrosis factor-binding protein purified to homogeneity from human urine protects cells from tumor necrosis factor toxicity. *J Biol Chem* 1989; 264:11974–11980.

41. Engelmann H, Novick D, Wallach D. Two tumor necrosis factor-binding proteins purified from human urine. Evidence for immunological cross-reactivity with cell surface tumor necrosis factor receptors. *J Biol Chem* 1990;265:1531–1536.

42. van Zee KJ, Kohno T, Fischer E, et al. Tumor necrosis factor soluble receptors circulate during experimental and clinical inflammation and can protect against excessive tumor necrosis factor-α in vitro and in vivo. *Proc Natl Acad Sci USA* 1992;89:4845–4849.

43. Lesslauer W, Tabuchi H, Gentz R, Brockhaus M. Recombinant soluble tumor necrosis factor receptor proteins protect mice from lipopolysaccharide-induced lethality. *Eur J Immunol* 1991;21:2883–2886.

44. Nicod LP, El Habre F, Dayer J-M. Natural and recombinant interleukin 1 receptor antagonist does not inhibit human T-cell proliferation induced by mitogens, soluble antigens or allogeneic determinants. *Cytokine* 1992;4:29–35.

45. Boraschi D, Villa L, Volpini G, et al. Differential activity of interleukin 1 alpha and interleukin 1 beta in the stimulation of the immune response in vivo. *Eur J Immunol* 1990;20:317–321.

46. Mertz W. The essential trace elements. *Science* 1981;213:1322–1338.

47. Weber PC, Leaf A. Cardiovascular effects of omega 3 fatty acids. Atherosclerosis risk factor modification by omega 3 fatty acids. *World Rev Nutr Diet* 1991;66:218–232.

48. Stenson WF, Cort D, Rodgers J, et al. Dietary supplementation with fish oil in ulcerative colitis. *Ann Intern Med* 1992;116:609–614.

49. Kremer JM, Lawrence DA, Jubiz W, et al. Dietary fish oil and olive oil supplementation in patients with rheumatoid arthritis. *Arthritis Rheum* 1990;33:810–820.

50. Bonaa KH, Bjerve KS, Straume B, Gram IT. Effect of eicosapentaenoic and docosahexaenoic acids on blood pressure in hypertension. *N Engl J Med* 1990;322:795–801.

51. Knapp HR, FitzGerald GA. The antihypertensive effects of fish oil. *N Engl J Med* 1989;320: 1037–1043.

52. Meydani SN, Dinarello CA. Influence of fatty acids on cytokine production and its clinical implications. *Nutr Clin Pract* 1993;8:65–72.

53. Endres S, Ghorbani R, Lonnemann G, et al. Measurement of immunoreactive interleukin-1β from human mononuclear cells: optimization of recovery, intrasubject consistency, and comparison with interleukin-1α and tumor necrosis factor. *Clin Immunol Immunopathol* 1988;49:424–438.

54. Endres S, Ghorbani R, Kelley VE, et al. The effect of dietary supplementation with n-3 polyunsaturated fatty acids on the synthesis of interleukin-1 and tumor necrosis factor by mononuclear cells. *N Engl J Med* 1989;320:265–271.

55. Meydani SN, Lichtenstein AH, Corwall S, et al. Immunologic effects of national cholesterol education panel step-2 diets with and without fish-derived N-3 fatty acids enrichment. *J Clin Invest* 1993;92: 105–113.

56. Meydani SN, Endres S, Woods MM, et al. Oral (n-3) fatty acid supplementation suppresses cytokine production and lymphocyte proliferation: comparison between young and older women. *J Nutr* 1991; 121:547–555.

57. Meydani S, Natiello F, Goldin B, et al. Effect of long-term fish oil supplementation on vitamin E status and lipid peroxidation in women. *J Nutr* 1991;121:484–491.

Organ Metabolism and Nutrition:
Ideas for Future Critical Care, edited by
J. M. Kinney and H. N. Tucker.
Raven Press, Ltd., New York © 1994.

10

Nutritional-Metabolic Support of the Intestine: Implications for the Critically Ill Patient

John L. Rombeau and John I. Lew

Department of Surgery, University of Pennsylvania Medical Center, Philadelphia,
Pennsylvania 19104; and Harrison Department of Surgical Research,
University of Pennsylvania Medical Center, Philadelphia, Pennsylvania 19104

Extensive research is ongoing in investigation of the effects of nutrients on intestinal cell growth and function. Improved in vitro and in vivo analytical techniques provide the opportunity to investigate the specific effects of malnutrition, bowel rest, and stress and disease on enterocyte and colonocyte kinetics. Moreover, prophylactic and therapeutic benefits of enteral nutrients on the gut epithelium of patients continue to be acknowledged.

This chapter reviews intestinal epithelial growth and function with particular emphasis on the effects of nutrient deficits and repletion. The relevance of these findings to the critically ill patient is presented. Additionally, the potential therapeutic utility of administering intestinal epithelial fuels and exogenous growth factors is discussed. It is anticipated that improved understanding of the interactions of nutrients, the gut epithelium, and stress and disease will provide further rationale for the use of enteral nutrients in the critically ill patient.

NORMAL INTESTINAL EPITHELIUM

Proliferation and Differentiation

Intestinal epithelial cells have one of the most rapid turnover rates of any tissue in the human body. Turnover of the intestinal epithelium involves proliferation and differentiation-maturation and eventual exfoliation of its component cells (Fig. 1). Renewal of mature intestinal epithelial cells depends on the continual division by proliferating stem cells deep within mucosal crypts. Stem cells of the small intestine and colon are undifferentiated cells capable of proliferation, self-maintenance, production of many types of differentiated functional progeny, and tissue regeneration

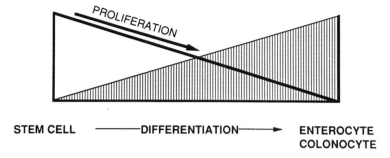

FIG. 1. Cell proliferation and differentiation in small intestine and colon.

after injury (1). Newly synthesized cells migrate from the lower half of crypts to the mucosal surface where they are, by this time, mature and eventually lost to the lumen. Under normal conditions, proliferation is balanced by exfoliation so that epithelial cell populations are preserved at a steady state (2).

Cell proliferation is a process that involves a consecutive pattern of changes in gene expression that ultimately leads to the physical division of cells (1). Traditionally, the initiation and termination of DNA synthesis and mitosis have been used as endpoints to identify proliferative cells (1). Certain precursor nucleic acid enzymes required in DNA synthesis serve as indices of cell proliferation. For example, thymidine kinase and thymidylate synthetase are nucleic acid enzymes that increase in activity as cell proliferation begins. These enzymes decrease in activity when cell proliferation decreases (3).

As proliferation ceases, intestinal epithelial cells move into the differentiative phase of the cell cycle. Cell differentiation is a process involving a qualitative change in cellular phenotype resulting from an onset of new gene product synthesis (1). Therefore, cell differentiation is often detected by the presence of a novel protein or characteristic usually identified by utilization of monoclonal antibodies (1). Additionally, differentiation is associated with a decrease in important cell constituents necessary for DNA synthesis. Although synthesis of protein and other substrates still occurs in differentiating cells, their ability to proliferate decreases and eventually ceases. Thus, changes in precursor nucleic acid enzyme activity, enzyme variability, and template stability are associated with cell differentiation and have a role in regulating the cessation of DNA synthesis before this phase (3).

Maturation is the quantitative change in cellular phenotype or constituent proteins leading to functional competence (1). Degree of cell maturation can be measured on a quantitative scale, such as weight of specific protein per cell.

As mentioned, specialized structures characteristic of certain cell types are associated with the later stages of cell differentiation and maturation. Villous columnar cells of the small intestine, for example, are highly polarized and possess well-developed brush borders. Additionally, the presence and quantity of hydrolases commonly found in the brush border also represent markers of differentiation and maturation.

Small Intestine

The epithelial cells of the small intestine (enterocytes) form an important lumenal interface with the outside environment. Absorption is greatly enhanced in the small bowel by mucosal villi that extend into the lumen. The surface that covers the villi is comprised mainly of three types of enterocytes: villous columnar cells, goblet cells, and enteroendocrine cells. These cells are bound together by tight junctions that maintain an impermeable barrier between the lumenal contents and intestinal submucosa (4). The cells of small-bowel crypts differ from the covering villi. The crypts contain four types of enterocytes: Paneth cells, crypt base columnar cells, immature goblet cells, and enteroendocrine cells.

The crypt base columnar cells of the small intestine are stem cells that differentiate into other constituent enterocyte types as they migrate up to the villi. Most of the enterocytes from crypt base to villi are absorptive columnar cells that become modified from crypt cell columnar cells to differentiated villous columnar cells. In humans, the time involved for columnar cells to reach the lumen and mature is 5 to 6 days in most of the small bowel and 3 days in the ileum (3).

The two kinds of mucus cells in the small intestine are immature goblet cells, found exclusively in the crypts, and mature mucus-secreting goblet cells located in the upper crypts and villi. These cells begin as immature goblet cells that migrate with the columnar cells to the villous tips where they mature to become mucus-secreting goblet cells. Additionally, Paneth cells do not divide and originate higher in crypts of the small intestine where they eventually degenerate and descend into the crypt base to be phagocytosed by macrophages. Renewal of these cells takes place after several weeks. Finally, enteroendocrine cells also migrate toward the villous tips, taking about 4 days to reach the surface. As these cells mature, they acquire a gradually increasing number of cytoplasmic granules and lose the ability to divide (3).

Large Intestine

In contrast to the small intestine, the human large intestine has no villi. The absorptive epithelium is planar and consists of straight tubular crypts that extend into the lamina propria. The colonic epithelial cells or colonocytes consist of three types: absorptive columnar cells, mucus secreting goblet cells, and enteroendocrine cells (5).

The colonic crypts consist primarily of mucus-releasing goblet cells with occasional enteroendocrine cells. The colonic surface is comprised mainly of absorptive columnar cells, which have microvilli on their lumenal surfaces found less abundantly than those in the small intestine. At colonic base crypts, there are stem cells that differentiate into the different colonocyte types. The stem cells of the ascending colon are small columnar cells, while those of the descending colon and rectum contain secretory vesicles and are called vacuolated cells. Before they reach the lumenal surface, these vacuolated cells lose their vesicles and mature into typical columnar cells with a brush border. The columnar, mucous, and enteroendocrine cells proliferate in the lower two thirds of colonic crypts. Migration of these cells to the lumenal surface takes about 3 to 8 days in humans (3,6).

Analytical Methods

A summary of analytical methods for proliferation and differentiation is included in Table 1. Cell proliferation has been analyzed traditionally by pulse labelling with [3H]thymidine, which measures the fraction or percentage of radiolabeled thymidine mitoses within a cell population (7–10). During the S phase (DNA synthesis phase) of the cell cycle, radiolabeled thymidine is incorporated into DNA. This method of radiolabeled analysis reveals the S and mitotic (M) phases of the cell cycle as well as the interphase gaps G1 and G2 before and after DNA synthesis.

TABLE 1. *Analytical methods for intestinal cell proliferation and differentiation: Partial listing.*

Method	Assay measures	Comments
Proliferation [^{3}H]-tritiated thymidine incorporation	DNA synthesis S phase and mitotic phase of cells	Advantages Relative ease in detection of incorporated modified nucleotide Extensive experience with assay and isotope Variety of radioactive isotopes available Disadvantages Isotopes expensive Assays can be prolonged and labor intensive. Kinetic analysis complex; dependent on factors difficult to standardize
Metaphase arrest technique or crypt cell proliferation rate (CCPR)	CCPR Number of cells per crypt per hour Fraction of cells in S and mitotic phase in all populations	Advantages Blocks cell cycle in mitosis and allows for metaphase structure accommodation Non-radioactive Use of colchicine or vincristine Disadvantages Labor-intensive assay Metaphase arrested mitotic figures postdistortion; difficult to distinguish
BrdUr incorporation	DNA synthesis S phase and mitotic phase of cell cycle	Advantages Non-radioactive thymidine analogue Detected by monoclonal antibody reactivity Rapid assay, kits available Relatively less expensive vs. radiolabelled isotopes Disadvantages Kinetic analysis complex; dependent on multiple factors to standardize
[^{14}C] leucine incorporation	Protein synthesis	Advantages Relative ease in detection of isotope Variety of isotopes available Disadvantages Nonspecific protein measurement Expensive Assays can be prolonged and labor intensive. Excess radioactive free isotope necessitates extreme caution and safety. Kinetic analysis complex; dependent on multiple factors; difficult to standardize

TABLE 1. *Analytical methods for intestinal cell proliferation and differentiation: Partial listing.*
(continued)

Method	Assay measures	Comments
Differentiation		
Immunocytochemistry	Direct, qualitative analysis and detection of novel or structured protein Characterizations of differentiated cell types (e.g., microvilli-columnar cell).	Use of monoclonal antibodies Several commerical kits available
Histochemistry	Indirect, qualitative analysis and detection of characteristic proteins (enzymes) of differentiated cell types (e.g., alkaline phosphatase), brush-border enzymes.	Nonspecific measurement of cellular proteins Specific tissue stains required Tissues must be maintained at 4°C or below. Frozen sections required
[^{14}C] glucosamine/ [^{14}C] leucine ratio	Direct measurement of glycoproteins (glycosaminoglycans) synthesis and protein synthesis (nonspecific) as a function of differentiated cells (e.g., goblet cells).	Glycoprotein synthesis more specific for differentiated cells than undifferentiated cells Both differentiated and undifferentiated cells have protein synthesis Increased glycoprotein synthesis or large G:P ratio is characteristic of differentiated cell population
In situ hybridization analysis	Abundance of mRNA for novel proteins characteristic of differentiated cell types (e.g., sucrase-isomaltase of brush border).	Higher levels of novel protein in mRNA may be found in differentiated cell types compared with undifferentiated cell types

Other methods for evaluating cell proliferation have been developed. One technique utilizes crypt cell production rate (CCPR) as a measure of epithelial cell proliferation (11,12). This method does not require the use of radioactive substances, but rather, the actions of drugs such as colchicine or vincristine sulphate which arrest cell mitosis at metaphase (13). Crypt cell production rate measures the number of cells produced per crypt per hour and the fraction of cells in the S and mitotic phase in a certain cell population. Yet another method of assessing cell proliferation involves the measurement of DNA synthesis by bromodeoxyuridine (BrdUr) incorporation (14). Bromodeoxyuridine is a nonradioactive thymidine analogue that can be detected by a monoclonal antibody. Under microscopic magnification, labelled (X) and unlabelled (Y) cells from the crypt base to the surface epithelium are counted to determine the labelling index (LI = X/X + Y) of each crypt. From several LI scores, cell proliferation can be measured (8,15).

Analysis of cell differentiation in intestinal epithelium can be determined by the presence of a novel structure characteristic of certain intestinal cells by monoclonal antibodies or by detection of certain hydrolases (e.g., sucrase, lactase) expressed in the well-developed brush borders of mature intestinal epithelial cells (16–18). Intestinal cell differentiation can also be determined by the ratio of [3H]glucosamine to [14C]leucine incorporated by these cells. This G:P ratio is a marker of glycoprotein synthesis and protein synthesis, respectively. An increase in glycoprotein synthesis is typical of differentiated intestinal epithelial cells (19,20).

NUTRIENTS AND INTESTINAL GROWTH AND FUNCTION

As mentioned, enterocyte and colonocyte renewal is dependent on the continued division of proliferating stem cells located deep within mucosal crypts. Mucosal growth is determined by the rates of epithelial cell proliferation and exfoliation. Normal mucosa is maintained at a steady state when cell proliferation is balanced by surface epithelial cell exfoliation. For mucosal growth to occur, the rate of cell production must be greater than the rate of cell loss. Growth may occur when the rate of cell proliferation increases and cell loss remains constant or when cell production remains the same and cell exfoliation decreases. Furthermore, mucosal atrophy or hypoplasia occurs when cell proliferation is insufficient and/or exfoliation increases. In contrast, mucosal hyperplasia results when cell production increases and/or cell life is prolonged. Thus, the rate of intestinal cell turnover determines mucosal growth, and any alteration in these processes will result in physiologic changes (2).

Since epithelial cell metabolic activity consumes most of the nutrient requirements of normal intestine, the most important stimulus for mucosal growth and function is the presence of lumenal (enteral) nutrients. Enteral nutrition (EN), the direct provision of nutrients into the intestinal lumen, mediates mucosal trophism by several mechanisms, namely, physical contact, stimulation of trophic gastrointestinal hormones, enhancement of intestinal blood flow, and incitement of the autonomic nervous system, as shown in Fig. 2.

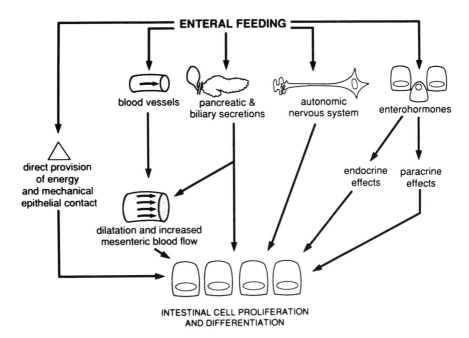

FIG. 2. Physiologic mechanisms by which enteral nutrients mediate intestinal cell proliferation and differentiation. From Lew and Rombeau (20a), with permission.

Physical Contact of Nutrients

The stimulatory effects of nutrients on mucosal growth is a result of two processes: by enteral nutrients and by dietary-induced trophic factors independent of nutritional value. Enteral nutrients in the form of digestible or indigestible material in the intestinal lumen directly stimulate mucosal growth by physical contact.

Several studies have demonstrated the importance of EN in the maintenance of intestinal mucosal growth, especially in intestinal adaptation after surgical resection (21–24). Enteral nutrition maintains cell proliferation consistently in the small intestinal mucosa after bypass surgery. Additionally, nonspecific esterase and α-glucosidase activity is elevated in villous columnar cells compared to control values (25). Enteral contents in the form of a fiber-free diet with poorly fermentable pure cellulose is capable of maintaining colonic mucosal growth. Cellulose causes a marked increase in crypt column height and may play a regulatory role in mucosal growth (26).

Certain enteral nutrients stimulate mucosal growth when converted into trophic factors by the action of digestive enzymes or bacteria within the intestinal lumen. Recent studies indicate that dietary fiber may belong in this category. Although dietary fiber is not digested by small intestinal secretions, there is significant fiber degradation in the ascending colon by bacterial fermentation (27). The extent of fermentation is determined by the type of fiber and bacterial flora. Numerous species of colonic bacteria have necessary enzymes required to digest or ferment dietary fiber. Metabolism of these fibers nourishes the colonic microflora and produces the major end-products of fermentation, namely, volatile short-chain fatty acids (SCFAs), which primarily include acetate, propionate, and n-butyrate in humans (28,29) (see the section on metabolic fuels).

Studies with [3H]thymidine show that animals on fiber-supplemented diets have increased crypt cell turnover and faster cell migration to the villous columns in the small intestine (30). Certain fibers, such as pectin and guar gum, alter the rate of cell turnover in small intestine as well. Rats fed pectin and guar gum–supplemented diets demonstrated faster rates of enterocyte turnover than those fed with oat bran and fiber-free diets (31). In the jejunum, pectin stimulated cell proliferation more than did guar gum. Similar effects were noted in the ileum. No significant effects were found in the duodenum.

Other studies have shown that fiber ingestion is important in the maintenance and growth of the colonic epithelium. Low-fiber diets produce atrophy as noted by mucosal hypoplasia and a decreased rate of colonocyte renewal (32). Although other dietary components such as cellulose may be important in sustaining colonic mucosal integrity (26), it is generally believed that the trophic effects in the colon are mediated by the fermentation products from dietary fiber and undigested starch (13).

Enterotrophic Gastrointestinal Hormones

The role of nutrient-induced production of gastrointestinal hormones in the regulation of intestinal mucosal growth has not been fully elucidated. Nevertheless, some studies reveal that gastrin and enteroglucagon have trophic effects in the small intestine and colon.

Gastrin, a peptide, is trophic for certain types of normal intestinal mucosa. This hormone stimulates cell proliferation and increases levels of DNA, RNA, and protein content in duodenal, ileal, and proximal colonic mucosa (2). Additionally, removal of the antrum with G cells that synthesize gastrin decreases DNA content in the colon (33). In an in vitro study with normal human colonic epithelial cells, pentagastrin caused a fivefold increase in cell number compared with a threefold increase in cells treated with saline (34). The extent of the effects of gastrin in intestinal growth, however, are still not entirely clear. While studies clearly demonstrate that gastrin stimulates gastric cell proliferation, similar effects in the small intestine and colon have been contradictory (35,36).

Endocrine cells in the ileum and colon produce enteroglucagon. Although there is a strong correlation between increased enteroglucagon levels and intestinal mucosal growth, to our knowledge, no studies have clearly demonstrated that enteroglucagon directly stimulates this growth (37,38). While glucagon has a small effect on colonocyte proliferation, enteroglucagon plays a larger role in enterocyte proliferation (39). Enteroglucagon was thought to stimulate cell proliferation in the small intestine after the finding of intestinal hypertrophy in a patient with an enteroglucagon-secreting tumor. After tumor resection, the small intestinal hypertrophy disappeared (40). Finally, other studies suggest intestinal resection and glucose perfusion increase intestinal cell proliferation and increase plasma levels of enteroglucagon (41–44).

Intestinal Blood Flow

Although reports on the effects of enteral nutrients on intestinal blood flow have been scarce, some studies suggest that SCFAs have a trophic effect on colonic mucosa by increasing blood flow to this organ (45,46). Intralumenal placement of SCFAs at postprandial concentrations increases colonic blood flow or hyperemia in dogs, suggesting these substances directly dilate colonic vasculature (45). Acetate appears to produce a greater increase of blood flow than to propionate and n-butyrate (45,47).

In an in vitro study with resected human colons, SCFAs, and not glutamine, individually and in combination caused concentration-dependent dilation of resistance arteries. This in vitro effect suggests SCFAs may improve colonic microcirculation, thereby providing a partial explanation for their trophic effect on colonic mucosa. Furthermore, such results might explain how modest doses of parenterally delivered SCFAs produce trophic effects on rat intestinal mucosa (48–50).

Autonomic Nervous System

Studies on the effects of the autonomic nervous system (ANS) on the gastrointestinal epithelium have been limited, except for the small intestine. Several studies suggest that stimulation of the ANS influences enterocyte proliferation. Sympathectomy inhibits DNA synthesis in intestinal crypts and decreases normal circadian rhythms in mitotic activity of undifferentiated cells in the small intestine (51–53). In small bowel mucosa, β-adrenergic stimulation with isoproterenol decreases enterocyte proliferation and, consequently, cell turnover (51). Noradrenergic fibers originate in the crypt base and rise into the villous tips (54). At the crypt base, these fibers make direct contact between epithelial cells and nerve terminals (55,56). Recent work from our laboratory suggests that the ANS is important in the mediation of enterotrophic effects of cecally produced SCFA (57). Rats with denervated ceca had significantly less SCFA-mediated enterotrophism when compared with animals with normal cecal innervation. When considered together, these findings strongly suggest that there are autonomic receptors that play an important role in nutrient-induced regulation and proliferation of epithelial cells in the small intestinal mucosa.

EFFECTS OF MALNUTRITION AND STARVATION ON INTESTINAL GROWTH AND FUNCTION

Several alterations in intestinal growth and function occur in malnourished and starved animal models, but the exact nature and significance of these nutritionally stressed states on the intestinal absorption of nutrients in humans remain to be studied. In malnutrition, gastric acid secretion decreases, thereby providing a milieu favorable for bacterial overgrowth in the proximal small intestine. Additionally, cell-mediated immunity and secretion of IgA may be reduced. These factors predispose the small bowel to propagation of microorganisms, which may lead to mucosal injury, diarrhea, and increased nutrient losses. Consequently, malnutrition alters the intestinal barrier to pathogens and increases the possibility of host infection (58).

Starvation causes several important changes in intestinal growth and function. During lengthened periods of starvation, gut mucosal atrophy occurs due to decreased CCPR and increased rates of cell exfoliation. These abnormal processes eventually shorten intestinal villi and decrease DNA and protein contents (59). Decreased enzyme function also occurs in starvation and is evaluated mainly by activity per unit length of intestine. Furthermore, the specific activity or enzyme activity per unit mucosal mass of certain enzymes can be measured and, under some conditions of starvation, may not indicate any significant changes (58). For instance, during starvation, disaccharidase activity per unit length is usually decreased. However, maltase and sucrase activities may not change, while lactase activity may be increased (58,60).

Several studies of small bowel in adult rats, infant rats, and infant rabbits reveal that nutritional deficits reduce villus height, change crypt depth, lower mucosal weight, decrease DNA, RNA, and protein contents, and alter disaccharidase activities (60–64). However, differences between animals and humans do exist, and whether these findings from animal models accurately explain these processes in humans remains unknown.

In infant rabbits, alterations in small-bowel growth and function caused by postnatal protein energy malnutrition are readily reversible with nutritional repletion or refeeding (64). Animals malnourished by litter expansion at 7 days postpartum demonstrated altered intestinal growth and function compared to *ad libitum* fed controls. Malnutrition in these young rabbits decreased jejunal and ileal mucosal mass as indicated by (a) lowered mucosal weight, DNA, and protein content; (b) decreased enterocyte proliferation and differentiation; (c) delayed cell maturation as measured by mucosal enzyme activity; and (d) increased glucose-stimulated sodium transport. Refeeding of these malnourished rabbits at 28 days led to rapid and complete recovery as shown by (a) restored jejunal and ileal mass within 4 days; (b) increased enterocyte renewal and differentiation by 7 days; (c) complete return of normal mucosal enzyme activity by 14 days; and (d) depressed glucose-sodium transport to control levels within 7 days (64). In malnourished infant rats, a similar effect occurs, as shown by recovery of disaccharidase activity and intestinal weight after 14 and 21 days of refeeding, respectively (60).

In adult rat small intestine, villus height, crypt cell depth, and mitotic pool decrease progressively during starvation (62). When adult rats are starved for several days and then refed, enterocyte proliferation and renewal occurs after 7 days (62,63). Furthermore, mucosal enzyme activity in adult rats returns to normal after 14 to 21 days of refeeding (61).

Marasmus and Kwashiorkor

In developed countries such as the United States, malnutrition associated with chronic illness, chronic hospitalization, or postsurgical recovery is more common than prolonged starvation. Although malnutrition is divided into two groups, namely marasmus and kwashiorkor, both forms often appear together in hospitalized patients (58).

In the small bowel of patients, marasmus causes increased presence of lymphocytes and plasma cells, reduced mucosal thickness, decreased mitotic indices, and depressed rate of cell differentiation. Structurally, the microvilli of the small intestine are short, sparse, and branched. Autophagic enzymes are widespread as is mitochondrial swelling. These findings are reversed within 4 months of refeeding (65). Functional abnormalities associated with marasmus in the small bowel are rare. Mild forms of steatorrhea can occur and may be the result of mucosal barrier injury. Furthermore, decreases in alkaline phosphatase, peptidases, and disaccharidases occur in patients with marasmus (66).

In kwashiorkor, mucosal injury of the small intestine is common with a majority of the patients having flat villous lesions. Other patients may reveal patchy, less severe lesions (58). Although mucosal thickness and mitotic indices are relatively normal in the small bowel, cell migration rate is noticeably decreased in kwashiorkor (65). The presence of increased amounts of intracellular lipid in enterocytes possibly reflects reduced apolipoprotein synthesis associated with severe protein malnutrition. In extreme cases, severe enterocyte destruction may occur with flat villus lesions (65). In contrast to marasmus, functional abnormalities are common in kwashiorkor.

Steatorrhea caused by mucosal injury involves the decreased uptake of fatty acids by small-bowel mucosa. Such lesions may depress chylomicron transport into villus lacteals. Reduced absorption of fat-soluble and water-soluble vitamins also often occurs. Furthermore, lack of disaccharidases and glucose transport proteins exacerbates preexisting conditions of carbohydrate malabsorption caused by mucosal injury. Fortunately, kwashiorkor patients quickly recover from all these abnormalities with nutritional repletion (58,65).

CRITICAL ILLNESS

Normal Intestinal Barrier

The normal intestinal epithelium allows for selective passage of nutrients into blood and lymph circulation, while serving as a protective physical barrier against the absorption of intralumenal bacteria and their toxins. The epithelial cell membranes prevent transcellular migration of such antigens, and the tight junctions hinder particle movement through paracellular channels. Furthermore, mucus cell secretions prevent the adherence and invasion of enteric bacteria and toxins.

The intestinal barrier is also characterized by several immunologic components. The mucosa and submucosa are replete with lymphocytes, macrophages, neutrophils, and Peyer's patches, which are lymphoid aggregates of the terminal ileum. Found abundantly in bile and intestinal secretions, IgA binds and mediates the recognition of such antigens as bacteria and their toxins. Moreover, Kupffer cells are in a key position to collect and detoxify antigens that penetrate beyond the intestinal wall and regional lymphatic tissue. The epithelium and its immunologic constituents are the major components of intestinal barrier function, although cell-mediated immunity may play a supportive role to the mucosa (67).

Alteration of the Intestinal Barrier in Critical Illness

The intestinal tract is one of several main target organs that are compromised in the critically ill patient. Stresses such as cardiogenic shock, hypovolemia, sepsis, and thermal injury can produce necrotic lesions in the intestinal mucosa. These conditions, with low mesenteric blood flow, disrupt the integrity of the intestinal barrier (68). In addition to these stresses, malnutrition, starvation, and altered intestinal flora, caused by broad-spectrum antibiotics, further impair intestinal absorption. Stress-induced lesions of the intestinal mucosa begin at the apices of the villi and progress downward to separate the epithelium from the lamina propria. If such lesions continue, destruction of the lamina propria, ulceration, and transmural necrosis of the intestinal barrier may occur. Such disruption of mucosal integrity allows for invasion by intralumenal constituents such as bacteria and endotoxin into the portal circulation (68). Thus, the eroded mucosa becomes an ineffective barrier, which allows disease processes to occur.

Hypoxia, associated with low blood flow, is an important cause of intestinal mucosal lesions during stress (69). Exfoliation of intestinal epithelial cells, decreased mucus production, and increased mucosal permeability to intralumenal particles occur with hemorrhagic shock. Furthermore, in such states of shock, lysosomal rupture renders the intestinal mucosa more susceptible to digestion by released enzymes. The lumenal presence of pancreatic enzymes such as elastase and trypsin also play an important role in the pathogenesis of barrier dysfunction in intestinal ischemia. Accordingly, preservation of blood flow and perfusion of the intestinal lumen with nutrients and oxygen may protect the mucosa from damage in the ischemic gut (68).

Although intestinal ischemia is a major cause of mucosal barrier lesions, past studies suggest reperfusion of such ischemic tissue promotes oxygen-free (superoxide) radical formation, which causes further barrier damage and eventual organ destruction. Generated by xanthine oxidase, superoxide radicals are eliminated by endogenous oxygen radical scavengers such as superoxide dismutase, catalase, and glutathione (68,70). Glutathione, a tripeptide and major antioxidant, consists of glutamate derived from glutamine, cysteine, and glycine. Recent studies suggest prophylactic administration of glutamine after intestinal shock and ischemia-reperfusion preserves glutathione stores which may enhance antioxidant protection (71,72).

Bacterial Translocation

Bacterial translocation is defined as the process by which bacteria migrate across the intestinal mucosal barrier to invade the liver, spleen, and mesenteric lymph nodes. Any combination of three conditions often found in critically ill patients will promote bacterial translocation. These conditions are physical disruption of mucosal barrier (i.e., hemorrhagic shock, sepsis), microflora imbalance resulting in bacterial overgrowth of enteric bacilli (i.e., broad-spectrum antibiotic therapy), and impaired host immune system (i.e., immunosuppressive drugs, protein deficiency) (67,73).

Intestinal barrier failure and bacterial translocation are not all or none phenomena (70). Disintegration of any one component of the intestinal barrier facilitates translocation of bacteria to the mesenteric lymph nodes, liver, and spleen. However, in the healthy host, translocated bacteria do not multiply and spread systemically. Microorganisms are localized in the aforementioned organs and eventually eliminated by tissue macrophages. In conditions of severe or complete intestinal barrier failure, translocating bacteria invade mesenteric lymph nodes, systemic organs, and the circulatory system. The majority of animal models with this condition usually survive. However, those animals with thermal injury or protein deficiency receiving nonlethal doses of endotoxin frequently die from the translocation of bacteria (70).

Although a physical mucosal barrier and host immune system are necessary for effective barrier function, an intact epithelial barrier will preclude bacterial translocation despite impaired cell-mediated immunity. Thus, the intestinal mucosal barrier may play a primary role in preventing bacterial translocation, while host immune defenses may serve a secondary role in intestinal barrier function (70).

Endotoxemia

Bacterial endotoxins may also cross an impaired intestinal barrier. Normally, endotoxins enter the portal system in small amounts and are detoxified rapidly by Kupffer cells. Intestinal ischemia markedly protentiates the systemic effects of endotoxemia. If the superior mesenteric artery is temporarily occluded in rabbits, fatal endotoxemia can occur. Interestingly, when the intestinal microflora of these animals is removed, fatal endotoxemia does not occur when the same artery is occluded (74). In mice, endotoxin enhances bacterial translocation from the intestinal lumen to the mesenteric lymph nodes in a dose-dependent fashion. Lethal doses of bacterial toxins disrupt intercellular tight junctions, increasing permeability to bacteria and maintaining or amplifying endotoxemia (75).

Endotoxemia occurs in critically ill patients with low blood flow (i.e., cardiogenic or hypovolemic shock). A large percentage of trauma patients in shock have endotoxemia without evidence of visceral perforations. Of those with systolic blood pressures less than 80 mmHg at hospital admission, 56% of patients have endotoxemia. Furthermore, of those with systolic blood pressures greater than 80 mmHg at admission, endotoxemia occurs in 9% of these patients (76). Thus, severe hypotension leads to marked increases in endotoxemia.

Multisystem Organ Failure Syndrome

Multisystem organ failure (MSOF) syndrome is a significant cause of morbidity and mortality in critically ill patients. Initially, MSOF was thought to be exclusively due to sepsis (70,77); however, recent evidence suggests it can occur in the absence of infection (78,79). Enteric bacteremia is found in some critically ill patients dying of MSOF and, in such cases, no septic focus can be found either clinically or by autopsy. Consequently, increasing attention has been directed to the investigation of gut-derived bacteria as translocating pathogens responsible for initiating sepsis and perpetuating MSOF.

In the gut-origin hypothesis of MSOF, translocated enteric bacteria and endotoxin travel to organs and tissues, causing sepsis, macrophage cytokine secretion, neutrophil protease stimulation, oxidant production, proinflammatory endothelial cell promotion, and complement and coagulation system activation. It has been hypothesized that these processes are self-sustaining and responsible for initiating MSOF (77,80).

There is no definitive evidence in humans to support the gut-origin sepsis as a cause of MSOF. In fact, evidence for this hypothesis rests primarily on laboratory experiments with animal models. In the opinion of one of the authors (JLR), gut-induced MSOF occurs only in a very small percentage of malnourished, critically ill patients who are severely septic and immunosuppressed with significantly compromised gut barrier function. While studies have demonstrated that increased bacterial translocation plays a major role in determining survival in animal models of critical illness, strong clinical evidence for this idea is lacking. Although increased gut barrier permeability to hydrophilic particles has been seen in both animal models and critically ill patients, the clinical significance of this finding is still unclear.

Enteral Nutrients in Critical Illness

Since most critically ill patients are unable to eat voluntarily, nutrients must be administered either enterally or parenterally. Although total parenteral nutrition (TPN) has contributed significantly to the management of critically ill patients, EN may be equally, if not more, beneficial to these patients. With improved methods of delivery, EN enhances intestinal structure and function. Although TPN may be used to maintain patients unable to receive EN, prolonged TPN administration leads to intestinal mucosal atrophy, enterocyte hypoplasia, and decreased intestinal enzyme activity. These combined effects may in turn contribute to intestinal barrier disruption, hypermetabolism, and other detrimental sequelae. Essential nutrients required for normal mucosal growth are usually not found in prolonged administrations of TPN used for treatment of critical illness. In fact, TPN is often associated with iatrogenic bowel malnutrition that impairs intestinal epithelial cell proliferation and mucosal repair (67).

The intestinal tract in critical illness has traditionally been considered to be inactive as a consequence of primary disease, infection, injury, or side effects of certain medications. Paralytic ileus usually occurs at some point in the course of treating critically ill patients. Different components of the intestinal tract are not equally susceptible to paralytic ileus. The small intestine is somewhat resistant to ileus development, and impaired absorption and dysmotility usually resolve within the first 24 hours following insult. The colon and stomach, however, may take more than 3 days to regain normal motility after injury (81). Consequently, early postoperative EN, which bypasses the stomach and delivers nutrients directly into the small bowel, is often used in critically ill patients (82,83).

Paralytic ileus also promotes enteric bacterial overgrowth. Thus, in addition to rapid repair or prevention of intestinal mucosal injury, control of microfloral overgrowth and mediation of the host immune system against translocating bacteria and endotoxins may be efficacious in treatment of critically ill patients. Accumulating evidence suggests that early administration of EN preserves intestinal barrier function by maintaining mucosal mass, preventing disruption of normal microflora balance and modulating host immune defenses (84).

In a recent comparative study, EN and TPN altered immunologic and metabolic response to endotoxemic injury in normal human volunteers (85). These subjects received either isocaloric, isonitrogenous EN or TPN for 7 days and were then given intravenous injections of *E. Coli* endotoxin. Total parenteral nutrition significantly worsened systemic manifestations of endotoxemia when compared with EN. Parenterally fed subjects demonstrated increased arterial and hepatic venous cachectin production (Fig. 3) consistent with activated reticuloendothelial cell response. Furthermore, TPN subjects showed greater adverse effects of endotoxemic injury, as

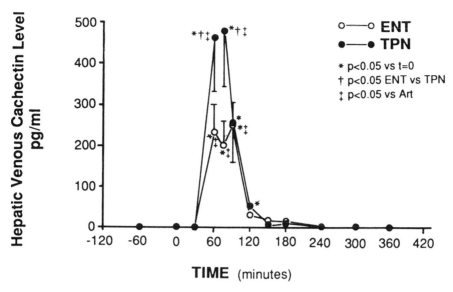

FIG. 3. Hepatic venous cachectin levels in normal human subjects following intravenous injection of *E. coli* endotoxin. Time 0, before endotoxin injection. From Fong et al. (85), with permission.

indicated by increased peripheral lactate production and increased peripheral amino acid release. This study suggests TPN or the lack of enteral nutrients impairs intestinal barrier function and increases hepatic and splanchnic host exposure to bacteria and endotoxin. These events may amplify cytokine response by increasing splanchnic and reticuloendothelial cell activation to subsequent injury. Cytokines produced and secreted by hepatic Kupffer cells and splanchnic lymphocytes also enhance production of counterregulatory hormones, which may transiently down-regulate cytokine production, increase output of hepatic-produced acute-phase proteins, and reduce gluconeogenesis (84). Thus, the antecedent route of nutritional support may influence immunologic and metabolic responses in critically ill patients to subsequent insults.

NEW THERAPIES

Metabolic Intestinal Fuels

Metabolic fuels of the intestinal tract have trophic effects on mucosal growth, and the small intestine and colon differ in fuel preference. Glutamine and butyrate are the preferred metabolic fuels, respectively, for rapidly proliferating enterocytes and colonocytes. When EN is ineffective and TPN is required in the critically ill, such nutritional support generally fails to provide these two essential intestinal nutrients. In fact, glutamine is absent in all currently available formulations of TPN in the United States. Furthermore, butyrate is not enterally administered to the colon in critically ill patients, and concomitant antibiotic therapy suppresses colonic microflora that produce butyrate from dietary fiber and undigested starch. Additionally, omega-3 fatty acids (fish oils), which may be important in maintaining gut immunocompetence, are not included in present nutritional therapy. Thus, at a time when the gut might conceivably benefit from appropriate feeding, the prescribed nutritional therapy paradoxically starves the intestinal tract and leads to mucosal atrophy. Current studies suggest that EN supplemented with intestinal metabolic fuels such as glutamine, butyrate, and fish oils may be more efficacious in critically ill patients with intestinal dysfunction when compared to providing formulations without these substrates.

Glutamine

Glutamine is a nonessential amino acid that plays a major role in the maintenance of intestinal metabolism, structure, and function. A principal fuel for enterocytes, glutamine may be especially important in critical illness when the intestinal barrier appears to be vulnerable (86,87). In the jejunum, enterocytes possess very active glutaminases that hydrolyze glutamine to glutamate and ammonia. Enterocytes use glutamine from the circulation as a metabolic fuel, and the majority of its nitrogen end-products appear in ammonia, alanine, and citrulline. Moreover, such nitrogen end-products are released into the portal circulation after enteral glutamine administration and are collected by the liver before reaching the systemic circulation. Thus, glutamine is metabolized when it enters enterocytes either across the lumenal brush border or through the basolateral membrane from the systemic circulation (86,87).

In critically ill patients, increased protein catabolism in skeletal muscle provides amino acids for systemic organs. Skeletal muscle, a source of body protein, is the primary organ of glutamine synthesis and storage. Accordingly, the concentration of this amino acid is 30 times higher in skeletal muscle than in the circulation (87). Although glutamine release from skeletal muscle markedly increases during critical illness, circulating concentrations of this amino acid are decreased, indicating its increased uptake by other tissues (67,87). In patients with multisystem trauma, increased and selective uptake of glutamine occurs in the intestinal tract (88). In stressed conditions, glutamine depletion surpasses that of all other amino acids and endures during recovery after all other amino acids have returned to normal levels (89).

Although included in some current EN formulations, these provisions of glutamine are probably administered in insufficient amounts to support intestinal mucosal growth. Furthermore, current TPN formulas do not contain glutamine, which may explain in part why the intestinal mucosa atrophies in patients receiving prolonged parenteral feeding. Additional causes for such mucosal disruption may be the result of decreased nutrient contact or insufficient production of enterotrophic gastrointestinal hormones. Elevated plasma glutamine levels above control values cause trophic effects on rat intestinal mucosa (90). Additionally, TPN with glutamine diminishes gut atrophy and stimulates small-bowel disaccharidase activity (91). Similar results occur when glutamine is administered enterally (92,93). Finally, both enteral and parenteral glutamine infusions significantly increase mucosal mass of intestinal grafts in rats receiving heterotopic small-bowel isografts compared to nonglutamine controls (94,95).

Current TPN formulas without glutamine promote bacterial translocation in rats. Bacterial translocation is reduced in rats orally fed glutamine, while it does not occur in those animals fed regular chow diets (96). Furthermore, EN and TPN glutamine-enriched formulas increased intestinal glutaminase activity and glutamine uptake. Accordingly, glutamine-supplemented TPN maintains immune cellularity better than do standard formulations (97,98). Glutamine-supplemented TPN maintains IgA at normal physiologic levels, which, in turn, prevent bacterial adherence to enterocytes. Thus, glutamine supplementation decreases bacterial translocation and preserves intestinal immune function during TPN.

Several studies suggest glutamine-enhanced EN and TPN benefit animals with intestinal mucosal injury due to chemotherapy. Glutamine-enriched EN preserves intestinal mass and improves survival of rats with methotrexate-induced enterocolitis (99). Similar results were found in rats on glutamine-enriched TPN after receiving 5-fluorouracil (5-FU). Increased villous height and mucosal DNA content were found in these rats. When the supplemented TPN was given before 5-FU administration, there was further increased mucosal cellularity and significantly lower mortality compared with controls (100).

As mentioned, glutathione (GSH) is a major antioxidant consisting of glutamate derived from glutamine. Although this tripeptide protects normal tissue from oxidant injury, GSH may also be a tumor tissue mechanism of resistance to chemotherapy and radiation. Oral glutamine supplementation may restore depleted GSH to normal levels in cancer patients thereby providing the intestinal tract and other organs a form of acquired resistance to oxygen-free radicals generated by chemotherapy and radiation therapy. Thus, enteral glutamine supplementation may enhance the selectivity of antitumor drugs by protecting normal tissue and sensitizing tumor cells to chemotherapy-related injury (101).

In a recent double-blind, randomized, controlled clinical trial, patients given glutamine-supplemented TPN after bone marrow transplantation demonstrated improved nitrogen balance, reduced infection, lower rates of microfloral overgrowth, and shortened hospital stay compared with patients receiving standard TPN (102). Although nutrient intake was similar in both groups, nitrogen balance improved in glutamine-supplemented TPN patients compared with controls (-1.4 ± 0.5 g/d vs. -4.2 ± 1.2; $p = 0.002$). Furthermore, fewer experimental patients (13%) developed fewer clinical infections in contrast to controls (43%). Finally, patients receiving glutamine had significantly lower incidences of microfloral colonization and shortened hospitalizations (29 ± 1 days vs. 36 ± 2 days; $p = 0.017$).

Although enteral diets supplemented with glutamine alone maintain intestinal mucosal integrity, the addition of epidermal growth factor has a synergistic effect on mucosal growth in the small intestine (103). Additionally, glucocorticoid hormones may increase intestinal glutamine utilization by increasing glutaminase expression, thereby providing more energy for enterocytes in stress-related states (104). Thus, growth factors and hormones may act as trophic factors in conjunction with glutamine to maintain the integrity of the intestinal mucosa.

Butyrate

Short-chain fatty acids, the most important of which in humans include acetate, n-butyrate, and propionate, are fermentation end-products of enzymatic breakdown of dietary fiber and undigested starch by the colonic microflora. They are essential for the metabolic welfare of colonocytes and are important regulators of the colonic milieu. Short-chain fatty acids increase colonocyte proliferation, stimulate mucosal growth, enhance blood flow, and improve energy metabolism. Numerous studies indicate increased mitotic indices and labelling index scores in crypts of colonic mucosa infused with SCFAs (13,105). Acetate, n-butyrate, and propionate account for the majority of SCFAs produced in the human colon. Of these, butyrate is preferentially oxidized by normal colonocytes when compared with such common fuels as glucose, glutamine, and ketone bodies (13,106,107). Butyrate has a sparing effect on glucose and glutamine oxidation. Accordingly, glucose or glutamine does not decrease the entry of butyrate carbons in the Krebs cycle (108).

Normal colonocytes depend on fatty acid oxidation (β-oxidation) for energy production, and SCFA availability strongly affects this oxidation process (108). When starved of SCFAs, colonocytes oxidize butyrate at a significantly diminished rate with decreased ketogenesis. Since butyrate is not synthesized by mammalian tissue, the colonic mucosa can only obtain it from bacterial fermentation of polysaccharides predominantly found in dietary fiber and undigested starch. In normal colonocytes, preferred activation of butyrate to its CoA derivatives by short-chain CoA synthetases leads to production of adenosine triphosphate (ATP) and acetyl CoA essential for cellular metabolism. Thus, butyrate deprivation, and consequently diminished β-oxidation, can cause severe functional consequences for colonocytes. Butyrate deficiency may lead to decreased absorption, diminished lipid synthesis, reduced mucus production, and impaired detoxification mechanisms in the colon. These conditions, in turn, may lead to colonocyte barrier breakdown and other detrimental sequelae (108).

Past studies demonstrate that butyrate is the most important SCFA in eliciting colonocyte proliferation (13,105). Dose response experiments in vivo demonstrate a dose-dependent stimulatory effect of SCFA on CCPR in the order of effectiveness: n-butyrate, propionate, and acetate in rats (13,106). Furthermore, intralumenal perfusion of butyrate concentrations of 20 mM, 40 mM, and 150 mM into cecectomized rat colon increases segmental DNA by 100%, 100%, and 50%, respectively. Infusion of 20 mM of butyrate stimulates colonic mucosal growth similarly to physiologic concentrations of acetate, butyrate, and propionate. Moreover, butyrate concentrations 7.5 times the normal colonic concentration (20 mM) do not significantly increase colonocyte proliferation and mucosal growth. Thus, butyrate is the primary fuel for colonocytes, and normal colonic concentrations of this fatty acid alone is optimal for colonocyte proliferation (107,109).

In a clinical study, seven patients with diversion colitis were treated with SCFA irrigations (butyrate, 40 mmol/l; propionate, 30 mmol/l; and acetate, 60 mmol/l) twice daily for 2 to 6 weeks. Endoscopic appearance of colonic mucosa of patients receiving SCFAs improved after 2 weeks and progressively improved after 4 to 6 weeks when compared with saline controls. Histologic degree of colonic inflammation decreased dramatically (110). In another study, butyrate enemas (100 mmol/l) given twice daily for 2 weeks to ten patients with distal ulcerative colitis returned colonocyte production to normal values and expanded proliferative zones within the mucosa. Stool frequency and rectal bleeding regressed in patients receiving butyrate enemas. Furthermore, endoscopic appearance of colonic mucosa improved considerably and histologic findings of inflammation decreased significantly (111).

Butyrate studies in vitro demonstrate paradoxical results to the in vivo studies. While some studies show that butyrate stimulates colonic epithelial cell proliferation in 25- and 60-mM concentrations in vitro, other cell studies show that butyrate concentrations of 2 to 8 mM has no effect or decreases cell proliferation (112–114). If these in vitro studies receive further confirmation, the possibility that butyrate acts via an intermediary found only in intact colonic mucosa appears likely. The paradoxical effects of butyrate in vitro merit further investigation.

In critically ill patients unable to eat voluntarily, prolonged TPN administration does not provide butyrate to the starving colon. Such fasting conditions decrease β-oxidation in colonocytes without compensation from other metabolic mechanisms. In past experimental models, when butyrate has been withheld from the colon, mucosal absorption of sodium and water is significantly reduced (108). Severe starvation of the colon may lead to mucosal alterations known as colitis, which is seen under famine conditions. Some detrimental effects of colonocyte starvation can be reversed by infusion of SCFA (i.e., butyrate), as demonstrated in dog colonic loops and human colon affected by diversion colitis (110,115). Orally administered butyrate is quickly and completely absorbed in the jejunum and does not reach the colon. Since a slow-release form of butyrate has not been developed, it is presently administered therapeutically by rectal irrigation (116).

In summary, there is conclusive evidence that butyrate metabolism is essential for normal colonocyte function. Colonocyte β-oxidation of butyrate is involved in such processes as ATP production, lipogenesis, sodium absorption, histone acetylation, and detoxification (108). Since butyrate is not synthesized in mammalian tissue, lack of enteral nutrients or suppressed colonic microflora due to antibiotic therapy may starve colonocytes and cause mucosal barrier breakdown. Theoretically, butyrate may prevent such functional and structural alterations within the colon in critical illness. Although initial clinical trials are encouraging, more extended human studies with butyrate are needed.

Omega-3 Fatty Acids (Fish Oils)

New immunoregulatory components in EN, such as omega-3 fatty acids (fish oils) may be important in stimulating the gut immune system and maintaining intestinal integrity in critically ill patients (117). Omega-3 fatty acids of fish oil alter inflammatory reactions by down-regulating eicosanoid production. Increased levels of eicosanoids elevate PGE2 production, which results in severe host immuosuppression. Excess PGE2 has been associated with postoperative infection, trauma, and sepsis. Following severe trauma or surgery, increased PGE2 production by host macrophages and monocytes results in diminished T-cell function, reduced T-cell proliferative response, and increased suppressor T-cell activity (118). This may explain in part why critically ill or postoperative patients, despite vigorous antibiotic therapy, have high infection rates sometimes accompanied by death due to sepsis. Recent studies in animals suggest omega-3 fatty acids ameliorate this immunosuppression by depressing eicosanoid production and action. In one study, high levels of dietary omega-3 fatty acids reduced PGE2 synthesis in rat spleen and thymus following immune challenge (119). Additionally, intravenously fed fish oil emulsions markedly improved survival in guinea pigs administered single doses of endotoxin (120). In rats administered fish oil–derived fatty acids for 50 days, decreased PGE2 production during the chronic phase of inflammation occurred after antigenic challenge (121). Thus, omega-3 fatty acid–supplemented enteral diets may be beneficial in down-regulating eicosanoid production in critically ill patients with severe sepsis.

Growth Factors

In recent years, the role of growth factors in intestinal growth and function has received considerable interest. Established methods of studying their effects in the gut include stimulation of endogenous growth factor production, administration of exogenous growth factor, and inhibition of growth factor synthesis (122). Furthermore, new approaches using molecular biologic techniques have improved our understanding in evaluating the relationship between growth factors and the gut. Identification of genes and cDNAs, which encode intestinal growth factors and their receptors, and nucleotide sequencing provide important mapping and structural information. Studies of gene expression by localization and measurement of mRNA may reveal changes in growth factor and/or receptor synthesis in intestinal growth. Direct information about growth factor effects in the gut can be obtained from transgenic mice that over- or underexpress growth factor and/or receptor genes (123).

Several growth factors help regulate mucosal growth in the small intestine and colon. Although some of their effects are tissue specific, alteration of cell proliferation is a common mechanism shared by all growth factors. Growth factors affecting cell proliferation in the intestinal mucosa include growth hormone (GH), insulin-like growth factor I (IGF-I), epidermal growth factor (EGF), neurotensin (NT), and transforming growth factors (TGFα and TGFβ) (Table 2).

Growth Hormone

The trophic effects of GH on intestinal mucosa are well known. However, there is still some uncertainty as to whether these effects are a direct consequence of GH

TABLE 2. *Summary and description of principle growth factors that influence intestinal cell proliferation and differentiation.*

Growth factor	Receptor/Location	Intestinal cell action	Comments

GH	GH receptors
	Small intestine
	  Crypt base columnar
	    cells
	  Villous columnar cells
	  Goblet cells
	  Enteroendocrine cells
	Colon
	  Crypt base cells
	  Surface columnar
	    cells
		Mucosal growth
		  Increases cell longevity.
		  Increases cell proliferation
		    (?)
			Probably mediated by IGF-I.

IGF-I,
IGF-II
	IGF-I, II receptors
	Small intestine
	  Crypt base cells
	  Villous columnar cells
	Colon
	  Crypt base cells
	  Apical columnar cells
	Binding activity
	  Colon > small
	    intestine
	Receptor density
	  Crypt > apex
		Mucosal Growth
		  Crypt cell proliferation
		    Increases DNA and
		    protein synthesis.
		  Increases postresection
		    adaptive hyperplasia.
			IGFBPs modulate
			IGF-receptor interaction.
			IGF-I ten times more potent
			than IGF-II.

EGF	EGF/TGFα receptors
	Small intestine and
	  colon
	Apical and basolateral
	  surfaces of cell
	  membranes
	Intrinsic protein-tyrosine
	  kinase activity.
		Mucosal growth
		  Increase crypt cell
		    production
		  Enhances cell maturation in
		    fetal intestine
		  Regulates water, sodium,
		    chloride, and glucose
		    transport
			Mediated by TGFα
			Parenteral effects > enteral
			effects

NT	NT receptors in small
	  intestine and colon
		Increases mucosal growth
		  Small intestine mostly
		    jejunum
		    Cell proliferation
		  Colon
		    Increases cell proliferation
		     in young.
		    Causes cell hypertrophy
		     in adult
		  Increases postresection
		    adaptive hyperplasia.
			NT mRNA found in small
			  intestine (mostly distal)
			  and colon
			Posttranscriptional
			  mechanism regulates NT
			  production in intestinal
			  mucosa.

TGFα	EGF/TGF receptor present
	  throughout small
	  intestine and colon.
		Increases mucosal growth
		  Increases cell proliferation
		  Increases cell migration
		    Enhances cell
		     differentiation.
		    Epithelial cell restituion
		     (wound healing).
			Similar in structure and
			  activity to EGF

TGFβ	Specific TGFβ receptor (?)
	  throughout small
	  intestine and colon
		Inhibits cell proliferation
		Cell migration
		  Induces cell
		    differentiation/
		    maturation
		  Enhances cell restitution
		    (wound healing)
			Production and function
			  apex > crypt base

or secondary to improved nutrition, hyperphagia, or nutrient-stimulated release of secondary hormones such as gastrin and somatostatin (124). In an early study, GH demonstrated a mitogenic effect on crypt cells of the duodenum in hypophysectomized rats (125). Subsequent studies showed that GH induced gastrointestinal tract hypertrophy in hypophysectomized rats as well as histogenesis in fetal rat intestinal transplants (126,127).

The growth-promoting effects of GH in the small intestine and colon have traditionally been considered to be mediated by IGF-I (128,129). One study, however, indicates that discrete epithelial cell subpopulations of the intestinal mucosa are directly responsive to GH (130). The crypt base columnar, villous columnar, goblet, and enteroendocrine cells of the small intestine and the crypt base and surface columnar cells of the colon all possess GH receptors of heterogeneous distribution (130). The localization of these specific GH receptors supports the importance of GH in the proliferation of intestinal epithelial cells (131,132). Thus, GH may act independently, via second messengers such as IGF-I or synergistically with IGF-I as a growth promoter in the small intestine and colon (130).

A model of chronic GH excess, transgenic mice with bovine GH gene linked to mouse metallothionein I promoter demonstrate increased growth of small-bowel mucosa (133). Chronic GH excess increases jejunal villus height, small-bowel weight, mucosal mass, and DNA protein content accompanied by an increase in intestinal IGF-I mRNA expression in mouse small intestine. Furthermore, this effect in transgenic mice appears not to be secondary to increased rate of enterocyte proliferation. This finding suggests GH may have a prolonging effect on the lifespan of intestinal mucosal cells (133).

Insulin-like Growth Factors I and II

Insulin-like growth factors I and II are polypeptides that play an important role in mucosal growth by modulating intestinal crypt cell proliferation. Insulin-like growth factor-I induces increased DNA and protein synthesis in intestinal crypt cells in vitro and enhances intestinal mucosal adaptation after gut resection (128,134–136). It interacts with its receptors throughout the small intestine and colon and is considered a primary mediator of postnatal trophic effects of GH (137,138). Similar to IGF-I, IGF-II stimulates DNA and protein synthesis in IEC-6 cells (135). In concentration response experiments, IGF-I is about ten times more potent than IGF-II in stimulating DNA and protein syntheses in IEC-6 cells (135).

Once considered to be primarily synthesized in the liver, IGFs are now known to be produced locally within many organs, including the gut (128,139). Studies with in situ hybridization and Northern blot techniques have revealed mRNA for IGF-I and IGF-II in fetal human and rat intestine (139,140). Intestinal synthesis of IGF as well as many of the binding proteins suggests that these growth factors function predominantly through either autocrine or paracrine mechanisms as well (135,138,141,142).

Despite intestinal synthesis of several types of IGF-binding proteins (IGFBPs)

(143–145), their roles have not been clearly determined. Several in vitro studies suggest that endogenous production of IGFBPs may facilitate or inhibit IGF action. However, most studies demonstrate an inhibitory role for IGFBPs that prevents IGFs from interacting with intestinal cell-surface IGF receptors (135,146). If these findings are correct, decreased IGF potency in vivo may correlate with binding with IGFBPs. In a recent animal study in vivo, decreased ileal synthesis of IGFBP-3 enhanced IGF-1 bioability to stimulate ileal cell proliferation and adaptation after massive small-bowel resection (147). Other research, however, indicates that the mitogenic effect of IGF-I is actually dependent on its ability to bind IGFBPs (148,149). Thus, the mitogenic effects of IGFs are most likely the result of complex interactions between IGFBPs and IGF cell receptors.

Receptors for IGF-I and IGF-II have higher expressions in proliferative crypt cells when compared to the apical cells of the rat small intestine and colon, although these receptors are present on a variety of cells in the intestinal epithelium (138). Additionally, heterogeneity among receptors exists between the small intestine and colon as well as among the various layers within each organ. Interestingly, binding activity to IGF receptors is higher in the colon than in the rest of the gastrointestinal tract in the rat (138). Receptor density in the intestinal epithelium is much greater in the crypts than in the villi, which suggests that IGF receptors modulate crypt cell proliferation and decrease in expression with intestinal cell differentiation (138,150). Insulin-like growth factor receptors are polarized on the apical membranes of proximal colon mucosa with apical colonocytes possessing only type I IGF receptors (151). Although abundant IGF-I and IGF-II receptors have been identified in the human colon, their role in mucosal growth and adaptation in both small intestine and colon is not fully understood (152,153).

Epidermal Growth Factor

Epidermal growth factor is a well-known mitogen that stimulates cell proliferation in vitro and in vivo. The trophic effects of EGF occur in many types of epithelial cells, especially in those of the intestinal mucosa (154,155). Although its underlying mechanisms are still unknown, recombinant human EGF (urogastrone) effectively stimulates intestinal cell production in adult rats and humans (156,157). Some of these EGF-induced effects may be mediated by the analogue TGFα (158,159). Since EGF and TGFα share the same intestinal cell-surface receptors (EGF/TGF α receptor), many effects of EGF may also apply to TGFα (160). Nevertheless, EGF is important in cell proliferation and maturation of pre- and postnatal intestine (161). In suckling mice, repeated injections of EGF stimulates intestinal DNA synthesis and production of certain absorptive enzymes (162). Furthermore, EGF promotes maturation of fetal small intestine and differentiation of brush border membranes in fetal mice (163,164).

While single dose of EGF does not affect cell proliferation, repeated daily injections or parenteral feeding with EGF greatly enhances this process in small intestine and colon (162,165). The effect of EGF differs when administered enterally or parenterally

(165,166). In one study, EGF given enterally did not stimulate cell proliferation in rat colon (167), whereas intravenous recombinant EGF reversed marked intestinal hypoplasia characteristically found in TPN-fed rats (168). Total parenteral nutrition with EGF restores CCPR in small intestine to levels found in orally fed rats and increases labelling (tritiated thymidine) per crypt in the colon more than twice that of enterally fed rats (168).

Epidermal growth factor receptors are present throughout the intestine and have been located on both basolateral and brush-border membranes (169,170). Such receptors with intrinsic protein-tyrosine kinase activity phosphorylate several endogenous proteins (171). While their role in signaling cell proliferation and mucosal growth remains unknown, EGF receptors may regulate water, sodium, chloride, and glucose transport in the gut. In vivo transport studies reveal that EGF-receptor interactions increase chloride, glucose, sodium, and water absorption in rabbit jejunum (172). Thus, EGF up-regulates electrolyte and nutrient absorption in the small bowel, which may partially explain its function in both normal and stressed intestine.

Neurotensin

Neurotensin is a tridecapeptide found in mucosal endocrine cells of the jejunum and ileum (173). It has a trophic effect in many tissues in the gastrointestinal tract, including small intestine and colon (174–176). Long-term NT administration stimulates colonic mucosal growth in both young and adult rats. Although NT increases colonocyte proliferation in young rats, it appears to only increase colonocyte size (hypertrophy) in adult rats (177). Subcutaneous injections of NT reverse small-bowel mucosal hypoplasia associated with liquid elemental diets in aged rats. Neurotensin apparently stimulates cell proliferation in rat small intestine that is most pronounced in the jejunum (177).

Neurotensin may also be important in the intestinal regeneration after small-bowel resection in rats (178,179). A recent study suggests NT augments adaptive hyperplasia in intestinal mucosa after small-bowel resection (180). Within 7 to 8 days after resection, maximal mucosal hyperplasia usually occurs in the residual small intestine. After 7 days of administration, NT increased DNA, RNA, and protein content in residual small intestinal mucosa after distal or proximal enterectomy. Thus, NT has the capability to promote cell proliferation usually stimulated solely by small-bowel resection (180).

Recent Northern blot analysis and hybridization of rat encoding gene for NT and neuromedin-N has been utilized to map the intestinal distribution of NT mRNA and to study the regulation of NT expression during periods of fasting and refeeding in rats (181). Neurotensin mRNA transcripts are distributed throughout rat small intestine and proximal colon with the greatest amount found in the distal small bowel. Furthermore, rats fasted for 72 hours have profoundly reduced NT intestinal tissue concentrations, while such animals refed for 24 hours return such NT concentrations to normal levels. Interestingly, the amount of NT mRNA and its rate of transcription are not affected by periods of fasting and feeding. Such results strongly suggest that a yet undefined posttranscriptional mechanism regulates NT production in intestinal mucosa (181).

Transforming Growth Factors α and β

Transforming growth factor α is expressed throughout the gastrointestinal tract with the highest amounts found in the colon (182). Similar to EGF in structure and activity, TGFα stimulates intestinal cell proliferation and may promote cell migration and modulate intestinal membrane transport (183–185). It promotes migration of many cell types, including intestinal epithelial cells. In the normal human adult, TGFα is localized in small intestinal villi and restricted to the upper third of colonic crypts (182,186,187). This pattern of distribution within the differentiated regions of the intestinal epithelium suggests TGFα, along with proliferative effects, may play an equally important role in cell differentiation. Such mediated migration may not only be important in cell differentiation from crypt to lumenal surface, but also in rapid restitution of the gut barrier after injury to the intestinal epithelium (188).

As mentioned, TGFα and EGF share the same intestinal cell-surface receptors (EGF/TGFα receptor) on intestinal epithelial cells. Because EGF is limited within the intestinal tract, TGFα is probably the natural ligand for this receptor (170,187). Indeed, coexpression of TGFα and EGF/TGFα receptor transcripts from morphologically normal human colonic epithelium has been reported (189). Nevertheless, how these TGFα-stimulated receptors signal or promote specific physiologic effects in the gut via an autocrine or paracrine mechanism remains to be determined.

In contrast to TGFα, TGFβ appears to inhibit cell proliferation in vitro and in vivo (190,191). Furthermore, TGFβ has the ability to induce differentiation and maturation by activating cells to develop into a nonproliferative state (191). In HT29 colon carcinoma sublines, TGFβ1 blocks or restricts cells in early G1 phase of the cell cycle where immature colonocytes begin to differentiate (192). Although initially thought to be greatest in crypt cells and least in columnar villous cells (186), recent studies have demonstrated that TGFβ activity and mRNA content are greatest in columnar villous cells and least in the crypt cells (191,193). In embryonic mice, isoform-specific antibodies intensely strain TGFβ1 in differentiated cells localized in villi and crypt surfaces of small intestine and colon, respectively (194).

As with TGFα, TGFβ may mediate rapid restitution of the gut barrier after injury to the intestinal epithelium. Although addition of this peptide inhibits cell proliferation in IEC-6 monolayers after "injury" with a razor blade, TGFβ nevertheless enhances restitution by quickening cell migration into the artificially induced wounds (195). Thus, TGFβ may accelerate healing of intestinal epithelial cells in vivo by inducing rapid cell migration into wounds.

CONCLUSION

The process of proliferation and differentiation maintain intestinal epithelial cell growth and function. These processes are enhanced by enteral nutrients and growth factors and retarded by malnutrition, bowel rest, and certain illnesses. As the result of these findings, scientific evidence is accruing to confirm the importance of providing some enteral nutrients to critically ill patients. Identification of the amount and type of nutrients to optimize gut structure and function remains to be elucidated.

ACKNOWLEDGMENTS

The authors gratefully acknowledge the secretarial assistance of Ms. Renée Seto.

REFERENCES

1. Potten CS, Loeffler M. Stem cells: attributes, cycles, spirals, pitfalls and uncertainties. Lessons for and from the crypt. *Development* 1990;110:1001–1020.
2. Johnson LR. Regulation of gastrointestinal growth. In: Johnson LR, ed. *Physiology of the Gastrointestinal Tract*. 2nd ed. New York: Raven Press, 1987;301–333.
3. Lipkin M. Proliferation and differentiation of normal and diseased gastrointestinal cells. In: Johnson LR, ed. *Physiology of the Gastrointestinal Tract*. 2nd ed. New York: Raven Press, 1987a;255–284.
4. Madara JL, Trier JS. Functional morphology of the mucosa of the small intestine. In: Johnson LR, ed. *Physiology of the Gastrointestinal Tract*. 2nd ed. New York: Raven Press, 1987;1209–1249.
5. Shamsuddin AM, Phelps PC, Trump BF. Human large intestinal epithelium: light microscopy, biochemistry, and ultrastructure. *Hum Pathol* 1982;13:790–803.
6. Colony PC. The identification of cell types in the normal adult colon. In: Augenlicht LH, ed. *Cell and Molecular Biology of Colon Cancer*. Boca Raton: CRC Press, 1989;2–21.
7. Lipkin M, Enker WE, Winawer SJ. Tritiated thymidine labelling of rectal epithelial cells in non prep biopsies of individuals at increased risk for colonic neoplasia. *Cancer Lett* 1987b;37:153–161.
8. Rozen P, Fireman Z, Fine N, et al. Oral calcium suppresses rectal epithelial proliferation of persons at risk of colorectal cancer. *Gut* 1989;30:650–655.
9. Gibson PR, van de Pol E, Maxwell LE, et al. The isolation of human colonic epithelial cells which maintain structural and metabolic viability *in vitro*. *Gastroenterology* 1989;96:283–291.
10. Whitehead RH, Nice EC, Lloyd CJ, et al. Detection of colonic growth factors using a human colonic carcinoma cell line (LIM 1215). *Int J Cancer* 1990;46:858–863.
11. Wimber DR, Lamerton LF. Cell population studies on the intestine of continuously irradiated rats. *Radiat Res* 1963;18:137–146.
12. Wright NA, Appleton DR. The metaphase arrest technique; a critical review. *Cell Tissue Kinet* 1980;13:643–663.
13. Sakata T. Stimulatory effect of short chain fatty acids on epithelial cell proliferation in the rat intestine: a possible explanation for trophic effects of fermentable fibre, gut miocrobes and luminal trophic factors. *Br J Nutr* 1987;58:94–103.
14. Darmon E, Pincu-Hornstein A, Rozen P. A rapid and simple *in vitro* method for evaluating human colorectal epithelial proliferation. *Arch Pathol Lab Med* 1990;114:855–857.
15. Lipkin M. Biomarkers of increased susceptiblity to gastrointestinal cancer: new application to studies of cancer prevention in human subjects. *Cancer Res* 1988;48:235–245.
16. Bell L, Williams L. Histochemical demonstration of alkaline phosphatase in human large intestine, normal and diseased. *Histochemistry* 1979;60:84.
17. Chung YS, Song IS, Erickson RH, et al. Effect of growth and sodium butyrate on brush border membrane associated hydrolases in human colorectal cancer cell lines. *Cancer Res* 1985;45:2976.
18. Higgins PJ. Antigenic and cytoarchitectural "markers" of differentiation pathways in normal and malignant colonic epithelial cells. In: Augenlicht LH, ed. *Cell and Molecular Biology of Colon Cancer*. Boca Raton: CRC Press, 1989;112–132.
19. Neutra MR, Grand RJ, Trier JS. Glycoprotein synthesis, transport and secretion by epithelial cells of human rectal mucosa. *Lab Invest* 1977;36:535.
20. Young GP, Gibson PR. Contrasting effects of butyrate on proliferation and differentiation of normal and neoplastic cells. In: Cummings J, Sakata T, Rombeau J eds. *Short-chain Fatty Acids: Metabolism*

and Clinical Importance. Report of the Ross Conference on Medical Research. Columbus: Ross Laboratories, 1991;50–55.

20a. Lew JI, Rombeau JL. The effects of nutrients on the intestine epithelium. In: Fürst P ed. *New Strategies in Clinical Nutrition.* Munich: W. Zuckschwerdt Verlag, 1993;64–84.

21. Feldman EJ, Dowling RH, McNaughton J, et al. Effects of oral versus intravenous nutrition on intestinal adaptation after small bowel resection in the dog. *Gastroenterology* 1976;70:712–719.

22. Reinken EO, Menge H. Nutritive effects of food constituents on the structure and function of the intestine. *Acta Hepatogastrenterol* 1977;24:388–399.

23. Ryan GP, Dudrick SJ, Copeland EM, et al. Effects of various diets on colonic growth in rats. *Gastroenterology* 1979;77:658–663.

24. Ecknauer R, Sicar B, Johnson LR. Effect of dietary bulk in small intestinal morphology and cell renewal in the rat. *Gastroenterology* 1981;81:781–786.

25. Rijike RPC, Plaisier HM, DeRuiter H, Galjaard H. Influence of experimental bypass on cellular kinetics and maturation of small intestinal epithelium in the rat. *Gastroenterology* 1977;72:896–901.

26. Cameron IL, Ord VA, Hunter KE, et al. Quantitative contribution of factors regulating rat colonic crypt epithelium: role of parenteral and enteral feeding, caloric intake, dietary cellulose level and the colon carcinogen DMH. *Cell Tissue Kinet* 1990;23:227–235.

27. Cummings JH, Branch WJ. Fermentation and the production of short chain fatty acids in the human large intestine. In: Vahouny GV, Kritchevsky D, eds. *Basic and Medical Aspects of Dietary Fiber.* New York: Plenum Press, 1986;131–149.

28. Cummings JH. Colonic absorption: the importance of short chain fatty acids in man. *Scand J Gastroenterol* 1984;19:90–99.

29. Vahouny GV. Effects of dietary fiber on digestion and absorption. In: Johnson LR, ed. *Physiology of the Gastrointestinal Tract.* 2nd ed. New York: Raven Press, 1987;1623–1648.

30. Vahouny GV, Cassidy MM. Dietary fiber and intestinal adaptation. In: Vahouny GV, Kritchevsky D, eds. *Basic and Medical Aspects of Dietary Fiber.* New York: Plenum Press, 1986;181–209.

31. Jacobs LR. Dietary fiber and the intestinal mucosa. In: Cummings JH, ed. *The Role of Dietary Fiber in Enteral Nutrition.* Abbott Park: Abbott International, 1989;24–35.

32. Bristol JB, Williamson CN. Large bowel growth. *Scand J Gastroenterol* 1984;19(S93):25–34.

33. Dembinski AB, Johnson LR. Growth of pancreas and gastrointestinal mucosa in antrectomy and gastrin treated rats. *Endocrinology* 1979;105:769–773.

34. Sirinek KR, Levine BA, Moyer MP. Pentagastrin stimulates *in vitro* growth of normal and malignant human colon epithelial cells. *Am J Surg* 1985;149:35–39.

35. Johnson LR. Regulation of gastrointestinal mucosal growth. *World J Surg* 1979;3:477–487.

36. Ryberg B, Axelson J, Hakanson R, et al. Trophic effects of continuous infusion of [Leu15]-gastrin-17 in the rat. *Gastroenterology* 1990;98:33–38.

37. Bloom SR, Polak JM. The hormonal pattern of intestinal adaptation. A major role for enteroglucagon. *Scand J Gastroenterol* 1982;17(S74):93–103.

38. Gornacz GE, Al Mukhtar MYT, et al. Pattern of cell proliferation and enteroglucagon response following small bowel resection in the rat. *Digestion* 1984;29:65–72.

39. Goodlad RA, Al Mukhtar MYT, Ghatei MA, et al. Cell proliferation, plasma enteroglucagon and plasma gastrin levels in starved and refed rats. *Virchows Arch Cell Pathol* 1983;43:55–62.

40. Gleeson MM, Bloom SR, Polak JK, et al. Endocrine tumor in kidney affecting small bowel structure, mobility and absorptive function. *Gut* 1971;122:773–782.

41. Sagor G, Ghatei M, Al-Mukhtar MYT, et al. Evidence for a humoral mechanism after small intestinal resection. *Gastroenterology* 1983;84:902–906.

42. Buchan A, Griffiths CJ, Morris JF, et al. Enteroglucagon cell hyperfunction in rat small intestine after gut resection. *Gastroenterology* 1985;88:8–12.

43. Miazza B, et al. Hyperenteroglucagonaemia and small intestinal mucosal growth after colonic perfusion of glucose in rats. *Gut* 1985;26:518–524.

44. Sagor G, Ghatei M, O'Shaughnessy DJ, et al. Influence of somatostatin and bombesin on plasma enteroglucagon and cell proliferation after intestinal resection in the rat. *Gut* 1985;26:89–94.

45. Kvietys PR, Granger ND. Effect of volatile fatty acids on blood flow and oxygen uptake by the dog colon. *Gastroenterology* 1981;80:962–969.

46. Demigné C, Remesy C. Stimulation of absorption of volatile fatty acids and minerals in the cecum of rats adapted to a very high fiber diet. *J Nutr* 1985;115:53–60.

47. Cummings JH, Pomare EW, Branch WJ, et al. Short chain fatty acids in human large intestine, portal, hepatic and venous blood. *Gut* 1987;28:1221–1227.

48. Sakata T. Effects of indigestible dietary fibre bulk and short-chain fatty acids on tissue and weight and epithelial proliferation rate of the digestive tract in rats. *J Nutr Sci Vitaminol* 1986;32:355–362.
49. Mortensen FV, Nielsen H, Mulvany MJ, Hessov I. Short chain fatty acids dilate isolated human colonic resistance arteries. *Gut* 1990;31:1391–1394.
50. Karlstad MD, Killeffer JA, Bailey JW, DeMichele SJ. Parenteral nutrition with short- and long-chain triglycerides: triacetin reduces atrophy of small and large bowel mucosa and improves protein metabolism in burned rats. *Am J Clin Nutr* 1992;55:1005–1011.
51. Tutton PJM, Helme RD. The influence of adrenoceptor activity on crypt cell proliferation in the rat jejunum. *Cell Tissue Kinet* 1974;7:125–136.
52. Tutton PJM. Absence of a circadian rhythm in crypt cell mitotic rate following chemical sympathetcomy in rats. *Virchows Arch [B]* 1975;19:151–156.
53. Klein RM. Analysis of intestinal cell proliferation after guanethidine-induced sympathectomy III. *Cell Tissue Kinet* 1980;13:153–162.
54. Thomas EM, Templeton D. Noradrenergic innervation of the villi of rat jejunum. *J Auton Nerv Syst* 1981;3:25–29.
55. Jacobowitz D. Histochemical studies of the autonomic innervation of the gut. *J Pharmacol Exp Ther* 1965;149:358–364.
56. Newson B, Ahlman H, Dahlstrom A, et al. On the innervation of the ileal mucosa in the rat-a synapse. *Acta Physiol Scand* 1979;105:387–389.
57. Frankel WL, Zhang W, Singh A, et al. Stimulation of autonomic nervous system mediates SCFA induced jejunal trophism. *Surg Forum* 1992;43:24–26.
58. Jackson WD, Grand RJ. The human intestinal response to enteral nutrients: a review. *J Am Coll Nutr* 1991;10:500–509.
59. Brown HO, Levine ML, Lipkin M. Inhibition of intestinal epithelial cell renewal and migration induced by starvation. *Am J Physiol* 1963;205:868–872.
60. Rossi TM, Lee PC, Young CM, et al. Effect of nutritional rehabilitation on the development of intestinal brush border disaccharidases of postnatally malnourished weanling rats. *Pediatr Res* 1986; 20:793–797.
61. Solimano G, Burgess EA, Levin B. Protein-calorie malnutrition: effect of deficient diets on enzyme levels of jejunal mucosa of rats. *Br J Nutr* 1967;21:55–68.
62. Altmann GG. Influence of starvation and refeeding on mucosal size and epithelial renewal in the rat small intestine. *Am J Anat* 1972;133:391–400.
63. Aldewachi HS, Wright NA, Appleton DR, Watson AJ. The effect of starvation and refeeding on cell population kinetics in the rat small bowel mucosa. *J Anat* 1975;119:105–121.
64. Butzner JD, Gall DG. Impact of refeeding on intestinal development and function in infant rabbits subjected to protein-energy malnutrition. *Pediatr Res* 1990;27:245–251.
65. Brunser O. Effects of malnutrition on intestinal structure and function in children. *Clin Gastroenterol* 1977;6:341–353.
66. James WPT. Effects of protein-calorie malnutrition on intestinal absorption. *Ann NY Acad Sci* 1971; 175:244–261.
67. Wilmore DW, Smith RJ, O'Dwyer ST, et al. The gut: a central organ after surgical stress. *Surgery* 1988;104:917–923.
68. Saadia R, Schein M, MacFarlane C, Boffard KD. Gut barrier function and the surgeon. *Br J Surg* 1990;77:487–492.
69. Jones WG, Minei JP, Barber AE, et al. Splanchnic vasoconstriction and bacterial translocation after thermal injury. *Am J Physiol* 1991;261:H1190–H1196.
70. Deitch EA. Bacterial translocation of the gut flora. *J Trauma* 1990;30:S184–S189.
71. Hong RW, Rounds JD, Helton WS, et al. Glutamine preserves liver glutathione after lethal hepatic injury. *Ann Surg* 1992;215:114–119.
72. Robinson MK, Rounds JD, Hong RW, et al. Glutathione deficiency increases organ dysfunction after hemorrhagic shock. *Surgery* 1992;112:140–149.
73. Berg RD. Translocation of indigenous bacteria from the intestinal tract lumen. In: Hentges DJ, ed. *Intestinal Microflora in Health and Disease.* New York: Academic Press, 1983;333–352.
74. Hammer-Hodges D, Woodruff P, Cuevas P, et al. Role of intraintestinal gram-negative bacterial flora in response to major injury. *Surg Gynecol Obstet* 1974;138:599–603.
75. Deitch EA, Berg R, Specian R. Endotoxin promotes the translocation of bacteria from the gut. *Arch Surg* 1987;122:185–190.
76. Rush BF, Sori AJ, Murphy TF, et al. Endotoxemia and bacteremia during hemorrhagic shock: the link between trauma and sepsis? *Ann Surg* 1988;207:549–554.

77. Deitch EA. Multiple organ failure: pathophysiology and potential future therapy. *Ann Surg* 1992; 216:117–134.
78. Goris RJA. Boekholtz WKF, van Bebber IPT, et al. Multiple organ failure and sepsis without bacteria: an experimental model. *Arch Surg* 1986;121:897–901.
79. Border JR. Multiple systems organ failure. *Ann Surg* 1992;216:111–116.
80. Zhi-Yong S, Yuan-Lin D, Xiao-Hong W. Bacterial translocation and multiple system organ failure in bowel ischemia and reperfusion. *J Trauma* 1992;32:148–153.
81. Rolandelli RH, Rombeau JL. Enteral nutrition in critically ill patients. *Perspect Crit Care* 1989;2: 1–16.
82. Ryan JA. Jejunal feeding. In: Fischer JE, ed. *Surgical Nutrition.* 1st ed. Boston: Little, Brown, 1983;757–777.
83. Muggia-Sullam M, Bower RH, Murphy RF, et al. Postoperative enteral versus parenteral nutritional support in gastrointestinal surgery. *Am J Surg* 1985;149:106–112.
84. Lowry SF. The route of feeding influences injury responses. *J Trauma* 1990;30:S10–S15.
85. Fong Y, Marano MA, Barber A, et al. Total parenteral nutrition and bowel rest modify the metabolic response to endotoxin in humans. *Ann Surg* 1989;210:449–457.
86. Windmueller HG. Glutamine utilization by the small intestine. *Adv Enzymol* 1982;53:201–237.
87. Souba WW, Herskowitz K, Austgen TR, et al. Glutamine nutrition: theoretical considerations and therapeutic impact. *J Parenter Enteral Nutr* 1990;14:237S–243S.
88. McAnena OJ, Moore FA, Moore EE, et al. Selective uptake of glutamine in the gastrointestinal tract: confirmation in a human study. *Br J Surg* 1991;78:480–482.
89. Herskowitz K, Souba WW. Intestinal glutamine metabolism during critical illness: a surgical perspective. *Nutrition* 1990;6:199–206.
90. O'Dwyer ST, Smith RJ, Hwang TL, Wilmore DW. Maintenance of small bowel mucosa with glutamine-enriched parenteral nutrition. *J Parenter Enteral Nutr* 1989;13:579–585.
91. Grant J, Snyder PJ. Use of L-glutamine in total parenteral nutrition. *J Surg Res* 1988;44:506–513.
92. Jacobs DO, Evans A, O'Dwyer ST, et al. Disparate effects of 5-fluorouracil on the ileum and colon of enterally fed rats with protection by dietary glutamine. *Surg Forum* 1987;38:45–49.
93. Smith RJ, O'Dwyer ST, Wang XD, et al. The gastrointestinal response to injury, starvation and enteral nutrition. Report of the Eighth Ross Conference on Medical Research, 1988;76.
94. Schroeder P, Schweizer E, Blomer A, Deltz E. Glutamine prevents mucosal injury after small bowel transplantation. *Transplant Proc* 1992;24:1104.
95. Frankel WL, Zhang W, Afonso J, et al. Glutamine enhancement of structure and function in the transplanted small intestine in the rat. *J Parenter Enteral Nutr* 1993;17:47–55.
96. Alverdy JC, Aoys E, Moss G. Total parenteral nutrition promotes bacterial translocation from the gut. *Surgery* 1988;104:185–190.
97. Burke D, Alverdy JC, Aoys E, Moss G. Glutamine supplemented TPN improves gut immune function. *Arch Surg* 1989;124:1396–1399.
98. Alverdy JC, Aoys E, Weiss-Carrington P, Burke D. The effect of glutamine-enriched TPN on gut immune cellularity. *J Surg Res* 1992;52:34–38.
99. Fox AD, Kripke SA, DePaula J, et al. Effect of a glutamine-supplemented enteral diet on methotrexate-induced enterocolitis. *J Parenter Enteral Nutr* 1988;12:325–331.
100. O'Dwyer ST, Scott T, Smith RJ, et al. 5-fluorouracil toxicity on small intestinal mucosa but not white blood cells is decreased by glutamine [abstract]. *Clin Res* 1987;35:369a.
101. Herskowitz K, Souba WW. Intestinal glutamine metabolism during critical illness: a surgical perspective. *Nutrition* 1990;6:199–206.
102. Ziegler TR, Young LS, Benfell K, et al. Clinical and metabolic efficacy of glutamine-supplemented parenteral nutrition after bone marrow transplantation. *Ann Intern Med* 1992;116:821–828.
103. Jacobs DO, Evans DA, Mealy K, et al. Combined effects of glutamine and epidermal growth factor (EGF) on GI mucosal cellularity. *Surgery* 1988;104:358–364.
104. Sarantos P, Abouhamze A, Souba WW. Glucocorticoids regulate intestinal glutaminase expression. *Surgery* 1992;112:278–283.
105. Sakata T, Yajima T. Influence of short chain fatty acids on the epithelial cell division of digestive tract. *Q J Exp Physiol* 1984;69:639–648.
106. Roediger WEW. Utilization of nutrients by isolated epithelial cells of the rat colon. *Gastroenterology* 1982;83:424–429.
107. Kripke SA, Fox AD, Berman JM, et al. Stimulation of intestinal mucosal growth with intracolonic infusion of short chain fatty acids. *J Parenter Enteral Nutr* 1989;13:109–116.

108. Roediger WEW. The place of SCFAs in colonocyte metabolism in health and ulcerative colitis: the impaired colonocyte barrier. In: Cummings JH, Sakata T, Rombeau JL, eds. *Physiologic and Clinical Aspects of Short-chain Fatty Acids*. Cambridge: Cambridge University Press, 1994; (in press).
109. Rombeau JL, Kripke SA, Settle RG. Short-chain fatty acids: production, absorption, metabolism and intestinal effects. In: Kritchevsky D, Bonfield C, Anderson JW, eds. *Dietary Fiber: Chemistry, Physiology and Health Effects*. New York: Plenum Press, 1990;317–337.
110. Harig JM, Soergel KH, Komorowski RA, Wood CM. Treatment of diversion colitis with short chain fatty acid irrigation. *N Engl J Med* 1989;320:23–28.
111. Scheppach WM, Sommer H, Kirchner T, et al. Effect of butyrate enemas on the colonic mucosa in distal ulcerative colitis. *Gastroenterology* 1992;103:51–56.
112. Friedman E, Lightdale C, Winawer S. Effects of psyllium fiber and short-chain organic acids derived from fiber breakdown on colonic epithelial cells from high risk patients. *Cancer Lett* 1988;43:121–124.
113. Young GP, Gibson PR. Contrasting effects of butyrate on proliferation and differentiation of normal and neoplastic cells. In: *Short-chain Fatty Acids: Metabolism and Clinical Importance*. Columbus: Ross Laboratories, 1991;50–55.
114. Scheppach WM. Short-chain fatty acids are a trophic factor for the human colonic mucosa in vitro. In: *Short-chain Fatty Acids: Metabolism and Clinical Importance*. Columbus: Ross Laboratories, 1991;90–93.
115. Roediger WEW, Rae DA. Trophic effect of SCFAs on mucosal handling of ions by the defunctioned colon. *Br J Surg* 1982;69:23–25.
116. Scheppach W, Bartram P, Richter F. Management of diversion colitis and other conditions. In: Cummings JH, Sakata T, Rombeau JL, eds. *Physiologic and Clinical Aspects of Short-chain Fatty Acids*. Cambridge: Cambridge University Press, 1994; (in press).
117. McClave SA, Lowen CC, Snider HL. Immunonutrition and enteral hyperalimentation of critically ill patients. *Dig Dis Sci* 1992;37:1153–1161.
118. Kinsella JE, Lokesh B, Broughton S, Whelan J. Dietary polyunsaturated fatty acids and eicosanoids: potential effects on the modulation of inflammatory and immune cells; an overview. *Nutrition* 1990; 6:24–44.
119. Marshall LA, Johnston PV. α-Linolenic and linoleic acids and the immune response. *Prog Lipid Res* 1982;20:731–734.
120. Mascioli E, Leader L, Flores E, et al. Enhanced survival to endotoxin in guinea pig fed IV fish oil emulsions. *Lipids* 1988;23:623–625.
121. Yoshino S, Ellis EF. Effect of a fish-oil-supplemented diet on inflammation and immunological processes in rats. *Int Arch Allergy Appl Immunol* 1987;84:233–240.
122. Vanderhoof JA. Regulatory peptides and intestinal growth. *Gastroenterology* 1993;104:1205–1208.
123. Lund PK, Ulshen MH, Rountree DB, et al. Molecular biology of gastrointestinal peptides and growth factors: relevance to intestinal adaptation. *Digestion* 1990;46(Suppl):66–73.
124. Konturek SJ. Role of growth factors in gastroduodenal protection and healing of peptic ulcers. *Gastroenterol Clin North Am* 1990;19:41–65.
125. Leblond CP, Carriere R. The effect of growth hormone and thyroxine on the mitotic rate of the intestinal mucosa of the rat. *Endocrinology* 1955;56:265.
126. Scow RO, Hagan SN. Effect of testerone propionate and growth hormone on growth and chemical composition of muscle and other tissues in hypophysectomized male rats. *Endocrinology* 1965;77: 852.
127. Cooke PS, Yonemura CU, Russel SM, Nicoll CS. Growth and differentiation of fetal rat intestine transplants: dependence on insulin and growth hormone. *Biol Neonate* 1986;49:211.
128. Daughaday WH, Rotwein P. Insulin-like growth factor I and II. Peptide, messenger ribonucleic acid and gene structures, serum and tissue concentration. *Endocrinol Rev* 1989;10:68–91.
129. Read LC, Lemmey AB, Howarth GS, et al. The gastrointestinal tract in one of the most responsive target tissues for IGF-1 and its potent analogs. In: Spencer EM, ed. *Modern Concepts of Insulin-like Growth Factors*. Amsterdam: Elsevier, 1991;225–234.
130. Lobie PE, Breipohl W, Waters MJ. Growth hormone receptor expression in the rat gastrointestinal tract. *Endocrinology* 1990;126:299–306.
131. Yeh KY, Moog F. Hormonal influences on the growth and enzymic differentiation of the small intestine of the hypophysectomized rat. *Growth* 1978;42:495.
132. Hart MH, Phares CK, Erdman SH, et al. Augmentation of postresection mucosal hyperplasia by pleroceroid growth factor. *Dig Dis Sci* 1987;32:1275.
133. Ulshen MH, Dowling RH, Fuller CD, et al. Enhanced growth of small bowel in transgenic mice overexpressing bovine growth hormone. *Gastroenterology* 1993;104:973–980.

134. Lemmey AB, Martin AA, Read LC, et al. IGF-I and the truncated analogue des-(1-3) IGF-I enhance growth in rats after gut resection. *Am J Physiol* 1991;260:E213–E219.
135. Park JHY, McCusker RH, Vanderhoof JA, et al. Secretion of insulin-like growth factor II (IGF-II) and IGF-binding protein-2 by intestinal epithelial (IEC-6) cells: implications for autocrine growth regulation. *Endocrinology* 1992;131:1359–1368.
136. Vanderhoof JA, McCusker RH, Clark R, et al. Truncated and native insulinlike growth factor I enhance mucosal adaptation after jejunoileal resection. *Gastroenterology* 1992;102:1949–1956.
137. Baxter RC. The somatomedins: insulin-like growth factors. *Adv Clin Chem* 1986;25:49–115.
138. Laburthe M, Rouyer-Fessard C, Gammeltoft S. Receptors for insulin-like growth factors I and II in rat gastrointestinal epithelium. *Am J Physiol* 1988;254:G457–G462.
139. Lund PK, Moats-Staats B, Hynes MA, et al. Somatomedin-C insulin-like growth factor I and insulin-like growth factor II mRNAs in rat fetal and adult tissues. *J Biol. Chem* 1986;262:14539–14544.
140. Han VKM, D'Ercole AJ, Lund PK. Cellular localization of somatomedin/insulin-like growth factor mRNAs in the human fetus. *Science* 1987;236:193–197.
141. Humbel RE. Insulin-like growth factors I and II. *Eur J Biochem* 1990;190:445–462.
142. Park JHY, Vanderhoof JA, Blackwood D, MacDonald RG. Characterization of type I and II insulin-like growth factor receptors in an intestinal epithelial cell line. *Endocrinology* 1990;126:2998–3005.
143. Shimasaki S, Koba A, Mercado M, et al. Complementary DNA structure of the high molecular weight rat insulin-like growth factor binding protein (IGF-BP3) and tissue distribution of its mRNA. *Biochem Biophys Res Commun* 1989;165:907–912.
144. Culouscou JM, Remaclebonnet M, Garrouste F, et al. Production of insulin-like growth factor II (IGF-II) and different forms of IGF-binding proteins by HT-29 human colon carcinoma cell line. *J Cell Physiol* 1990;143:405–415.
145. Orlowski CC, Brown AL, Ooi GT, et al. Tissue, developmental and metabolic regulation of messenger ribonucleic acid encoding a rat insulin-like growth factor-binding protein. *Endocrinology* 1990; 126:644–652.
146. Gopinath R, Watson PE, Etherton TD. An acid-stable insulin-like growth factor (IGF)-binding protein from pig secrum inhibits binding of IGF-I and IGF-II to vascular endothelial cells. *J Endocrinol* 1989;120:231–236.
147. Albiston AL, Taylor RG, Herington AC, et al. Divergent ileal IGF-I and IGFBP-3 gene expression after small bowel resection: a novel mechanism to amplify IGF action? *Mol Cell Endocrinol* 1992; 83:R17–R20.
148. Elgin RG, Busby WH, Clemmons DR. An insulin-like growth factor binding protein enhances the biologic response to IGF-I. *Proc Natl Acad Sci* 1987;84:3254–3258.
149. Blum WF, Jenne EW, Reppin F, et al. Insulin-like growth factor I (IGF-I) binding protein complex is a better mitogen than free IGF-I. *Endocrinology* 1989;125:766–772.
150. Termanini B, Nardi RV, Finam TM, et al. Insulin-like growth factor I receptors in rabbit gastrointestinal tract. Characterization and autoradiographic localization. *Gastroenterology* 1990;99:51–60.
151. Pillion DJ, Haskell JF, Atchison JA, et al. Receptors for IGF-I, but not for IGF-II, on proximal colon epithelial cell apical membranes. *Am J Physiol* 1989;257:E27–E34.
152. Rouyer-Fessard C, Gammeltoft S, Laburthe M. Expression of two types of receptor for insulinlike growth factors in human colonic epithelium. *Gastroenterology* 1990;98:703–707.
153. Grey V, Rouyer-Fessard C, Gammeltoft S, et al. Insulin-like growth factor II/mannose-6-phosphate receptors are transiently increased in the rat distal intestinal epithelium after resection. *Mol Cell Endocrinol* 1991;75:221–227.
154. Al Nafussi AI, Wright NA. The effect of epidermal growth factor (EGF) on cell proliferation of the gastrointestinal mucosa in rodents. *Virchows Arch Cell Pathol* 1982;40:63–69.
155. Conteas CN, Majumdar APN. The effects of gastrin, epidermal growth factor, and somatostatin on DNA synthesis in a small intestinal crypt cell line (IEC-6). *Proc Soc Exp Biol Med* 1987;184:307–311.
156. Walker-Smith JA, Phillips AD, Walford N, et al. Intravenous epidermal growth factor/urogastrone increases small intestinal cell proliferation in congenital microvillous atrophy. *Lancet* 1985;11:1239.
157. Sullivan PB, Brueton MJ, Tabara Z, et al. Epidermal growth factor in necrotising enteritis. *Lancet* 1991;338:53.
158. Marquardt H, Hunkapillar MW, Hood LE, et al. Rat transforming growth factor type I: Structure and relation to epidermal growth factor. *Science* 1984;223:1079–1082.
159. Derynck R. Transforming growth factor α. *Cell* 1988;43:593–595.
160. Downward J, Yarden Y, Mayes E, et al. Close similarity of epidermal growth factor receptor and v-erb-B oncogene protein sequences. *Nature* 1984;307:521–527.

161. Weaver LH, Walker WA. Epidermal growth factor and the developing human gut. *Gastroenterology* 1988;94:845–847.
162. Malo C, Menard D. Influence of epidermal growth factor on the development of suckling mouse intestinal mucosa. *Gastroenterology* 1982;83:28–35.
163. Malo C, Menard D. Epidermal growth factor accelerates the maturation of intestinal brush border membranes. *J Cell Biol* 1980;87:13A.
164. Beaulieu JF, Calvert R. The effect of epidermal growth factor on the differentiation of the rough endoplasmic reticulum in fetal mouse small intestine in organ culture. *J Histochem Cytochem* 1981; 29:765–770.
165. Goodlad R, Wilson TJ, Lenton W, et al. Intravenous but not intragastric urogastrone EGF is trophic to the intestine of parenterally fed rats. *Gut* 1987;28:573–582.
166. Ulshen MH, Lyn-Cook L, Roasch R. Effects of intraluminal epidermal growth factor on mucosal proliferation in the small intestine of adult rats. *Gastroenterology* 1986;91:1134–1140.
167. Foster HM, Whitehead RH. Intravenous but not intracolonic epidermal growth factor maintains colonocyte proliferation in defunctioned rat colorectum. *Gastroenterology* 1990;99:1710–1714.
168. Goodlad RA, Lee CY, Wright NA. Cell proliferation in the small intestine and colon of intravenously fed rats: effects of urogastrone-epidermal growth factor. *Cell Prolif* 1992;25:393–404.
169. Thompson J. Specific receptors for epidermal growth factor in rat intestinal microvillus membranes. *Am J Physiol* 1988;254:G429–G435.
170. Scheving LA, Shiurba RA, Nguyen TD, Gray GM. Epidermal growth factor receptor of the intestinal enterocyte. *J Biol Chem* 1989;264:1735–1741.
171. Carpenter G. Receptors for epidermal growth factor and other polypeptide mitogens. *Annu Rev Biochem* 1987;56:881–914.
172. Opleta-Madsen K, Hardin J, Gall DG. Epidermal growth factor upregulates intestinal electrolyte and nutrient transport. *Am J Physiol* 1991;260:G807–G814.
173. Helmstaedter V, Feurle GE, Forssmann WG. Ultrastructural identification of a new cell type the N-cell as the source of neurotensin in the gut mucosa. *Cell Tissue Res* 1977;184:445–452.
174. Wood JG, Hoang HD, Bussjaeger LJ, et al. Neurotensin stimulates growth of small intestine in rats. *Am J Physiol* 1988;255:G812–G817.
175. Izukura M, Parekh D, Evers BM, et al. Neurotensin stimulates colon growth in rats. *Gastroenterology* 1990;98:A416.
176. Evers BM, Izukura M, Townsend CM Jr, et al. Neurotensin prevents intestinal mucosal hypoplasia in rats fed an elemental diet. *Dig Dis Sci* 1992a;37:425–431.
177. Evers BM, Izukura M, Chung DH, et al. Neurotensin stimulates growth of colonic mucosa in young and aged rats. *Gastroenterology* 1992b;103:86–91.
178. Olsen PS, Pedersen JH, Poulsen SS, et al. Neurotensin-like immunoreactivity after intestinal resection in the rat. *Gut* 1987;28:1107–1111.
179. Evers BM, Izukura M, et al. Molecular mechanisms of intestinal adaptation after resection. *Surg Forum* 1991a;42:130–132.
180. Izukura M, Evers BM, Parekh D, et al. Neurotensin augments intestinal regeneration after small bowel resection in rats. *Ann Surg* 1992;215:520–527.
181. Evers BM, Beauchamp RD, Ishizuka J, et al. Posttranscriptional regulation of neurotensin in the gut. *Surgery* 1991b;110:247–252.
182. Cartlidge SA, Elder JB. Transforming growth factor α and epidermal growth factor levels in normal human gastrointestinal mucosa. *Br J Cancer* 1989;60:657–660.
183. Blay J, Brown KD. Epidermal growth factor promotes the chemotactic migration of cultured rat intestinal epithelial cells. *J Cell Physiol* 1985;125:107–112.
184. Knickelbein RG, Aronson PS, Dobbins JW. Membrane distribution of sodium-hydrogen and chloride-bicarbonate exchangers in crypt and villus cell membranes from rabbit ileum. *J Clin Invest* 1988;82:2158–2163.
185. Suemori S, Ciacci C, Podolsky DK. Regulation of transforming growth factor expression in rat intestinal epithelial cell lines. *J Clin Invest* 1991;87:2216–2221.
186. Koyama SY, Podolsky DK. Differential expression of transforming growth factors α and β in rat intestinal epithelial cells. *J Clin Invest* 1989;83:1768–1773.
187. Thomas DM, Nasim MM, Gullick WJ, Alison MR. Immunoreactivity of transforming growth factor α in the normal adult gastrointestinal tract. *Gut* 1992;33:628–631.
188. Moore R, Carlson S, Madara JL. Rapid barrier restitution in an in vitro model of intestinal epithelial injury. *Lab Invest* 1989;60:237–244.

189. Markowitz SD, Molkentin K, Gerbic C, et al. Growth stimulation by coexpression of transforming growth factor α and epidermal growth factor-receptor in normal and adenomatous human colon epithelium. *J Clin Invest* 1990;86:356–362.
190. Roberts AB, Anzano MA, et al. Type β transforming growth factor: A bifunctional regulator of cellular growth. *Proc Natl Acad Sci USA* 1985;82:119–123.
191. Barnard JA, Beauchamp RD, Coffey RJ, Moses HL. Regulation of intestinal epithelial cell growth by transforming growth factor type β. *Proc Natl Acad Sci USA* 1989;86:1578–1582.
192. Hafez MM, Hsu S, Yan Z, et al. Two roles for transforming growth factor β1 in colon enterocytic cell differentiation. *Cell Growth Differ* 1992;3:753–762.
193. Barnard JA, Beauchamp RD, Coffey RJ, et al. Transforming growth factors and intestinal epithelia: more questions than answers. *Gastroenterology* 1989a;97:1587–1588.
194. Pelton RW, Saxena B, Jones M, et al. Immunolocalization of TGF-β1, TGF-β2 and TGF-β3 in the mouse embryo: expression patterns suggest multiple roles during embryonic development. *J Cell Biol* 1992;115:1091–1105.
195. Mahida YR, Ciacci C, Podolsky DK. Peptide growth factors: role in epithelial-lamina propria cell interactions. *Ann NY Acad Sci* 1992;664:148–156.

Organ Metabolism and Nutrition:
Ideas for Future Critical Care, edited by
J. M. Kinney and H. N. Tucker.
Raven Press, Ltd., New York © 1994.

11

The Gut as an Immune Organ: Intestinal Antiendotoxin Antibodies

Anne Ferguson, Jamal Sallam, Laura McLintock, Nicholas Croft, and
*Ian Poxton

Department of Medicine, University of Edinburgh, Western General Hospital, Edinburgh
EH4 2XU, United Kingdom; and *Department of Medical Microbiology, University of
Edinburgh, Edinburgh EH8 9AG, United Kingdom

THE IMMUNE SYSTEM OF THE GUT

The immune system of the gut (i.e., gut-associated lymphoid tissue [GALT]) is separate and distinct from the systemic immune system in many respects: the cells and immunoglobulin isotypes involved, various effector functions, and its immunoregulation. Several different tissues and organs combine to make up the GALT (Table 1), and they are linked in their functions, e.g., by lymphocyte traffic routes, with lymphoid tissues of other mucosae.

Much research on GALT has been conducted in mice. It is likely that the general principles derived from the results of such experimental work are also applicable in humans, but this has been proven for only a few aspects of immunity. Good clinical studies of the physiology and regulation of the human GALT are urgently required.

INDUCTION AND EXPRESSION OF IMMUNITY

Overall, mucosal immune functions can be separated into induction and effector phases. The *induction* of a specific immune response is critically dependent on the situation of the individual at the time antigen is first encountered. Factors such as age, dose, route of encounter, and physicochemical form of antigen critically influence the type of immune response that will predominate for the rest of the life of the individual. The state of activation of antigen-processing cells and T cells in the tissues where antigen is first encountered are also important factors.

When antigen is first delivered via the gut, the normal immune responses are:

1. An active intestinal antibody response, present throughout the mucosa associated lymphoid tissues but probably with a higher density of specific immunocytes in areas where antigen persists after the initial encounter. This antibody is initially of IgM and subsequently of IgA class.

TABLE 1. *Constituents of the gut-associated lymphoid tissues.*

Small intestine	Peyer's patches, appendix, disseminated cells of mucosae
Colon	Organized lymphoid nodules, disseminated cells
Anus	Anal lymphoid aggregates
Lymphatics, lymph, lymph nodes, thoracic duct	
Portal vein, liver (important filtering function)	

2. Antigen-specific suppression of most facets of the systemic immune repertoire, including T-cell immunity, IgG, and IgE antibody. This phenomenon is called "oral tolerance," and is a critically important homeostatic function, protecting the individual from the effects of potentially damaging hypersensitivity reactions and food allergy.

Expression of immunity in the gut occurs when an individual who is already actively immunized is reexposed to the same antigenic determinant. Antibody-mediated or specific cell-mediated immune reactions may occur in any of the organs of the gastrointestinal (GI) tract, and the location of the immune reaction may be at the luminal surface, within the epithelium, in the lamina propria, lymphatics, capillaries, or in deeper tissues.

Such active immune responses may be host protective, e.g., conferring resistance to bacterial infection, neutralizing viruses, or toxins; the immune responses may occur but may be completely irrelevant to any protective or other function of the

TABLE 2. *Range of potential functions of molecular and cellular immune reactions in the gut.*

	Physiologic	Potentially protective	Producing tissue damage
Immunoglobulins			
IgA	*	*	
IgM	*	*	*
IgG		?	*
IgE		Parasites	*
Cells			
Delayed-type hypersensitivity T cells		Parasites ? cancer	*
Other T effectors		*	?
Polymorphonuclears		*	*
Tissue macrophages (various subsets)	*	*	*
Molecules			
Immunoregulatory cytokines	*	*	
Inflammatory cytokines		*	*
Other molecular mediators (e.g., prostaglandins)	?	?	*

gut (as in most reactions between antibodies and food antigens); and, from time to time, the immune responses cause tissue damage, e.g., delayed-type hypersensitivity (DTH) reactions and IgG- or IgM-mediated complement-fixing hypersensitivity. Hypersensitivity may be entirely inappropriate, and thus a primary cause of disease (e.g., to gluten in coeliac disease), but also may be an unavoidable side effect of a protective immune response, as is well recognized in tuberculosis and leprosy, and in the elimination phase of helminth parasite expulsion from the gut.

Table 2 illustrates, for a variety of immune effector molecules and cells, the overlapping occurrence of physiologic functions, potentially protective properties, and those capable of producing tissue damage.

INVESTIGATION OF THE HUMAN GALT

Ideally, in order to study the mucosal immune system in clinical situations, a range of components should be assessed (Table 3). Animal and clinical studies show that with very few exceptions tests on components of the systemic immune system (blood antibodies and circulating cells and cytokines) are virtually useless as indices of mucosal immunity at gut level. Some general information on the function of the mucosa-associated lymphoid tissues can be obtained from studies of saliva or tears but these materials cannot provide organ-specific information relevant to the gut.

There have been a number of studies on fluid aspirated from the proximal jejunum. If appropriately processed by addition of protease inhibitors, this is a valuable source of material. In theory, jejunal fluid could be obtained readily from any patient with a nasoenteric tube in situ, but we are not aware of any studies using this material for investigation of mucosal immunity in a critical care setting.

Many papers have been published in which influences regarding the immune functions of the gut have been based on fecal immunoglobulins and on specific antibodies (including IgE antibodies) and cytokines in feces. There is now good evidence that data based on analysis of feces will be highly misleading, and despite the apparent ease of specimen collection, such studies should be discouraged.

TABLE 3. *Studies required for comprehensive investigation of the human gut-associated lymphoid tissue.*

Specific IgA antibodies
Potentially immunopathogenic but also potentially useful IgM, IgG, IgG antibodies
Antigen-specific T cells (currently the only method available is based on intestinal antigen challenge, multiple biopsies, and morphometric analysis of these biopsies)
T-cell and macrophage activation by immunologic marker studies or measurement of activation products
Polymorphonuclear activation
Immunoregulatory molecular signals
Inflammatory cytokines
Other molecular mediators of inflammation

RATIONALE AND EVIDENCE AGAINST THE USE OF FECAL EXTRACTS TO STUDY GALT

Even on theoretical grounds, there are many potential problems in the interpretation of results based on fecal samples. There may be mechanical or biological interference in immunoassays by substances present in feces. The reference measure, often per gram feces, will be profoundly affected by fecal water content. Intestinal transit time is also relevant, as this will influence the time available within the lumen of the GI tract for molecules of interest to be destroyed by digestive enzymes and bacterial proteases. An additional complicating factor is that some of the substances in feces (and also in intestinal fluids) may be derived from plasma that is leaked into the gut lumen through ulcerated or inflamed sections of intestinal mucosa.

Paired samples of feces and whole gut lavage fluid (WGLF; see next section) have been examined from ten patients with various GI diseases. Total IgA and sIgA (with secretory component) were assayed in WGLF and in a saline extract of feces (1 g of prefrozen feces homogenized in 10 ml of saline, filtered, and centrifuged). Results of assays of IgA by ELISA in the two sets of specimens are shown in Fig. 1. In gut lavage, the whole gut is perfused at a rate of approximately 20 ml/min, so daily production of IgA can be calculated as

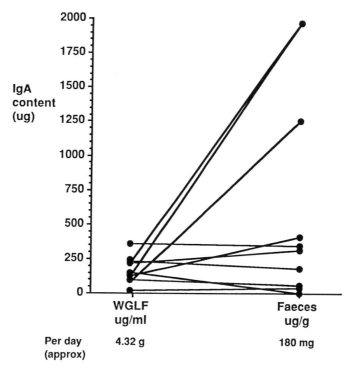

FIG. 1. Content of IgA in samples of WGLF (perfusion rate approximately 20 ml/min) and feces (daily fecal output approximately 200 g daily) from ten patients with GI diseases.

$$WGLF = (IgA \text{ concentration in } \mu g/ml) \times 20 \times 60 \times 24$$

The mean value obtained, 4.3 g/d, is close to the generally accepted value for intestinal production of IgA in humans of 40 mg/kg body weight per day. In contrast, if fecal weight is assumed to be 200 g daily, a value of only 160 mg daily is obtained for our ten patients, again similar to the ranges reported in the literature, e.g., a range 6 to 173 mg/d in 16 healthy adults. In other words, fecal IgA comprises only some 4% of the amount produced in the GI tract. This is likely to be selectively depleted of some molecular forms of IgA.

USE OF WHOLE GUT LAVAGE FLUID TO STUDY GUT IMMUNITY

The technique of whole gut lavage with nonabsorbable polyethyleneglycol–based solution has been widely applied in clinical practice for cleansing of the bowel prior to barium enema, colonoscopy, or colonic surgery. This is also a radical but excellent technique for the treatment of intractable constipation.

After gut cleansing is complete, the clear fluid passed per rectum, WGLF, is essentially a whole gut perfusate. Our studies in adults and children have shown that this material can readily be used for biochemical and immunochemical assays to assess intestinal immunity, inflammation, and gut losses of protein and blood (1–10).

It is unlikely that whole gut lavage would be clinically acceptable in a critical care setting, although this is theoretically an excellent route for delivery for nonabsorbable antibiotics, for cleansing the colon of feces, and reducing the gut bacterial load. However, studies in the convalescent phase would certainly be feasible and would rapidly answer questions as to the presence or absence of mucosal immunodeficiency in otherwise immunocompromised individuals.

APPLICATIONS OF WGLF TESTS IN CLINICAL RESEARCH

GI Protein Loss: Index of Activity in Inflammatory Bowel Disease

Fluid obtained by whole gut lavage normally contains traces of IgG, albumin, and alpha-1-antitrypsin (AAAT). Normal values, based on results for 63 immunologically normal patients or volunteers, are IgG (by ELISA) <1 to 10 μg/ml; albumin (by immunoturbidimetry) <1 to 26 μg/ml; A1AT (by immunoturbidimetry) <1 to 19 μg/ml (5). In our initial technical appraisal of the technique we had found that higher concentrations of these proteins were found in WGLF from patients with inflammatory bowel disease (IBD) (2,6). Our further experience has shown that assay of these proteins in WGLF cannot be used as a diagnostic test for IBD; normal results are obtained in patients with unequivocal radiological or endoscopic abnormalities, if the disease is clinically inactive. However, this approach clearly has potential as an objective means of grading "disease activity" in patients with IBD—until now, a phenomenon that is clearly recognized by clinicians but has proved very difficult to measure.

We carried out a prospective study in which 53 lavages were performed in 45 well-characterized IBD patients (27 Crohn's disease, 18 ulcerative colitis) in whom disease activity was simultaneously assessed by using the Crohn's Disease Activity Index or the Powell Tuck index (7). For IgG, concentrations in lavage fluid correlated closely with activity indices: in Crohn's disease, $r = 0.723$ ($p < 0.0001$); in ulcerative colitis, $r = 0.714$ ($p < 0.0001$). Results for lavage fluid albumin and alpha-1-antitrypsin concentrations were generally similar to those for IgG, but less sensitive in detecting active disease.

Because the high concentrations of WGLF IgG, albumin, and A1AT probably reflect plasma leakage, we assessed to what extent this occurs in conditions other than active IBD (5). High concentrations of one or more proteins were present in 15 of 142 patients with diseases other than IBD; in the majority, the existence of GI protein loss was consistent with the clinical picture (one lymphangiectasia, seven colorectal cancers, one gut lymphoma, one perforated diverticulitis, one pouchitis, and one lymphocytic colitis).

Studies of gut lavage fluid proteins provide a new approach to the screening of clinically complex patients with IBD and other ulcerating and inflammatory lesions. This simple technique offers an alternative to fecal isotope excretion in the diagnosis and quantitation of protein-losing enteropathy.

Measurement of GI Blood Loss

Occult GI bleeding can be measured by using a highly sensitive technique, Hemo-Quant, for assay of hemoglobin (Hb) in WGLF (8). In patients with a normal GI tract, WGLF Hb concentration ranged from 0.5 to 5.1 µg/ml, equating to an estimated daily occult blood loss of 0.1 to 1.2 ml. High values for WGLF Hb were found in patients with colorectal cancer, severe diverticular disease, rectal varices, in seven of 16 patients with active IBD, in one of seven patients with benign colonic polyps (a patient on anticoagulants), and in four patients with iron deficiency anemia thought to be due to occult GI bleeding. In these four patients, estimated blood loss ranged from 2.6 to 24.5 ml per day.

Intestinal Antibody Responses to Oral Vaccines

Strangely, in the development of oral typhoid vaccines, extensive and expensive field trials have been performed to measure protective efficacy of candidate vaccines in the absence of any knowledge of the intestinal antibody status of vaccines. The only published data on the capacity of the vaccine strain (Ty21a) to induce local mucosal immunity are those of Forrest et al. (11), who studied healthy Australian volunteers and specifically excluded individuals with a history of Salmonella infection or food poisoning. Most of his volunteers received doses of the organism one or two logs greater than those used in the vaccine formulation that is sold in many countries.

In a work in progress, we are using enteric vaccines as oral immunogens in protocols for the investigation, in humans, of intestinal immunity and its regulatory mechanisms. Our experience with the oral Ty21a vaccine is limited, but the results are showing that well under 50% of healthy individuals develop intestinal antibodies after a course of vaccine.

We pointed out, in a letter to the *Lancet* (9), that mucosal immunity is quite separate from systemic immunity in the types of cells and isotypes of antibody involved and in the factors that regulate its induction and expression. We suggested that appropriate intestinal antibody tests should be used to define the baseline intestinal antibody status of a study population, changes in antibody levels after vaccination and the relationship (if any) between serum antibody levels, intestinal secretory antibody titers, and clinical protection.

In the course of oral vaccine development, influences of malnutrition or previous antigen exposure on mucosal immune responses should be measured rather than assumed.

Studies in African Children

In view of the potential roles of intestinal immunodeficiency and hypersensitivity in the infection-diarrhea-malnutrition cycle, a safe and ethical method to study intestinal immunity in children is needed. Guidelines for nontherapeutic research in children suggest that any investigative technique "subjects the child to no more than minimal risk as a result of his or her participation" (12). Gut lavage seemed an ideal approach.

In collaboration with Dr. Mary Hodges, Director of the St Andrew's Clinic for Children, and with the approval of the Ministry of Health Research and Ethics Committee, Sierra Leone, gut lavage was successfully performed in 24 of 25 "normal" children, aged 6 to 9 years, from Freetown, Sierra Leone, with parental informed consent (10). WGLF was treated with protease inhibitors, stored at $-20°C$, and transferred to Edinburgh for laboratory studies. These showed that no child had occult blood loss, but four had evidence of protein-losing enteropathy. When compared with values for Scottish adults, WGLF from the Sierra Leonean children had significantly higher concentrations of IgA and IgM and of IgA and IgM antibodies to dietary antigens and to *Salmonella typhi* lipopolysaccharide (LPS). In three children, very low levels of IgA and IgA antibody were present. Clearly, substantial information on childrens' intestinal immunity can be obtained by this method.

INTESTINAL IgA DEFICIENCY

Figure 2 illustrates concentrations of IgA measured by ELISA in WGLF from 16 normal adults studied in Edinburgh and from 24 healthy children recruited from the population of Freetown, Sierra Leone (10). Overall, the African children had significantly higher concentrations of IgA in WGLF than did the Scottish adults, but a subset had very low concentrations, with virtual absence in three cases. Positive

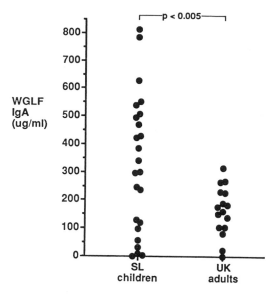

FIG. 2. Concentration of IgA in WGLF from 24 healthy Sierra Leonean children and 16 U.K. adults (from 10).

results in assays for polyethylene glycol and low but definitely positive levels of other immunoglobulins and antibodies in these cases confirmed that the specimens were indeed lavage fluid and not some other substance.

In the two cases of U.K. adults with low levels of WGLF IgA, serum levels of IgA were normal, but counts of IgA plasma cells in morphologically normal gut mucosal biopsies were 13% and 17% of the mean of the reference range for adults. This indicates that low values for IgA in WGLF are not due to technical problems (as we had earlier assumed) but may be evidence of a new immunodeficiency state, intestinal IgA deficiency.

Immunoglobulin A content has been assayed in a further 140 specimens from Edinburgh adult patients: 52 with Crohn's disease, 14 with ulcerative colitis, and 74 with various other GI symptoms or diseases. Low levels of WGLF IgA were found in six of the 140 specimens. In two patients, serum IgA was also undetectable (a man with common variable hypogammaglobulinemia and a 12-year-old girl with Crohn's disease), but serum levels of IgA were normal in the other four (three with Crohn's disease and one with collagenous colitis). We have preliminary evidence that, at least in the cases of Crohn's disease, the intestinal IgA deficiency is transient.

Other interesting observations arose from this descriptive study. There were two cases with diarrhea due to small-bowel bacterial overgrowth; intestinal IgA levels were normal in both. Two of the 140 cases had extremely high levels of WGLF IgA (1,575 and 1,455 µg/ml). They both had had colectomy with creation of a pelvic ileal reservoir (pouch) and had clinical pouchitis at the time of lavage. Four other pouch patients, studied when healthy, had normal WGLF IgA levels, in the range of 92 to 350 µg/ml.

Currently we are setting up methods to assay cytokines in WGLF and will test the hypothesis that intestinal IgA deficiency is due either to deficiency of IL4, IL5, or IL6, the cytokines responsible for maturation and differentiation of IgA B cells, or to the overproduction of proinflammatory cytokines IL1, IL2, or gamma interferon, potentially immunosuppressive to mucosal B cells.

INTESTINAL ANTIBODIES TO BACTERIAL ENDOTOXIN

There are complex interrelationships between the normal gut flora, intestinal infection, invasion of the tissues by gut bacteria or their products, sepsis syndrome, shock, and multiorgan failure. As viewed by gut immunologists, a central role for bacterial "translocation" across the gut wall, rather than for endotoxin effects in shock, is not particularly convincing. There are many specific and nonspecific factors that constrain bacterial metabolism, multiplication, and invasive properties within the lumen of the gut as they cross the bowel wall and certainly within the milieu of draining lymph nodes and within the liver. Increased recovery of bacteria from lymph nodes or even the bloodstream could be due to failure of these normally efficient housekeeper operations, rather than be caused by changes in intestinal permeability and ingress of bacteria into the tissues (Fig. 3).

The presence of bacterial endotoxin (LPS) in the tissues and bloodstream might be due to absorption of greatly increased quantities from a larger than normal load of small intestinal bacteria or to abnormally increased permeability, perhaps with some local tissue invasion, which allows a surge of LPS to be absorbed. Shock is variously attributed to the effects of endotoxin directly (which might then be neutralized by antiendotoxin antibody) or to the effects of other mediators including tumor necrosis factor (TNF), whose secretion is stimulated by LPS into the tissues and whose effects might equally be neutralized by anti-TNF antibodies.

In Edinburgh there has been considerable interest in the structure and immunogenicity of bacterial endotoxin, the properties of serum antiendotoxin antibody, and the separation of antibodies, for therapeutic use, from blood donor plasma (13–17).

Figure 4 illustrates the structure of LPS. Variations in the structure (and thus antigenicity) of the long carbohydrate O-polysaccharide chain allow serotyping of bacteria and aid their classification in bacterial taxonomy. However, there is also antigenic crossreactivity between gram-negative organisms due to the existence of highly conserved core region antigens. "Rough" mutants of gram-negative bacteria lack the long polysaccharide chain, and the core glycolipid antigens are exposed (Fig. 5). ELISAs for IgG antibodies in blood donor sera have shown that Rc and Re antigens are immunodominant for humans (13), and antibodies to these core LPS forms, reacting with many bacterial species, can neutralize endotoxin activity (17).

We have measured IgA antibodies to LPS core antigens in matched specimens of serum and WGLF from 14 patients. Three patients, with trivial disorders, were

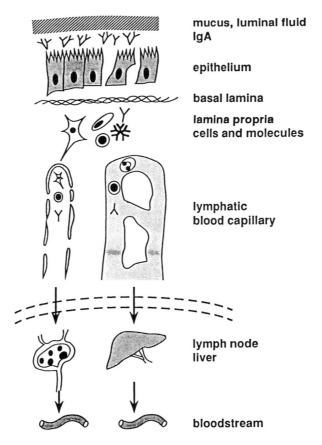

mucus, luminal fluid
IgA

epithelium

basal lamina

lamina propria
cells and molecules

lymphatic
blood capillary

lymph node
liver

bloodstream

FIG. 3. Components of the immune system encountered by bacteria in transit between the lumen of the gut and the blood stream.

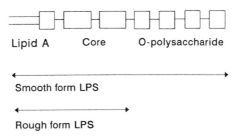

Lipid A   Core   O-polysaccharide

Smooth form LPS

Rough form LPS

FIG. 4. Diagrammatic representation of LPS. The O-polysaccharide is a chain of heterogeneous length consisting of repeating oligosaccharide units that specify a vast range of serotype antigens. The outer region of the core oligosaccharide, which consists of five hexoses (see Fig. 5), has a degree of antigenic variability but is more conserved in the inner KDO/heptose region. Lipid A, the endotoxic part of the molecule, has a structure that is largely conserved in all gram-negative bacteria. If the O-polysaccharide is lost through mutation, the LPS is termed "rough," compared to the "smooth" wild-type parent. Rough-form LPS is found naturally in some species of bacteria.

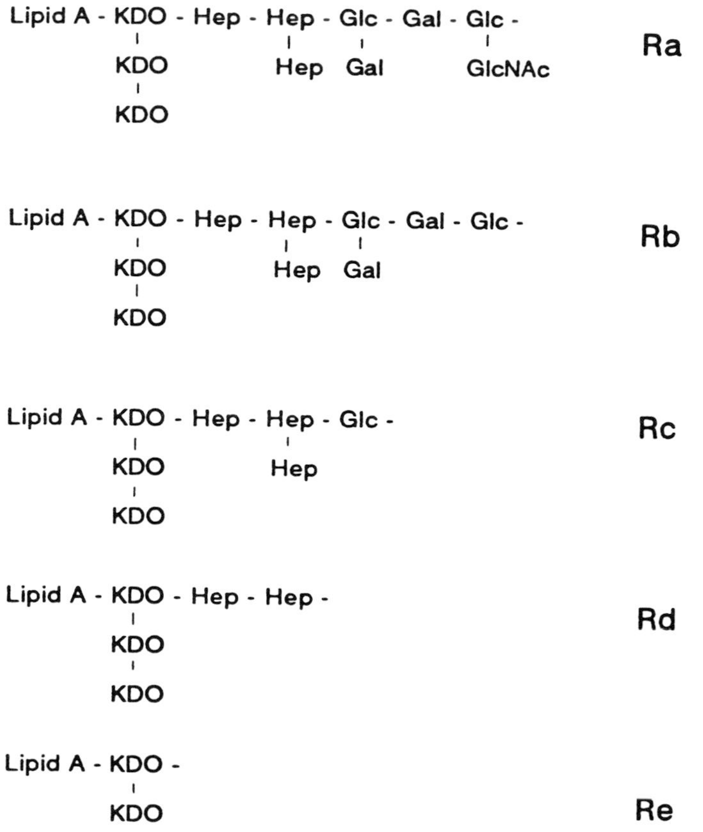

```
Lipid A - KDO - Hep - Hep - Glc - Gal - Glc -
           |                |     |          |        Ra
          KDO              Hep   Gal       GlcNAc
           |
          KDO
```

```
Lipid A - KDO - Hep - Hep - Glc - Gal - Glc -
           |                |     |              Rb
          KDO              Hep   Gal
           |
          KDO
```

```
Lipid A - KDO - Hep - Hep - Glc -
           |                             Rc
          KDO              Hep
           |
          KDO
```

```
Lipid A - KDO - Hep - Hep -
           |                       Rd
          KDO
           |
          KDO
```

```
Lipid A - KDO -
           |                   Re
          KDO
```

FIG. 5. Rough mutants of Salmonella. The Ra mutant produces LPS with a complete core but no O-polysaccharide. Other R-mutants are available that produce only partial cores. These are termed Rb-Re. The Re mutant is the minimum LPS structure that permits viability. The Rc-Re structures carry a series of epitopes that are common to many gram-negative bacteria. Phosphate and other non-sugar substituents are not shown to aid clarity. KDO, 3-deoxy-D-manno-2-octulosonic acid (keto-deoxy-octonic acid); Hep, heptose; Glc, glucose; Gal, galactose; GlcNAc, N-acetyl glucosamine.

considered to be immunologically normal, but there were four patients with ulcerative colitis, six with Crohn's disease, and one with pouchitis. The pattern of results in a typical case is illustrated in Fig. 6. Just as has been reported for IgG antibodies in serum, the Rc (and in some cases the Re) regions are immunodominant for IgA antibody responses at the mucosal level. Results for antibodies to Rc in the 14 patients, expressed as empirical units, are shown in Fig. 7. Both in serum and in WGLF, levels of antibody were strikingly higher in Crohn's patients than in those with ulcerative colitis or in normals. The patient with pouchitis had undetectable serum levels of antibody to this antigen but high intestinal antibody levels. Although ELISA data,

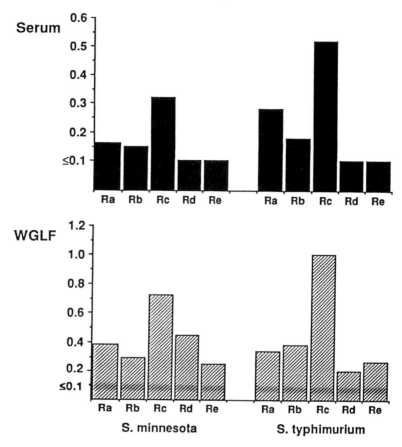

FIG. 6. Profiles of serum *(open columns)* and WGLF *(closed columns)* IgA antibody to the Ra-Re antigens of *Salmonella minnesota* and of *Salmonella typhimurium.* Values are expressed as arbitrary units; serum was diluted 1/200 and WGLF 1/2 before analysis. In this patient (who had ulcerative colitis), the Rc region is immunodominant in both compartments.

being expressed as arbitrary units, are difficult to translate into absolute amounts of antibody, the values obtained show that intestinal secretion of IgA antibody to Rc LPS per day is equivalent to the IgA antibody content of around 500 ml blood.

Clearly a vital question, which could readily be answered by direct studies of mucosal immunity, is whether patients with sepsis syndrome and multiorgan failure have adequate intestinal mucosal antibody to bacterial endotoxin or whether there is transient or prolonged mucosal antibody failure in this situation.

Passive administration of antibody via the gut could be theoretically most attractive, cheaper, and safer than parenteral administration of antibody. It might not even be necessary to use human antibodies for this purpose.

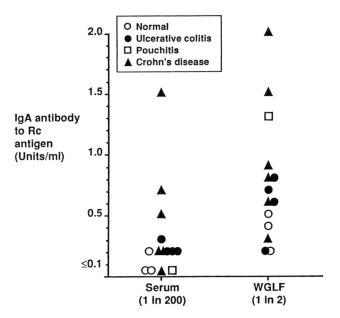

FIG. 7. Serum WGLF IgA-class antibodies to the Rc (rough mutant) antigen of *Salmonella minnesota*. Values given are arbitrary units of IgA antibody activity to the various antigens. Serum was diluted 1/200 and WGLF 1/2 before analysis.

CONCLUSIONS

Methods for safe and noninvasive investigation of gut mucosal immunity are now available, based either on the use of jejunal fluid or on WGLF. Simple descriptive studies of humoral immunity have already revealed a new disease entity, intestinal IgA deficiency; the clinical relevance of this phenomenon, and its underlying immunopathogenesis, remain to be explored.

ACKNOWLEDGMENTS

We thank our consultant colleagues for allowing us to study their patients, and Dr. Robin Barclay for his collaboration; we gratefully acknowledge the skilled assistance in specimen collection by Helen Brian and Sister Sheila Crichton; and we thank Norman Anderson, Kenneth Humphreys, and Diane Edmond for technical support.

REFERENCES

1. Gaspari MM, Brennan PT, Soloman SM, Elson CO. A method of obtaining, processing, and analysing human intestinal secretions for antibody content. *J Immunol Methods* 1988;110:85–91.

2. O'Mahony S, Barton JR, Crichton S, Ferguson A. Appraisal of gut lavage in the study of intestinal humoral immunity. *Gut* 1990;31:1341–1344.
3. O'Mahony S, Arranz E, Barton JR, Ferguson A. Dissociation between systemic and mucosal humoral immune responses in coeliac disease. *Gut* 1991;32:29–35.
4. Arranz E, O'Mahony S, Barton JR, Ferguson A. Immunosenescence and mucosal immunity: significant effects of old age on serum and secretory IgA concentrations and on intraepithelial lymphocyte counts. *Gut* 1992;33:882–886.
5. Brydon WG, Choudari CP, Ferguson A. Relative specificity for active inflammatory bowel disease of plasma-derived proteins in gut lavage fluid. *Eur J Gastroenterol Hepatol* 1993;5:269–273.
6. O'Mahony S, Choudari CP, Barton JR, et al. Gut lavage fluid proteins as markers of activity of inflammatory bowel disease. *Scand J Gastroenterol* 1991;26:940–944.
7. Choudari CP, O'Mahony S, Brydon G, et al. Gut lavage fluid protein concentrations: objective measures of disease activity in inflammatory bowel disease. *Gastroenterology* 1993;104:1064–1071.
8. Brydon WG, Ferguson A. Haemoglobin in gut lavage fluid as a measure of gastro-intestinal blood loss. *Lancet* 1992;340:1381–1382.
9. Sallam J, Ferguson A. Mucosal immunity to oral vaccines. *Lancet* 1992;339:179.
10. Hodges M, Kingstone K, Brydon WG, Sallam J, Ferguson A. Use of whole gut lavage to measure intestinal immunity in healthy Sierra Leonean children. *J Pediatr Gastroenterol Nutr* (in press).
11. Forrest BD, LaBrooy JT, Beyer L, et al. The human humoral immune response to *Salmonella typhi* Ty21a. *J Infect Dis* 1991;163:336–345.
12. Working Party on Research on Children. The ethical conduct of research on children. London: Medical Research Council, 1991.
13. Barclay GR, Scott BB. Serological relationships between *Escherichia coli* and *Salmonella* smooth- and rough-mutant lipopolysaccharides as revealed by enzyme-linked immunosorbent assay for human immunoglobulin G antiendotoxin antibodies. *Infect Immun* 1987;55:2706–2714.
14. Scott BB, Barclay GR. Endotoxin-polymyxin complexes in an improved enzyme-linked immunosorbent assay for IgG antibodies in blood donor sera to gram-negative endotoxin core glycolipids. *Vox Sang* 1987;52:272.
15. Barclay GR. Antibodies to endotoxin in health and disease. *Rev Med Microbiol* 1990;1:133–142.
16. Scott BB, Barclay GR, Smith DGE, et al. IgG antibodies to gram-negative endotoxin in human sera. I. Lipopolysaccharide (LPS) cross-reactivity due to antibodies to LPS core. *Serodiag Immunother Infect Dis* 1990;4:25–38.
17. Di Padova FE, Brade H, Barclay GR, et al. A broadly cross-protective monoclonal antibody binding to *Escherichia coli* and *Salmonella* lipopolysaccharide. *Infect Immun* 1993;61:3863–3872.

Organ Metabolism and Nutrition:
Ideas for Future Critical Care, edited by
J. M. Kinney and H. N. Tucker.
Raven Press, Ltd., New York © 1994.

12

The Role of Arginine and Related Compounds in Intestinal Functions

Luc A. Cynober

Departments of Biochemistry, Molecular Biology, and Nutrition, Faculte de Medecine-Pharmacie, Laboratoire de Biochimie, Clermont-Ferrand 63000, France.

As discussed in other chapters of this book, the intestinal tract plays a major role in the protection of the body against invasion by microorganisms present in the lumen. This role is performed by two components: the first is the intestinal wall and the second is immunologic protection by gut-associated lymphoid tissue (GALT).

Maintenance of intestinal trophicity and GALT function is dependent on numerous factors, some nutritional (1,2). Some amino acids play a special role either because they are a major fuel for these cells or because they generate metabolites, which mediate functionality. Glutamine is in the first category but falls outside of the scope of this review; the reader may wish to read recent reviews on this subject (3,4). The second category includes two related amino acids, arginine and ornithine, which form nitric oxide (NO°) and aliphatic polyamines (putrescine, spermine, and spermidine), respectively (5,6).

Although few studies discuss the action of arginine and ornithine on the intestine, these amino acids may play a key role in maintaining intestinal function by their effect on immunoregulation and in the growth of rapidly dividing cells (e.g., in wound healing).

The effects of arginine and ornithine on immunity and on intestinal trophicity are discussed here, keeping in mind that these amino acids exert other nutritional effects, e.g., improving nitrogen balance in catabolic situations (7,8).

METABOLISM OF ARGININE AND RELATED COMPOUNDS IN THE GUT

Arginine and ornithine are linked by a series of enzymes: arginase (converts arginine into ornithine with urea release), ornithine carbamoyltransferase, arginosuccinate synthetase, and arginosuccinate lyase (forms arginine via citrulline and arginosuccinate). Only periportal hepatocytes and certain brain areas possess all the enzymes required for arginine recycling and urea synthesis (9).

The gut uses arginine because enterocytes possess argininase and ornithine carbamoyltransferase (10). The gut thus releases urea and citrulline (11). In addition, enterocytes contain ornithine decarboxylase (ODC) (6) and an $NADPH_2$-dependent arginine deiminase (12,13), which produce aliphatic polyamines and nitric oxide, respectively, the importance of which is discussed later.

However, arginine and ornithine are not equally potent in producing citrulline or polyamines because of a certain degree of compartmentalization of the metabolic pathways:

Arginine flux is directed preferentially toward citrulline production because arginase (located at the outer face of the mitochondrial membrane), ornithine translocase (which transports ornithine from the cytoplasm to mitochondria), ornithine carbamoyltransferase (closely associated with the inner face of the mitochondria membrane), and citrulline translocase (which transports citrulline from mitochondria to the cytoplasm) seem to operate as a multienzyme complex (9).

Ornithine is paradoxically a poor precursor of citrulline in the gut (14); this could be due to the fact that ornithine translocase (required to convert ornithine to citrulline) is closely related to arginase. This probably explains why ornithine is the preferential precursor of polyamines in the cytoplasm.

IMMUNOLOGIC EFFECTS

Arginine

According to Rose's classification, arginine is a semiessential amino acid: in adults, arginine provided by alimentation and *de novo* synthesis is sufficient to meet requirements; however, when requirements increase (e.g., during growth and in hypermetabolic situations), arginine becomes an essential amino acid. This has been documented (15,16) in stressed rats, where arginine is required for healing and survival. In the course of these studies, a possible role for arginine as an immunomodulator was proposed because arginine administration inhibited the thymus involution induced by stress.

The effect of arginine on GALT has not been studied. However, studies discussed in the next section are relevant because 70% to 80% of all immunoglobulin-producing cells are located in the intestinal mucosa (1) and the immunologic effects of arginine have been shown in athymic mice (17).

Experimental and Clinical Data

Arginine administration has been shown to improve the immunologic status of various animal models. In rats given total parenteral nutrition (TPN) for seven days, thymus weight, the number of lymphocytes contained in the thymus, and the response of lymphocytes to mitogenic agents (concanavalin A and phytohemagglutinin) were higher in rats treated with arginine-enriched TPN (1.8 g/kg/d) than in rats receiving conventional TPN (0.37 g/kg/d) (18). Similar results were obtained in rats traumatized

TABLE 1. *Immunomodulatory effects of arginine: Experimental studies.*

Reference	Model	Nutrition	Arginine intake	Treatment time (days)	Nitrogen balance	Immunologic parameters
18	Rat	TPN	1.8 g/kg/24 h	7	=	↗ Thymus weight
19	Rat (femoral fracture)	TPN	1.9 g/kg/24 h	5	↗	↗ Thymus lymphocyte nb ↗ reponse to PHA and Con A
20	Guinea pig (burn)	Enteral	1.1 g/kg/24 h	14	=	↗ Delayed hypersensitivity (DNFB)
21	Rat (sepsis)	Oral	1 g/kg/24 h	15		↗ Response to PHA and ConA ↗ Delayed hypersensitivity (DNBF)

TPN, total parenteral nutrition; PHA, phytohemagglutinin; Con A, concanavalin A; DNFB, dinitrofluoro-benzene.

by a femoral fracture (19). In burned guinea pigs, arginine-enriched enteral nutrition increased the delayed hypersensitivity to dinitrofluorobenzene and decreased mortality (20). This latter action has also been found in septic rats (21) (Table 1).

In tumor-bearing rats, arginine-supplemented diets decreased tumor growth and increased thymus weight, the response of spleen lymphocytes to mitogenic agents, the production of interleukin-2 (IL-2) by lymphocytes, and the lytic capacity of activated natural killer cells (22,23). However, arginine has no effect on immune dysfunction in the elderly (24).

Some of these results have been confirmed in studies involving humans. For example, arginine administration (25 g/d) for 2 weeks to healthy volunteers (25) or to surgical patients (26) increased the lymphocyte response to mitogenic agents; however, IL-2 production by these cells was not modified (25). It is noteworthy that the effects of arginine are no longer found when this amino acid is the only nitrogen supply in hypocaloric parenteral nutrition (27).

The most recent approach consists of including arginine at high concentrations in ready-to-use commercial formulas (Impact [Sandoz]). Critically ill (28) and surgical (29) patients treated with Impact show an improved response to mitogenic agents, fewer infectious complications, and shorter hospital stay. Finally, mice challenged with *Listeria monocytogenes* showed lower mortality when fed with Impact (30). However, this formula is also enriched with RNA and omega-3 fatty acids, which both could have immunoregulatory properties (31), and this makes it impossible to ascribe its beneficial effects solely to arginine. In addition, in one of the clinical studies cited (29), daily nitrogen intake was clearly different in the Impact-treated and control patients (respectively, 15.6 ± 2.8 and 9.0 ± 2.8 gN/d; $p < 0.001$). In the same way, it is not clear whether nitrogen intakes were similar in the experimental study (30).

The effects of arginine on immunologic status have been described as dose dependent (18,19) (Table 2), although this is controversial (20,32). In severe stress (20,32),

TABLE 2. *Dose-dependent effects of arginine on immunity.*

	Solution A (1.55 g/l)	Solution B (4.05 g/l)	Solution C (7.5 g/l)
Thymus weight (mg)	345 ± 27[a]	445 ± 34[b]	438 ± 26[b]
Lymphocyte number (10^6/gland)	93 ± 12[a]	137 ± 18[b]	146 ± 15[b]
Response to PHA (cpm)	9,558 ± 3,798[a]	20,085 ± 5,890[a]	37,234 ± 6,209[b]

Adapted from Barbul, et al. (18).
[a,b] Indicates different $p < 0.05$.

high arginine intake (above 2 g/kg/d) is less efficient than moderate intake (20) and may even increase mortality (32). This deleterious effect could be explained by the excessive production of nitric oxide.

It is noteworthy that the arginine-mediated improvement in the nitrogen balance is never dose dependent, which suggests that the immunologic and anabolic effects of this amino acid involve different mechanisms (7).

Mechanism of Action: A Possible Role for Nitric Oxide

The mechanism of action of arginine on immunity is only now being elucidated, mainly by Salvatore Moncada's group (see ref. 33 for a review). It seems that arginine's effect is mediated through its metabolism into nitric oxide in the reaction arginine → citrulline + NO°, catalyzed by arginine deiminase (also called "nitric oxide synthase"). This enzyme has been identified in various cells, and at least two types of arginine deiminase have been characterized, which differ by their dependency on calcium and their sensitivity to glucocorticoids (Table 3). The first is constitutive and present in the brain, vascular endothelium, and platelets (34). The second is inducible and is present in many cells, including macrophages, polymorphonuclear neutrophils, lymphocytes, hepatocytes, and enterocytes (13,35–37).

TABLE 3. *Similarities and differences between the two NO° syntheses*

Endothelial cells		Macrophages
	Cytosolic NADPH-dependent inhibited by L-arginine analogues	
Constitutives Ca^{2+}/calmodulin-dependent picomoles NO released; short-lasting release unaffected by glucocorticoids		Inducible Ca^{2+}/calmodulin-independent nanomoles NO released; long-lasting release; induction inhibited by glucocorticoids

Adapted from Moncada, et al. (33).

The half-life of NO° is very short: It is inactivated by oxidation to form nitrite and nitrate. It is now possible to delineate the various roles of NO° by using inhibitors of arginine deiminase: N^G-monomethyl-L-arginine, N^G-amino-L-arginine, and N^G-nitro-L-arginine (38). Nitric oxide triggers the cytotoxic activity of phagocytic cells. For example, it has been shown (39) that IL-1β–mediated cytotoxicity for pancreatic islets is due to NO° formation. Nitric oxide also plays a major role in the lysis of tumor cells (40), an action relevant to the effects of arginine administration in tumor-bearing rats (see previous section). Nitric oxide may play a role in the microbicidal activity of macrophages (36) and is likely a primary defense mechanism against pathogens such as fungi and helminths that are too large to be phagocytosed (33). Finally, it is interesting to note that cytokines produced by Kupffer cells induce the expression of arginine deiminase in hepatocytes, leading to production of NO°, which inhibits protein synthesis (41,42). All these actions are thought to be primarily mediated through the metabolic inhibition of the targets that results from the NO°-dependent degradation of enzymes containing Fe-S groups in the electron transport chain and the tricarboxylic acid cycle (36).

Nitric oxide also induces vascular smooth muscle relaxation (43) by activating guanylate cyclase, thereby forming cyclic GMP, which therefore acts as the second messenger of NO°. It is now evident that the relaxing factor endothelium-derived relaxing factor (EDRF) is in fact NO°.

Lipopolysaccharide, IL-1 IL-6, and tumor necrosis factor are strong inducers of NO° synthesis (35,44–46), while interferon-γ acts synergistically with these cytokines (44). In addition, LPS and interferon-γ synergistically promote the transport of arginine into macrophages (47), which further increases substrate availability for arginine deiminase. Nitric oxide production in response to LPS is blocked by cycloheximide (an inhibitor of protein synthesis) and dexamethasone (46). The fact that NO° production is blocked by antiinflammatory steroids (46,48) further indicates that the NO° pathway is a key component of the inflammatory reaction.

There is some evidence that synthesis of NO° from L-arginine has a role in maintaining the macrovascular integrity of the intestinal mucosa following acute endotoxin challenge in the rat (49). However, in some cases, under the action of cytokines this reaction becomes excessive and is detrimental (50): large production of NO° is probably involved in the fatal hypotension that occurs in the septic shock syndrome (51). These data probably explain the deleterious effects of arginine when administered at high doses in sepsis (32). An experimental study supports this idea: in LPS-treated rats, aortic rings present an increase in cyclic GMP content and a decrease in the maximal contractile response to norepinephrine, which can be prevented by the presence of N^G-nitro-L-arginine; in contrast, incubation of aortic rings from LPS-treated rats with L-arginine leads to a relaxation and a parallel increase in cyclic GMP (52).

Ornithine

Ornithine is not a component of proteins and, until recently, was viewed solely as the starter of ureagenesis. However, this amino acid is the precursor of important molecules, especially polyamines, which play a key role in the control of cell differentiation and protein synthesis (6).

Experimental and Clinical Data

A low concentration of ornithine (10 μM) in the incubation medium of lymphocytes increases their response to mitogenic agents (53). Administration of ornithine to traumatized (54), chemically immunosuppressed mice (55) or LPS-treated rats (56) restores thymus weight (54,56) and its lymphocyte content (54) and increases the response to mitogenic agents (55).

Mechanism of Action

From the data presented, it appears that ornithine displays the same immunologic actions as arginine; therefore, the simplest explanation for ornithine's action on immunity is its conversion to arginine followed by the formation of NO°. In fact, except for periportal hepatocytes, no tissue possesses all the enzymes required (9). Furthermore, it has been demonstrated (J. Albina, et al., unpublished data) that activated macrophages incubated in the presence of ornithine do not produce more NO° than controls.

An alternative hypothesis can be drawn from the observation that the full response of lymphocytes to mitogenic agents requires the expression of ODC (57). This suggests that ornithine could exert its immunologic properties through polyamine synthesis.

Ornithine and Arginine: Metabolic and Intercellular Cooperation

As discussed, arginine could modulate immunity through NO° production and ornithine could do so through polyamine synthesis. Although all of the enzymes required to produce polyamines from arginine and NO° from ornithine may not be present in a given tissue, we must keep in mind that both amino acids display important interorgan exchanges and are metabolites of each other. Thus, arginine administration by the oral (20,23,25,28) or parenteral (18,27) route leads to a dramatic increase in plasma ornithine concentrations, and ornithine administration (as an alpha-ketoglutarate salt, Cétornan) increases plasma arginine levels (58,59). Thus, it is virtually impossible to determine which is the true immunomodulator. However, it seems certain that this property is not shared by citrulline (7).

In fact, it seems that both ornithine and arginine play a role in regulating immunity and may act cooperatively. Indeed, the activated macrophage synthesizes NO° and, at the moment of its lysis (60), releases arginase into the extracellular fluid surrounding the inflammatory site (61). As a result, arginine is actively transformed to ornithine, which is transported into lymphocytes for polyamine synthesis (62) (Fig. 1).

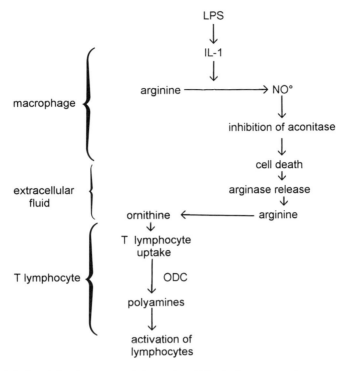

FIG. 1. Metabolic relation between arginine and ornithine in the context of macrophage-lympho-cyte cooperation. ODC, ornithine decarboxylase. Adapted from Cynober L, et al. *Nutr Clin Metab* 1993;7:183–189. with permission.

Therefore, the production of ornithine from arginine may be a signal sent by macro-phages to lymphocytes (63).

EFFECTS ON INTESTINAL TROPHICITY

Ornithine is the precursor of polyamines, which may play an important role in the control of hypo- and hyperplasia in the intestine. Ornithine decarboxylase in the mucosa of the small intestine has a high basal activity relative to most tissues (6). Ornithine decarboxylase is associated with mature cells of the villus type as well as with proliferating crypt cells, suggesting that polyamines are involved in both intes-tinal cell differentiation and proliferation (64).

Intestinal polyamine content falls after fasting (65) or 8 days of TPN in rats (65), then increases during refeeding (66). The fall in the level of polyamines during fasting is due to a simultaneous decrease in their synthesis (i.e., a decrease in ODC content) and an increase in their degradation (i.e., an increase in diamine oxidase content). The reverse is true during refeeding (67). This effect is strong in the jejunum and ileum, moderate in the duodenum, and weak in the proximal colon (68).

Likewise, during intestinal adaptation in response to jejunectomy (69) or to parasite-induced inflammation (70), intestinal levels of polyamines and ODC increase in parallel with mucosal proliferation indices. This is obvious in the distal segment of the intestine, where the polyamine content is lowest at the basal state (71). With the administration of difluoromethylornithine (DFMO), an inhibitor of ODC synthesis, the increase in ODC and polyamines is suppressed and intestinal adaptation is abrogated (69).

Ornithine and arginine are also potent stimulators of growth hormone secretion (7,8), which could have trophic effects on the intestine. Theoretically, it seems likely that ornithine and arginine can support gut trophicity, but what has been demonstrated in practice?

Arginine

The effect of arginine administration on gut trophicity has not been studied and it is not certain that exogenous arginine is a suitable precursor of polyamines (72). The fact that a large fraction of metabolized arginine is released from the enterocyte as citrulline (see previous discussion) argues against the significant involvement of arginine in gut polyamine synthesis.

Ornithine

Only one study is available (73) in which rats were starved for 3 days and then refed for 4 days by continuous enteral nutrition supplemented with ornithine (0.32 g/kg/d) as the alpha-ketoglutarate salt. The rats were then sacrificed and intestinal morphology and enzyme content were studied; ornithine administration led to a significantly higher crypt height in the jejunum and ileum and a higher total villous height in the ileum. In addition, sucrase and lactase levels were higher in the ileum of ornithine alpha-ketoglutarate–supplemented rats.

The relation of this effect of ornithine to polyamine generation is unclear; however, an association is supported by results obtained in cultured human fibroblasts, which are also rapidly dividing cells: fibroblasts incubated with OKG exhibited higher thymidine incorporation into DNA than controls and this effect was blocked when DFMO was also present in the incubation medium (74).

REFERENCES

1. Laissue JA, Gebbers JO. The intestinal barrier and the gut-associated lymphoid tissue. In: Cottier H, Kraft R, eds. *Gut-derived Infectious Toxic Shock*. Basel: Karger, 1992;19–43.
2. Alverdy JC. The effect of enteral and parenteral nutrition on gut-barrier function to bacteria. In: Bounous G, ed. *Uses of Elemental Diets in Clinical Situations*. Boca Raton: CRC Press, 1993;91–100.
3. Souba WW, Klimberg VS, Plumley DA, et al. The role of glutamine in maintaining a healthy gut and supporting the metabolic response to injury and infection. *J Surg Res* 1990;48:383–391.

4. Newsholme EA, Newsholme D, Curi R, et al. A role for muscle in the immune system and its importance in surgery, trauma, sepsis and burns. *Nutrition* 1988;4:261–268.
5. Moncada S, Palmer RMJ, Higgs EA. Biosynthesis of nitric oxide from L-arginine. A pathway for the regulation of cell function and communication. *Biochem Pharmacol* 1989;38:1709–1715.
6. Pegg AE. Recent advances in the biochemistry of polyamines in eukaryotes. *Biochem J* 1986;234: 249–262.
7. Barbul A. Arginine: biochemistry, physiology and therapeutic implications. *JPEN* 1986;10:227–238.
8. Cynober L. Ornithine alpha-ketoglutarate in nutritional support. *Nutrition* 1991;7:313–322.
9. Meijer AJ, Lamers WH, Chamuleau RAFM. Nitrogen metabolism and ornithine cycle function. *Physiol Rev* 1990;70:701–748.
10. Herzfeld A, Raper SM. The heterogeneity of arginases in rat tissues. *Biochem J* 1976;153:469–478.
11. Windmueller HG, Spaeth AE. Metabolism of absorbed aspartate, asparagine, and arginine by rat small intestine in vivo. *Arch Biochem Biophys* 1976;175:660–676.
12. Blachier F, M'Rabet-Touil H, Darcy-Vrillon B, et al. Stimulation by D-glucose of the direct conversion of arginine to citrulline in enterocytes isolated from pig jejunum. *Biochem Biophys Res Commun* 1991;177:1171–1177.
13. Blachier F, Darcy-Vrillon B, Sener A, et al. Arginine metabolism in rat enterocytes. *Biochim Biophys Acta* 1991;1092:304–310.
14. Vaubourdolle M, Jardel A, Coudray-Lucas C, et al. Fate of enterally administered ornithine in healthy animals: interactions with alpha-ketoglutarate. *Nutrition* 1989;5:183–187.
15. Seifter E, Rettura G, Barbul A, Levenson SM. Arginine: an essential amino acid for injured rats. *Surgery* 1978;84:224–230.
16. Chyun JH, Griminger P. Improvement of nitrogen retention by arginine and glycine supplementation and its relation to collagen synthesis in traumatized mature and aged rats. *J Nutr* 1984;114:1697–1704.
17. Kirk SJ, Regan MC, Wasserkrugh HL, et al. Arginine enhances T-cell responses in athymic nude mice. *JPEN* 1992;16:429–436.
18. Barbul A, Wasserkrug HL, Penberthy LT, et al. Optimal levels of arginine in maintenance intravenous hyperalimentation. *JPEN* 1984;8:281–284.
19. Barbul A, Wasserkrug HL, Yoshimura N, et al. High arginine levels in intravenous hyperalimentation abrogate post-traumatic immune suppression. *J Surg Res* 1984;36:620–624.
20. Saito H, Trocki O, Wang SL, et al. Metabolic and immune effects of dietary arginine supplementation after burn. *Arch Surg* 1987;122:784–789.
21. Madden HP, Breslin RJ, Wasserkrug HL, et al. Stimulation of T cell immunity by arginine enhances survival in peritonitis. *J Surg Res* 1988;44:658–663.
22. Reynolds JV, Thom AKT, Zhang SM, et al. Arginine, protein malnutrition and cancer. *J Surg Res* 1988;45:513–522.
23. Reynolds JV, Daly JM, Shou J, et al. Immunologic effects of arginine supplementation in tumor-bearing and non-tumor-bearing hosts. *Ann Surg* 1990;211:202–210.
24. Ronnenberg AG, Gross KL, Hartman WJ, et al. Dietary arginine supplementation does not enhance lymphocyte proliferation or interleukin-2 production in young and aged rats. *J Nutr* 1991;121: 1270–1278.
25. Barbul A, Lazarou SA, Efron BA, et al. Arginine enhances wound healing and lymphocyte immune responses in humans. *Surgery* 1990;108:331–337.
26. Daly JM, Reynolds J, Thom A, et al. Immune and metabolic effects of arginine in the surgical patient. *Ann Surg* 1988;205:512–523.
27. Sigal RK, Shou J, Daly JM. Parenteral arginine infusion in humans: nutrient substrate or pharmacologic agent. *JPEN* 1992;16:423–428.
28. Cerra FB, Lehmann S, Konstantinides N, et al. Improvement in immune function in ICU patients by enteral nutrition supplemented with arginine, RNA, and menhaden oil is independent of nitrogen balance. *Nutrition* 1991;7:193–199.
29. Daly JM, Leberman MD, Goldfine J, et al. Enteral nutrition with supplemental arginine, RNA, and omega-3 fatty acids in patients after operation; immunologic, metabolic, and clinical outcome. *Surgery* 1992;112:56–67.
30. Chandra RK, Baker M, Whang S, Au B. Effect of two feeding formulas on immune responses and mortality in mice challenged with Listeria monocytogenes. *Immunol Lett* 1991;27:45–48.
31. Cerra FB. Role of nutrition in the management of malnutrition and immune dysfunction of trauma. *J Am Coll Nutr* 1992;11:512–518.
32. Gonce SJ, Peck MD, Alexander W, Miskell PW. Arginine supplementation and its effect on established peritonitis in guinea pigs. *JPEN* 1990;14:237–244.

33. Moncada S, Palmer RMJ, Higgs EA. Nitric oxide: physiology, pathology and pharmacology. *Pharmacol Rev* 1991;43:109–142.
34. Radomski MW, Palmer RMJ, Moncada S. Modulation of platelet aggregation by an L-arginine-nitric oxide pathway. *Trends Pharmacol Sci* 1991;12:87–88.
35. Pittner RA, Spitzer JA. Endotoxin and TNF-α directly stimulate nitric oxide formation in cultured rat hepatocytes from chronically endotoxemic rats. *Biochem Biophys Res Commun* 1992;185:430–435.
36. Albina JE, Henry WL. Suppression of lymphocyte proliferation through the nitric oxide synthesizing pathway. *J Surg Res* 1991;50:403–409.
37. Schmidt HHHW, Seifert R, Bohme E. Formation and release of nitric oxide from human neutrophils and HL-60 cells induced by a chemotactic peptide, platelet activating factor and leukotriene B4. *FEBS Lett* 1989;244:357–360.
38. Lambert LE, Whitten JP, Baron BM, et al. Nitric oxide synthesis in the endothelium and macrophages differs in the sensitivity to inhibition by arginine analogues. *Life Sci* 1990;48:69–75.
39. Bergmann L, Kroncke KD, Suschek C, et al. Cytotoxic action of IL-1β against pancreatic islets is mediated via nitric oxide formation and is inhibited by N^g-mono methyl-L-arginine. *FEBS Lett* 1992; 299:103–106.
40. Li L, Kilbourn RG, Adams J, Fidler IJ. Role of nitric oxide in lysis of tumor cells by cytokine-activated endothelial cells. *Cancer Res* 1991;51:2531–2535.
41. Billiar TR, Curran RD. Kupffer cell and hepatocyte interactions: a brief overview. *JPEN* 1990;14: 175S–180S.
42. Curran RD, Billiar TR, Stuehr DJ, et al. Multiple cytokines are required to induce hepatocyte nitric oxide production and inhibit protein synthesis. *Ann Surg* 1984;212:462–471.
43. Sakuma I, Stuehr DJ, Gross SS, et al. Identification of arginine as a precursor of endothelium-derived relaxing factor. *Proc Natl Acad Sci* 1988;85:8664–8667.
44. Marletta MA. Nitric oxide: biosynthesis and biological significance. *TIBS* 1989;14:488–492.
45. Stuehr DJ, Marletta MA. Mammalian nitrate biosynthesis: mouse macrophages produce nitrite and nitrate in response to *Escherichia coli* lipopolysaccharide. *Proc Natl Acad Sci USA* 1985;82: 7738–7742.
46. Moncada S. Nitric oxide gas: mediator, modulator, and pathophysiologic entity. *J Lab Clin Med* 1992;120:187–191.
47. Bogle RG, Baydoun AR, Pearson JD, et al. L-arginine transport is increased in macrophages generating nitric oxide. *Biochem J* 1992;284:15–18.
48. Di Rosa M, Radomski M, Carnuccio R, Moncada S. Glucocorticoids inhibit the induction of nitric oxide synthase in macrophages. *Biochem Biophys Res Commun* 1990;172:1246–1252.
49. Hutcheson IR, Whittle BJR, Boughton-Smith NK. Role of nitric oxide in maintaining vascular integrity in endotoxin-induced acute intestinal damage in the rat. *Br J Pharmacol* 1990;101:815–820.
50. Kilbourn RG, Gross SS, Jubran A, et al. NG-methyl-L-arginine inhibits tumor necrosis factor-induced hypotension: implications for the involvement of nitric oxide. *Proc Natl Acad Sci USA* 1990;87: 3629–3632.
51. Ochoa JB, Uderkwu AO, Billiar TM, et al. Nitrogen oxide levels in patients after trauma and during sepsis. *Ann Surg* 1991;214:621–626.
52. Fleming I, Julou-Schaeffer G, Gray GA, et al. Evidence than an L-arginine/nitric oxide dependent elevation of tissue cyclic GMP content is involved in depression of vascular reactivity by endotoxin. *Br J Pharmacol* 1991;103:1047–1052.
53. Pasquali JL, Urlacher A, Storck D. La stimulation lymphocytaire in vitro par le pockeweed mitogène chez les sujets normaux et les sujets dénutris; influence des sels d'ornithine. *Pathol Biol* 1983;31: 191–194.

54. Rettura G, Barbul A, Levenson SM, Seifter E. Citrulline does not share the thymotropic properties of arginine and ornithine. *Fed Proc* 1979;38:289 (abstract).
55. Limborg J. Contribution à l'étude de l'influence de l'α-cétoglutarate d'ornithine sur la réponse immunitaire chez la souris. Thèse: Maison-Alfort, France, 1983.
56. Lasnier E, Le Boucher J, Jardel A, et al. Efficacité de l'α-cétoglutarate d'ornithine chez le rat endotoxémique. *Nutr Clin Metabol* 1992;6(Suppl 4):(abstract).
57. Endo Y, Matsushima K, Onozaki K, Oppenheim JJ. Role of ornithine decarboxylase in the regulation of cell growth by IL-1 and tumor necrosis factor. *J Immunol* 1988;141:2342–2348.
58. Cynober L, Coudray-Lucas C, De Bandt JP, et al. Action of ornithine alpha-ketoglutarate, ornithine hydrochloride and calcium alpha-ketoglutarate on plasma amino acid and hormonal patterns in healthy subjects. *J Am Coll Nutr* 1990;9:9–12.

59. Grimble GK, Coudray-Lucas C, Payne-James JJ, et al. Augmentation of plasma arginine and gluta-mine by ornithine alpha-ketoglutarate in healthy enterally-fed volunteers. *Proc Nutr Soc* 1991 (ab-stract).
60. Albina JE, Mills CD, Barbul A, et al. Arginine metabolism in wounds. *Am J Physiol* 1988;254: E459–E467.
61. Albina JE, Mills CD, Henry WL Jr, Caldwell MD. Temporal expression of different pathways of L-arginine metabolism in healing wounds. *J Immunol* 1990;144:3877–3880.
62. Albina JE, Caldwell MD, Henry WL Jr, Mills CD. Regulation of macrophage functions by L-arginine. *J Exp Med* 1989;169:1021–1029.
63. Daly JM, Reynolds J, Sigal RK, et al. Effect of dietary protein and amino acids on immune function. *Crit Care Med* 1990;118:S86–S93.
64. Johnson LR, Tseng CC, Wang P, et al. Mucosal ornithine decarboxylase in the small intestine: localization and stimulation. *Am J Physiol* 1989;256:G624–G630.
65. Alarcon P, Lin CH, Lebenthal E, Lee PC. Interaction of malnutrition and difluoromethylornithine induced intestinal mucosal damage: degree of severity and subsequent recovery. *Digestion* 1988;41: 68–77.
66. Hosomi M, Stace NH, Lirussi F, et al. Role of polyamines in intestinal adaptation in the rat. *Eur J Clin Invest* 1987;17:375–385.
67. D'Agostino L, Daniele B, Pignata S, et al. Modifications in ornithine decarboxylase and diamine oxidase in small bowel mucosa of starved and refed rats. *Gut* 1987;28(Suppl 1):135–138.
68. Jain R, Eikenburg BE, Johnson LR. Stimulation of ornithine decarboxylase activity in digestive tract mucosa. *Am J Physiol* 1987;253:G303–G307.
69. Luk GD, Yang P. Polyamines intestinal and pancreatic adaptation. *Gut* 1987;28(Suppl 1):95–101.
70. Wang JY, Johnson LR, Tsai YH, Castro GA. Mucosal ornithine decarboxylase, polyamines, and hyperplasia in infected intestine. *Am J Physiol* 1991;23:G45–G51.
71. Hosomi MM, Smith SM, Murphy GM, Dowling RH. Polyamine distribution in the rat intestinal mucosa. *J Chromatogr* 1986;375:267–275.
72. Cynober L. Can arginine and related compounds support gut functions? *Gut* 1994;Suppl 1:S42–S49.
73. Hasselman M, Gosse F, Galluser M, Raul F. Effets d'une supplémentation entérale en alpha-cétoglu-tarate d'ornithine sur la trophicité et les hydrolases intestinales. *Nutr Clin Metab* 1992;6(Suppl):30 (abstract).
74. Vaubourdolle M, Salvucci M, Coudray-Lucas C, et al. Action of ornithine alpha-ketoglutarate on DNA synthesis by human fibroblasts. *In Vitro Cell Develop Biol* 1990;26:187–192.

Organ Metabolism and Nutrition:
Ideas for Future Critical Care, edited by
J. M. Kinney and H. N. Tucker.
Raven Press, Ltd., New York © 1994.

13

Interorgan Exchange of Amino Acids after Trauma

Peter B. Soeters and Nicolaas E.P. Deutz

Academical Hospital Maastricht, 6229 NL Maastricht, The Netherlands

The past decade has witnessed an enormous increase in interest in the role of glutamine as a conditionally essential amino acid. Of all amino acids glutamine is most abundantly present in its free form in many tissues and in plasma, both in health and disease.

It has been well established for more than two decades that during muscle protein degradation, the resulting free amino acids do not appear in the circulation as such but largely donate their amino groups to pyruvate and α-ketoglutarate, yielding alanine and, eventually, glutamine, which then are released in the circulation. In the old days it was claimed that the advantage of this process is that, first, glutamine and alanine can furnish carbon skeletons that can act as precursors for gluconeogenesis in the liver and, second, that the flux of these amino acids can vary substantially without untoward side effects because both are nontoxic in a wide range of concentrations. In this manner amino and amide nitrogen can be transported in the circulation without side effects and taken up by organs able to process alanine and glutamine. Alternatively, release as such of the free amino acids derived from proteolysis in differing quantities would have harmful effects on protein synthesis and degradation, neurotransmitter synthesis, and so on.

It has been hypothesized that in addition to the role of glutamine as a nontoxic nitrogen carrier and precursor for gluconeogenesis, glutamine may have beneficial effects on muscle protein synthesis, gut mucosa morphology and protein content, and immune system function, and may play a role in acid-base homeostasis.

Clinical studies initially focused on overall nitrogen economy, and in several patient studies. A reproducible but rather modest improvement in nitrogen balance could be demonstrated when parenteral nutrition was enriched with glutamine (peptide) in an isonitrogenous manner and administered to patients undergoing a standard operation (1,2). This improvement, however, can be largely explained by the preservation of free glutamine levels in muscle of the enriched group, leaving little room for net protein retention. The finding might therefore be insignificant if the modest net protein retention that may have been achieved would only apply to muscle. On the other hand, even small net increases in protein retention in the gut mucosa or in immune cells may have significant effects on function.

After trauma, splanchnic tissues have been found to take up more glutamine (3,4). This increased uptake has been hypothesized to regulate the production of glutamine in peripheral tissues (5). Souba et al. have postulated that after trauma also the gut mucosa require and utilize more glutamine, and that a relative lack of glutamine might induce villous atrophy and increased permeability of the gut, which in turn might hypothetically lead to harmful endotoxin resorption and bacterial translocation (6). Indeed, in experimental animals glutamine addition to the parenteral nutrition regimen had beneficial effects on gut morphology, protein and DNA content, and some clinical parameters (7–9).

The finding that the intestine itself utilizes more glutamine after trauma has been demonstrated in two human studies, in which leg muscle glutamine release diminished after enterectomy (10,11).

The exact mechanism operative in this setting is difficult to establish. First, removal of a diseased intestine may diminish the catabolic rate and thus glutamine production. Second, it is still a matter of debate to what extent gut consumption of glutamine regulates glutamine production of peripheral tissues, or, vice versa, that peripheral glutamine production determines gut utilization. Third, the suggestions put forward by Souba et al. on the basis of the human studies are based on changes in leg muscle release of glutamine after enterectomy without quantitation of uptake by splanchnic tissues. In experimental and human studies, uptake of substrates across the splanchnic tissues have been measured by determining arterohepatic fluxes. In experimental animals also, arterioportal fluxes have been measured. Both types of measurement still do not distinguish fluxes across the intestine, itself, and the spleen. The assumption, that total arterioportal fluxes reflect largely metabolism in the intestinal mucosa, may be questioned.

We therefore studied flux of metabolites separately across the spleen and across the portal drained viscera after trauma (12), and studied the influence of excision of a large part of the healthy small intestine (13).

FLUXES OF AMINO ACIDS AND AMMONIA ACROSS SPLANCHNIC TISSUES AFTER TRAUMA

Cannulation of the venous effluent of the hindquarter, the hepatic, portal, and splenic vein, and the arterial circulation allows flow measurements across these organs by means of indicator dilution methods and flux measurements of metabolites by simultaneous measurement of transorgan concentration differences of these metabolites (12). Such flux measurements can be performed in the awake, nonrestrained experimental animal. We have employed young growing pigs because they are cheap, can be handled easily, and have many metabolic similarities with humans.

We specifically were interested in the metabolite fluxes after standard trauma. For this purpose we used the major operative procedure, during which the catheters were inserted as standard trauma, and measured fluxes across the separate organs 1, 2, 3, and 4 days after operation. Pretrauma values at time zero could, by necessity,

TABLE 1. *Portal drained viscera fluxes.*

	Control	POD 1	POD 2	POD 3	POD 4
Plasma flow (ml min^{-1} kg^{-1} body weight)	34 ± 6	21 ± 4	24 ± 5	25 ± 4	23 ± 7[b]
HCO$_3^-$ (μmol min^{-1} kg^{-1} body weight)	53 ± 14[a]	19 ± 8[b]	29 ± 5[a]	8 ± 13[a,b]	37 ± 13[a]
O$_2$ consumption (μmol min^{-1} kg^{-1} body weight)	−38 ± 6[a]	−17 ± 3[a,c]	−24 ± 4[a,b]	−31 ± 1[a,b]	−23 ± 2[a,b]
Ammonia[e] (nmol min^{-1} kg^{-1} body weight)	5217 ± 524[a]	877 ± 250[a,d]	2744 ± 515[a,b]	2950 ± 562[a,b]	2263 ± 720[a,b]
Gln[e] (nmol min^{-1} kg^{-1} body weight)	−1944 ± 145[a]	−614 ± 98[a,d]	−1064 ± 284[a,b]	−1024 ± 230[a,c]	−1137 ± 167[a,c]

Values are means ± SEM.
[a] Wilcoxon test: significantly different from zero.
[b] Mann-Whitney U-test vs. normal: $p < 0.05$.
[c] Mann-Whitney U-test vs. normal: $p < 0.01$.
[d] Mann-Whitney U-test vs. normal: $p < 0.001$.
[e] Analysis of variance of controls, POD 1, POD 2, POD 3, POD 4: $p < 0.001$.

only be measured after insertion of the catheters. For this purpose, measurements were performed after 7 days when animals had fully recovered and resumed their normal life pattern.

Immediately after operation, exchange of metabolites and oxygen across the portal drained viscera was decreased, indicating a lowered metabolic rate (Table 1), but at day 2, HCO$_3$ production by the liver increased concomitantly with increased glucose and urea production, reflecting increased gluconeogenesis (Table 2). After operation, liver glutamine production reverted to consumption. In contradistinction with the findings of Souba et al. (6), glutamine uptake of total portal drained viscera decreased to 30% to 50% of control (Table 1). As expected, portal drained viscera ammonia production balanced liver uptake at all time points.

Glutamine and alanine production by the hindquarter increased after operation, parallelled by an increased efflux of amino acids that cannot be degraded in peripheral tissues (tyrosine, phenylalanine, methionine, tryptophan, lysine) and also the BCAAs (not shown). This reflects increased net protein degradation. Net efflux of these amino acids normalized at day 3 (Table 3).

Splenic ammonia production increased strikingly after operation in parallel with an increase in glutamine consumption, glucose uptake, and lactate production (Table 4, Fig. 1). In control animals, glutamine was released by the spleen, whereas after operation, release reverted to uptake despite similar delivery to the spleen (arterial

TABLE 2. *Liver fluxes.*

	Control	POD 1	POD 2	POD 3	POD 4
Plasma flow (ml min^{-1} kg^{-1} body weight)	41 ± 8	27 ± 4	42 ± 8	52 ± 10	32 ± 9
HCO$_3^-$ [e] (μmol min^{-1} kg^{-1} body weight)	16 ± 18	−15 ± 16[b]	42 ± 14[a]	65 ± 16[a]	30 ± 14[a,b]
O$_2$ consumption[e] (μmol min^{-1} kg^{-1} body weight)	−49 ± 8[a]	−26 ± 4[a,b]	−52 ± 20[a]	−73 ± 17[a]	−48 ± 6[a,b]
Ammonia[f] (nmol min^{-1} kg^{-1} body weight)	−5308 ± 492[a]	−814 ± 382[d]	−3082 ± 542[a,b]	−3269 ± 735[a,b]	−2319 ± 637[a,c]
Urea (nmol min^{-1} kg^{-1} body weight)	1786 ± 2955	600 ± 835	3702 ± 374[a]	4534 ± 2201[a]	1578 ± 667[a]
Glucose[f] (nmol min^{-1} kg^{-1} body weight)	8940 ± 3046[a]	348 ± 3369	21083 ± 2001[a,b]	14626 ± 4132[a]	168 ± 7181
Gln[f] (nmol min^{-1} kg^{-1} body weight)	676 ± 266[a]	−788 ± 268[a,d]	−1907 ± 887[b]	−1284 ± 539[a,b]	−1395 ± 305[a,c]

Values are means ± SEM.
[a] Wilcoxon test: significantly different from zero.
[b] Mann-Whitney U-test vs. normal: $p < 0.05$.
[c] Mann-Whitney U-test vs. normal: $p < 0.01$.
[d] Mann-Whitney U-test vs. normal: $p < 0.001$.
[e] Analysis of variance of controls, POD 1, POD 2, POD 3, POD 4: $p < 0.05$.
[f] Analysis of variance of controls, POD 1, POD 2, POD 3, POD 4: $p < 0.01$.

TABLE 3. *Hindquarter fluxes.*

	Control	POD 1	POD 2	POD 3	POD 4
Plasma flow (ml min^{-1} kg^{-1} body weight)	20 ± 2	16 ± 4	16 ± 4	19 ± 3	22 ± 7
Gln (nmol min^{-1} kg^{-1} body weight)	685 ± 167[a]	1140 ± 115[a,b]	1301 ± 339[a]	645 ± 140[a]	1299 ± 470[a]
Ala[g] (nmol min^{-1} kg^{-1} body weight)	397 ± 105[a]	1862 ± 277[a,d]	896 ± 266[a]	239 ± 92[a]	571 ± 406

Values are means ± SEM.
[a] Wilcoxon test: significantly different from zero.
[b] Mann-Whitney U-test vs. normal: $p < 0.05$.
[c] Mann-Whitney U-test vs. normal: $p < 0.001$.
[d] Mann-Whitney U-test vs. normal: $p < 0.001$.
[e] Analysis of variance of controls, POD 1, POD 2, POD 3, POD 4: $p < 0.05$.
[f] Analysis of variance of controls, POD 1, POD 2, POD 3, POD 4: $p < 0.01$.
[g] Analysis of variance of controls, POD 1, POD 2, POD 3, POD 4: $p < 0.001$.

TABLE 4. *Splenic fluxes.*

	Control	POD 1	POD 2	POD 3	POD 4
Plasma flow (ml min^{-1} kg^{-1} body weight)	11 ± 7	13 ± 4	16 ± 7	11 ± 3	9 ± 4
Ammonia[e] (nmol min^{-1} kg^{-1} body weight)	288 ± 104[a]	579 ± 201[a]	1988 ± 691[a,b]	913 ± 357[a]	565 ± 355[a]
Glucose[g] (nmol min^{-1} kg^{-1} body weight)	−964 ± 632	−4960 ± 1463[a,b]	−3933 ± 1524[b]	−1352 ± 710[c]	1406 ± 1417
Lactate[g] (nmol min^{-1} kg^{-1} body weight)	−158 ± 469	747 ± 544	3294 ± 642[a,c]	1325 ± 276[a]	919 ± 275[a]
Gln[g] (nmol min^{-1} kg^{-1} body weight)	391 ± 143[a]	−423 ± 54[a,d]	−752 ± 169[a,d]	−350 ± 113[d]	−457 ± 52[a,d]
Ala (nmol min^{-1} kg^{-1} body weight)	−181 ± 66[a]	−21 ± 166[b]	20 ± 69	9 ± 23[b]	−90 ± 72[a,d]

Values are means ± SEM.
[a] Wilcoxon test: significantly different from zero.
[b] Mann-Whitney *U*-test vs. normal: $p < 0.05$.
[c] Mann-Whitney *U*-test vs. normal: $p < 0.01$.
[d] Mann-Whitney *U*-test vs. normal: $p < 0.001$.
[e] Analysis of variance of controls, POD 1, POD 2, POD 3, POD 4: $p < 0.05$.
[f] Analysis of variance of controls, POD 1, POD 2, POD 3, POD 4: $p < 0.01$.
[g] Analysis of variance of controls, POD 1, POD 2, POD 3, POD 4: $p < 0.001$.

Gln concentration × flow). This implies that after trauma, Gln extraction by the spleen is significantly stimulated. The availability of these data and the fluxes across the total portal drained viscera allowed computations of the pure intestinal fluxes (Table 5). Glutamine uptake across the intestine proved to be modest and lower than across the spleen on days 1 and 2 after operation.

To address the question of whether splanchnic tissues in some way regulate post-traumatic glutamine release by peripheral tissues, glutamine fluxes and fluxes of related compounds were studied in enterectomized and sham operated rats (13). Specifically, hindquarter, liver, and portal drained visceral fluxes were measured 24 hours after operation.

Hindquarter production of glutamine was similar in enterectomized and sham operated rats, whereas glutamine uptake across splanchnic tissues decreased after enterectomy. Specifically, uptake across the intestine decreased (23% of uptake in sham rats), whereas uptake by the liver increased (Fig. 2). However, uptake of glutamine per gram tissue increased in the remaining intestine after enterectomy compared to sham operated controls.

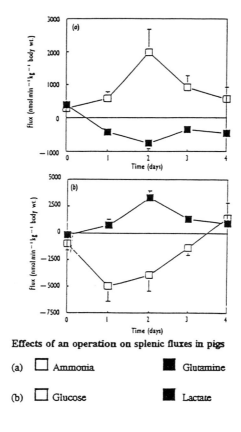

Effects of an operation on splenic fluxes in pigs

(a) ☐ Ammonia   ■ Glutamine

(b) ☐ Glucose   ■ Lactate

Values are means ± SEM.

FIG. 1.

POSTTRAUMATIC METABOLISM

Many of the findings in the aforementioned studies confirm what is already known. After injury, there is an increased release from peripheral tissues of amino acids mainly consisting of glutamine and alanine but also including amino acids that are not degraded in peripheral tissues, i.e., most essential amino acids. The flux is quantitatively so important that it must be the consequence of protein degradation. Simultaneously, HCO_3, urea, and glucose production by the liver is increased, reflecting increased gluconeogenesis.

In the literature, the enhanced production of glutamine and alanine by peripheral tissues was offset by increased uptake of glutamine by the intestine and of glutamine and alanine by the liver (4). We confirmed increased uptake of glutamine and alanine by the liver after operative trauma but found a decreased uptake of glutamine and decreased release of ammonia by the portal drained splanchnic tissues. Uptake by the

TABLE 5. *Intestinal fluxes.*

	Control	POD 1	POD 2	POD 3	POD 4
O$_2$ consumption (μmol min^{-1} kg^{-1} body weight)	-27 ± 6^a	$-7 \pm 4^{a,b}$	$-10 \pm 5^{a,b}$	-22 ± 2^a	-14 ± 3^a
Ammonia^g (nmol min^{-1} kg^{-1} body weight)	5212 ± 566^a	305 ± 407^c	484 ± 980^c	$2037 \pm 571^{a,c}$	$1539 \pm 523^{a,c}$
Gln^g (nmol min^{-1} kg^{-1} body weight)	-2397 ± 217^a	$-231 \pm 125^{a,d}$	-313 ± 229^c	-596 ± 337^c	$-680 \pm 125^{a,d}$
Ala (nmol min^{-1} kg^{-1} body weight)	211 ± 76^a	-253 ± 277	322 ± 199	192 ± 50^a	135 ± 146
α-AN^e (nmol min^{-1} kg^{-1} body weight)	4210 ± 907^a	-444 ± 1097	1966 ± 1320	-919 ± 1376	-537 ± 1462

Values are means ± SEM.
[a] Wilcoxon test: significantly different from zero.
[b] Mann-Whitney U-test vs. normal: $p < 0.05$.
[c] Mann-Whitney U-test vs. normal: $p < 0.01$.
[d] Mann-Whitney U-test vs. normal: $p < 0.001$.
[e] Analysis of variance of controls, POD 1, POD 2, POD 3, POD 4: $p < 0.05$.
[f] Analysis of variance of controls, POD 1, POD 2, POD 3, POD 4: $p < 0.01$.
[g] Analysis of variance of controls, POD 1, POD 2, POD 3, POD 4: $p < 0.001$.

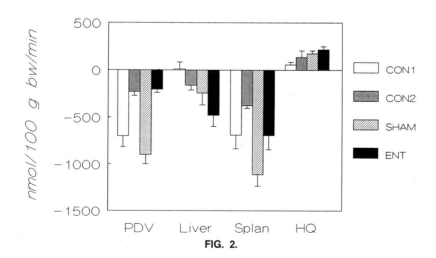

FIG. 2.

intestine of glutamine was even less because splenic uptake increased substantially, whereas also glucose uptake and ammonia and lactate release across the spleen increased.

These findings may be viewed in the light of activation of the immune system. Although flux measurements, as performed in this type of study, do not allow us to pinpoint cellular systems that utilize glutamine, the in vitro finding that lymphocytes utilize more glutamine and glucose when activated and produce more ammonia supports the possibility that enhanced uptake of glutamine and release of ammonia by the spleen is actually performed by lymphocytes and macrophages, allowing them to be activated (14,15). A similar reasoning may, in part, apply to the liver.

Immune system activation has been demonstrated to occur after injury, and our data suggest that in this process enhanced glutamine release by peripheral tissues plays an important role. It has been hypothesized that glutamine release by peripheral tissues is generated by consumption by the immune system. Our data show that more than 60% of the glutamine released from the periphery is taken up by liver (Kupffer cells?) and spleen (lymphocytes?) and that, in fact, a minor proportion is taken up by the intestine itself.

The studies do not allow us to distinguish between uptake of immune cells in the wall of the intestine and the mucosal cells, but if there is an increased uptake in these cells, parallel with increased uptake by liver and spleen, uptake by the mucosal cells is even less than indicated by the values obtained for total uptake by the portal drained viscera.

GLUTAMINE METABOLISM IN THE INTESTINE

This decreased intestinal uptake, in our view, casts doubt on the proposed role of the intestine as a key regulator of nitrogen handling following surgical stress (6). The data rather support the possibility that, indeed, immune system activation generates peripheral amino acid release (16,17). The type of data presented cannot furnish conclusive proof that this mechanism actually exists. In our view, it strongly supports the hypothesis that to generate an immune response after trauma, glutamine is required. The diminished uptake of glutamine by the intestine after trauma suggests that even in previously well-fed growing pigs, after operative trauma, there is no mechanism to preserve metabolic rate, glutamine uptake, and related flux of metabolites in the intestine when the gut is (semi)starved. This does not imply that this arrangement is beneficial to the gut, as evidenced by e.g., posttraumatic atrophy and gut permeability. The experimental findings that addition of glutamine (peptide) to parenteral nutrition in a multitude of experimental settings has beneficial effects on gut morphology, protein, and DNA content, and on some aspects of clinical outcome (7–9), suggest that when glutamine is administered in abundance, beneficial effects on gut morphology and function can be achieved.

In a study in patients, we found that isonitrogenous glutamine peptide enrichment of the parenteral nutrition regimen preserved villus height and gut integrity, as measured by the lactulose-mannitol ratio, in patients that did not receive enteral nutrition (18). In the patients receiving isonitrogenous, conventional, parenteral nutrition, both villus height and gut integrity deteriorated.

After trauma, an increased net efflux of glutamine, alanine, and most essential amino acids from peripheral tissues occurs. This efflux is counterbalanced largely by uptake by the splanchnic tissues and results in increased urea production and glucose production in the liver. Specifically, the liver and spleen take up more glutamine after trauma, whereas, in contradistinction with findings in the literature, the intestine takes up lesser amounts of glutamine. In the spleen, increased posttraumatic uptake of glutamine coincides with increased ammonia production, glucose uptake, and lactate release. These findings are consistent with in vitro findings demonstrating increased glutamine and glucose uptake and ammonia and lactate release when lymphocytes are activated. They therefore furnish supportive evidence for the possibility that posttraumatic activation of the immune system, including lymphocytes and macrophages in spleen (and possibly Kupffer cells in the liver), requires glutamine and may be an important glutamine flux–generating event. In contradistinction with earlier hypotheses, the intestine does not appear to play such a role because enterectomy and decreased uptake by the remaining intestine did not induce diminished release of glutamine by peripheral tissues. The finding that increased gut permeability and villous atrophy occur after trauma and enteral starvation suggests that the metabolic arrangement described is harmful for the gut. There is now preliminary evidence in humans that these harmful effects may be prevented by parenteral administration of supraphysiologic quantities of glutamine (peptide).

REFERENCES

1. Stehle P, Zander J, Mertes N, et al. Effect of parenteral glutamine peptide supplements on muscle glutamine loss and nitrogen balance after major surgery. *Lancet* 1989;1:231–233.
2. Hammarqvist F, Wernerman J, All R, et al. Addition of glutamine to total parenteral nutrition after elective abdominal surgery spares free glutamine in muscle, counteracts the fall in muscle protein synthesis, and improves nitrogen balance. *Ann Surg* 1989;209:455–461.
3. Clowes G. Aminoacid transfer between muscle and the visceral tissues in man during health and disease. In: Odessey R, ed. *Problems and Potential of Branched-chain Aminoacids in Physiology and Medicine*. Amsterdam: Elsevier Science Publishers, 1986;299–334.
4. Souba W, Wilmore D. Postoperative alteration of arteriovenous exchange of amino acids across the gastrointestinal tract. *Surgery* 1983;94:342–350.
5. Souba W, Roughneen P, Goldwater D, et al. Postoperative alterations in interorgan glutamine exchange in enterectomized dogs. *J Surg Res* 1987;42:117–125.
6. Souba W, Klimberg V, Plumley D, et al. The role of glutamine in maintaining a healthy gut and supporting the metabolic response to injury and infection. *J Surg Res* 1990;48:383–391.
7. Tamada H, Nezu R, Imamura I, et al. The dipeptide alanylglutamine prevents intestinal mucosal atrophy in parenterally fed rats. *JPEN* 1992;16:110–116.
8. O'Dwyer S, Smith R, Hwang T, Wilmore D. Maintenance of small bowel mucosa with glutamine-enriched parenteral nutrition. *JPEN* 1989;13:579–585.
9. Rombeau J. A review of the effects of glutamine-enriched diets on experimentally induced enterocolitis. *JPEN* 1990;14:100S–105S.
10. Fong Y, Tracey K, Hesse D, et al. Influence of enterectomy on peripheral tissue glutamine efflux in critically ill patients. *Surgery* 1990;107:321–326.

11. Darmaun D, Messing B, Just B, et al. Glutamine metabolism after small intestinal resection in humans. *Metabolism* 1991;40:42–44.
12. Deutz N, Reijven P, Athanasas G, Soeters P. Post-operative changes in hepatic, intestinal, splenic and muscle fluxes of aminoacids and ammonia in pigs. *Clin Sci* 1992;83:607–614.
13. Deutz N, Dejong C, Athanasas G, Soeters P. Partial enterectomy in the rat does not diminish muscle glutamine production. *Metabolism* 1992;41:1343–1350.
14. Ardawi M. Glutamine and glucose metabolism in human peripheral lymphocytes. *Metab Clin Exp* 1988;37:99–103.
15. Ardawi M, Newsholme E. Glutamine metabolism in lymphocytes of the rat. *Biochem J* 1983;212: 835–842.
16. Newsholme E, Crabtree B, Ardawi M. Glutamine metabolism in hymphocytes: its biochemical, physiological and clinical importance. *Q J Exp Physiol* 1985;70:473–489.
17. Newsholme E, Newsholme P, Curi R. The role of the citric acid cycle in cells of the immune system and its importance in sepsis, trauma and burns. *Biochem Soc Symp* 1987;54:145–161.
18. van der Hulst R, von Meyenfeldt M, Arends J-W, et al. Glutamine and the preservation of gut integrity. *Lancet* 1993;1, accepted for publication.

Organ Metabolism and Nutrition:
Ideas for Future Critical Care, edited by
J. M. Kinney and H. N. Tucker.
Raven Press, Ltd., New York © 1994.

14

Essential and Conditionally Essential Nutrients in Clinical Nutrition

George K. Grimble

*Department of Gastroenterology and Nutrition, Central Middlesex Hospital,
London NW10 7NS, United Kingdom*

"When I use a word," Humpty Dumpty said in a scornful tone, "it means just what I chose it to mean—neither more nor less."
Lewis Carroll, *Alice Through the Looking Glass*

WHAT CONSTITUTES AN ESSENTIAL NUTRIENT?

Definitions, as Alice found, can be as slippery as a 10-foot snake and this is as true in clinical nutrition as elsewhere. With the advent of novel substrates, proposed as clinically useful adjuncts, a new class of definitions has entered the scientific and medical literature. These substrates, which include glutamine, arginine, ornithine α-ketoglutarate, nucleotides, and the short-chain fatty acids, have been variously described as conditionally essential nutrients, functional nutrients, nutraceutics, pseudonutrients, or even as agents "supporting" some aspect of body metabolism. It is clear that, regardless of the definition used, a final judgment of their usefulness will be on the grounds of clinical and nutritional efficacy. The semantics do, however, have force because they tend to drive clinical perceptions, even when the evidence for essentiality may be quite weak.

One example is inappropriate terminology used to describe glutamine as "conditionally essential." The data shown in Fig. 1 is taken from a study in which patients who were undergoing colonic resection received either standard total parenteral nutrition (TPN) solutions or TPN in which part of the amino acids had been replaced with ornithine α-ketoglutarate (OKG) (1). Supplementation moderated the normal catabolic response to this type of surgery, as it did following cholecystectomy (2). Glutamine supplementation had effects of similar magnitude (3). As can be seen, the excess outpouring of urinary nitrogen after injury was inhibited by OKG supplementation, which maintained patients in slight positive nitrogen balance (Fig. 1, upper panel). What is especially intriguing is that the pattern of nitrogen excretion was more akin to that of nontraumatized patients, and clearly there was a reversal of the

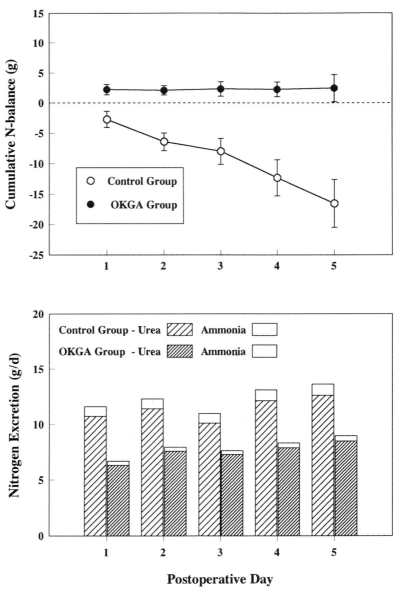

FIG. 1. Effect of OKG on postoperative nitrogen excretion in patients undergoing colonic resection. All patients received an isonitrogenous, isoenergetic TPN regime supplemented with 2.5 g of nitrogen as OKG or mixed L-amino acids. **Upper panel:** Cumulative nitrogen balance; OKG *(solid symbols)*, controls *(open symbols)*. **Lower panel:** Pattern of nitrogen excretion; OKG *(fine hatching)*, controls *(coarse hatching)*; unshaded area, NH_4^+; shaded area, urea. Data adapted from Leander et al. (1).

mild metabolic acidosis (increased NH_4^+ excretion), which is a consequence of injury. Other indicators of trauma, such as depletion of intracellular muscle glutamine concentration and the number of ribosomes engaged in protein synthesis, were also partially reversed (2,4).

Despite the common description of glutamine as a conditionally essential nutrient in the catabolic patient (5), if its action can be mimicked by other metabolically related substrates that have not been considered nutrients, then this definition is clearly wrong. In the case of OKG, neither of its two moieties are found in the normal diet except in the sense that braised liver would contain trace amounts of Kreb's (α-ketoglutarate) or urea cycle (ornithine) metabolites.

An interpretation of the term "functional" nutrient is the case of minor nutrients that are found in breast milk and due to this presence are thus assumed to have specific positive biological value for the suckling infant. Nucleotides in breast milk comprise 0.1% to 0.15% of total milk nitrogen (6). In the weaning rat, they have been shown to increase the rate of intestinal maturation and alter red blood cell membrane fatty-acid profiles (7). Similarly, polyamines that are found as very minor components of mother's milk (6 to 10 μmol/d) increase the rate of intestinal maturation if the diet is modestly supplemented (8). The polyamine content of milk is maintained for 2 months after birth and then falls precipitously (9). Finally, the casomorphin peptide, a sequence found in casein in mother's milk has been shown to stimulate electrolyte uptake in the ileum, to slow gastric emptying, and to have immunostimulatory properties (10–13). Because of this, all could be classed as functional nutrients in the newborn. However, this teleological argument has obvious pitfalls. Many compounds diffuse from the maternal circulation into milk and can have effects on the infant gastrointestinal tract. Thus capsaicin (8-methyl-N-vanillyl-6-nonenamide) from peppers will be found in breast milk from Asian mothers and can increase gastric motility (14,15). Is it therefore a functional nutrient?

Since Rose first classified amino acids into essential and nonessential categories, there has been continuing debate about this division (16). According to the original scheme, some amino acids were essential for growth because their carbon skeleton they could not be synthesized endogenously, whereas those that could be synthesized from other amino acids or metabolites were classified as nonessential, or dispensable. This clear division of amino acids has been refined over the years (17–19) for several reasons.

The first relates to the basic criterion used to define essentiality. The most sensitive indicator of nutritional adequacy of any diet is that it will allow a normal rate of weight gain in infants or young animals or maintain the body weight and nitrogen balance of adults. Animal models allow the possibility to study the adequacy of individual nutrients in parenteral nutrition solutions. Thus, for example, sulphur amino acid adequacy of different regimen can be measured simply by comparing the growth characteristics of young animals (20). Measurements of dietary amino acid adequacy in healthy volunteers or patients are more difficult for technical and ethical reasons. Thus, to take the apparently simple example of protein requirements, technical issues would include the length of the study period (adaptation responses), the range of protein intakes investigated (inadequate to adequate?), the impact of biological variability on final estimates of a global value, and most importantly, the effect of age-related changes on amino acid requirements (18,19). It is not the intention of this review to enter into this debate, merely to point out the difficulty of assessing amino acid requirements under ideal experimental conditions with well-motivated volunteers. In the clinical setting, such estimates are much more difficult to obtain.

The second reason for refinement in the classification, is that some amino acids that are nonessential in the adult may become rate-limiting for growth in the young. Growth is accompanied by net deposition of tissue protein. In the young, there is a higher relative requirement for the essential amino acids in dietary protein, as described elsewhere (18). However, there may be an inability of pathways of interconversion or biosynthesis to provide sufficient supply of some amino acids (e.g., cysteine, tyrosine) for net deposition in tissue protein. Thus, in the neonatal infant receiving standard parenteral amino acid solutions, imbalances in the ratio of plasma methionine and cysteine have been observed (21). This can be related to poor conversion of methionine to cysteine because of low tissue levels of the enzyme cystathionase in the neonate (22). There is no evidence that cysteine is a semiessential amino acid in the adult. The issue of age-related changes in semiessential amino acid requirements is complicated also by species differences. Growth retardation and poor nitrogen balance will occur if arginine is omitted from the diet of young cats (23) and the young of a group of other species (see ref. 24), which does not include humans (25). Thus, some species may not be an ideal model for assessing whether deficiency of any of the "novel substrates" has an impact on clinically significant parameters.

According to the original classification of amino acids, the inability to synthesize the carbon skeleton of some amino acids *de novo* conferred on them their essential nature. As argued elsewhere, this view does not take into account the likelihood of whether the amino group can be incorporated from other amino acids (26). Thus, if dietary branched-chain amino acids are provided in the form of their α-ketoacids (e.g., in renal disease), transamination will result in endogenous synthesis of a sufficient supply of the branched-chain amino acids to meet requirements (27). The argument can be taken further in the case of methionine, which comprises the aminogroup, carbon-skeleton plus sulphur, and a methyl group. Of these, only the carbon skeleton and sulphur is truly essential; the amino group can be provided by transamination and the methyl group via the 1-carbon pool (e.g., tetrahydrofolic acid, dietary choline) through methylation of homocysteine to methionine. Thus, as du Vigneaud and Rachele showed several years ago, rats fed on a diet in which methionine was replaced by homocysteine and choline grew as well as their methionine-fed controls (28). This was an entirely artificial situation, which highlights the virtuosity of metabolic pathways for interconversion of amino acids and may help explain our ability to adapt to a wide range of protein intakes of varying quality. In absolute terms, only lysine and threonine can be considered essential with regard to their carbon-skeleton and amino groups together (Table 1)(26). The fact that an enzymic pathway for transamination of essential amino acids or synthesis of nonessential amino acids exists, does not necessarily mean, however, that it is sufficient to meet demand under all

TABLE 1. *Classification of amino acids according to essentiality.*

| Amino group | Carbon skeleton | |
	Essential	Nonessential
Essential	Lysine	Serine
	Threonine	Glycine*
		Cysteine*
Nonessential	Branched-chain amino acids	Glutamate
	Tryptophan	Alanine
	Phenylalanine	Aspartate
	Methionine	Glutamine
		Asparagine
		Proline*
		Tyrosine*
		Histidine*
		Arginine*
		Serine*
		Taurine*

Adapted from refs 18,29,241.
* May become conditionally-essential because of limitations in rate of synthesis.

dietary or clinical circumstances. As discussed elsewhere (29), some of the nonessential amino acids can also be classified as conditionally essential according to the ease with which they can be synthesized in humans (Table 1).

As the foregoing discussion suggests, the concept of essentiality is complex but an attempt should be made to define it in terms that can be applied to the clinical situation. A possible set of criteria is given in Table 2.

TABLE 2. *Criteria for conditionally essential nutrients.*

Deficiency will result in	
Growth limitation or failure to maintain nitrogen balance	In the young or the malnourished, traumatized, or septic patient
	Regardless of species used as the experimental model
Organ dysfunction	In healthy subjects or malnourished, traumatized, or septic patients
	Regardless of species used as the experimental model
Delayed recovery	After trauma or sepsis
	Regardless of species used as the experimental model
Metabolic abnormalities	In healthy subjects or malnourished, traumatized, or septic patients
	Regardless of species used as the experimental model
Clinical abnormalities	In malnourished, traumatized, or septic patients
	Regardless of species used as the experimental model

GLUTAMINE, ARGININE, ORNITHINE, AND α-KETOGLUTARATE

Role in Nitrogen Homeostasis

Nitrogen homeostasis is dependent on acid-base balance. This can be demonstrated by comparing the effects of metabolic acidosis consequent on surgical injury (1) or infusion with a triple-hormone regime of glucagon, cortisol, and adrenalin (30) or experimental acidosis (31) or urinary nitrogen excretion, especially in respect to the increased contribution of NH_4^+ to the total (32). The common features that accompany this are a reduction in the blood concentration of the major interorgan nitrogen carrier glutamine (33) and a corresponding decrease in its concentration in skeletal muscle (34,35). As has been argued elsewhere (36), these are biochemical aspects of a shift in patterns of glutamine consumption and production, the rapid fall in arterial glutamine concentration being mirrored by increased renal glutamine consumption, and urinary NH_4^+ production (33). It has been suggested that renal glutamine consumption in the rat, *controls* acid-base balance by luminal excretion of NH_4^+ and renal vein excretion of HCO_3^- (from α-ketoglutarate metabolism). However, this model is very species dependent, the rat is exquisitely sensitive to NH_4^+-loading, whereas humans are less so (37), and the dog (a widely used model) seems to be hardly responsive (31,38).

The quantitative effect of renal glutamine consumption and ammoniagenesis on acid-base balance is small compared to that exerted by respiratory CO_2 loss and it may only produce a partial counterregulatory supply of HCO_3^- to balance pulmonary loss and act as a dampening mechanism (39). However, the converse is not true: Metabolic acidosis profoundly increases renal ammoniagenesis from glutamine—normally 2% of total glutamine synthesis in humans (40)—to approximately four times this value (37). In acidotic humans this would account for up to 5g/d of nitrogen excreted as urinary NH_4^+. Despite this, there is abundant evidence that this does not affect whole-body glutamine turnover (41).

These considerations help explain the, almost obligatory, loss of glutamine from tissue and plasma pools following surgery and trauma and the switches in patterns of glutamine consumption and production by different organs (36,42–45). It is possible to reconstruct a situation in which metabolic acidosis consequent on even the least invasive forms of surgery (e.g., laparoscopic endoscopy) will increase glutamine consumption (46). The common pattern that has been observed is of a net efflux of intracellular glutamine and other amino acids from skeletal muscle, increased uptake by the kidney, and a net uptake by the splanchnic bed (see ref. 47). Careful dissection of increased splanchnic glutamine consumption has localized it to the spleen and the liver, rather than the intestine (48). It is therefore no longer possible to sustain the teleological argument that the reciprocal relationship between muscle efflux and increased splanchnic uptake of glutamine represents the requirement for a "preferred fuel" for the intestine after uncomplicated elective surgery (49,50). What is more likely is that the perturbation in glutamine metabolism is a consequence of transient acidosis, which accompanies the perioperative and recovery phases of surgery.

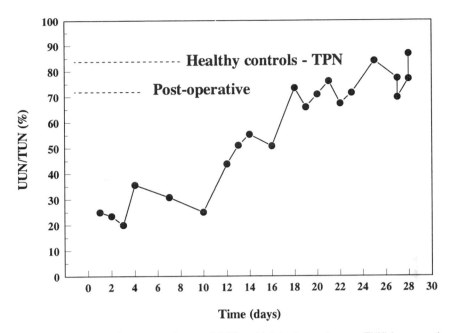

FIG. 2. Evolution of urinary urea nitrogen (UUN) and total urinary nitrogen (TUN) in one patient on TPN. Diagnosis: abdominal mass and pyrexia. days; Y-axis "UUN/TUN (%); major interval 10%. From Grimble et al, (32) and unpublished data.

The evidence for this is surprisingly strong. First, if the hallmark of metabolic acidosis is a high urinary NH_4^+ excretion rate, then many malnourished or postoperative patients are acidotic. This can be inferred from the reduced ratio of urinary ureanitrogen to total urine nitrogen (UUN/TUN), which may persist for some time after operation or which develops during ketoacidosis consequent on 3 to 5 days starvation (32,51–53). It is often assumed that nitrogen balance can be calculated from urinary urea excretion but this has been shown to be an unreliable index in hospitalized patients (32,51), as shown in Fig. 2, for a patient receiving prolonged TPN. Second, several studies have shown that net muscle protein catabolism will occur after mild respiratory acidosis (54) or metabolic acidosis (55–57) or acidosis consequent on chronic renal failure (58,59). Intracellular acidosis after ischemic injury very markedly depresses protein synthesis and disaggregates polyribosome profiles in proportion to the severity of intracellular acidosis (60,61). This is similar to the effects of surgery on muscle polyribosome profiles (35,62).

If this analysis is true, it has three consequences. First, the immediate postoperative period is the worst model in which to attempt to demonstrate the conditional essentiality of any amino acid on the grounds of improved nitrogen balance. Second, the overriding metabolic "set" determined by acidosis would explain why several different intermediary metabolites have the same effect on nitrogen balance after cholecystectomy or major abdominal surgery (2–4,63–65). It is likely that each restores acid-base balance, by different mechanisms, and thus ameliorates the consequences of acidosis. It is possible that intravenous glutamine supplementation reverses the consequences of metabolic acidosis on skeletal muscle by suppressing net glutamine efflux (66), thus reducing net nitrogen loss. α-Ketoglutarate, OKG, and arginine may reduce hyperammonemia by relieving the renal requirement for glutamine-derived generation of α-ketoglutarate and NH_4^+ (38,39,44,67–69) or by increasing the efficiency of ureagenesis, in the case of ornithine and arginine (70). It should be noted that of these intermediary metabolites, only OKG, not glutamine or protein, has been shown to normalize acid-base balance in starved rats (71). The third consequence of this analysis relates to the ability of urea, which diffuses into the intestinal lumen, to be hydrolyzed by bacterial urease to NH_4^+, which provides a source of nitrogen for resynthesis of the α-NH_2 of amino acids, via the following reaction:

$$(NH_2)_2CO + H_2O \longrightarrow 2NH_3 + CO_2$$
Urea

Ammonia is reincorporated into the general amino acid pool via the transaminase reaction. The extent of this cycle in humans has been shown by stable-isotope studies with $^{15}N^{15}N$-urea, which demonstrated its resynthesis into $^{14}N^{15}N$-urea. Thus, it was shown that permeation of urea from the lumen across the colonic wall is significant (72,73) and in reverse when $^{15}N^{15}N$-urea was intravenously infused (74). The flux of urea nitrogen that is processed by this route is not inconsiderable and has been estimated at 2.6 g N/d (of which 1.4 g N/d is recycled into amino acids) in comparison to a daily urea production rate of 8.5 g N from 14 g N protein intake (73,75,76). Part will be incorporated into the amino acid pool via glutamate dehydrogenase or glutamine synthetase in bacteria (see ref. 77) or into the host after absorption across the colonic mucosa. This is not an insignificant pathway because in infants and adults, at low dietary nitrogen intakes that will not support growth or nitrogen balance, supplementation with urea has been shown to restore positive nitrogen balance (78,79). This is clearly a significant contribution to blood NH_4^+ flux in addition to that derived from metabolic consumption of glutamine. It is also enhanced by the presence of fermentable material in the colonic lumen (80,81).

In the fasted intravenously fed patient, receiving concurrent antibiotic therapy, this route of nitrogen recycling will be markedly reduced (82). It would be tempting to speculate that glutamine supplementation will partly replace this route of NH_4^+ recycling, since intestinal consumption is proportional to arterial load (83) and part of the NH_4^+ produced will diffuse freely into the lumen and back into the portal circulation (84).

Effects on Growth Kinetics of Whole Animals

As defined by Rose, essentiality can be determined by the effect of omission of an amino acid from the diet on growth and nitrogen balance. It is highly unlikely that glutamine is essential because it can be readily formed from oral glutamate (85) in humans. In the growing rat, replacement of casein in the diet with an amino acid mixture simulating it, but lacking glutamine (glutamate and NH_4^+ substitution) had no effect on any growth parameters (86). In addition, during TPN support of the piglet, addition of glutamine or glutamate had no effect on any nutritional parameter or aspect of gut morphology (87). This suggests that in vivo glutamine synthesis is large (40) and that it may be produced from a variety of metabolic precursors, as we have shown before (88). Changes in plasma and muscle intracellular glutamine concentrations consequent on injury, sepsis, or acidosis may therefore reflect a shift in interorgan flow of glutamine but with no overall change in the rate of whole-body glutamine synthesis. This can clearly be seen in the case of the acidotic rat (41). The concentration of a plasma amino acid is not necessarily related to its rates of disposal or synthesis or effects on biosynthetic processes in specific organs. Thus, reduced arterial glutamine concentrations following surgery or acidosis do not alter the rate of glutamine extraction by the kidney (42,47). This confusion may underly the new definition of glutamine as a conditionally essential amino acid in sick patients.

Arginine has also been claimed to be an essential amino acid for growth, but this effect is very species dependent (24). This is best seen in the cat, an obligate carnivore, for which arginine is hyperessential (23,70,89). Presumably, this relates to a poor capacity to synthesize arginine from citrulline in the kidney (45,90) in order to compensate for citrulline and ornithine production from dietary arginine in the liver and intestine (91). In adult humans, this situation does not pertain because, as suggested by Lund, "synthesis of citrulline from glutamine is interesting from the nutritional point of view, because it provides an explanation as to why arginine is not an essential amino acid in the adult" (90). Whatever the therapeutic mode of action of arginine in stimulating responsiveness of human lymphocytes to mitogens, after trauma (92) it does not relate to any question of essentiality because the same effect can be seen in healthy adult volunteers (93). Arginine has potent druglike effects on anabolic hormone secretion, nitric oxide generation, and control of plasma ammonia concentrations, which are reviewed elsewhere (see Chapter 12).

Gastrointestinal Absorption of Arginine and Plasma Kinetics

Of the four major Na^+-dependent group-specific, active transport systems in the mammalian enterocyte, that for the dibasic amino acid has been most studied. This is partly because of the existence of an inborn error of metabolism, cystinuria, which is characterized by high urinary excretion of all dibasic amino acids and cystine. The lesion occurs at the level of the intestine and renal transporter protein and has several foci (94). We have confirmed that at high perfused concentrations, the major component of ornithine uptake in the jejunum is by passive uptake (95), as may be inferred from the text of a similar study of lysine and arginine absorption (96). Amino acids that do not share the same transporter at apical or basolateral enterocyte membranes can stimulate uptake of the dibasic amino acids via countertransport or allosteric effects (97,98). This feature is common to other tissues where marked transport interactions between ornithine and polyamines (99) or α-ketoglutarate (95) have been noted.

All dibasic amino acids stimulate net water secretion in the perfused jejunum (95,100). Arginine is the most potent secretagogue and can convert glucose-stimulated net water and electrolyte absorption into profound net secretion at modest (5 to 10 mmol/l) perfused arginine concentrations. The effect is local, not shared by D-arginine, and is rather puzzling (100). An explanation may lie in the fact that luminal arginine will appear as ornithine and citrulline in portal blood, suggesting that the intestine has a unique adaptation for arginine metabolism (91). It is tempting to propose that this is an effect of nitric oxide on intestinal motility and regional blood flow (101,102). Perhaps, rapid metabolic conversion of arginine by the intestine represents an adaptive response to excessive stimulation of local motility via the noninducible nitric oxide synthetase pathway, after an oral *bolus*. However, the effect may be a general property of the dibasic amino acids since 20-g bolus doses of OKG (103), lysine (104), and arginine (93) all promote gastrointestinal symptoms of diarrhea and distension. This is probably of secretory origin with secondary malabsorption and may explain the higher incidence of diarrhea noted in postoperative patients receiving an enteral diet supplemented with arginine (105), especially because concurrent antibiotics promote dibasic amino acid malabsorption (104).

We have investigated plasma kinetics of arginine indirectly in healthy volunteers to 12 hours of enteral feeding with additional infusion or bolus of 10 g or 20 g of OKG (88). Feeding, per se, had little effect on plasma ornithine or arginine but resulted in a persistent rise in citrulline concentration (Fig. 3A). Infusion of OKG abolished citrullinemia and increased ornithine and glutamine (Fig. 3B), but, as expected, an oral bolus of OKG (Fig. 3C) resulted in a marked peak of plasma ornithine with a small but significant secondary peak of arginine that crossed over with a depression of citrulline concentration (88). Thus, supplements of individual urea cycle intermediates can markedly alter the plasma concentration of the other intermediates, as was shown in the trial described earlier, where arginine and ornithine concentrations were raised by enteral diet supplementation with arginine (105).

This point has been labored because it underlines the metabolic versatility of humans in interconverting amino acids that can be transaminated. According to the criteria set out in Tables 1 and 2, none of the metabolites described can be considered essential or conditionally essential from the nutritional point of view. The group of amino acids that may be more profitable to study are those whose nitrogen could theoretically come from this group, but does not, as shown by ^{15}N-studies (106). In particular, glycine, which is overrepresented in acute-phase proteins, may require reevaluation in critically ill patients (107,108).

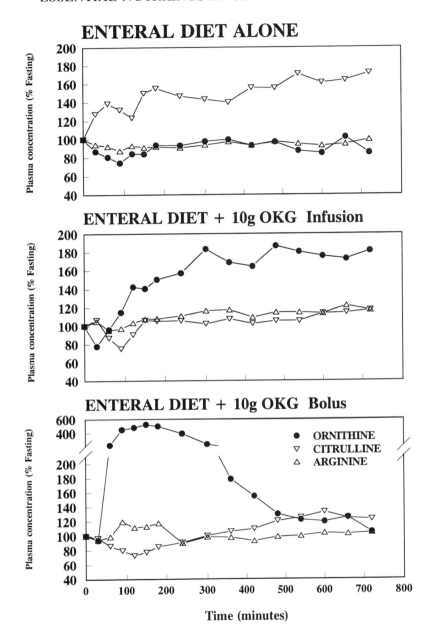

FIG. 3. Effect of OKG on evolution of plasma amino acids in healthy subjects receiving nasoenteral nutrition support. Data adapted from ref. 88.

NUCLEIC ACIDS

Nucleic acids are not thought to be essential nutrients because pathways exist for synthesis of purines and pyrimidines *de novo*. Most research into nucleic acid metabolism has related to "informational" rather than metabolic aspects. Examples would include modulation of cytokine mRNA levels (109) or muscle ribosome levels (2,110) as mediators of growth-induced (111) or posttraumatic changes (4) in protein synthesis.

Nevertheless, three questions can be addressed. How are synthetic pathways for purine and pyrimidines affected by the dietary intake of purines and pyrimidines? What is the nature of purine and pyrimidine requirements and can endogenous purine and pyrimidine supply ever be exceeded by demand in the acutely ill patient? Will organ function be impaired by *no* intake of purines and pyrimidines, as occurs for most patients fed with most current enteral and parenteral formulae?

Purine and Pyrimidine Biosynthesis

Endogenous purines and pyrimidines are synthesised *de novo* from amino acids and other small molecules. The pathways for purines differ fundamentally from that for pyrimidines in that the ribose moiety of purine nucleosides is incorporated as 5-phosphoribosyl-1-phosphate (PRPP) in the first reaction of purine synthesis, not at the end-stage after ring formation of the pyrimidines (112–114).

Pyrimidines are synthesized from NH_3, CO_2, and aspartate, the latter being synthesized from glutamine in lymphocytes (115). The ribose and phosphate moieties are derived from glucose and adenosine triphosphate (ATP), respectively. In contrast, purines incorporate the γ-NH_2 group of glutamine [2], nitrogen from glycine and aspartate [1 or 2], and carbon from CO_2, formate, glycine, and aspartate. The sugar and phosphate moieties are as for pyrimidines.

Salvage and Catabolism of Purines and Pyrimidines

Degradation of the 5'-mono, di-, and triphosphates occurs through the stepwise removal of phosphate and ribose (or 2'-deoxyribose) to form the nucleobases, uracil, cytosine (pyrimidines), or hypoxanthine (purines). Salvage of the nucleobases occurs by a single-step addition of PRPP to form the 5'-monophosphate [hypoxanthine-guanosine phosphoribosyl transferase (HGPRTase)]. Degradation products of orotic acid, uracil, and cytosine include β-alanine and β-aminoisobutyric acid. Purine catabolism appears to be controlled by three factors, namely intracellular PRPP levels, the activity of the phosphoribosylamidotransferase (PRPP + gln $\longrightarrow$ 5'-P ribosylamine + glu), and the intracellular concentrations of IMP, AMP, and GMP (114). An adequate intracellular concentration of nucleotide monophosphates will inhibit the first step in purine synthesis; an adequate supply of the precursor PRPP will activate it.

The Relationship between Salvage and *De Novo* Synthesis

Evidence from Whole-Animal Studies

A surprisingly small amount of radiolabelled dietary nucleotides are incorporated into tissue RNA, DNA, and nucleotide pools (112). Although there are efficient intestinal transport mechanisms for all four purine-pyrimidine bases and nucleosides in the small and large intestine, their capacity is limited and excess oral intake is malabsorbed and metabolized by colonic luminal microflora (116–119). In one study (120) with ^{14}C-labelled purines, the ratio of label-incorporated tissue RNA from oral and IV routes was always highest in those tissues most actively involved in nucleic acid synthesis (e.g., salivary, adrenal, thyroid, thymus and pituitary glands, and lymph tissue, 25:1 to 59:1). Similar results have been obtained in rats infused with nucleoside-nucleotide mixtures (121). Thus the gut is capable of quite markedly modifying dietary intake because adenine could be taken up intact by the gut, whereas guanine, hypoxanthine, and xanthine were extensively catabolized in their passage from mucosa to serosa, implying that the gut is unable to synthesize significant amounts of adenine *de novo* (122). The different fates of oral or IV purines may result from the gut mucosa's high requirement for exogenous purines because first passage of absorbed purines through gut and liver would result in preferential extraction and metabolism (123).

A reciprocal relationship between purine intake and *de novo* synthesis exists in the gut (124,125) because dietary supplementation with pyrimidines suppressed [^{14}C]glycine incorporation into mucosal RNA, suggesting that under normal circumstances the *de novo* pathway was relatively inactive and could only be stimulated by omission of purines and pyrimidines from the diet (124,125). This relationship, however, relies on an adequate dietary protein intake to supply substrate for *de novo* synthesis (126,127).

Evidence from Cell Culture Studies

Measurements of RNA synthesis in cultured cells, with [^{14}C]uridine and [^{14}C]orotic acid are difficult because not only is the intracellular pool compartmented but RNA is also synthesized in two separate compartments (mRNA, tRNA-nucleoplasm and rRNA-nucleolus) and these precursors feed into the salvage and *de novo* pools, respectively. The measured specific radioactivity of the intracellular nucleotide pool may not represent that of the precursor for RNA synthesis. These problems can be circumvented by using [^{14}C-*methyl*]methionine to label intracellular S-adenosylmethionine (SAM), the donor for methylation of rRNA during synthesis (110,128). Fortunately, these difficulties have provided much information on compartmentation of the intracellular pool and the contribution of *de novo* and salvage pathways to synthesis of each RNA species. Thus, there are different precursor pools for mRNA and rRNA synthesis (small-nonexpandable and large-expandable) in Ehrlich ascites cells (129),

HeLa S3 cells (130) regenerating rat liver (131), and rat hepatoma cells (132). The small pool is nucleolar (rRNA synthesis) and supplied mainly by *de novo* synthesis (130,133,134). The large pool is under metabolic control in the sense that *de novo* synthesis is suppressed by exogenous supply (135).

Evidence from Studies of Ribosome Turnover

In growth or dietary restriction studies, it has been consistently noted that the time course of changes in cellular ribosome content or ribosome synthesis usually precede those of protein, often by a considerable margin (128,136–138). Ribosomal RNA is the most abundant species and accounts for the largest requirement for *de novo* and salvage of purines and pyrimidines.

It is synthesized in the nucleolus by RNA polymerase I, which is separately regulated from the other nuclear polymerases. The primary transcript, 45 S pre-rRNA, is cleaved by specific nucleolar nucleases to 18S and 28S rRNA species, which exit the nucleus as mature 40S and 60S ribosomal subunits (Fig. 4). A significant proportion of the pre-rRNA is degraded during processing and these correspond to the unmethylated "spacer" region. As such, their nucleotides can enter the salvage pathway for subsequent reutilisation in RNA synthesis (for reviews, see refs. 139,140). In nongrowing tissues, a further proportion (up to 50%) of the 45S pre-RNA is degraded completely, termed "wastage."

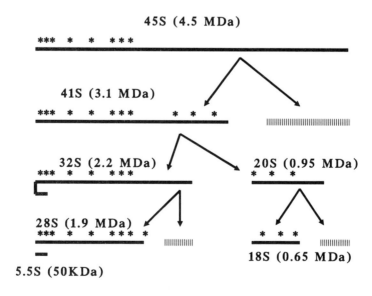

* = *Methylnucleosides conserved during processing*

FIG. 4. Outline of nucleolar ribosomal RNA synthesis and processing. Adapted from ref. 140.

The supply of rRNA and ribosomal proteins is coordinated because if rRNA synthesis is inhibited, degradation of nucleolar rProteins increase (141,142), whereas if rProtein synthesis is inhibited, there is increased degradation of 45S pre-rRNA (133,143,144). This apparently expensive process (wastage) is loosely coupled to rProtein synthesis, but may give exquisite control of cytoplasmic ribosome appearance rates. Warner (140,141) has aptly called the inhibitory modulation of excess rRNA and rProtein levels (through degradation) "fine-tuning" of ribosome supply. The level of "coarse-tuning" would be supplied by gross coordinate changes in rProtein and rRNA synthesis in response to growth or nutritional depletion.

Control of Ribosome Production in Response to Growth Stimuli

Liver

The regenerating liver has been widely studied because two growth phases can be discerned (days 1 to 5, "proliferative"; days 6 to 12, "postproliferative"). During proliferative growth, appearance of new cytoplasmic ribosomes increases fivefold but 45S pre-rRNA synthesis increases only twofold, and degradation of cytoplasmic ribosomes remains unaltered (145–147). This implies that in the resting liver, nearly 60% of 45S-pre-rRNA was "wasted" and because processing results in the loss of nearly 50% of 45S pre-rRNA of nucleotides incorporated into 45S pre-rRNA only 20% ever reaches the cytoplasm. In addition, processing of 45S pre-rRNA is altered in the proliferative phase, the length of time taken being shorter (148).

Turpentine injection, which results in an acute-phase response, has been shown to increase transport of mature ribosomes from nucleolus to cytoplasm increases, preceding the large increase in rRNA synthesis that occurs *before* activation of the the acute-phase protein response (149,150).

Kidney

Unilateral nephrectomy (UNI) causes compensatory hypertrophic growth of the contralateral kidney, which will reach about 75% of the weight of both kidneys within 2 weeks. Within 48 hours, however, rRNA content-cell increases by 40% (151). Two mechanisms are responsible for this: an increase in the efficiency of processing of 45S pre-rRNA (151,152) *and* an increase in rDNA transcription and 45S pre-rRNA synthesis within a few hours of surgery (153).

Growing Muscle: Normal and Rapid Growth

During "catch-up" growth of protein-depleted animals, the number of ribosomes in skeletal muscle doubles, as does the efficiency of ribosome use in protein synthesis

(154). Severe protein-energy malnutrition results in coordinated loss of cellular ribosomes and cell muscle protein (155), whereas energy deficiency reduces efficiency of ribosome use in protein synthesis (111,156). There are thus two mechanisms for modulating muscle protein synthesis, through changes in the *number* of ribosomes and their *efficiency* of use. During accelerated growth, this relationship is perturbed, as was demonstrated during weight-induced hypertrophy of the anterior and posterior latissimus dorsi muscles of chicken (136). Although muscle protein increased steadily over 50 days, RNA levels doubled within 3 days. The major factor that mediated increased muscle protein synthesis was therefore the number of ribosomes, not their efficiency of use, as also occurs during hypertrophy of the heart, which follows aortic stenosis (157–159).

Normal-Transformed Cell Lines

Normal cells are responsive to exogenous growth signals in a way not shared with transformed cell lines. A "competence signal" initiates recruitment into the cell cycle, while a "progression signal" is essential for effective expression of growth (160,161). Normal 3T3 cells do not enter the cell cycle until their ribosome content reaches a certain threshold, in contrast to transformed 3T6 (162). Thus, during stimulated cell growth, ribosome content should double before recruitment (163). A proliferative signal for cells of the immune system must therefore be accompanied by increased ribosome synthesis before division and immunoglobulin synthesis can occur.

Resting and Growing Cells in Culture

Following stimulation of cultured lymphocytes with phytohaemagglutin (PHA), the cells enlarge, increase their ribosome number, replicate DNA after 24 to 48 hours, and finally divide. The increase in rate of rRNA synthesis is large, ten to 50 times that seen in resting lymphocytes (164). This model thus represents an extreme anabolic stress. Pulse, or continuous labelling with [methyl-^{14}C]methionine, established that in resting cells approximately half of the 45S pre-rRNA was "wasted" but that this had ceased 20 hours after PHA stimulation. As described, this mechanism allows for rapid increases in ribosome production at the least energetic cost. *De novo* synthesis provides most of the nucleotide flux for increased RNA and DNA synthesis in the PHA-stimulated lymphocyte, as suggested by the limited ability of exogenous nucleobases and nucleosides (salvage pathway) to relieve inhibition of growth by limiting amounts of glutamine in the culture medium (*de novo* pathway) (165).

Exogenous Nucleotides in Growth: Essential or Not?

Where protein intake is adequate, *de novo* synthesis provides the main source of nucleotides for nucleic acid synthesis. Although it can be suppressed by dietary purine and pyrimidine supply, the degree to which this occurs depends on the tissue type. Liver and gut behave differently; in the former case, dietary purines increase the activity of salvage and catabolism pathways simultaneously, while the gut, which has only a low capacity for *de novo* synthesis, is dependent on the liver for its supply of nucleotides. Where protein intake is reduced, the salvage pathway assumes a greater importance as a means of recycling purines and pyrimidines released by nucleic acid catabolism. Lack of dietary purines and pyrimidines will switch on *de novo* synthesis in the gut to a limited extent.

Within the cell itself, the split between *de novo* and salvage pathways differs for each species of RNA. Ribosomal RNA production appears to rely more heavily on *de novo* synthesis than does mRNA or tRNA synthesis. In this sense, a major component of protein synthesis (the ribosome) can be seen to be under the same general nutritional controls as protein synthesis itself, i.e., the dietary amino acid supply.

The importance of an adequate increase in cellular ribosome synthesis during production and maturation can only be inferred from the known effects of malnutrition on mucosal architecture and cell kinetics. As described, this relationship holds true for many other cell types and there is no reason to believe that the enterocyte is an exception. Indeed, it could be argued that because of the reliance of rRNA synthesis on *de novo* pathways, and the low levels of these pathways in the enterocyte, cell turnover should be particularly sensitive to any limitation of purine and pyrimidine supply.

Evidence for a Positive Role for Dietary Nucleotides in Clinical Nutrition

Dietary supplementation with nucleotides, nucleosides, or nucleobases can improve growth rates and nitrogen retention in young animals (166,167). Furthermore, four lines of evidence suggest that supplementation with dietary or parenteral nucleotides-nucleosides may be of clinical significance.

Infection

The ability of IV-injected *Candida albicans* to induce candidiasis in mice was tested in animals receiving a nucleotide-free diet or one with additions of yeast-RNA or individual nucleobases. Mean survival time was significantly increased in RNA-supplemented animals (168,169).

Immune Function

Following suggestions that nucleotides were essential factors for T-lymphocyte function (see also ref. 165), Kulkarni and colleagues investigated the effects of nucleotide-free diets in impairing fatal graft-vs-host (g-v-h) reactions in irradiated mice. The mirror to these experiments was to determine the proliferative potential of transplanted lymphocytes in animals receiving nucleotide-free and nucleotide-supplemented diets (170). Surprisingly, nucleotide-free diets were immunosuppressive, as mortality from g-v-h reactions was significantly reduced. Conversely, nucleotide-free diets reduced the responsiveness of lymphocytes to PHA to a very marked extent. High dietary nucleotide content (i.e., 0.35-g to 100-g diet) inhibits natural killer (NK) cell activity of macrophages from weaning mice. At the lowest intake (0.035 mg to 100 g), however, there was a transient increase in NK activity that returned to control levels by 6 weeks (171).

As has been discussed, a nucleotide-free diet appears to increase the activity of *de novo* pathway enzymes at the expense of salvage, whereas nucleotide supplementation has the opposite effect. It is possible that in vitro activation assays are inappropriate unless carried out in media designed to simulate precursors either for *de novo* or salvage pathways. Thus, where the diet is nucleotide-free (i.e., animals adapted to *de novo* synthesis), the in vitro medium should contain only salvage precursors. Where the animals receive a nucleotide-containing diet (i.e., salvage adapted), the medium should contain only *de novo* precursors. I suspect that cellular responsiveness would be as poor in each group.

Overall, the effects of nucleotide supplementation on immune cell responsiveness have been difficult to relate to the clinical setting, just as it has proved difficult to show clinically significant effects of nutritional status on immune function (172). However, the whole-animal studies that show reduced mortality after nucleotide supplementation are highly suggestive.

Liver Regeneration

Using the 70% hepatectomy model in rats, supplementation of TPN regimes with nucleotides and nucleosides (as 10% of amino acid nitrogen) significantly increased postoperative nitrogen balance (became positive) and whole-body protein turnover and synthesis (173,174). Supplementation also reduced the extent of galactosamine-induced liver injury, as judged by histology and circulating concentrations of the liver enzymes GOT and GPT (121). These data suggest that repair and growth in a major organ of purine and pyrimidine biosynthesis can be improved by providing an external supply of preformed nucleotides and nucleosides.

Intestinal Repair

In order to model mucosal damage during infective diarrhea, Nunez and colleagues (175) induced chronic diarrhea in rats by substituting the maltodextrins in the enteral diet with lactose. Two diets were used (± nucleotides) and it was observed that supplementation partially restored the biochemical atrophy of the small intestine at proximal and distal sites. There were significant increases in protein content and brush-border saccharidases, although the changes were not large.

Exogenous Nucleotides in Clinical Situations: Essential or Not?

Because the gut is uniquely dependent on salvage and exogenous supplies of purines and pyrimidines, limitation in supply may impair maintenance of the barrier function in the malnourished, stressed or septic patient. A teleological argument has been advanced recently to explain why glutamine consumption by the liver increases greatly during endotoxaemia, whilst gut consumption falls. Increased liver uptake reflects the need to supply nucleotide precursors and glutathione for cell repair in the gut and liver (176). Normal diets probably provide sufficient purines and pyrimidines to allow for any such limitation, indeed 'requirements' are probably quite modest given the tight metabolic control of purine synthesis and degradation and low utilisation of dietary sources. TPN or Enteral Nutrition is unusual in that no purine/pyrimidine intake is given even though the patient's pre-existing diet would have conditioned purine and pyrimidine metabolism to 'salvage' rather than *de novo* synthesis.

The few, relevant studies cited above are quite persuasive and can only serve to promote further studies. It would be particularly fruitful to investigate animal models of stress in which there is known to be involvement of the gut (barrier function) or immune system.

SHORT-CHAIN FATTY ACIDS

Development of Colonic Fermentation Capacity in Humans

The colonic luminal bacteria have been described as an "organ-within-an-organ" that develops slowly during the first 2 years of life in human infants (177). This type of longitudinal study of colonic function has a particular power because, in this case, the baby is born germ-free but will adapt to an adult intestinal function that remains stable for prolonged periods of time (178). These luminal functions of the colon are bacterial and comprise mucin breakdown, the regulation of fecal tryptic activity, the conversion of bilirubin to urobilinogen, cholesterol catabolism, and finally the generation of short-chain fatty acids (SCFA) and other organic acids. Adaptation is clearly driven by the diet because marked differences in the evolution of luminal organic acids occurs between breast-fed and formula-fed infants. The process is complete by 1 month in formula-fed infants because of malabsorption of components of the diet; in contrast it takes up to 9 months in breast-fed infants because better absorption of the macronutrients in breast milk leads to a relative lack of colonic luminal nutrients. In contrast, indicators of fermentation of malabsorbed protein (*iso-* and *n*-valeric acids) are not complete until 16 months of life (177). The entire process can be described in two ways. First, establishment of butyrate-producing bacteria is at the expense of acetate production. With time, there is also the establishment of an acetate buffer in the colonic lumen that is strongly bacteriostatic for some gram-negative bacteria. The process may be retarded by antibiotic treatment in early life, which allows the establishment of *Clostridium difficile* colonies, which may be detected by the presence of *iso*-caproic acid in fecal samples. Malabsorption of components of formula diet, because of their strong buffering capacity, will tend to oppose establishment of an acetate buffer and thus allow establishment of coliform and streptococcal colonies.

Symbiosis between Colonic Luminal Fermentation and the Host

Before discussing the interrelationship between generation of SCFAs by luminal bacteria and the metabolic needs of the colon itself, two factors need to be discussed. The first is that SCFAs may not necessarily be the major organic anion group generated within the colonic lumen. This has often been overlooked because analysis of luminal organic acids has usually been accomplished by gas chromatography, which will only detect the volatile SCFAs, not lactate and the dicarboxylic acids. Anion exclusion HPLC techniques will, however, resolve all major organic acids in fecal samples (Fig. 5). Although SCFAs make a substantial contribution to the tonicity of luminal contents—260 mOsm/l and 180 mOsm/l in the cecum and rectum, respectively (179)—and fecal output is isotonic (180,181). However, colonic fermentation and absorption patterns may be so disrupted by the patchy lesions of inflammatory bowel disease (IBD) that SCFA becomes the minor component of the fecal stream, and lactate, fumarate, succinate, and malate (Fig. 5) make the major contribution to osmolarity (181).

The second factor is that the relationship between bacteria and the colon is truly symbiotic. Thus, luminal bacteria derive the nitrogen necessary for growth from fermentation of endogenous and dietary protein, which is not completely absorbed in the small intestine (182–184). In addition, transfer of urea from circulation into the intestinal lumen results in liberation of NH_4^+ after hydrolysis by bacterial urease (previously discussed).

The host therefore makes a significant contribution to the growth of luminal bacteria by providing fermentable carbohydrate (dietary sources, mucins) and nitrogen (urea, endogenous proteins). Two studies have defined the synergistic relationship between carbohydrate and nitrogen in promoting colonic bacterial growth (185,186). This approach to the issue may explain the discrepancy between estimated dietary "fiber" intakes and the amount of fermentable substrate that is consumed by luminal bacteria. Thus, approximately 70 g/d of fermentable carbohydrate would be required to produce the bacterial mass present in an average daily stool output (77).

The interrelationship between bacterial species that hydrolyse fiber (187) and ferment monosaccharides to produce SCFAs and substrates (acetate, H_2) for subsequent production of CH_4 and CO_2 is described elsewhere (77,188–190).

Short-chain Fatty Acids and Colonic Water and Electrolyte Uptake

Three kinetic studies have demonstrated that jejunal and colonic mucosal transport of SCFAs is accompanied by water and Na^+ uptake. There appear to be two mechanisms involved: The first is an active process in which protonated SCFAs and Na^+

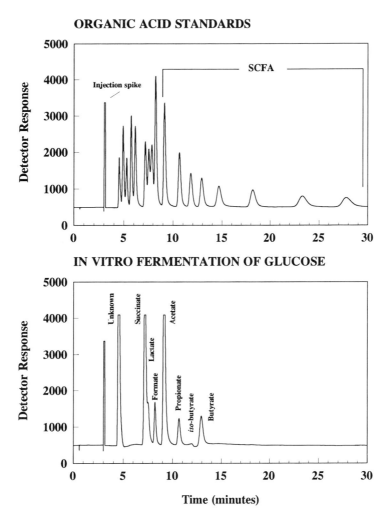

FIG. 5. High-performance liquid chromatography of organic acids produced during in vitro fermentation of glucose with fecal innoculates. From Grimble and Aimer, unpublished data.

are exchanged for H^+ and Cl^- exchanges with butyrate. The second mode of uptake is probably by passive diffusion of protonated SCFA down a concentration gradient (191–193). The latter may explain why inflammatory bowel disease, which reduces colonic uptake of organic anions, markedly depresses absorption of lactate, fumarate, malate, and succinate, which are predominantly absorbed by active transport processes, but has a lesser impact on SCFA uptake (181). The capacity of the colonic luminal bacteria to ferment nonabsorbed disaccharides such as lactulose (180) and lactitol (194) and for the colon to absorb SCFAs is limited (approximately 80 g/d), and above this level of intake osmotic diarrhea will ensue. Thus, at lower levels of intake of fermentable carbohydrate, SCFAs, generated by luminal bacteria, aid the process of dehydrating the fecal stream and salvage 90% of the water and electrolytes that enter the colon from the small intestine (ca. 1,350 ml/d).

Some antibiotics interfere with this process. Thus in healthy volunteers, 20-g intake of lactulose had no effect on stool output, but preadministration of ampicillin reduced fermentation of lactulose and increased the incidence of diarrhoeal symptoms (195). This may explain the relationship between concurrent antibiotic therapy and the incidence of diarrhea in patients receiving enteral nutrition support (196), which we described some years ago (197,198). Some antibiotics (most notably ampicillin, erythromycin, clindamycin, and metronidazole) can suppress indices of colonic bacterial fermentation, such as breath-H_2 output (195), acidification of the cecum (199), urinary excretion of D-amino acids derived from colonic bacteria (200), and in vitro production of SCFAs by fecal innoculates (201). In addition, metronidazole therapy has been shown to be of significant clinical benefit in reducing the colonic production of SCFAs in children with inborn errors of methylmalonate and propionate metabolism (202).

Short-chain Fatty Acids and Colonic Metabolism

Of the SCFAs, butyrate has the most pronounced effects on the epithelial cells of the cecum and colon. It provides the function of a precursor for ketone production, which is not shared with acetate and propionate (203,204), and of the possible metabolic fuels (e.g., glucose and glutamine), it appears to be preferentially used by co-lonocytes (205). This specificity has been confirmed for colonic cells in culture. In particular, butyrate promotes proliferation and differentiation of colonic epithelial crypt cells toward the mature, highly polarized forms that express apical membrane hydrolases at the top of the crypt (206–209). In vivo studies in rats have confirmed that it is the fermentation products of dietary fiber (i.e., SCFAs) and not its effects in lowering luminal pH (210) or the presence of bulk in the intestinal lumen that increases crypt cell proliferation rates in the rat colon (211,212). Butyrate also appears to modulate the cell cycle at the level of gene transcription because it can downregulate N-ras oncogene expression and the proliferative potential of cultured human colon tumor cell lines (207,213,214). In addition, addition of butyrate to the medium induces greater differentiation in terms of expression of surface hydrolases and glyco-sylated cell-surface components (215), while reducing expression of surface tumour-specific antigens (207).

The route by which the colonocyte receives SCFA is important. In an outstanding series of studies, Rombeau and colleagues carefully investigated factors that would promote healing of the colon in a rat model of surgical resection and re-anastomosis. Chronic intraluminal delivery of SCFAs, butyrate in particular, increased the cellularity of the colonic epithelium and improved burst-strength of the anastomotic wound

(216,217). Intravenous delivery of SCFAs, however, were trophic to the small intestinal but not the colonic mucosa (218). This is one aspect of luminal SCFAs that is unique. Their presence in the colonic lumen has marked effects on the epithelial cells in contrast to other luminal nutrients such as glucose (219,220), amino acids (221), and glutamine (83), which appear to be supplied for metabolism by absorptive cells from arterial blood rather than from the intestinal lumen.

In contrast, acetate, the major SCFA produced-by fermentation, has the most marked stimulatory effects on colonic blood flow (80,222,223). In general, absorption of luminal nutrients is accompanied by increased regional blood flow to the intestine (224,225). In particular, a 50% increase in superior mesenteric artery blood has been demonstrated during the period corresponding to peak glucose absorption after an oral glucose (but not lactulose) meal in humans (226) or the hypovolaemic or septic rat (227,228). Luminal glutamine will also exert the same effect (227). It is therefore difficult to disentangle the contribution of direct metabolic trophism of the SCFAs and the consequences of regional stimulation of the intestine through increased blood flow.

The Clinical Significance of Short-chain Fatty Acid Supplementation of Colonic Luminal Contents

The most recent prospective trials have shown that supplementation of enteral formulae with fermentable fiber has little effect on the incidence of diarrhea. Concurrent antibiotic therapy was the most significant predictor of diarrhea (196,229). However, it all depends on the definition of diarrhea that is used. Thus in a small prospective study (230), definitions from lenient (i.e., >1 stool/d) to rigorous (>5 stools/d) yielded an incidence of 72% and 21%, respectively. There was no correlation between diarrhea and hypoalbuminemia (i.e., fluid secretion into the intestinal lumen), as has been proposed before (231). A second factor that may also relate to incidence of diarrhea after gastrointestinal surgery is abnormally rapid small intestinal motility in the immediate postoperative period, which leads to dumping of nutrients into the colon. This has been suggested by one study that showed this to be the case 3 but not 7 days postoperatively (232). A similar mechanism can be inferred from one study in 24 patients fed by needle-catheter jejunostomy after gastrointestinal surgery, in which the onset of diarrhea (mostly on the first postoperative day) could be predicted by an increase in breath-H_2 production (233).

Benefits from the presence of luminal SCFAs may, however, relate to the maintenance of normal mucosal cellularity. The concept of "bowel rest" following surgery or during inflammatory episodes of Crohn's disease was developed to suppress the activity of luminal aggressive factors such as bile and pancreatic secretions on inflamed or healing tissue. However, it has been noted that where part of the large intestine is diverted from the intestinal luminal stream by surgery, yet circulation is maintained, even though these aggressive factors are absent from the lumen, diversion colitis can occur. Restoration of the continuity of the fecal stream by re-anastomosis has been shown to reduce colitis in the affected segment (234). This has led to the suggestion that the key luminal factor, whose absence may lead to colonic "starvation," is butyrate, since its instillation into the diverted loop of intestine has been shown to reduce inflammation, as reviewed elsewhere (235). In the intact gut, Kasper and colleagues have demonstrated that 2 weeks of treatment with rectal enemas of 100 mmol/l sodium butyrate normalized the histological appearance of the distal colon in patients with steroid resistant ulcerative colitis (236). It was of interest that this treatment also halved the frequency of defecation, presumably because the absorptive function of the mucosa was restored. There is a clear need for studies of this type in patients undergoing large bowel surgery to determine if luminal irrigation at the time of surgery and postoperatively will influence outcome.

CONDITIONALLY ESSENTIAL?

According to the criteria defined in Table 2, glutamine, arginine, and related metabolite supply, as part of nutrition support, can only be defined as conditionally essential if they correct clinical abnormalities. An attempt has been made to integrate the confusing picture that current clinical trials of supplemented feeds presents (237–239). The confusion in terminology has led to their definition as conditionally essential nutrients when the human frame is capable of producing them in abundance. Thus, in describing the influence of reduced intracellular glutamine on muscle protein synthesis, it is remarkable that the concentration of a nonessential amino acid can affect the disposal of clearly essential amino acids (240). Careful reading of that particular study suggests that glutamine depletion is consequent on the effects of trauma and does not cause them. Glutamine flow will follow the direction given to it by metabolic acidosis and alterations in the ratio of intracellular and plasma Na^+ and K^+; in other words, it is part of the epiphenomonology of the disease process. This does not preclude its use (and that of arginine, OKG, or α-ketoglutarate itself) in correcting the underlying acidosis of injury and trauma metabolism. The appropriate frame of reference is as pharmaceutical agents, not essential nutrients.

Purine and pyrimidine requirements are more difficult to define. There is little evidence to suggest essentiality in view of the capacity for *de novo* synthesis. However, it is conceivable that in the period after injury, it would be prudent to continue providing purines and pyrimidines as nutrients on the grounds that prior nutrient intake has not lead to full expression of the enzymes of the *de novo* pathway. A number of studies suggest that this has beneficial effects on tissues that are undergoing rapid cell division or repair.

Short-chain fatty acids are the only nutrients that can be classed as essential on the grounds that organ function is impaired by their absence. This relates to the fact that no alternative pathway for butyrate synthesis exists apart from that provided by colonic luminal bacteria. The use of antibiotics and parenteral or low-residue enteral nutrition in hospitalized patients will all lead to reduced SCFA production compared to preadmission levels. As has been described, this can lead to impairment of one aspect of organ function, water, and electrolyte handling, and may be implicated in the etiology of inflammatory bowel disease.

REFERENCES

1. Leander U, Furst P, Vesterberg K, et al. Nitrogen sparing effect of Ornicetil® in the immediate postoperative state: clinical biochemistry and nitrogen balance. *Clin Nutr* 1985;4:43–51.
2. Wernerman J, Hammarqvist F, von der Decken A, et al. Ornithine-alpha-ketoglutarate improves skeletal muscle protein synthesis as assessed by ribosome analysis and nitrogen use after surgery. *Ann Surg* 1987;206:674–678.
3. Hammarqvist F, Wernerman J, Ali R, et al. Addition of glutamine to total parenteral nutrition after elective abdominal surgery spares free glutamine in muscle, counteracts the fall in muscle protein synthesis and improves nitrogen balance. *Ann Surg* 1989;209:455–461.
4. Wernerman J, Hammarqvist F, Vinnars E. α-ketoglutarate and post-operative muscle catabolism. *Lancet* 1990;335:701–703.
5. Souba WW. Intestinal glutamine metabolism and nutrition. *J Nutr Biochem* 1993;4:2–9.
6. Janas L, Picciano M. The nucleotide profile of human milk. *Pediatr Res* 1982;16:659–662.
7. Jimenez J, Boza J Jr, Suarez MD, et al. Changes in fatty acid profiles of red blood cell membranes mediated by dietary nucleotides in weanling rats. *J Pediatr Gastroenterol Nutr* 1992;14:293–299.
8. Romain N, Jeusette DF, Forget P. Polyamine concentration in rat milk and food, human milk, and infant formulas. *Pediatr Res* 1992;32:58–63.
9. Pollack PF, Koldovsky O, Nishioka K. Polyamines in human and rat milk and in infant formulas. *Am J Clin Nutr* 1992;56:371–375.
10. Jaziri M, Migliore-Samour D, Casabianca-Pignède M-R, et al. Specific binding sites on human phagocytic blood cells for Gly-Leu-Phe and Val-Glu-Pro-Ile-Pro-Tyr, immunostimulating peptides from human milk proteins. *Biochem Biophys Acta Protein Struct Mol Enzymol* 1992;1160:251–261.
11. Hautefeuille M, Brantl V, Dumontier AM, et al. In vitro effects of beta-casomorphins on ion transport in rabbit ileum. *Am J Physiol* 1986;250:G92–G97.
12. Daniel H, Vohwinkel M, Rehner G. Effect of casein and beta-casomorphins on gastrointestinal motility in rats. *J Nutr* 1990;120:252–257.
13. Teschemacher H, Koch G. Opioids in the milk. *Endocr Regul* 1991;25:147–150.
14. Castonguay TW, Bellinger LL. Capsaicin and its effects upon meal patterns, and glucagon and epinephrine suppression of food intake. *Physiol Behav* 1987;40:337–342.
15. Raybould HE. Capsaicin-sensitive vagal afferents and CCK in inhibition of gastric motor function induced by intestinal nutrients. *Peptides* 1991;12:1279–1283.
16. Rose WC. The nutritive significance of the amino acids and certain related compounds. *Science* 1937;86:298–300.
17. Munro HN. An introduction to nutritional aspects of protein metabolism. In: Munro HN, Allison JB, eds. *Mammalian Protein Metabolism, volume II.* New York: Academic Press, 1964;3–39.
18. Millward DJ, Jackson AA, Price G, et al. Human amino acid and protein requirements: current dilemmas and uncertainties. *Nutr Res Rev* 1989;2:109–132.
19. Young VR, Pellet PL. How to evaluate dietary protein. In: Barth CA, Schlimme E, eds. *Milk Proteins in Human Nutrition.* Darmstadt: Steinkopff, 1989;7–36.
20. Bjelton L, Fransson G-B. Availability of cysteine and L-2-oxo-thiazolidine-4-carboxylic acid as a source of cysteine in intravenous nutrition. *J Parenter Enteral Nutr* 1990;14:177–182.
21. Helms RA, Christensen ML, Mauer EC, et al. Comparison of a pediatric versus standard amino acid formulation in preterm neonates requiring parenteral nutrition. *J Pediatr* 1972;110:466–470.
22. Gaull G, Sturman JA, Raiha NCR. Development of mammalian sulfur metabolism: absence of cystathionase in human fetal tissue. *Pediatr Res* 1972;6:538–547.
23. MacDonald ML, Rogers QR, Morris JG. Nutrition of the domestic cat, a mammalian carnivore. *Annu Rev Nutr* 1984;4:521–562.
24. Barbul A. Arginine, biochemistry, physiology and therapeutic implications. *J Parenter Enteral Nutr* 1986;10:227–238.
25. Nakagawa J, Takahashi T, Suzuki T, et al. Amino acid requirements of children: minimal needs of tryptophan, arginine and histidine based on nitrogen balance method. *J Nutr* 1963–80:305–310.
26. Jackson AA. Optimizing amino acid and protein supply and utilization in the newborn. *Proc Nutr Soc* 1989;48:293–301.
27. Walser M. Rationale and indications for the use of α-keto analogues. *J Parenter Enteral Nutr* 1984; 8:37–41.
28. du Vigneaud V, Rachele JR. In: Shapiro SK, Schlenk F, etds. *Transmethylation and Methionine Biosynthesis.* Chicago, London: University of Chicago Press, 1965;1–20.

29. Laidlaw SA, Kopple JD. Newer concepts of the indispensible amino acids. *Am J Clin Nutr* 1987; 46:593–605.
30. Bessey PQ, Watters JM, Aoki TT, et al. Combined hormonal infusion simulates the metabolic response to injury. *Ann Surg* 1984;199:264–281.
31. Fine A, Bennett FI, Alleyne GAO. Effects of acid-base alterations on glutamine metabolism and renal ammoniagenesis in the dog. *Clin Sci Mol Med* 1978;54:503–508.
32. Grimble BK, West MFE, Acuti ABC, et al. Assessment of an automated chemiluminescence nitrogen analyser for routine use in clinical nutrition. *J Parenter Enteral Nutr* 1988;12:100–106.
33. Owen EE, Robinson RR. Amino acid extraction and ammonia metabolism by the human kidney during prolonged administration of ammonium chloride. *J Clin Invest* 1963;42:263–276.
34. Roth E, Funovics J, Muhlbacher F, et al. Metabolic disorders in severe abdominal sepsis: glutamine deficiency in skeletal muscle. *Clin Nutr* 1982;1:25–42.
35. Petersson B, Vinnars E, Waller S-O, et al. Long-term changes in muscle free amino acid levels after elective surgery. *Br J Surg* 1992;79:212–216.
36. Welbourne TC. Interorgan glutamine flow in metabolic acidosis. *Am J Physiol* 1987;253: F1069–F1076.
37. Tizianello AG, Deferrari G, Garibotto G, et al. Effects of chronic renal insufficiency and metabolic acidosis on glutamine metabolism in man. *Clin Sci Mol Med* 1978;55:391–397.
38. Vinay P, Allignet E, Pichette C, et al. Changes in renal metabolite profile and ammoniagenesis during acute and chronic metabolic acidosis in dog and rat. *Kidney Int* 1980;17:312–325.
39. Kurtz I, Dass PD, Cramer S. The importance of renal ammonia metabolism to whole body acid-base balance: a reanalysis of the pathophysiology of renal tubular acidosis. *Miner Electrolyte Metab* 1990;16:331–340.
40. Golden MHN, Jahoor P, Jackson AA. Glutamine production rate and its contribution to urinary ammonia in normal man. *Clin Sci* 1982;62:299–305.
41. Squires EJ, Brosnan JT. Measurements of the turnover rate of glutamine in normal and acidotic rats. *Biochem J* 1983;210:277–280.
42. Tamarappoo BK, Joshi S, Welbourne TC. Interorgan glutamine flow regulation in metabolic acidosis. *Miner Electrolyte Metab* 1990;16:322–330.
43. Haussinger D, Lamers WH, Moorman AF. Hepatocyte heterogeneity in the metabolism of amino acids and ammonia. *Enzyme* 1992;46:72–93.
44. Tannen RL, Sahai A. Biochemical pathways and modulators of renal ammoniagenesis. *Miner Electrolyte Metab* 1990;16:249–258.
45. Brosnan JT. The 1986 Borden award lecture. The role of the kidney in amino acid metabolism and nutrition. *Can J Physiol Pharmacol* 1987;65:2355–2362.
46. Liu SY, Leighton T, Davis I, et al. Prospective analysis of cardiopulmonary responses to laparoscopic cholecystectomy. *J Laparoendosc Surg* 1991;1:241–246.
47. Wernerman J, Vinnars E. The effect of trauma and surgery on interorgan fluxes of amino acids in man. *Clin Sci* 1987;73:129–133.
48. Deutz NEP, Reijven PLM, Athanasas G, et al. Post-operative changes in hepatic, intestinal, splenic and muscle fluxes of amino acids in pigs. *Clin Sci* 1992;83:607–614.
49. Lund J, Stjernstrom H, Vinnars E, et al. The influence of abdominal surgery on the splanchnic exchange of amino acids. *Acta Chir Scand* 1986;152:191–197.
50. Souba WW, Wilmore DW. Postoperative alterations of arteriovenous exchange of amino acids across the gastrointestinal tract. *Surgery* 1982;94:342–350.
51. Konstantanides FN, Konstantanides NM, Li JC, et al. Urinary urea nitrogen: too insensitive for calculating nitrogen balance studies in surgical clinical nutrition. *J Parenter Enteral Nutr* 1991;15: 189–193.
52. Steinhorn D, Radmer W. Urea synthesis is not consistent throughout the acute phase of stress. *J Parenter Enteral Nutr* 1986;10(Suppl):11S.
53. Owen OE, Felig P, Morgan AP, et al. Liver and kidney metabolism during prolonged starvation. *J Clin Invest* 1969;48:574–583.
54. Preedy VR, Garlick PJ. The influence of restraint and infusion on rates of muscle protein synthesis in the rat. Effect of altered respiratory function. *Biochem J* 1988;251:577–580.
55. Jeevanandam M, Long CL, Birkhahn RH, et al. Evaluation of whole body nitrogen kinetics in acute metabolic acidosis. *Am J Clin Nutr* 1983;37:201–210.
56. May RC, Masud T, Logue B, et al. Chronic metabolic acidosis accelerates whole body proteolysis and oxidation in awake rats. *Kidney Int* 1992;41:1535–1542.

57. Reaich D, Channon SM, Scrimgeour CM, et al. Ammonium chloride-induced acidosis increases protein breakdown and amino acid oxidation in humans. *Am J Physiol* 1992;263:E735–E739.
58. Garibotto G, Russo R, Sala MR, et al. Muscle protein turnover and amino acid metabolism in patients with chronic renal failure. *Miner Electrolyte Metab* 1992;18:217–221.
59. May RC, Kelly RA, Mitch WE. Mechanisms for defects in muscle protein metabolism in rats with chronic uremia. Influence of metabolic acidosis. *J Clin Invest* 1987;79:1099–1103.
60. Metter EJ, Yanagihara T. Protein synthesis in rat brain in hypoxia, anoxia and hypoglycemia. *Brain Res* 1979;161:481–492.
61. Holstein SB, Myers RE. Asphyxia-induced disaggregation of cerebral polyribosomes in rhesus monkey fetuses. *J Neurophathol Exp Neurol* 1978;38:85–94.
62. Petersson B, Wernerman J, Waller S-O, et al. Elective abdominal surgery depresses muscle protein synthesis and increases subjective fatigue: effects lasting more than 30 days. *Br J Surg* 1990;77: 796–800.
63. Elsair J, Poey J, Isaad H, et al. Effect of arginine chlorhydrate on nitrogen balance during the three days following surgery in man. *Biomedecine* 1978;29:312–317.
64. Vesterberg K, Vinnars E, Leander U, et al. Nitrogen sparing effect of Ornicetil in the immediate post-operative state: plasma and muscle amino acids. *Clin Nutr* 1987;6:213–219.
65. Stehle P, Zander J, Mertes N, et al. Effect of parenteral glutamine peptide supplements on muscle glutamine loss and nitrogen balance after major surgery. *Lancet* 1989;i:231–233.
66. Adibi SA, Lochs H, Abumrad NN, et al. Removal of glycylglutamine from plasma by individual tissues: mechanism and impact on amino acid fluxes in postabsorption and starvation. *J Nutr* 1993; 123:325–331.
67. Martin M, Ferrier B, Baverel G. Transport and utilization of alpha-ketoglutarate by the rat kidney in vivo. *Pflugers Arch* 1989;413:217–224.
68. Lowry M, Ross BD. Activation of oxoglutarate dehydrogenase in the kidney in response to acute acidosis. *Biochem J* 1980;190:771–780.
69. Batshaw ML, Walser M, Brusilow SW. Plasma α-ketoglutarate in urea cycle enzymopathies and its role as a harbinger of hyperammonemic coma. *Pediatr Res* 1980;14:1316–1319.
70. Milner JA. Metabolic aberrations associated with arginine deficiency. *J Nutr* 1985;115:516–523.
71. Ziegler F, Coudray-Lucas C, Jardel A, et al. Ornithine α-ketoglutarate and glutamine supplementation during refeeding of food-deprived rats. *J Parenter Enteral Nutr* 1992;16:505–510.
72. Moran BJ, Jackson AA. Metabolism of 15N-labelled urea in the functioning and defunctioned human colon. *Clin Sci* 1990;79:253–258.
73. Moran BJ, Jackson AA. 15N-urea metabolism in the functioning human colon: luminal hydrolysis and mucosal permeability. *Gut* 1990;31:454–457.
74. Hibbert JM, Forrester T, Jackson AA. Urea kinetics: comparison of oral and intravenous dose regimens. *Eur J Clin Nutr* 1992;46:405–409.
75. Jackson AA, Picou D, Landman J. The non-invasive measurement of urea kinetics in normal man by a constant infusion of 15N15N-urea. *Hum Nutr Clin Nutr* 1984;38:339–354.
76. Danielsen M, Jackson AA. Limits of adaptation to a diet low in protein in normal man: urea kinetics. *Clin Sci* 1992;83:103–108.
77. Smith CJ, Bryant MP. Introduction to metabolic activities of intestinal bacteria. *Am J Clin Nutr* 1979;32:149–157.
78. Snyderman SE, Holt LE Jr, Davies J, et al. "Unessential" nitrogen: a limiting factor for human growth. *J Nutr* 1962;78:1–15.
79. Kies C. Nonspecific nitrogen in the nutrition of human beings. *Fed Proc* 1972;41:1172–1177.
80. Remesy C, Demigne C. Specific effects of fermentable carbohydrates on blood urea flux and ammonia absorption in the rat cecum. *J Nutr* 1989;119:560–565.
81. Langran M, Moran BJ, Murphy JL, et al. Adaptation to a diet low in protein: effect of complex carbohydrate upon urea kinetics in normal man. *Clin Sci* 1992;82:191–198.
82. van Berlo CL, van Leeuwen PA, Soeters PB. Procine intestinal ammonia liberation. Influence of food intake, lactulose and neomycin treatment. *J Hepatol* 1988;7:250–257.
83. Windemueller HG. Glutamine utilisation by the small intestine. *Adv Enzymol* 1982;53:201–238.
84. Soeters PB, van Leeuwen PA. [Ammonia and glutamine metabolism of the intestine. The effect of lactulose and neomycin]. *Infusionsther Klin Ernahr* 1986;13:186–190.
85. Johnson AW, Berrington JM, Walker I, et al. Measurement of the transfer of the nitrogen moiety of intestinal glutamic acid after oral ingestion of 1-[^{15}N]glutamic acid. *Clin Sci* 1988;75:499–502.
86. Itoh H, Kishi T, Chibata I. Comparative effects of casein and amino acid mixture simulating casein on growth and food intake in rats. *J Nutr* 1973;103:1709–1715.

87. Burrin DG, Shulman RJ, Storm MC, et al. Glutamine or glutamic acid effects on intestinal growth and dissaccharidase activity in infant piglets receiving total parenteral nutrition. *J Parenter Enteral Nutr* 1991;15:262–266.
88. Grimble GK, Coudray-Lucas C, Payne-James JJ, et al. Augmentation of plasma arginine and glutamine by ornithine α-ketoglutarate in healthy enterally-fed volunteers. *Proc Nutr Soc* 1992;51:119A (abst).
89. Buddington RK, Diamond J. Ontogenetic development of nutrient transporters in cat intestine. *Am J Physiol* 1992;263:G605–G616.
90. Lund P. Glutamine metabolism in the rat. *FEBS Lett* 1980;117(Suppl):K86–K92.
91. Rerat A, Simoes-Nunes C, Mendy F, et al. Amino acid absorption and production of pancreatic hormones in non-anaesthetised pigs after duodenal infusions of a milk enzymic hydrolysate or of free amino acids. *Br J Nutr* 1988;60:121–136.
92. Barbul A, Lazarou SA, Efron DT, et al. Arginine enhances wound healing and lymphocyte immune responses in humans. *Surgery* 1990;108:331–337.
93. Barbul A, Sisto DA, Wasserkrug HL, et al. Arginine stimulates lymphocyte immune responses in healthy humans. *Surgery* 1981;90:244–251.
94. Milliner DS. Cystinuria. *Endocrinol Metab Clin North Am* 1990;19:889–907.
95. Payne-James J, Grimble G, Cahill E, et al. Jejunal absorption of ornithine-oxoglutarate (OKGA) in man. *J Parenter Enteral Nutr* 1989;13(suppl):22S.
96. Hellier MD, Holdsworth CD, Perrett D. Dibasic amino acid absorption in man. *Gastroenterology* 1973;65:613–618.
97. Lawless K, Maenz D, Cheeseman C. Is leucine an allosteric modulator of the lysine transporter in the intestinal basolateral membrane? *Am J Physiol* 1987;253:G637–G642.
98. Cheeseman C. Role of intestinal basolateral membrane in absorption of nutrients. *Am J Physiol* 1992;263:R482–R488.
99. Medina MA, Urdiales JL, Nunez de Castro I, et al. Diamines interfere with the transport of L-ornithine in Ehrlich-cell plasma-membrane vesicles. *Biochem J* 1991;280:825–827.
100. Hegarty JE, Fairclough PD, Clark ML, et al. Jejunal water and electrolyte secretion induced by L-arginine in man. *Gut* 1981;22:108–113.
101. Calignano A, Whittle BJR, Di Rosa M, et al. Involvement of endogenous nitric oxide in the regulation of rat intestinal motility in vivo. *Eur J Pharmacol* 1992;229:273–276.
102. Palmer RMJ, Ferrige AG, Moncada S. Nitric oxide release accounts for the biological activity of endothelium-derived relaxing factor. *Nature (Lond)* 1987;327:524–526.
103. Payne-James JJ, Grimble GK, Cahill E, et al. Enteral administration of ornithine-oxoglutarate (OKG) in man: effects on hormone profiles and nitrogen (N) metabolism. *J Parenter Enteral Nutr* 1989; 13S:105.
104. Milne MD, Asatoor AM, Edwards KDJ, et al. The intestinal absorption defect in cystinuria. *Gut* 1961;2:323–337.
105. Daly JM, Lieberman MD, Goldfine J, et al. Enteral nutrition with supplemental arginine, RNA and omega-3 fatty acids in patients after operation: immunologic, metabolic, and clinical outcome. *Surgery* 1992;112:56–67.
106. Jackson AA, Golden MH. [15N]Glycine metabolism in normal man: the metabolic alpha-amino-nitrogen pool. *Clin Sci* 1980;58:517–522.
107. Grimble RF, Jackson AA, Persaud C, et al. Cysteine and glycine supplementation modulate the metabolic response to tumor necrosis factor alpha in rats fed a low protein diet. *J Nutr* 1992;122: 2066–2073.
108. Jackson AA. The glycine story. *Eur J Clin Nutr* 1991;45:59–65.
109. Heinrich PC, Castell JV, Andus T. Interleukin-6 and the acute phase response. *Biochem J* 1990; 265:621–636.
110. Grimble GK, Millward DJ. The measurement of ribosomal ribonucleic acid synthesis in rat liver and skeletal muscle in vivo. *Biochem Soc Trans* 1977;5:913–916.
111. Millward DJ, Nnanyelugo DO, James WP, et al. Protein metabolism in skeletal muscle: the effect of feeding and fasting on muscle RNA, free amino acids and plasma insulin concentrations. *Br J Nutr* 1974;32:127–142.
112. D'Mello JPF. Utilization of dietary purines and pyrimidines by non-ruminant animals. *Proc Nutr Soc* 1982;41:301–308.
113. Giesecke D, Tiemeyer W. Availability and metabolism of purines of single-cell proteins in monogastric anuimals. *Proc Nutr Soc* 1982;41:319–327.

114. Zollner N. Purine and pyrimidine metabolism. *Proc Nutr Soc* 1982;41:329–342.
115. Wu G, Greene LW. Glutamine and glucose metabolism in bovine blood lymphocytes. *Comp Biochem Physiol B* 1992;103:821–825.
116. Roden M, Paterson AR, Turnheim K. Sodium-dependent nucleoside transport in rabbit intestinal epithelium. *Gastroenterology* 1991;100:1553–1562.
117. Schanker LS, Jeffrey JJ, Tocco DJ. Interaction of purines with the pyrimidine transport process of the small intestine. *Biochem Pharmacol* 1963;12:1047–1053.
118. Scharrer E, Stubenhofer L, Tiemeyer W, et al. Active pyrimidine absorption by chicken colon. *Comp Biochem Physiol A* 1984;77:85–88.
119. Griefe HA, Molnar S. 14C-Tracerstudien zum Nukleinsauren-Stoffwechsel von Jungratten, Kuken und Ferkeln. 1: Mitteilung. Untersuchungen zum Purinestoffwechsel der Jungratte. *Z Tierphysiol Tierernahr Futtermittelkd* 1983;50:79–91.
120. Savaiano DA, Ho CY, Chu V, et al. Metabolism of orally and intravenously administered purines in rats. *J Nutr* 1980;110:1793–1804.
121. Ogoshi S, Iwasa M, Kitagawa S, et al. Effects of total parenteral nutrition with nucleoside and nucleotide mixture on D-galactosamine-induced liver injury in rats. *J Parenter Enteral Nutr* 1988; 12:53–57.
122. Savaiano DA, Clifford AJ. Adenine, the precursor of nucleic acids in intestinal cells is unable to synthesise purines ne novo. *J Nutr* 1981;111:1816–1822.
123. Sonoda T, Tatibana M. Metabolic fate of pyrimidines and purines in dietary nucleic acids ingested by mice. *Biochim Biophys Acta* 1978;521:55–66.
124. Leleiko NS, Bronstein AD, Baliga BS, et al. De novo purine nucleotide synthesis in the rat small and large intestine: effect of dietary protein and purines. *J Pediatr Gastroenterol Nutr* 1983;2: 313–319.
125. Leleiko NS, Bronstein AD, Munro HN. Effect of dietary purines on de novo synthesis of purine nucleotides in the small intestinal mucosa. *Pediatr Res* 1979;13:403.
126. Gross CJ, Stiles JE, Savaiano DA. Effect of nutritional state and allopurinol on purine metabolism in the rat small intestine. *Biochim Biophys Acta* 1988;966:168–175.
127. Ghiggeri GM, Ginevri F, Cercignani G, et al. Effect of dietary protein restriction on renal purines and purine-metabolizing enzymes in adriamycin nephrosis in rats: a mechanism for protection against acute proteinuria involving xanthine oxidase inhibition. *Clin Sci* 1990;79:647–656.
128. Grimble GK. *RNA Metabolism in Skeletal Muscle*. University of London: PhD Thesis, 1981.
129. Genchev DD, Kermechiev MB, Hadjiolov AA. Free pyrimidine nucleotide pool of Ehrlich Ascites-tumour cells. *Biochem J* 1980;188:85–90.
130. Wiegers U, Kramer G, Klapproth K, et al. Separate pyrimidine-nucleotide pools for messenger-RNA and ribosomal-RNA synthesis in HeLa S3 cells. *Eur J Biochem* 1976;64:535–540.
131. Ove P, Adams RLP, Abrams R, et al. Liver uridine triphosphate after partial hepatectomy. *Biochim Biophys Acta* 1966;123:419–421.
132. Losman MJ, Harley EH. Evidence for compartmentation of uridine nucleotide pools in rat hepatoma cells. *Biochim Biophys Acta* 1978;521:762–769.
133. Grummt I, Grummt F. Control of nucleolar RNA synthesis by the intracellular pool sizes of ATP and GTP. *Cell* 1976;7:447–453.
134. Grummt I, Smith VA, Grummt F. Amino acid starvation affects the initiation frequency of nucleolar RNA polymerase. *Cell* 1976;7:439–445.
135. Goody HE, Ellem KAO. Nutritional effects on precursor uptake and compartmentalization of intracellular pools in relation to RNA synthesis. *Biochim Biophys Acta* 1975;383:30–39.
136. Laurent GJ, Sparrow MP, Millward DJ. Turnover of muscle protein in the fowl. 2. changes in rates of protein synthesis and breakdown during hypertrophy of the anterior and posterior latissimus dorsi muscles. *Biochem J* 1978;176:407–417.
137. Bates PC, Grimble GK, Sparrow MP, et al. Myofibrillar protein turnover. Synthesis of protein bound 3-methyl histidine, actin, myosin heavy-chain and aldolase in rat skeletal muscle in the fed and fasted state. *Biochem J* 1983;214:593–605.
138. Ashford AJ, Pain VM. Insulin stimulation of growth in diabetic rats. Synthesis and degradation of ribosomes and total tissue protein in skeletal muscle and heart. *J Biol Chem* 1986;261:4066–4070.
139. Warner JR. The nucleolus and ribosome formation. *Curr Opin Cell Biol* 1990;2:521–527.
140. Warner JR. The nucleolus and ribosome formation. In: Nomura M, Tissieres A, Lengyel P, eds. *The Ribosomes*. New York: Cold Spring Harbor Laboratory, 1974;461–488.
141. Warner JR. In the absence of ribosomal RNA synthesis, the ribosomal proteins of HeLa cells are synthesised normally and degraded rapidly. *J Mol Biol* 1977;115:315–333.

142. Tsurugi K, Ogata K. Degradation of newly synthesised ribosomal proteins and histones in regenerating rat liver with and without treatment with a low dose of Actinomycin D. *Eur J Biochem* 1979; 101:205–213.
143. Stoyanova BB, Hadjiolov AA. Alteration in the processing of rat-liver rRNA caused by cycloheximide inhibition of protein synthesis. *Eur J Biochem* 1979;96:357–362.
144. Karagyozov LK, Stoyanova BB, Hadjiolov AA. Effect of cycloheximide on the in vitro synthesis of ribosomal RNA in rat liver. *Biochim Biophys Acta* 1980;607:295–303.
145. Loeb JN, Yeung LL. Synthesis and degradation of ribosomal RNA in regenerating liver. *J Exp Med* 1975;142:575–587.
146. Nikolov EN, Dabeva MD. Turnover of ribosomal 28S and 18S rRNA during rat liver regeneration. *Biosci Rep* 1983;15:1255–1260.
147. Nikolov EN, Dabeva MD, Nikolov TK. Turnover of ribosomes in regenerating rat liver. *Int J Biochem* 1983;14:1255–1260.
148. Dudov KP, Dabeva MD. Post-transcriptional regulation of ribosome formation in the nucleus of regenerating rat liver. *Biochem J* 1983;210:183–192.
149. Aletti MG, Picolletti R, Bernelli-Zazzera A. Release of rRNA from liver nuclei during the early stages of the acute-phase reaction. *Biochim Biophys Acta* 1984;783:179–182.
150. Piccoletti R, Aletti MG, Bernelli-Zazzera A. Inflammation associated events in liver nuclei during acute-phase reaction. *Inflammation* 1986;10:109–117.
151. Hill JM, Ab G, Malt RA. Ribonucleic acid labelling and nucleotide pools during compensatory renal hypertrophy. *Biochem J* 1974;144:447–453.
152. Hill JM. Ribosomal RNA metabolism during renal hypertrophy. Evidence of decreased degradation of newly synthesized ribosomal RNA. *J Cell Biol* 1975;64:260–265.
153. Ouellette AJ, Moonka R, Zelenetz AD, et al. Regulation of ribosome synthesis during compensatory renal hypertrophy in mice. *Am J Physiol* 1987;253:C506–C513.
154. Millward DJ, Garlick PJ, Stewart RJ, et al. Skeletal-muscle growth and protein turnover. *Biochem J* 1975;150:235–243.
155. Spence CA, Hansen Smith FM. Comparison of the chemical and biochemical composition of thirteen muscles of the rat after dietary protein restriction. *Br J Nutr* 1978;39:647–658.
156. Millward DJ, Garlick PJ, James WP, et al. Relationship between protein synthesis and RNA content in skeletal muscle. *Nature (Lond)* 1973;241:204–205.
157. Mezzetti G, Ferrari S, Davilli P, et al. Peptide chain initiation and analysis of in vitro translation products in rat heart undergoing hypertrophic growth. *J Mol Cell Cardiol* 1983;15:629–635.
158. Morgan HE, Siehl D, Chua BH, et al. Faster protein and ribosome synthesis in hypertrophying heart. *Basic Res Cardiol* 1985;80(Suppl 2):115–118.
159. Ray A, Aumont MC, Ausseday J, et al. Protein and 28S ribosomal RNA fractional turnover rates in the rat heart after abdominal aortic stenosis. *Cardiovasc Res* 1987;21:587–592.
160. Mercer WE, Avignolo C, Galanti N, et al. Cellular DNA replication is independent of the synthesis or accumulation of ribosomal RNA. *Exp Cell Res* 1984;150:118–130.
161. Seuwen K, Steiner U, Adam G. Cellular content of ribosomal RNA in relation to the progression and competence signals governing proliferation of 3T3 and SV40-3T3 cells. *Exp Cell Res* 1984;154: 10–24.
162. Kleuzer B, Adam G. Interrelation between cellular rRNA content and regulation of the cell cycle of normal and transformed mouse cell lines. *Cell Biol Int Rep* 1985;9:985–992.
163. Johnson LF, Abelson HT, Green H, et al. Changes in RNA in relation to growth of the fibroblast. I: amounts of mRNA, rRNA and tRNA in resting and growing cells. *Cell* 1974;1:95–100.
164. Cooper HL. Studies on RNA metabolism during lymphocyte activation. *Transplant Rev* 1972;11: 3–38.
165. Szondy Z, Newsholme EA. The effect of various concentrations of nucleobases, nucleosides or glutamine on the incorporation of [³H]thymidine into DNA in rat mesenteric-lymph-node lymphocytes stimulated by phytohaemagglutinin. *Biochem J* 1990;270:437–440.
166. Gyorgy P. The uniqueness of human milk: biochemical aspects. *Am J Clin Nutr* 1971;24:970–975.
167. Greife HA, Molnar S, Bos T, et al. N-stoffwechsel wachsender Schweine bei Austach von Sojaextraktionsschrot durch einen bakteriellen Proteintrager *(Alcaligenes eutrophus). Arch Tierernahr* 1984;34:179–190.
168. Fanslow WC, Kulkarni AD, Van Buren Ct, et al. Effect of nucleotide restriction and supplementation on resistance to experimental murine candidiasis. *J Parenter Enteral Nutr* 1988;12:49–52.
169. Kulkarni AD, Fanslow WC, Rudolph FB, et al. Effect of dietary nucleotides on bacterial infections. *J Parenter Enteral Nutr* 1986;10:169–171.

170. Kulkarni SS, Bhateley DC, Zander AR, et al. Functional impairment of T-lymphocytes in mouse radiation chimeras by a nucleotide-free diet. *Exp Hematol* 1984;12:694–699.
171. Carver JD, Cox WI, Barness LA. Dietary nucleotide effects upon murine natural killer cell activity and macrophage activation. *J Parenter Enteral Nutr* 1990;14:18–22.
172. Christou N. Perioperative nutritional support: immunologic defects. *J Parenter Enteral Nutr* 1990; 14:186S–192S.
173. Ogoshi S, Iwasa M, Mizobuchi S, et al. Effect of a nucleoside and nucleotide mixture on protein metabolism in rats given total parenteral nutrition after 70% hepatectomy. In: Tanaka T, Okada A, eds. *Nutritional Support in Organ Failure.* Amsterdam: Elsevier Science Publishers, 1990;309–317.
174. Ogoshi S, Iwasa M, Tamiya T. Effect of nucleotide and nucleoside mixture on rats given total parenteral nutrition after 70% hepatectomy. *J Parenter Enteral Nutr* 1985;9:339–342.
175. Nunez MC, Ayudarte MV, Morales D, et al. Effect of dietary nucleotides on intestinal repair in rats with experimental chronic diarrhea. *J Parenter Enteral Nutr* 1990;14:598–604.
176. Austgen TR, Chen MK, Flynn TC, et al. The effects of endotoxin on the splanchnic metabolism of glutamine and related substrates. *J Trauma* 1991;31:742–751.
177. Midtvedt A-C, Midtvedt T. Production of short chain fatty acids by the intestinal microflora during the first 2 years of human life. *J Pediatr Gastroenterol Nutr* 1992;15:395–403.
178. Weaver GA, Krause JA, Miller TL, et al. Constancy of glucose and starch fermentations by two different human faecal microbial communities. *Gut* 1989;30:19–25.
179. Cummings JH, Pomare EW, Branch WJ, et al. Short chain fatty acids in human large intestine, portal, hepatic and venous blood. *Gut* 1987;28:1221–1227.
180. Hammer HF, Santa Ana CA, Schiller LR, et al. Studies of osmotic diarrhea induced in normal subjects by ingestion of polyethylene glycol and lactulose. *J Clin Invest* 1989;84:1056–1062.
181. Vernia P, Gnaedinger A, Hauck W, et al. Organic anions and the diarrhea of inflammatory bowel disease. *Gastroenterology* 1988;33:1353–1358.
182. Chacko A, Cummings JH. Nitrogen losses from the human small bowel: obligatory losses and the effect of physical form of food. *Gut* 1988;28:809–815.
183. MacFarlane GT, Cummings JH, Allison C. Protein degradation by human intestinal bacteria. *J Gen Microbiol* 1986;132:1647–1656.
184. Grimble GK, Silk DBA. Peptides in human nutrition. *Nutr Res Rev* 1989;2:87–108.
185. Mortensen PB, Clausen MR, Bonnen H, et al. Colonic fermentation of Ispaghula, wheat bran, glucose and albumin to short-chain fatty acids and ammonia evaluated in vitro in 50 subjects. *J Parenter Enteral Nutr* 1992;16:433–439.
186. Mueller KJ, Crosby LO, Oberlander JL, et al. Estimation of fecal nitrogen in patients with liver disease. *J Parenter Enteral Nutr* 1983;7:266–269.
187. Salyers AA, Leedle JAZ. Carbohydrate metabolism in the human colon. In: Hentges DJ, ed. *Human Intestinal Microflora in Health and Disease.* New York, London: Academic Press, 1983;129–146.
188. Grimble GK. Leading Article: Fibre, fermentation, flora and flatus. *Gut* 1989;30:6–13.
189. Flourie B, Pellier P, Florent C, et al. Site and substrates for methane production in human colon. *Am J Physiol* 1991;260:G752–G757.
190. Gibson GR, MacFarland GT, Cummings JH. Occurrence of sulphate-reducing bacteria in human faeces and the relationship of dissimilatory sulphate reduction to methanogenesis in the large gut. *J Appl Bacteriol* 1988;64:103–111.
191. Ruppin H, Barr-Meir S, Soergel KH, et al. Absorption of short chain fatty acids in the colon. *Gastroenterology* 1980;78:1500–1507.
192. Binder HJ, Metha P. Short-chain fatty acids stimulate active sodium chloride absorption in vitro in the rat distal colon. *Gastroenterology* 1989;96:989–996.
193. Watson AJ, Elliott EJ, Rolston DD, et al. Acetate absorption in the normal and secreting rat jejunum. *Gut* 1990;31:170–174.
194. Patil DH, Grimble GK, Silk DB. Lactitol, a new hydrogenated lactose derivative: intestinal absorption and laxative threshold in normal human subjects. *Br J Nutr* 1987;57:195–199.
195. Rao SS, Edwards CA, Austen CJ, et al. Impaired colonic fermentation of carbohydrate after ampicillin. *Gastroenterology* 1988;94:928–932.
196. Guenter PA, Settle RG, Perlmutter S, et al. Tube-feeding related diarrhea in acutely-ill patients. *J Parenter Enteral Nutr* 1991;15:277–280.
197. Koehane PP, Attrill H, Jones BJM, et al. The roles of lactose and *Clostridium difficile* in the pathogenesis of enteral feeding associated diarrhoea. *Clin Nutr* 1983;1:259–264.
198. Rees RGP, Koehane PP, Grimble GK, et al. Tolerance of elemental diet administered without starter regimen. *Br Med J* 1985;290:1869–1870.

199. Patil DH, Westaby D, Mahida YR, et al. Comparative modes of action of lactitol and lactulose in the treatment of hepatic encephalopathy. *Gut* 1987;28:255–259.
200. Konno R, Niwa A, Yasumura Y. Intestinal bacterial origin of D-alanine in urine of mutant mice lacking D-amino-acid oxidase. *Biochem J* 1990;268:263–265.
201. Clausen MR, Bonnen H, Tvede M, et al. Colonic fermentation to short-chain fatty acids is decreased in antibiotic-associated diarrhea. *Gastroenterology* 1991;101:1497–1504.
202. Thompson GN, Chalmers RA, Walter JH, et al. The use of metronidazole in management of methylmalonic and propionic acidaemias. *Eur J Pediatr* 1990;149:792–796.
203. Windemueller HG, Spaeth AE. Identification of ketone bodies and glutamine as the major respiratory fuels in vivo for postabsorptive rat small intestine. *J Biol Chem* 1978;253:69–76.
204. Henning SJ, Hird FJR. Concentrations and metabolism of volatile fatty acids in the fermentative organs of two species of kangaroo and the guinea-pig. *Br J Nutr* 1970;24:145–155.
205. Roediger WEW. Role of anaerobic bacteria in the metabolic welfare of the colonic mucosa in man. *Gut* 1980;21:793–798.
206. Young GP, Gibson P. Contrasting effects of butyrate on proliferation and differentiation of normal and neoplastic cells. In: Roche AF, ed. *Short-chain Fatty Acids: Metabolism and Clinical Importance. Report of 10th Ross Conference on Medical Research.* Columbus, Ohio: Ross Laboratories, 1991;50–55.
207. Niles RM, Wilhelm SA, Thomas P, et al. The effect of sodium butyrate and retinoic acid on growth and CEA production in a series of human colorectal tumor cell lines representing different states of differentiation. *Cancer Invest* 1988;6:39–45.
208. Scheppach W, Bartram P, Richter A, et al. Effect of short-chain fatty acids on the human colonic mucosa in vitro. *J Parenter Enteral Nutr* 1992;16:43–48.
209. Sakata T. Stimulatory effect of short-chain fatty acids on epithelial cell proliferation in the rat intestine: a possible explanation for trophic effects of fermentable fibre, gut microbes and luminal trophic factors. *Br J Nutr* 1987;58:95–103.
210. Lupton JR, Coder DM, Jacobs LR. Influence of luminal pH on rat large bowel epithelial cell cycle. *Am J Physiol* 1985;249:G382–G388.
211. Goodlad RA, Lenton W, Ghatei MA, et al. Effects of an elemental diet, inert bulk and different types of dietary fibre on the response of the intestinal epithelium to refeeding in the rat and relationship to plasma gastrin, enteroglucagon and PYY concentrations. *Gut* 1987;28:171–180.
212. Goodlad RA, Ratcliffe B, Fordham JP, et al. Does dietary fibre stimulate intestinal epithelial cell proliferation in germ free rats? *Gut* 1989;30:820–825.
213. Kruh J, Defer N, Tichonicky L. Molecular and cellular effects of sodium butyrate. In: Roche AF, ed. *Short-chain Fatty Acids: Metabolism and Clinical Importance. Report of the 10th Ross Conference on Medical Research.* Columbus, Ohio: Ross Laboratories, 1991;45–50.
214. Tanaka Y, Bush KK, Klauck TM, et al. Enhancement of butyrate-induced differentiation of HT-29 human colon carcinoma cells by 1,25-dihydroxyvitamin D_3. *Biochem Pharmacol* 1989;38:3859–3865.
215. Siddiqui B, Kim YS. Effects of sodium butyrate, dimethyl sulfoxide, and retinoic acid on glycolipids of human adenocarcinoma cells. *Cancer Res* 1984;44:1648–1652.
216. Rolandelli RH, Koruda MJ, Settle RG, et al. Effects of intraluminal short-chain fatty acids on the healing of colonic anastomoses in the rat. *Surgery* 1986;100:198–203.
217. Kripke SA, Fox AD, Berman JM, et al. Stimulation of intestinal mucosal growth with intracolonic infusion of short-chain fatty acids. *J Parenter Enteral Nutr* 1989;13:109–116.
218. Koruda MJ, Rolandelli RH, Settle RG, et al. Effect of parenteral nutrition supplemented with short-chain fatty acids on adaptation to massive small bowel resection. *Gastroenterology* 1988;95:715–720.
219. Fernandez Lopez JA, Casado J, Argiles JM, et al. In the rat, intestinal lymph carries a significant amount of ingested glucose into the bloodstream. *Arch Int Physiol Biochim Biophys* 1992;100:231–236.
220. Fernandez Lopez JA, Casado J, Argiles JM, et al. Intestinal handling of a glucose gavage by the rat. *Mol Cell Biochem* 1992;113:43–53.
221. Egan CJ, Rennie MJ. Relative importance of luminal and vascular amino acids for protein synthesis in rat jejunum. *J Physiol [Lond]* 1986;378:49P(abstr).
222. Mortensen FV, Nielsen H, Mulvany MJ, et al. Short chain fatty acids dilate isolated human colonic resistance arteries. *Gut* 1990;31:1391–1394.
223. Kvietys PR, Granger DN. Effect of volatile fatty acids on blood flow and oxygen uptake by the dog colon. *Gastroenterology* 1981;80:962–969.
224. Crissinger KD, Burney DL. Influence of luminal nutrient composition on hemodynamics and oxygenation in developing intestine. *Am J Physiol* 1992;263:G254–G260.

225. Buckley NM, Frasier ID. Regional circulatory responses to intestinal work in developing swine. *Am J Physiol* 1990;258:H1119–H1125.
226. Qamar MI, Read AE, Mountford R. Increased superior mesenteric artery blood flow after glucose but not lactulose ingestion. *Q J Med* 1986;60:893–896.
227. Flynn WJJ, Gosche JR, Garrison RN. Intestinal blood flow is restored with glutamine or glucose suffusion after hemorrhage. *J Surg Res* 1992;52:499–504.
228. Lang CH, Obih JC, Bagby GJ, et al. Increased glucose uptake by intestinal mucosa and muscularis in hypermetabolic sepsis. *Am J Physiol* 1991;261:G287–G294.
229. Hart GK, Dobb GJ. Effect of a faecal bulking agent on diarrhoea during enteral feeding in the critically ill. *J Parenter Enteral Nutr* 1988;12:465–468.
230. Bliss DZ, Guenter PA, Settle RG. Defining and reporting diarrhea in tube-fed patients—what a mess. *Am J Clin Nutr* 1992;55:753–759.
231. Brinson RR, Curtis WD, Singh M. Diarrhea in the intensive care unit: the role of hypoalbuminemia and the response to a chemically defined diet (case reports and review of the literature). *J Am Coll Nutr* 1987;6:517–523.
232. Miholic J, Vogelsang H, Schlappack O, et al. Small bowel function after surgery for chronic radiation enteritis. *Digestion* 1989;42:30–38.
233. Homann H-H, Kemen M, Mumme A, et al. The role of carbohydrate malabsorption in the pathogenesis of diarrhea during postoperative enteral nutrition. *J Clin Nutr Gastroenterol* 1992;7:54–59.
234. Korelitz BI, Cheskin LJ, Sohn N, et al. Proctitis after fecal diversion in Crohn's disease and its elimination with reanastomosis: implications for surgical management. *Gastroenterology* 1984;87:710–713.
235. Roediger WEW. The starved colon—diminished mucosal nutrition, diminished absorption and colitis. *Dis Colon Rectum* 1990;33:858–862.
236. Scheppach W, Sommer H, Kirchner T, et al. Effect of butyrate enemas on the colonic mucosa in distal ulcerative colitis. *Gastroenterology* 1993;103:51–56.
237. Souba WW, Klimberg VS, Plumley DA, et al. The role of glutamine in maintaining a healthy gut and supporting the metabolic response to injury and infection. *J Surg Res* 1990;48:383–387.
238. Adibi SA. Intravenous use of glutamine in peptide form: clinical applications of old and new observations. *Metabolism* 1989;38:89–92.
239. Kirk SJ, Barbul A. Role of arginine in trauma, sepsis and immunity. *J Parenter Enteral Nutr* 1990;14:226S–229S.
240. Rennie MJ, Hundal HS, Babij P, et al. Characteristics of a glutamine carrier in skeletal muscle have important consequences for nitrogen loss in injury, infection and chronic disease. *Lancet* 1986;ii:1008–1012.
241. Jackson AA. Aminoacids: essential and non-essential? *Lancet* 1983;1:1034–1037.

Organ Metabolism and Nutrition: Ideas for Future Critical Care, edited by J. M. Kinney and H. N. Tucker. Raven Press, Ltd., New York © 1994.

Overview: Intestinal Function

John M. Kinney

The Hirsch-Leibel Laboratories, Rockefeller University, New York, New York 10021

The clinical attitude toward the function of the gastrointestinal (GI) tract in the patient with acute illness, not suffering from local disease or injury of the gut, has undergone considerable change during the past 50 years. During the 1940s the metabolic response to a major injury was centered on muscle protein breakdown and a negative nitrogen balance. Organs such as the intestinal tract were assumed to remain passively uninvolved in the systemic response and to resume normal function whenever the response in the involved tissues had subsided.

Clinical practice regarding nutrition and the gut has also undergone shifting attitudes in regard to the acutely ill patient. It was assumed for many years that in the absence of vomiting, ileus, or diarrhea, conventional food should be given to the patient as tolerated. Nevertheless, varying degrees of partial starvation were expected during any acute illness. The introduction of total parenteral nutrition (TPN) in the 1960s was thought to remove the concern about inadequate nutrient intake during acute illness. The unspoken assumption was that the GI mucosa would remain essentially unchanged during periods of TPN. In the presence of inflammatory bowel disease, the use of TPN allowed total "bowel rest," which was thought to be of therapeutic benefit. However, TPN is no longer recommended as the primary modality in inflammatory bowel disease (1). There has been increasing attention to the atrophy of the intestinal mucosa that occurs during intravenous nutrition, with nutrient absorption becoming impaired. The unresolved question is the degree to which such atrophy, especially if associated with some mucosal ischemia, may predispose to translocation of toxins or bacteria during acute stress states. The increased clinical study of nonocclusive intestinal ischemia has led to the recent suggestion that endotoxemia may contribute to three out of every 100 deaths in the United States (2).

The intestinal tract has received increasing attention from another perspective, that of immune function and the inflammatory state. It is now accepted that the gut represents one of the largest concentrations of immune cells in the body. These cells may influence intestinal requirements for blood supply and specific nutrients. Experimental evidence has been accumulating regarding the important role that the gut may play in systemic immune responses and perhaps in initiating generalized inflammatory states.

The 1980s saw the rapid evolution of inflammatory cytokines and growth factors, which are adding an entirely new dimension to our understanding of convalescence from either injury or sepsis. The 1990s have brought the septic counterpart of the metabolic response to injury in the systemic inflammatory response syndrome (SIRS). There is intense interest in whether the gut may play a major role in the profound changes that lead to the multiple organ failure syndrome with its persistently high mortality. Therefore the intestinal tract is now considered a "vital organ," in ways that are relatively recent and emphasize the potential importance of improved nutritional support in the critically ill patient.

This overview presents selected material in three areas: intestinal function and nutrition, the intestine as an immune organ, and the intestinal role in inflammation.

INTESTINAL FUNCTION AND NUTRITION

Development, Architecture, and Function

The morphology of the small intestine is uniquely designed at the organ and at the cellular level for maximizing epithelial absorption of enteral nutrients. The presence of folds, villi, and microvilli results in a 600-fold increase in surface area compared with the surface area of a simple cylindrical tube (3). This indicates that the surface area of the small intestine available for absorption is approximately 100 times larger than the surface area of the human body.

Polarized epithelial cells, such as those of the intestinal mucosa, have tight junctions that separate the apical and basolateral domains. These two domains have completely different sets of integral proteins and different lipid compositions (4). Most protein and all lipids in the plasma membrane, as well as in the internal membranes, are laterally mobile. Some proteins are immobile, probably because they are anchored to parts of the cytoskeleton.

Research on epithelial cells, such as those of the intestinal mucosa, has been aided by the development of cell lines that form polarized cell monolayers in cell culture (4). These cell layers form a barrier to the passage of most small molecules and ions, which cannot pass readily through the cells themselves, or cross the cell layer via the spaces between cells. Impermeable, tight junctions seal off the lumen of the intestine from the fluid that flows past the basolateral surface of the cells from the surrounding blood. Gap junctions are distributed along the lateral surfaces of cells and allow them to exchange small molecules. These gap junctions help to integrate the metabolic activities of all cells in the tissue by assuring that they share a common pool of metabolites.

Drs. Rombeau and Lew (Chapter 10) have reviewed the cell types in the small intestine and colon and traced the steps in cellular turnover, separating the processes of proliferation from differentiation and maturation. Enteral feeding can contribute to intestinal cell proliferation and differentiation by providing both substrates for mucosal metabolism and mechanical epithelial contact. They have separated the trophic influences into those of the microcirculation, the pancreatic and biliary secretions, the autonomic nervous system, and enterohormones. Recent evidence is reviewed regarding nutrients with unique metabolic roles for the gut, including arginine, glutamine, and butyrate.

Arginine

The growing interest in arginine relates to its special properties beyond its conventional role as a constituent of proteins and as a central part of the urea cycle. It is now recognized to play an important part in host defense as well as a special role in rapidly dividing cells such as the intestinal mucosa.

Dr. Cynober (Chapter 12) notes that the enterocyte contains the appropriate enzymes to release urea and citrulline from arginine. The enterocyte uses arginine to produce both aliphatic polyamines and nitric oxide (NO). The arginine flux is preferentially toward citrulline production in the enterocyte as a result of unique intracellular location of particular enzymes. This is in contrast to ornithine in the enterocyte cytoplasm, which is the preferential precursor of polyamines.

Arginine has been proposed as an immunomodulator because its administration in the rodent inhibited the thymus involution induced by stress. Arginine administration has been shown to improve lymphocyte responsiveness to mitogens after arginine administration in both animals and humans. Barbul (5) observed that the arginine-mediated improvement in N balance is not dose dependent, which suggests that the immunologic and anabolic effects of this amino acid involve different mechanisms.

The recent recognition that nitric oxide may have many and diverse functions in the body lends importance to arginine, which appears to be the primary source of NO. Nitric oxide synthase, which catalyzes the reaction yielding NO from arginine, has been identified in two forms, which differ in their dependency on calcium and their sensitivity to glucocorticoids. One form is present in brain, endothelium, and platelets, while the other is inducible in many cells, particularly white blood cells, hepatocytes, and enterocytes. Lipopolysaccharide (LPS), IL-1, IL-6, and tumor necrosis factor (TNF) all induce NO synthesis, while interferon-gamma acts synergistically with these cytokines. Nitric oxide production can be blocked by antiinflammatory steroids, indicating that the NO pathway is a key component of the inflammatory reaction. There is animal evidence that NO is important in maintaining vascular integrity, but that large concentrations of NO may cause fatal hypotension, such as in the septic shock syndrome.

Dr. Cynober observes that arginine can modulate immunity in two ways: through NO production and via ornithine, which can effect immunity through polyamine synthesis. He proposes that trophic effects on the gut occur more from ornithine than arginine, although both stimulate growth hormone secretion.

Glutamine

Glutamine is abundantly present in its free form in many tissues and in plasma, both in health and disease. It has been recognized for two decades that glutamine is a nontoxic nitrogen carrier and precursor for gluconeogenesis as well as ammoniagenesis. More recently, glutamine has been reported to influence muscle morphology, protein synthesis and protein content of the gut mucosa, and cells of the immune system.

An increase in proteolysis and the resultant negative nitrogen balance is a hallmark of the metabolic response to injury and sepsis. It is commonly thought to be largely at the expense of skeletal muscle. Dr. Rennie (Chapter 2) has reviewed current approaches to the study of synthesis and breakdown of muscle protein and notes that much more is understood about amino acid metabolism than protein kinetics in muscle. The same observation applies even more to nitrogen metabolism in the gut.

Nearly two decades have passed since establishing that the intestine contributes an important part to the uptake of the glutamine released from muscle and yields alanine for gluconeogenesis in the liver (6). After trauma, the splanchnic tissues have been reported to take up more glutamine. This increased uptake has been hypothesized to regulate the production of glutamine in peripheral tissues. Souba et al. (7) have postulated that after trauma the gut mucosa requires more glutamine, that a relative lack of glutamine might induce villous atrophy, and that such changes might cause increased permeability leading to translocation of endotoxin or bacteria.

Previous studies of substrate flux across splanchnic tissues have not distinguished between the intestine and the spleen. Dr. Soeters and Deutz (Chapter 13) have presented new evidence on the role of glutamine in the gut after trauma. Catheterization studies in the pig allowed the flux of metabolites to be measured separately across the spleen and across the portal drained viscera. Their data indicate that the gut demand for glutamine does not increase after trauma in this model and that the gut does not signal muscle to increase glutamine release after trauma. Their data also indicate that the spleen has an increase in glutamine uptake after trauma, which they attribute to the increased requirements of activated white cells.

Drs. Molina and Abumrad (Chapter 4) bring new attention to the nitrogen metabolism of the intestine, studying the effect of hypoglycemia in chronically catheterized dogs. Acute hypoglycemia is found to result in gut proteolysis as evidenced by leucine release. This is shown to be a brain response by selective catheterization, however the mediators of this response are not known and which part of the gut wall is responding with proteolysis remains to be elucidated.

Short-chain Fatty Acids

The short-chain fatty acids (SCFAs) are essential for the metabolism of the colonocytes and also may regulate the colonic microflora. The three principal SCFAs (acetate, N-butyrate, and propionate) increase colonocyte proliferation, stimulate mucosal growth, enhance blood flow, and improve energy metabolism. Of these, butyrate appears to be of greatest importance and is preferentially oxidized by normal colonocytes when compared with glucose, glutamine, and ketone bodies. Butyrate is not synthesized by mammalian tissue, thus the colonic mucosa can obtain it only from bacterial fermentation, which is predominantly from dietary fiber and undigested starch.

Butyrate deficiency may lead to decreased absorption, diminished lipid synthesis, reduced mucus production, and impaired detoxification mechanisms in the colon. Theoretically, these factors could each contribute to loss of mucosal barrier function in the critically ill patient.

Hormonal Effects on Metabolism

Drs. Matthews and Battezzati (Chapter 1) review the role of insulin versus the catabolic hormones, noting the rapidity of onset of hormone effects. Catecholamines will cause metabolic changes in seconds, while insulin and glucagon produce metabolic effects in minutes, while growth hormone and cortisol have effects that require 6 to 12 hours to become evident. They note that proteolysis was seen too soon with combined hormone infusions in normal humans for the effect to be due to cortisol alone.

Growth hormone infusions in humans increase protein synthesis without changing rates of proteolysis, while IGF-1 and insulin decrease proteolysis. Growth hormone induces glucose intolerance and increased lipolysis. Whether it can be used as therapy in the future to ameliorate the protein breakdown of cortisol remains to be studied.

Drs. Carlson and Little (Chapter 3) summarize the evidence for possible mechanisms of insulin resistance in sepsis and injury. The normal anabolic actions of insulin are impaired in the setting of hypermetabolism, with increased gluconeogenesis at a time of increased availability of glucose, lipid, and amino acids.

Fong et al. (8) emphasized that epinephrine, either alone or together with cortisol, did not produce acute loss of nitrogen from the extremity. Epinephrine infusions did produce an acute decrease in plasma amino acids. Cortisol was considered to play the major role in insulin resistance. Hormonal changes in glucose and fat metabolism are nearly always greater in magnitude than what is seen in protein metabolism. Insulin infusion produced a more than 200% increase in glucose disposal compared with a suppression of proteolysis of only approximately 25%.

"Conditionally Essential" Nutrients

Dr. Grimble (Chapter 14) presented a provocative discussion of the current semantic problem concerning certain nutrients, which have been designated as "conditionally essential." He has approached the subject of conditionally essential nutrients by emphasizing that for a nutrient to qualify, a deficiency of the nutrient must cause a growth limitation, a negative nitrogen balance, organ dysfunction, delayed recovery, or metabolic abnormalities. Such changes should be demonstrable in healthy subjects, a variety of patients, and in experimental models, regardless of species.

Dr. Grimble challenges glutamine as conditionally essential on the basis that its action in the catabolic patient can be produced by other metabolically related substrates, such as ornithine and ornithine-ketoglutarate, which have never been considered nutrients. He notes that nitrogen homeostasis is dependent on acid-base balance and that metabolic acidosis produces a similar change in urinary nitrogen excretion as the combined infusion of glucagon, cortisol, and epinephrine in normal humans, or after surgical injury. Each of these conditions causes a decrease in glutamine concentration in plasma and in skeletal muscle. It is proposed that the alteration in glutamine metabolism is a consequence of transient acidosis, which accompanies stress states. This view of glutamine metabolism has certain consequences. The nitrogen balance of the early postoperative period is not suitable for demonstrating the conditional essentiality of glutamine or any other amino acid. The metabolism associated with metabolic acidosis accounts for several different metabolites having the same effect on nitrogen balance. In addition, urea can diffuse into the gut lumen and be hydrolyzed to provide ammonia, which is reincorporated into the general amino acid pool.

Whatever the therapeutic mode of action of arginine in stimulating responsiveness of human lymphocytes to mitogens after trauma, it does not relate to any question of essentiality because the same effect can be seen in healthy adult volunteers.

Purine and pyrimidine requirements are difficult to define. The obvious capacity for *de novo* synthesis argues against essentiality. However, it is noted that in a catabolic state, it might be useful to provide dietary nucleotides on the grounds that prior nutrient intake had not produced a full expression of the enzymes of the *de novo* pathway.

Short-chain fatty acids are the only nutrients that are considered as essential on the grounds that organ function is impaired by their absence. Butyrate is a central fuel for the colonic mucosa, and there is no alternative pathway for butyrate synthesis apart from that provided by colonic luminal bacteria.

THE GUT AS AN IMMUNE ORGAN

The adaptive significance of the intestinal immune system relates to serving as the first line of defense against foreign invasion at a strategic interface between the body and the outside world. The digestive tract contains an extensive immune system with a total number of immune cells equal to the number found in the entire rest of the body (8). Immune reactions of the gut may be divided into immunoglobulins, white blood cells, and inflammatory mediators. The gut-associated lymphoid tissue (GALT) is separate and distinct from the systemic immune system. Dr. Ferguson and colleagues (Chapter 11) emphasize that much of the research on GALT has been conducted in mice and that clinical studies of the physiology and regulation of human GALT are greatly needed.

The lymphocyte traffic routes assume importance because mature lymphocytes recirculate continuously between the blood and lymphoid organs. Lymphocytes are thought to freely migrate through different organs until they are activated by an encounter with antigen, which determines where they will ultimately migrate (9). This cellular movement has lead to the concept of a common mucosal immune system.

In the gut, the lymphocytes differentiate in Peyer's patches, drain into the intestinal lymphatics, pass via the mesenteric nodes, and enter the thoracic duct and the systemic circulation. Finally, they will leave the blood at mucosal sites, distributing cells sensitized at one mucosal surface to other mucosal sites (10). When entering the intestinal area, most B cells localize in the lamina propria where they further proliferate and differentiate. In contrast, many T cells migrate further into the intestinal epithelium. Luminal antigens are thought to determine the magnitude of the epithelial migration. Castro (11) has reviewed the evidence that gut epithelium, as a secretor of IgA and as an antigen processor and T-cell regulator, functions in the afferent and efferent arms of the mucosal immune system, suggesting that GALT might also be called the gut-associated lymphoepithelial tissue.

Exposure of the gut to foreign antigens in food or organisms sensitizes the enteric mucosal immune system. When this occurs, a second exposure to the same antigen triggers predictable cooperative activity of the intestinal effector systems. Integrative activity of the musculature, mucosa, and intramural blood circulation results in organized behavior of the whole organ, resulting in expulsion of the offending antigen. Signalling between the enteric immune system and the enteric minibrain initiates this behavior (9).

An alteration of GALT function has been observed with protein-calorie malnutrition (PCM), vitamin A deficiency, and glutamine deprivation. Protein-calorie malnutrition alters the return of stimulated lymphocytes from within mesenteric lymph nodes to the intestine. Lymphocytes from animals suffering from both PCM and vitamin A deficiencies travel to the intestine in even fewer numbers than are seen with malnutrition alone (12).

Dr. Ferguson and colleagues (Chapter 11) emphasize that measurement of systemic immune function on antibodies, cells, or mediators in the blood are virtually useless as indices of mucosal immunity at the gut level. Likewise, clinical studies on fecal extracts may be misleading for many reasons. Therefore, whole-gut lavage with a nonabsorbable solution can provide biochemical and immunochemical assays of gut function that are not otherwise available. Dr. Cynober (Chapter 12) observed that 70% to 80% of all immunoglobulin-producing cells are located in the intestinal mucosa. Evidence has been presented by Dr. Ferguson for a new human immunodeficiency state, that of intestinal IgA deficiency. A vital question is whether patients with sepsis syndrome or multiorgan failure have adequate intestinal mucosal antibody production.

In recent years, the whole concept of neuroimmune regulation has come to the fore. The intestine is characterized by a large lymphoid mass and a large neural component. Furness and Costa (13) have calculated that there are as many nerve cell bodies in the GI tract as are found in the spinal cord. This innervation is recognized as a specialized third division of the autonomic nervous system and is referred to as the enteric nervous system. There is growing evidence for direct communication between neural elements and immune cells. As with the central nervous system, the enteric nervous system is an independently functional system that works like a little brain (9). The neurons of the enteric minibrain consist of sensory neurons, interneurons, and motorneurons that are synaptically connected into microcircuits. These neural networks process information locally and are responsible for programming the digestive function of the specialized regions found along the digestive tract. There are submucosal microcircuits that program mucosal secretion, absorption, and local blood flow. The enteric minibrain not only determines the activity of these separate effector systems but also coordinates the behavior of each part to ensure normal physiologic behavior at the level of the integrated organ system.

Nerves and neuropeptides, such as substance P, have been shown to affect a variety of gut immune functions in vivo and/or in vitro (14). Nerves and mast cells are known to interact in neurogenic inflammation. When a pain stimulus is transmitted via pain sensory receptors, local communication with mast cells may occur and mediators are released which stimulate nerves and thus amplify the original signal.

Dr. Colten (Chapter 7) reviews the role of complement protein synthesis in establishing tissue-specific regulation of inflammation. Tissue injury or infection elicits changes in expression of these acute phase proteins by an elaborate system of cell-to-cell communication mediated by a complex network of cytokines. Dr. Hechtman (Chapter 20) has reviewed the activation of complement factors leading to the adhesion of polymorphonuclear cells to endothelial cells. A review by Brandtzaeg et al. (15) emphasizes the central role of complement activation in the intestinal immune response and its possible role in bowel inflammation. An important source of information concerning the central importance of the intestine in a chronic generalized immune response comes from the study of graft-vs.-host disease.

Graft-versus-Host Disease

The enteropathy caused by acute graft-versus-host disease (GVH) is an important clinical problem in patients receiving allogeneic bone marrow transplants. Intestinal damage is also a common feature of most animals models of GVH disease (16). Graft-versus-host disease is a systemic immunologic disorder that occurs after transfer of immunocompetent T lymphocytes into a genetically disparate, immunoincompetent host. The earliest description came from Billingham et al. (17) in which the majority of newborn mice given allogeneic lymphocytes developed a wasting disease characterized by weight loss, skin lesions, and diarrhea.

The intestine is particularly susceptible to the effector mechanisms of GVH disease, producing diarrhea, malabsorption, and protein-losing enteropathy. Crypt cells are the principal targets of intestinal GVH disease (16). Initial increased crypt cell proliferation, migration, and differentiation is followed by cessation of crypt cell mitotic activity and crypt necrosis with the onset of villous atrophy. A depletion of mucosal lymphoid cells is followed by mucosal invasion of T lymphocytes preceding obvious mucosal damage. Gut-associated lymphoid tissue shows a similar biphasic pattern of damage from early T-cell lymphoblast infiltration to depletion of all cell types. The depletion of local lymphoid cells in established GVH disease is associated with mucosal immunodeficiency, which is manifested by reduced levels of both secretory and serum IgA levels. Total secretory IgA responses may be increased early in murine GVH disease before later reduction. Mucosal lymphocytes isolated from mice with acute GVH disease produce several cytokines, including IL-2, IL-3, and interferon-g (IFN-g), while acute GVH disease in mice and humans is associated with increased levels of TNF-a in serum. Interferon-g may be important for initiating the early proliferating phase and TNF-a being responsible for the later, destructive lesions.

An additional way in which cytokines could damage the gut directly is by interfering with the function of mesenchymal cells such as endothelial cells and fibroblasts. Both of these cell types are known to be targets for cytokines such as TNF-a, and mesenchymal function is essential for maintenance of normal mucosal architecture. The intestinal crypt abscess is a characteristic lesion of acute intestinal inflammation (18). Pericryptal fibroblasts seem particularly likely to be important intermediate targets of cytokine effects, and their involvement could include production of further inflammatory mediators.

THE INTESTINE AND INFLAMMATORY STATES

Gut Perfusion and Absorption in Sepsis

Mucosal ischemia, ulceration, inflammation, and increased intestinal permeability have all been reported in septic patients. Sympathetic nervous stimulation can evoke a redistribution of blood flow within the wall of the gut such that mucosal perfusion diminishes and muscular blood flow increases about equally. The result is that enterocytes may become necrotic at the tips of the intestinal villi, while there is angiographic evidence of normal blood flow in the superior mesenteric artery. Small intestinal ischemia has been associated with experimental bacteria and endotoxemia. Morphologic changes in the intestine are a common feature after endotoxin injection. Sepsis may also diminish intestinal function by the release of oxygen-free radicals, cytokines, platelet activating factor (PAF), or thromboxane A2. Intravenous injection of PAF produces macroscopic and microscopic intestinal changes similar to those produced after endotoxin administration.

Horton and Walker (19) have developed a model of temporary occlusion of the superior mesenteric artery in the rat in which to study the role of intestinal hypoperfusion. Hypoxanthine is known to accumulate during intestinal ischemia and catalyze the production of toxic oxygen metabolites via xanthine oxidase promoting lipid peroxidation of cell membranes. An alternate source of damage is from endotoxin activation of neutrophils with the release of reactive oxygen species.

Singh and coworkers (20) have demonstrated that the loss of gut absorptive capacity following a standardized experimental hemorrhage is reversed by the administration of heparan sulfate. These investigators propose that the benefit is due to an unexplained improvement in the microcirculation of the gut that is unrelated to any anticoagulant effect.

Activities of various enzymes within the enterocyte are reduced in sepsis with evidence that the mucosal barrier is impaired, and translocation of enteric bacteria may occur. Gardiner and Barbul (21) have noted that during sepsis, anorexia results in decreased dietary intake of amino acids at a time when demand is increased because of insulin resistance, leukocyte activity, and acute-phase protein synthesis. These authors demonstrated the in vivo decreases in intestinal disappearance and circulatory appearance of arginine, leucine, proline, and α-aminoisobutyric acid within 24 hours after induction of peritoneal sepsis in the rat. Diminished amino acid absorption after sepsis was also demonstrated by using in vitro everted gut sacs. Such studies emphasize the potential advantages of enteral feeding when compared with parenteral feeding.

A reduction in the number or affinity of transport proteins of the enterocyte has been suggested during sepsis (21). It has also been proposed that there may be a reprioritization of protein synthesis by the enterocyte similar to that occurring in the hepatocyte during sepsis. These ideas have led to the suggestion that during sepsis, the enterocyte may undergo a redirection of available energy and substrates toward more acute synthetic needs at the expense of the synthesis of transporter proteins. This could lead to a vicious cycle of reduced transporter proteins, less substrate absorption, further decrease in intracellular availability of substrate, and declining protein synthesis. This could be aggravated by reduced microcirculatory flow to the enterocyte.

There is good evidence to suggest that T-cell–mediated immune reactions can cause gut damage (22). Activated T cells that secrete lymphokines are seen in increased numbers in the lamina propria and among intraepithelial T lymphocytes of such diverse conditions as coeliac disease, cows milk protein intolerance, and inflammatory bowel disease. An important question in current immunology is whether these T lymphocytes are of primary importance in mediating intestinal damage or merely a secondary phenomenon.

Stress, Cytokines, and Systemic Inflammatory Response Syndrome

Cuthbertson (23) divided the metabolic response to injury into an early "ebb" phase requiring circulatory support followed by a "flow" phase associated with hypermetabolism and a negative nitrogen balance. This general metabolic response was often attributed to either injury or sepsis. It now appears that the term "systemic inflammatory response syndrome" may represent a more specific nomenclature to describe the events when sepsis is involved. The most severe form of SIRS is the shock syndrome associated with gram-negative bacteremia, but patients with less severe or noninfectious forms of the syndrome may benefit from the same therapies. Certain cytokines stimulate endothelial cells from their normal anticoagulant state to a procoagulant state with increased adhesiveness for leukocytes and platelets.

Dinarello and coworkers (24) have summarized current evidence concerning the role of cytokines in SIRS. They consider the syndrome as a generalized activation of the endothelium that can lead to septic shock in its most severe form. They suggest that IL-1 and TNF stimulate platelet-activating factor, prostaglandin F, and nitric oxide synthesis, which causes vasodilation and hypotension. This is associated with poor organ perfused, acidosis, and organ failure. Interleukin-1 and TNF stimulate the synthesis of endothelial adhesion molecules, which facilitate the adherence of neutrophils to the endothelial surface. These adhesion molecules are discussed by Dr. Hechtman (Chapter 20) and by Dr. Cerra (Chapter 23). The cytokines also induce interleukin-8 production from the endothelium, which attracts neutrophils that are adhering to the endothelial surface to emigrate into the extravascular space where tissue is damaged by the released enzymes and oxygen-free radicals. New understanding of the role of the proinflammatory cytokines in producing endothelial cell activation in the intestine, appears to depend on developing the ability to grow endothelial cells from the gut in culture.

Translocation Revisited

A single layer of cells on the intestinal mucosa separates the external environment from the interior of the body. The maintenance of this balance across the intestinal wall depends on the integration of a variety of immunologic processes involving the epithelial cell layer, the natural gut flora, and the intestinal immune cells. Translocation has been reported to occur from either direct injury to enterocytes, reduced mucosal blood flow, or increased numbers of bacteria or fungi in the lumen. Patients with critical illness are prime candidates for translocation because they often have conditions that are associated with underperfusion of the intestine, while frequently receiving antibiotics that cause bacterial overgrowth in the intestine. These reports have lead to new enthusiasm for early enteral nutrition following injury, particularly for the major burn where experimental evidence has indicated that the expected hypermetabolism and loss of intestinal mass could be inhibited by prompt enteral nutrition (25).

Fong et al. (26) reported a study in normal male subjects in which it was shown that endotoxin injections caused enhanced counterregulatory hormones and splanchnic cytokine responses after 7 days of TPN when compared with the same interval of enteral nutrition. This study provides additional evidence that the intestinal tract is an important site for the immune and metabolic processes that interact to support normal homeostasis.

The route and the timing of nutrition may influence the metabolic response to both injury and disease. However, Eyer et al. (27) have reported that starting aggressive enteral feeding within 24 hours after major blunt trauma offered no advantage in terms of biochemical measurements of the stress response or any improvement in patient outcome.

Most clinical attention to the possibility of translocation has centered on conditions in which the enterocyte might be damaged from altered mucosal blood flow, such as in major burns (28). However St. John and coworkers (29) studied acid-induced lung injury in cats and demonstrated acute permeability changes in the intestine that could be prevented by pretreatment with antileukocyte adherence antibody. Thus, acute structural and functional changes can occur in the intestine via leukocyte effects as a result of distant damage to an organ such as the lungs.

Despite the broad clinical interest in translocation, both Drs. Rombeau and Ferguson have suggested in their chapters that caution is needed regarding any conclusion that translocation plays a central role in most clinical sepsis, noting that much of the evidence to date is from selected animal studies.

The function of the intestinal tract in the critically ill patient appears to be highly variable, presumably as a result of factors that are only slowly being recognized and remain difficult to measure. New information is being sought that can be expected to greatly expand our understanding of two separate aspects of intestinal function. One aspect is the unique perfusion, metabolism, and nutrition of the enterocyte and how each of these may contribute to mucosal atrophy. This new information will enlarge our understanding of the role of specific nutrients for the gut and whether they can be made as effective when given by the parenteral as the enteral route. The other large aspect of intestinal function relates to appreciation of the gut as an immune organ and how enteric immune mechanisms may play important roles in SIRS. This new knowledge is most important in order to establish the true incidence of translocation in critical illness and, therefore, the most effective therapeutic program for preventing its occurrence and specific approaches to counteract its effects when it does occur.

REFERENCES

1. Sitzmann JV, Pitt HA, The Patient Care Committee of the American Gastroenterological Association. Statement on guidelines for total parenteral nutrition. *Dig Dis Sci* 1989;34:489–496.
2. Jacobson ED. The splanchnic circulation. In: Johnson LR, ed. *Gastrointestinal Physiology*. 4th ed. St. Louis: Mosby Year Book, 1991;142–161.
3. Caspary WF. Physiology and pathophysiology of intestinal absorption. *Am J Clin Nutr* 1992;55:299S–308S.
4. Darnell J, Lodish H, Baltimore D. *Molecular Cell Biology*. 2nd ed. New York: American Scientific Books, 1990;521.
5. Barbul A. Arginine: biochemistry, physiology and therapeutic implications. *JPEN* 1986;10:227–238.
6. Felig P. Amino acid metabolism in man. *Annu Rev Biochem* 1975;44:933.
7. Souba W, Klimberg V, Plumley D, et al. The role of glutamine in maintaining a healthy gut and supporting the metabolic response to injury and infection. *J Surg Res* 1990;48:383–391.
8. Fong Y, Albert JD, Tracey K, et al. The influence of substrate background on the acute metabolic response to epinephrine and cortisol. *J Trauma* 1991;31:1467–1476.
9. Wood JD. Enteric neuroimmune interactions. In: Walker WA, Harmatz PR, Wershil BK, eds. *Immunophysiology of the Gut*. San Diego: Academic Press, 1993;207–227.
10. Salami M, Jalkanen S. Molecular basis of cell migration into normal and inflamed gut. In: MacDonald TT, ed. *Immunology of Gastrointestinal Disease*. Dordrecht, The Netherlands: Kluwer Academic Publishers, 1992;151–171.
11. Castro GA. Immunological regulation of epithelial function. In: Walker WA, Harmatz PR, Wershil BK, eds. *Immunophysiology of the Gut*. San Diego: Academic Press, 1993;7–23.

12. Langkamp-Henken B, Glezer JA, Kudsk KA. Immunologic structure and function of the gastrointestinal tract. *Nutr Clin Pract* 1992;7:100–108.
13. Furness JB, Costa M. Types of nerves in the enteric nervous system. *Neuroscience* 1980;5:1–20.
14. Bienenstock J. Neuroimmune interactions in the regulation of mucosal immunity. In: Walker WA, Harmatz PR, Wershil BK, eds. *Immunophysiology of the Gut*. San Diego: Academic Press, 1993; 171–181.
15. Brandtzaeg P, Halstenen TS, Helgeland L, Kett K. The mucosal immune system in inflammatory bowel disease. In: MacDonald TT, ed. *Immunology of Gastrointestinal Disease*. Dordrecht, The Netherlands: Kluwer Academic Publishers, 1992;19–39.
16. Mowat A.Mcl. Intestinal graft-versus-host disease. In: MacDonald TT, ed. *Immunology of Gastrointestinal Disease*. Dordrecht, The Netherlands: Kluwer Academic Publishers, 1992;105–136.
17. Billingham RE, Brent L, Medawar PB. Acquired tolerance of skin homografts. *Ann NY Acad Sci* 1955;59:409–498.
18. Madara JL, Nash S, Parkos C. Modeling the intestinal crypt abscess—A Characteristic lesion of acute intestinal inflammation. In: Walker WA, Harmatz PR, Wershil BK, eds. *Immunophysiology of the Gut*. San Diego: Academic Press, 1993;119–127.
19. Horton JW, Walker PB. Oxygen radicals, lipid peroxidation, and permeability changes after intestinal ischemia and reperfusion. *J Appl Physiol* 1993;74(4):1515–1520.
20. Singh G, Chaudry KI, Chaudry IH. Restoration of gut absorptive capacity following trauma-hemorrhagic shock by the adjuvant use of heparan sulfate. *J Trauma* 1993;34:645–652.
21. Gardiner K, Barbul A. Intestinal amino acid absorption during sepsis. *J Parenter Enterol Nutr* 1991; 17:277–283.
22. James SP, Zeitz M, Mullin GE, Braun-Elwert L. Role of lymphokines in function of gastrointestinal mucosal T cells. In: Walker WA, Harmatz PR, Wershil BK, eds. *Immunophysiology of the Gut*. San Diego: Academic Press, 1993;129–143.
23. Cuthbertson DP. Post-shock metabolic response. *Lancet* 1942;i:433–437.
24. Dinarello CA, Gelfand JA, Wolff SM. Anticytokine strategies in the treatment of the systemic inflammatory response syndrome. *JAMA* 1993;269:1829–1835.
25. Cerra FB. Nutrient modulation of inflammatory and immune function. *Am J Surg* 1991;161:230.
26. Fong Y, Marano MA, Barber A, et al. Total parenteral nutrition and bowel rest modify the metabolic response to endotoxin in humans. *Ann Surg* 1989;210:193–201.
27. Eyer SD, Micon LT, Konstantinides FN, et al. Early enteral feeding does not attenuate metabolic response after blunt trauma. *J Trauma* 1993;34:639–644.
28. Tokyay R, Zeigler ST, Traber DL, et al. Postburn gastrointestinal vasoconstriction increases bacterial and endotoxin translocation. *J Appl Physiol* 1993;74(4):1521–1527.
29. St. John RC, Mizer LA, Kindt GC, et al. Acid aspiration-induced acute lung injury causes leukocyte-dependent systemic organ injury. *J Appl Physiol* 1993;74(4):1994–2003.

Organ Metabolism and Nutrition:
Ideas for Future Critical Care, edited by
J. M. Kinney and H. N. Tucker.
Raven Press, Ltd., New York © 1994.

15

Glutamine and Hepatic Metabolism

Dieter Häussinger

Department of Internal Medicine, The University of Freiburg, D-79106 Freiburg, Germany

The early work of Hans Krebs identified the liver as having a particular role not only in urea synthesis, but also in glutamine metabolism, thereby already emphasizing the different properties of hepatic and renal glutaminases, respectively (1). Much effort has been devoted since then to the understanding of glutamine metabolism in the liver and its relation to ammonia and acid-base homeostasis (for reviews, see refs. 2,3). A fundamental conceptional change in the field of hepatic glutamine metabolism was derived from the understanding of the unique regulatory properties of liver glutaminase, the discovery of hepatocyte heterogeneities in nitrogen metabolism with metabolic interactions between differently localized subacinar hepatocyte populations, and the role of an intercellular cycling of glutamine in the liver acinus for the maintenance of ammonia and bicarbonate homeostasis. Another important aspect of glutamine and hepatic metabolism arose from the finding that the concentrative uptake of glutamine into liver cells induces an increase of the hepatocellular hydratation state, which in turn triggers a variety of metabolic hepatocellular functions, even those that are unrelated to glutamine metabolism, such as protein turnover or transcellular bile acid transport. Thus, the glutamine transporting system N in the hepatocyte plasma membrane acts like a signaling system that regulates hepatocellular function. This chapter briefly reviews some modern aspects of hepatic glutamine metabolism and its functional implications. The reader is referred to more extensive reviews (2–4).

STRUCTURAL AND FUNCTIONAL ORGANIZATION OF HEPATIC GLUTAMINE METABOLISM

Hepatocyte Heterogeneity in Glutamine Metabolism

In the liver acinus, periportal (at the sinusoidal inflow) and perivenous (at the sinusoidal outflow) hepatocytes differ in their enzyme equipment and metabolic function. This functional hepatocyte heterogeneity is remarkably developed with respect to ammonium and glutamine metabolism. The enzymes of the urea cycle and glutaminase are present in periportal hepatocytes, whereas glutamine synthetase is found only in perivenous hepatocytes. This was shown in metabolic flux studies (5), in experiments on zonal cell damage (6), by immunohistochemistry (7–9), in situ hybridization (10,11), and more recently with hepatocyte preparations enriched in periportal and perivenous cells (12). The borderline between the periportal urea-synthesizing compartment and the perivenous glutamine-synthesizing compartment is rather strict: Glutamine synthetase is exclusively found in a small hepatocyte population (about 6% to 7% of all hepatocytes of an acinus) surrounding the terminal hepatic venules at the outflow of the sinusoidal bed (so-called scavenger cells). These scavenger cells are virtually free of urea cycle enzymes and exhibit remarkable transport features compared to periportal hepatocytes. Evidence has been presented that vascular glutamate, aspartate, α-ketoglutarate, malate, and related dicarboxylates are almost exclusively taken up by scavenger cells, where they can serve as precursors for glutamine synthesis (13–15). On the other hand, uptake of these compounds does not occur into periportal cells under the conditions yet studied. Whereas glutaminase and glutamine synthetase are heterogeneously distributed in the liver acinus, glutamine transaminases are present in the periportal as well as in the perivenous area of the acinus (16).

Glutamine Synthetase as an Ammonia Scavenger

Several functional implications arise from the reciprocal acinar distribution of the two ammonia detoxication systems, urea and glutamine synthesis. The sinusoidal blood stream first contacts cells capable of urea synthesis before the glutamine-synthesizing compartment is reached. In the intact perfused rat liver, the affinity of urea synthesis for ammonium ions is lower than that of glutamine synthesis, with $K_{0.5}$ values of about 0.6 and 0.1 mM, respectively; ie., similar to the differences in the $K_m(NH_4^+)$ values for isolated carbamoylphosphate synthetase and glutamine synthetase. This may explain why detoxication of a physiologic portal ammonia load in the isolated perfused rat liver occurs by about two thirds through urea synthesis and by about one third through glutamine synthesis, although the urea cycle capacity is by far not exceeded under these conditions. From a structural-functional point of view, urea and glutamine synthesis represent in the intact liver acinus the sequence of a periportal low-affinity, but high-capacity system (urea synthesis) and a perivenous high-affinity system (glutamine synthesis) for ammonia detoxication (5). The role of perivenous glutamine synthetase is that of a scavenger for the ammonia that escaped periportal urea synthesis, before the sinusoidal blood stream enters the systemic circulation (4). The importance of this scavenger function for ammonia homeostasis is underlined by the finding that efficient hepatic ammonia extraction at physiologically low ammonia concentrations requires an intact glutamine synthetase activity: After destruction of the perivenous area by CCl_4 treatment, glutamine synthesis is virtually abolished and hyperammonemia ensues, although, simultaneously, periportal urea synthesis is not affected (6). An impairment of perivenous glutamine synthesis is also an important pathogenetic factor for the development of hyperammonemia in cirrhotic humans; here a scavenger cell defect has been demonstrated with an 80% decrease of the capacity to synthesize glutamine (17). A considerable fraction of the ammonia generated during the breakdown of amino acids in the periportal hepatocytes is released into the sinusoidal space, despite the high urea cycle enzyme activity in this compartment. These ammonium ions, however, are taken up by perivenous hepatocytes and utilized there for glutamine synthesis (6). This not only demonstrates metabolic interactions between different subacinar hepatocyte populations (ammonia flow from periportal to perivenous hepatocytes), but also underlines the comparatively low affinity of periportal urea synthesis for ammonia. The structural and functional organization of the ammonia-detoxicating pathways in the liver acinus also implies that with a constant ammonia supply via the portal vein, flux through the urea cycle in the whole periportal compartment will determine the amount of NH_4^+ reaching perivenous hepatocytes, thereby setting the substrate (ammonia) supply for perivenous glutamine synthetase. Accordingly, all factors regulating urea cycle flux will indirectly exert control on the more downstream-located hepatic glutamine synthetase. This is of special importance, for example, in metabolic acidosis. Under these conditions, periportal urea synthesis is switched off in order to spare bicarbonate (for regulatory and mechanistic details, see refs. 3,18) and ammonia is increasingly delivered to the perivenous hepatocytes. Here, ammonia homeostasis is maintained by an increased glutamine synthesis ("ammonia scavenging") (3,18). Thus, the structural and functional acinar organization of the ammonia-detoxicating pathways, including the scavenger role of perivenous glutamine synthetase, allows modulation of urea synthesis (for example, according to the requirements of acid-base homeostasis) without the threat of hyperammonemia.

Hepatic Glutaminase: Properties and Amplifier Function

Phosphate-dependent glutaminase (in the following, referred to as glutaminase) is the major glutamine-degrading enzyme in the liver. It has a joint localization together with carbamoylphosphate synthetase I inside the mitochondria of the periportal hepatocytes. The enzyme is both immunologically and kinetically different from kidney glutaminase (for reviews, see ref. 19). Liver glutaminase is not inhibited by its product glutamate (1), but requires its other product, ammonia, as an essential and obligatory activator, features clearly differing from those of the kidney enzyme. In the absence of ammonia, the enzyme is virtually inactive (20). In the intact liver, half-maximal and maximal activation of glutaminase is observed with ammonia concentrations of 0.2 and 0.6 mM, respectively, indicating that the portal ammonia concentration within physiologic limits is an important regulator of hepatic glutamine breakdown (21,22). Regarding the gut-liver axis, intestinal ammonia production was soon recognized as an important signal for glutamine degradation in the liver (the so-called interorgan feed-forward activation [21]). Flux through hepatic glutaminase is very sensitive to small pH changes with inhibition at low pH (18,20,22–24), due to a diminished ammonia activation of the enzyme (22,23) and an inhibition of glutamine transport across the plasma and mitochondrial membrane, resulting in a decreased mitochondrial steady-state concentration of glutamine (24). The pH-sensitivity of hepatic glutaminase markedly differs from the kidney enzyme: Whereas kidney glutaminase is activated in acidosis, the liver enzyme is inhibited and an inverse regulatory pattern for both enzymes is found in alkalosis.

Flux through hepatic glutaminase is an important factor regulating urea cycle flux (4) because of its structural and functional link to the first enzyme of the urea cycle, i.e., carbamoylphosphate synthetase. This occurs at the level of ammonia provision inside the mitochondria for carbamoylphosphate synthesis, the rate-controlling step of the urea cycle (25) with its K_m(ammonia) far above the physiologic ammonia concentrations (26). The unique regulatory properties of glutaminase (i.e., activation by its product ammonia and pH sensitivity) enable this enzyme to function as a pH- and hormone-modulated ammonia amplifying system (3) inside the mitochondria (Fig. 1). This amplification allows the urea cycle to operate efficiently even at physiologically low portal ammonia concentrations, otherwise impossible in view of the high K_M(ammonia) of carbamoylphosphate synthetase: Ammonia is generated from glutamine inside the mitochondria in parallel to the ammonia delivered via the portal vein (4). Accordingly, a comparatively high urea cycle flux, despite the low ammonia affinity of carbamoylphosphate synthetase, can be maintained physiologically. In perfused rat liver and with physiologic portal ammonia and glutamine concentrations, up to 30% of the urea produced is due to intramitochondrial ammonia formation by periportal glutamine breakdown. In addition, some evidence for a direct channeling of glutamine-amide–derived nitrogen into carbamoylphosphate synthetase has been presented (27). The outstanding role of glutamine as a substrate for ureogenesis is also underlined by the finding that glutamine-derived nitrogen, in contrast to portal ammonia, is incorporated into urea without requirement of a mitochondrial carbonic anhydrase (28). A further increase in the efficiency of delivery of glutamine-derived ammonia into carbamoylphosphate synthetase is obtained by the fact that N-acetylglutamate stimulates glutaminase as well as carbamoylphosphate synthetase (29).

The Intercellular Glutamine Cycle

In the intact liver acinus, periportal glutaminase and perivenous glutamine synthetase are simultaneously active (4,21,22), resulting in an intercellular glutamine cycle (4) with periportal glutamine consumption and perivenous resynthesis of glutamine. Intercellular glutamine cycling also occurs in vivo (30,31) and the flux through both enzymes underlies a complex regulation (by hormones, pH, ammonia, and glutamine concentrations; see ref. 22), resulting in either a net glutamine uptake or release by the liver or no net glutamine turnover at all, depending on experimental and nutritional conditions. In the special case of a well-balanced pH situation, intercellular glutamine

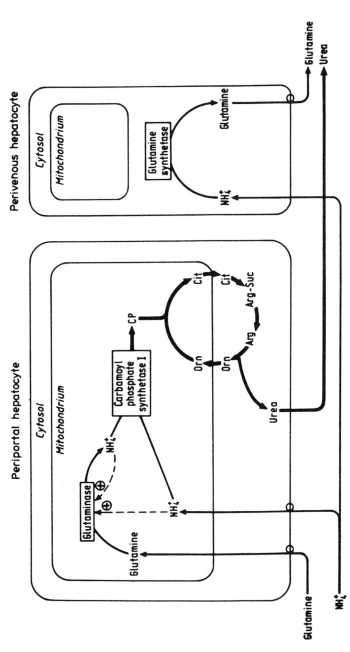

FIG. 1. Functional hepatocyte heterogeneity in glutamine and ammonia metabolism: the intercellular glutamine cycle. Periportal glutamine breakdown by ammonia-activated glutaminase (GlNase) increases flux through the urea cycle by amplifying the mitochondrial ammonia supply for carbamoylphosphate synthetase (CPS). Periportally consumed glutamine is resynthesized perivenously from the ammonia that escaped periportal urea synthesis (low affinity system for ammonia detoxication). With a well-balanced acid-base, status flux through glutaminase matches glutamine synthetase flux (intercellular glutamine cycling); there is no net turnover of glutamine; however, portal ammonia is completely converted into urea despite the low affinity of CPS for ammonia. Perivenous glutamine synthetase (GS) acts as a scavenger for ammonia at the sinusoidal outflow and allows modulation of urea cycle flux without threat of hyperammonemia. Periportal glutaminase acts as a pH- and hormone-modulated ammonia amplifier, thereby adjusting urea cycle flux (as well as other mechanisms, which were omitted from the scheme for clarity) according to the requirements of the hormonal and acid-base status. From Häussinger (3) with permission.

cycling is an effective means for the complete conversion of portal ammonia into urea (4,18) (for review see ref. 32), and the net glutamine balance across the liver is close to zero. These events, however, include simultaneous glutamine consumption for ammonia amplification in the periportal compartment and glutamine resynthesis by perivenous scavenger cells from the ammonia that escaped the periportal low affinity system urea synthesis: The net effect is a complete conversion of portal ammonia into urea without net glutamine turnover (4). These relationships are schematically depicted in Fig. 1. In line with the important role of intercellular glutamine cycling for effective ammonia detoxication via the urea cycle is also the finding that flux through the intercellular glutamine cycle increases under conditions known to stimulate urea synthesis, such as glucagon treatment or an increase of the portal ammonia load. In acidosis, however, the ammonia amplifier glutaminase is switched off. Accordingly, flux through the urea cycle and periportal glutamine consumption decrease. This results in an increased ammonia delivery to the perivenous glutamine synthesizing cells in a net production of glutamine by the liver (18) and explains the rapid switching of hepatic ammonia detoxication from urea to net glutamine synthesis when the extracellular pH drops (for a detailed description on the role of hepatic nitrogen metabolism in systemic acid-base homeostasis, see ref. 18).

GLUTAMINE TRANSPORT AND CELL VOLUME

Glutamine is transported across the plasma membrane and the inner mitochondrial membrane by specific transport systems (32–36). Glutamine transport across the plasma membrane occurs via system N (33), is Na^+-dependent, and represents another major site of control of hepatic glutamine degradation (35,36). The activity of the transporter is controlled by the acid-base status and the nutritional state (35–37). The Na^+-dependent glutamine transporter can build up intra/extracellular amino acid concentration gradients of up to 20. Na^+ entering the hepatocyte, together with the amino acid, is extruded in exchange for K^+ by the electrogenic Na^+/K^+ ATPase.

The accumulation of glutamine and K^+ into the cells leads to hepatocyte swelling. This increase of the hepatocellular hydratation state in turn triggers a volume regulatory K^+ efflux (38,39). The volume-regulatory mechanisms that are activated during isoosmotic (e.g., cumulative substrate transport-induced) cell swelling are probably identical to those involved in anisoosmotic cell volume regulation (for review, see ref. 40). As illustrated in Fig. 2, addition of glutamine to isolated perfused rat liver creates within about 12 minutes an intra/extracellular glutamine concentration gradient of about 12. During the first 2 minutes of glutamine accumulation, liver mass increases rapidly due to hepatocellular swelling, as validated by measurements of intracellular water space. Hepatic net K^+ uptake during this phase is probably due to extrusion of cotransported Na^+ by Na^+/K^+ ATPase. Thereafter, no further increase in cellular water content is observed, despite continuing accumulation of glutamine inside the cell. This is achieved by a volume-regulatory K^+ efflux from the liver, which occurs until the steady-state intracellular glutamine concentration of

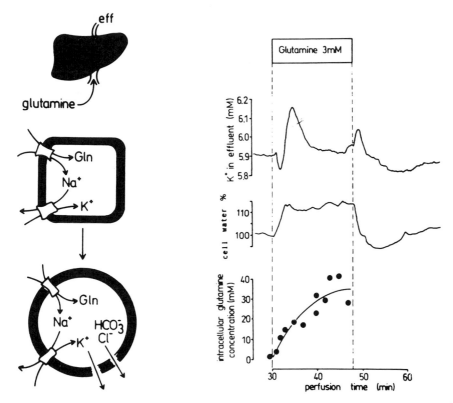

FIG. 2. Effect of glutamine (3 mM) addition to influent perfusate of isolated, single-pass perfused rat liver on intracellular glutamine accumulation, cell volume, and volume-regulatory K$^+$ fluxes. Addition of glutamine to portal perfusate leads to rapid cell swelling due to cumulative, Na$^+$-dependent uptake of glutamine into liver cells. The initial net K$^+$ uptake is explained by exchange of cotransported Na$^+$ against K$^+$ by Na$^+$/K$^+$ ATPase. Glutamine-induced cell swelling during the first 2 minutes of glutamine infusion activates volume regulatory K$^+$ (plus Cl$^-$ and HCO$_3^-$) efflux. This volume-regulatory response prevents further cell swelling, despite continuing glutamine accumulation inside the cell, until a steady-state intracellular glutamine concentration of about 35 mM is reached. However, the liver cell remains in a swollen state as long as glutamine is infused. This degree of cell swelling modifies cellular function. For further details, see Häussinger et al. (38).

about 35 mM is reached (Fig. 2). During the rapid washout of glutamine following its withdrawal from the influent perfusate, the swollen hepatocytes shrink rapidly, as is evident from the respective decrease of liver mass and a secondary volume-regulatory net K$^+$ uptake, which lasts for more than 10 minutes and restores cell volume to the starting level (Fig. 2). It became clear that amino acid-induced cell swelling and volume-regulatory responses occur on exposure to glutamine in the physiologic concentration range. Glutamine-induced cell swelling is half-maximal at a concentration of 0.6 to 0.8 mM, i.e., the concentration normally found in portal venous blood, and is maximal at 2 mM (39). Accordingly, physiologic fluctuations of the portal glutamine concentration are accompanied by parallel alterations of liver cell volume. Cell swelling and volume-regulatory K^+ fluxes were shown not only to occur on addition of glutamine, but also in response to other amino acids that are concentrated inside the liver cells, such as alanine, proline, serine, and glycine (39,41–45). However, in our experience, glutamine turned out to be the amino acid with the highest swelling potency. This may, at least in part, explain why glutamine received much attention in the past as an anabolic compound.

GLUTAMINE-INDUCED CELL SWELLING TRIGGERS CELLULAR FUNCTIONS

In recent years, evidence has accumulated that the hepatocellular hydratation state, i.e., "cell volume" in the present context, is one important determinant of hepatocellular function (4,40,46). Many amino acids, preferably glutamine but also hormones such as insulin and glucagon, can trigger metabolic liver function at least in part by altering the hepatocellular hydratation state (4,46,47). That glutamine-induced cell swelling is responsible for the functional alterations of the cell is evidenced by the fact that many of the glutamine-induced metabolic responses are quantitatively mimicked by equipotent hypoosmotic cell swelling. Several long-known, but mechanistically poorly understood, effects of glutamine that could not be related to its metabolism, such as stimulation of glycogen synthesis (48,49), inhibition of proteolysis (50–54), or a stimulation of amino acid uptake (55), can simply be mimicked by hypoosmotic swelling of hepatocytes just to the extent that the amino acid does (45,56–60). Thus, the aforementioned amino acid effects are probably mediated by glutamine-induced cell swelling. Table 1 lists the effects of glutamine on hepatocellular function, which can, at least in part, be ascribed to a glutamine-induced increase of the hepatocellular hydratation state. When the metabolic pattern triggered by cell swelling is seen as a whole (Table 1), it appears that cell swelling acts like an anabolic

TABLE 1. *Liver cell swelling as an anabolic signal.*

* Stimulation of protein synthesis	* Inhibition of oxidized glutathione (GSSG) efflux
* Inhibition of proteolysis	
* Stimulation of glycogen synthesis	* Stimulation of taurocholate excretion into bile
Inhibition of glycogenolysis and glycolysis	
* Stimulation of amino acid uptake	* Stimulation of pentose phosphate pathway
Stimulation of glutaminase	
* Stimulation of glycine oxidation	* Stimulation of actin polymerization
Stimulation of ketoisocaproate oxidation	* Increased inositol-1,4,5-trisphosphate formation
Stimulation of urea synthesis from amino acids	
Stimulation of sinusoidal glutathione efflux	* Increase of mRNA levels for β-actin and tubulin

The table lists metabolic alterations following hypoosmotic liver cell swelling; (*) denotes effects that have been shown to be induced also by glutamine-induced cell swelling.

proliferative signal for the cell, whereas cellular shrinkage is catabolic and antiproliferative (4,46,47). Apparently, glutamine can set this anabolic signal simply by increasing the hepatocellular hydratation state. It is likely that glutamine-induced swelling also occurs in skeletal muscle, which could explain the repeatedly suggested anabolic actions of glutamine in muscle tissue (61–65). Because the activity of the Na^+-dependent glutamine transport systems in the plasma membrane is now recognized to exert marked effects on cellular function via alterations of the cellular hydratation state, the glutamine transporter in the plasma membrane can no longer be viewed as a simple glutamine-translocating system; instead it acts as transmembrane signaling system, which triggers hepatocellular function via alterations of the hepatocellular hydratation state (4).

As mentioned, hepatic proteolysis is under the control of amino acids and hormones, such as insulin and glucagon, but the underlying mechanisms remain obscure (52). A strict relationship between the changes of the cellular hydratation state induced by these effectors and their effects on proteolysis was recognized (60). This is shown in Fig. 3: Proteolysis is inhibited by cell swelling and stimulated by cell shrinkage. This relationship is maintained regardless of whether cell volume is modified by insulin, glucagon, cAMP, inhibitors of Na-K-2Cl-cotransport, glutamine, glycine, Ba^{2+}, or hypoosmotic exposure. Apparently, the alteration of the cellular hydratation state is the common denominator of all these effectors on proteolysis. Thus, the known antiproteolytic action of glutamine, glycine, or insulin can be mimicked quantitatively simply by swelling the hepatocytes in hypotonic environments to the same extent as these agents do in normotonic media. These findings suggest that glutamine- and hormone-induced cell volume changes are largely responsible for their effects on hepatic proteolysis. In line with this and observations regarding other metabolic pathways (for review, see ref. 23), it was concluded that alterations of the cellular hydratation state under the influence of glutamine and hormones act like a "second messenger" of amino acid and hormone action (19). Amino acids distinct from glutamine or glycine exert their antiproteolytic effect not exclusively via alterations of the cellular hydratation state. For example, in the case of proline, and serine, only 50% of the antiproteolytic action can be explained on the basis of cell volume changes; here apparently other mechanisms come into play. Glutamine-induced cell swelling not only inhibits proteolysis in liver but also stimulates protein synthesis when the pathway was preinhibited by shrinking maneuvers (66). Thus, glutamine favors a protein-anabolic state via cell swelling.

Another example for the functional consequences of glutamine-induced liver cell swelling is the stimulation of transcellular bile acid transport under these conditions. Cell swelling, induced by either glutamine, hypoosmotic exposure, or tauroursodeoxycholate, increases within minutes the v_{max} of taurocholate excretion into bile (67) in a colchicine-sensitive way (68). It has been hypothesized that this effect is due to the rapid insertion of previously latent, intracellularly stored bile acid transporter molecules into the canalicular membrane following cell swelling under the influence of glutamine or other agents known to induce cellular swelling (67).

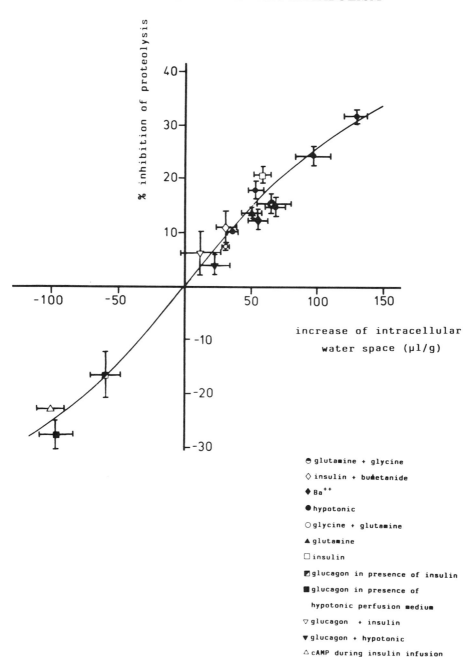

Glutamine-induced cell swelling also increases the flux through the pentose phosphate shunt (68). To what extent such a response is cytoprotective against oxidative stress remains to be established.

HOW DOES GLUTAMINE-INDUCED CELL SWELLING MODIFY CELLULAR METABOLISM?

The mechanisms by which glutamine-induced alterations of the hepatocellular state modify liver cell function are largely obscure. It is likely that the multiple effects of cell swelling on metabolic functions will involve different mechanisms. Glutamine-induced cell swelling is accompanied by membrane stretching and may, as with hypo-osmotic cell swelling, activate membrane-associated signaling systems, leading to an increased formation of inositol-1,4,5-triphosphate, a transient rise of intracellular Ca^{2+}, lowering of pH_i, and hyperpolarization of the membrane following cell swelling (70–73). However, the significance of these alterations for the observed effects on hepatic metabolism is doubtful. There is some evidence that cytoskeletal alterations are involved in mediating swelling-induced metabolic responses. Indeed, glutamine-induced cell swelling leads to a rapid polymerization of actin, increases β-actin and tubulin mRNA levels and microtubule stability (74,75). Intact microtubules are a conditio sine qua non for the regulation of bile acid excretion and proteolysis by cellular hydration (68,75): after disruption of microtubules by colchicine the swelling-induced inhibition of proteolysis and stimulation of bile acid excretion are abolished. Although evidence has been presented for a role of microfilaments in regulating protein synthesis (76), little is known about their role in mediating the swelling-induced stimulation of protein synthesis. Like proteolysis, mRNA breakdown has been suggested to involve the autophagic pathway and to underlie a control by amino acids and hormones similar to proteolysis (77,78). Thus, it is feasible that mRNA breakdown may also be controlled by cell volume. Another interesting observation is that cell swelling interferes with the acidfication of intracellular vesicular compartments, such as lysosomes (79). Alkalinization of these compartments occurs in response to cell swelling and may contribute to the swelling-induced inhibition of autophagic proteolysis. Cellular hydration also affects gene expression. In line with this, cell swelling increases the mRNA levels for tubulin and β-actin (74,75), but

---

FIG. 3. Relationship between cell volume and proteolysis in liver. Cell volume in perfused liver was determined as intracellular water space and proteolysis was assessed as [³H]leucine release in effluent perfusate from perfused livers from rats, which were prelabelled in vivo by intraperitoneal injection of [³H]leucine 16 hours prior to the perfusion experiment. Cell shrinkage stimulates proteolysis, whereas cell swelling inhibits. It should be noted that proteolysis is already maximally activated in the absence of hormones and amino acids and cannot be further stimulated by hyperosmotic or glucagon-induced cell shrinkage. The proteolysis-stimulating effect of these cell-shrinking maneuvers, however, becomes apparent when proteolysis is preinhibited by either amino acids or insulin. Cell volume changes were induced by insulin, cAMP, glucagon, amino acids, Ba^{2+} or anisoosmotic exposure. From Häussinger et al. (60).

lowers the mRNA levels of phosphoenolpyruvate carboxykinase (PEPCK) (80). Conversely, cell shrinkage increases the mRNA levels for PEPCK, largely due to a stimulation of transcription. This may be due to modification of gene expression by changes of the intracellular ionic strength (81) or to activation of transcription factors. Indeed, cell swelling increases the levels of c-jun mRNA (82) and there is cumulating evidence for alterations of protein phosphorylation in response to cell swelling/shrinkage (80,83). It is hoped that this article will stimulate future research in this exciting area.

ACKNOWLEDGMENTS

Our own studies reported herein were supported by Deutsche Forschungsgemeinschaft, Sonderforschungsbereich 154, the Heisenbergprogramm, the Fonds der Chemischen Industrie, and the Leibniz-Price.

REFERENCES

1. Krebs HA. Metabolism of amino acids. The synthesis of glutamine from glutamic acid and the enzymatic hydrolysis of glutamine in animal tissues. *Biochem J* 1935;29:1951–1959.
2. Häussinger D, Sies H, eds. *Glutamine Metabolism in Mammalian Tissues.* Heidelberg: Springer Verlag, 1984.
3. Häussinger D, ed. *pH Homeostasis—Mechanisms and Control:* San Diego: Academic Press London, 1988.
4. Häussinger D, Lang F. Cell volume in the regulation of hepatic function: a mechanism for metabolic control. *Biochim Biophys Acta* 1991;1071:331–350.
5. Häussinger D. Hepatocyte heterogeneity in glutamine and ammonia metabolism and the role of an intercellular glutamine cycle during ureogenesis in perfused rat liver. *Eur J Biochem* 1983;133:269–275.
6. Häussinger D, Gerok, W. Hepatocyte heterogeneity in ammonia metabolism: impairment of glutamine synthesis in CCl_4 induced liver cell necrosis with no effect on urea synthesis. *Chem Biol Interact* 1984;48:191–194.
7. Gebhardt R, Mecke D. Heterogeneous distribution of glutamine synthetase among rat liver parenchymal cells in situ and in primary culture. *Embo J* 1983;2:567–570.
8. Gaasbeek-Janzen JW, Lamers WH, Moorman AFM, et al. Immunohistochemical localization of carbamoyl-phosphate synthetase (ammonia) in adult rat liver; evidence for a heterogeneous distribution. *J Histochem Cytochem* 1984;32:557–564.
9. Saheki T, Yagi Y, Sase M, et al. Immunohistochemical localization of argininosuccinate synthetase in the liver of control and citrullinemic patients. *Biomed Res* 1984;4:235–238.
10. Watford M, Smith EM. Distribution of hepatic glutaminase activity and mRNA in perivenous and periportal hepatocytes. *Biochem J* 1990;267:265–267.
11. Gebhardt R, Ebert A, Bauer G. Heterogeneous expression of glutamine synthetase mRNA in rat liver parenchyma revealed by in situ hybridization and Northern blot analysis of mRNA from periportal and perivenous hepatocytes. *FEBS Lett* 1988;241:89–93.
12. Pösö AR, Penttilä KE, Suolinna EM, Lindros KO. Urea synthesis in freshly isolated and in cultured periportal and perivenous hepatocytes. *Biochem J* 1986;239:263–267.
13. Stoll B, Stehle T, Häussinger D. Functional hepatocyte heterogeneity: vascular oxoglutarate is almost exclusively taken up by perivenous glutamine-synthetase-containing hepatocytes. *Eur J Biochem* 1989;181:709–716.
14. Stoll B, Häussinger D. Hepatocyte heterogeneity in uptake and metabolism of malate and related dicarboxylates in perfused rat liver. *Eur J Biochem* 1991;195:121–129.
15. Stoll B, McNelly S, Buscher HP, Häussinger D. Functional hepatocyte heterogeneity in glutamate, aspartate and α-ketoglutarate uptake: a histoautoradiographic study. *Hepatology* 1991;12:247–253.
16. Häussinger D, Stehle T, Gerok W. Glutamine metabolism in isolated perfused rat liver. The transamination pathway. *Biol Chem Hoppe-Seyler* 1985;366:517–536.

17. Häussinger D, Steeb R, Gerok W. Ammonium and bicarbonate homeostasis in liver cirrhosis. *Klin Wochenschr* 1989;68:175–182.
18. Häussinger D, Gerok W, Sies H. Hepatic role in pH regulation: role of the intercellular glutamine cycle. *Trends Biochem Sci* 1984;9:300–302.
19. McGivan JD, Bradford MN, Verhoeven AJ, Meijer AJ. Liver glutaminase. In: Häussinger D, Sies H, eds. *Glutamine Metabolism in Mammalian Tissues*. Heidelberg: Springer Verlag, 1984;122–137.
20. Verhoeven AJ, van Iwaarden JF, Joseph SK, Meijer AJ. Control of rat liver glutaminase by ammonia and pH. *Eur J Biochem* 1983;133:241–244.
21. Häussinger D, Sies H. Hepatic glutamine metabolism under the influence of the portal ammonia concentration in the perfused rat liver. *Eur J Biochem* 1979;101:179–184.
22. Häussinger D, Gerok W, Sies H. Regulation of flux through glutaminase and glutamine synthetase in isolated perfused rat liver. *Biochim Biophys Acta* 1983;755:272–278.
23. McGivan JD, Bradford MN. Characteristics of the activation of glutaminase by ammonia in sonicated rat-liver mitochondria. *Biochim Biophys Acta* 1983;759:296–302.
24. Lenzen C, Soboll S, Sies H, Häussinger D. pH control of hepatic glutamine degradation. Role of transport. *Eur J Biochem* 1987;166:483–488.
25. Meijer AJ, Lof C, Ramos IC, Verhoeven AJ. Control of ureogenesis. *Eur J Biochem* 1985;148:189–196.
26. Cohen NS, Kyan FS, Kyan SS, et al. The apparent K_m of ammonia for carbamoylphosphate synthetase (ammonia) in situ. *Biochem J* 1985;229:205–211.
27. Meijer AJ. Channeling of ammonia from glutaminase into carbamoylphosphate synthetase in rat liver mitochondria. *FEBS Lett* 1985;191:249–251.
28. Häussinger D. Urea synthesis and $CO_2/HCO_3{}^-$ compartmentation in isolated perfused rat liver. *Biol Chem Hoppe-Seyler* 1986;367:741–750.
29. Meijer AJ, Verhoeven AJ. Regulation of hepatic glutamine metabolism. *Biochem Soc Trans* 1986;14:1001–1004.
30. Welbourne TC. Hepatic glutaminase flux regulation of glutamine homeostasis: studies in vivo. *Biol Chem Hoppe-Seyler* 1986;367:301–305.
31. Cooper AJ, Nieves E, Filc-DeRicco S, Gelbard AS. Short-term metabolic fate of ^{13}N-ammonia, ^{13}N-alanine, ^{13}N-glutamate and amide-^{13}N-glutamine in normal rat liver in vivo. In: Soeters PB, Wilson JHP, Meijer AJ, Holm E, eds. *Advances in Ammonia Metabolism and Hepatic Encephalopathy*. Amsterdam: Elsevier Science, 1988;11–25.
32. Kovacevic Z, McGivan JD. Glutamine transport across biological membranes. In: Häussinger D, Sies H, eds. *Glutamine Metabolism in Mammalian Tissues*. Heidelberg: Springer Verlag, 1984;47–58.
33. Kilberg MS, Handlogten ME, Christensen HN. Characteristics of an amino acid transport system in rat liver for glutamine, asparagine, histidine and closely related analogues. *J Biol Chem* 1980;255:4011–4109.,
34. Fafournoux P, Demigne C, Remesy C, LeCam A. Bidirectional transport of glutamine across the cell membrane in rat liver. *Biochem J* 1983;216:401–408.
35. Häussinger D, Soboll S, Meijer AJ, et al. Role of plasma membrane transport in hepatic glutamine metabolism. *Eur J Biochem* 1985;152:597–603.
36. Remesy C, Morand C, Demigne C, Fafournoux P. Control of hepatic utilization of glutamine by transport processes or cellular metabolism in rats fed a high protein diet. *J Nutr* 1988;118:569–578.
37. Hayes MR, McGivan JD. Differential effects of starvation on alanine and glutamine transport in isolated rat hepatocytes. *Biochem J* 1982;204:365–368.
38. Häussinger D, Lang F, Bauers K, Gerok W. Interactions between glutamine metabolism and cell volume regulation in perfused rat liver. *Eur J Biochem* 1990;188:689–695.
39. Wettstein M, vom Dahl S, Lang F, et al. Cell volume regulatory responses of isolated perfused rat liver: the effect of amino acids. *Biol Chem Hoppe-Seyler* 1990;371:493–501.
40. Lang F, Häussinger D. *Interactions between Cell Volume and Cell Function*. Heidelberg: Springer Verlag, 1993.
41. Bakker-Grunwald T. Potassium permeability and volume control in isolated rat hepatocytes. *Biochim Biophys Acta* 1983;731:239–242.
42. Kristensen LO. Energization of alanine transport in isolated rat hepatocytes. *J Biol Chem* 1980;255:5236–5243.
43. Kristensen LO, Folke M. Volume-regulatory K^+ efflux during concentrative uptake of alanine in isolated rat hepatocytes. *Biochem J* 1984;221:265–268.
44. Kristensen LO, Folke M. Effects of perturbation of the Na^+-electrochemical gradient on influx and efflux of alanine in isolated rat hepatocytes. *Biochim Biophys Acta* 1986;855:49–57.

45. Hallbrucker C, vom Dahl S, Lang F, Häussinger D. Control of hepatic proteolysis by amino acids: the role of cell volume. *Eur J Biochem* 1986;197:717–724.
46. Häussinger D. The hepatocellular hydratation state: a regulator of liver cell function. *Hepatology Rapid Lit Revs* 1992;22:V–XIII.
47. Häussinger D, Lang F. Cell volume and hormone action. *Trends Pharmacol Sci* 1992;13:371–373.
48. Katz J, Golden S, Wals PA. Stimulation of hepatic glycogen synthesis by amino acids. *Proc Natl Acad Sci* 1976;73:3433–3437.
49. Lavoinne A, Baquet A, Hue L. Stimulation of glycogen synthesis and lipogenesis by glutamine in isolated rat hepatocytes. *Biochem J* 1987;248:429–437.
50. Mortimore GE, Pösö AR. Mechanisms and control of deprivation-induced protein degradation in liver: role of glucogenic amino acids. In: Häussinger D, Sies H, eds. *Glutamine Metabolism in Mammalian Tissues.* Heidelberg: Springer Verlag, 1984;138–157.
51. Pösö AR, Schworer CM, Mortimore GE. Acceleration of proteolysis in perfused rat liver by deletion of glucogenic amino acids: regulatory role of glutamine. *Biochem Biophys Res Commun* 1982;107: 1433–1439.
52. Mortimore GE, Pösö AR. Intracellular protein catabolism and its control during nutrient deprivation and supply. *Annu Rev Nutr* 1987;7:539–564.
53. Seglen PO, Gordon PB, Poli A. Amino acid inhibition of the autophagic/lysosomal pathway of protein degradation in isolated rat hepatocytes. *Biochim Biophys Acta* 1980;630:103–118.
54. Seglen PO, Gordon PB. Amino acid control of autophagic sequestration and protein degradation in isolated rat hepatocytes. *J Cell Biol* 1984;99:435–444.
55. Weissbach L, Kilberg MS. Amino acid activation of amino acid transport system N early in primary cultures of rat hepatocytes. *J Cell Physiol* 1984;121:133–138.
56. Baquet A, Hue L, Meijer AJ, et al. Swelling of rat hepatocytes stimulates glycogen synthesis. *J Biol Chem* 1990;265:955–959.
57. Baquet A, Lavoinne A, Hue L. Comparison of the effects of various amino acids on glycogen synthesis, lipogenesis and ketogenesis in isolated rat hepatocytes. *Biochem J* 1991;273:57–62.
58. Bode B, Kilberg M. Amino acid dependent increase of hepatic system N activity is linked to cell swelling. *J Biol Chem* 1991;266:7376–7381.
59. Häussinger D, Hallbrucker C, vom Dahl S, et al. Cell swelling inhibits proteolysis in perfused rat liver. *Biochem J* 1990;272:239–242.
60. Häussinger D, Hallbrucker C, vom Dahl S, et al. Cell volume is a major determinant of proteolysis control in liver. *FEBS Lett* 1991;283:70–72.
61. MacLennan PA, Brown RA, Rennie MJ. A positive relationship between protein synthetic rate and intracellular glutamine concentration in perfused rat skeletal muscle. *FEBS Lett* 1987;215:187–191.
62. MacLennan PA, Smith K, Weryk B, et al. Inhibition of protein breakdown by glutamine in perfused rat skeletal muscle. *FEBS Lett* 1988;237:133–136.
63. Rennie MJ, Hundal HS, Babij P, et al. Characteristics of a glutamine carrier in skeletal muscle have important consequences for nitrogen loss in injury, infection and chronic disease. *Lancet* 1986;ii: 1008–1012.
64. Roth E, Karner J, Ollenschläger G. Glutamine: an anabolic effector? *JPEN* 1990;14:130S–136S.
65. Häussinger D, Roth E, Lang F, Gerok W. The cellular hydratation state: a major determinant for protein catabolism in health and disease. *Lancet* 1993;341:1330–1332.
66. Stoll B, Gerok W, Lang F, Häussinger D. Liver cell volume and protein synthesis. *Biochem J* 1992; 287:217–222.
67. Häussinger D, Hallbrucker C, Saha N, et al. Cell volume and bile acid excretion. *Biochem J* 1992; 288:681–689.
68. Häussinger D, Saha N, Hallbrucker C et al. Involvement of microtubules in the swelling-induced stimulation of transcellular taurocholate transport in perfused rat liver. *Biochem J* 1993;291:355–360.
69. Saha N, Stoll B, Lang F, Häussinger D. Effect of anisotonic cell volume modulation on glutathione-S-conjugate release, t-butylhydroperoxide metabolism and the pentose phosphate shunt in perfused rat liver. *Eur J Biochem* 1992;209:437–444.
70. vom Dahl S, Hallbrucker C, Lang F, Häussinger D. Role of eicosanoids, inositol phosphates and extracellular Ca^{++} in cell volume regulation of rat liver. *Eur J Biochem* 1991;198:73–83.
71. Corasanti JG, Gleeson D, Gautam A, Boyer JL. Effects of osmotic stresses on isolated rat hepatocytes: ionic mechanisms of cell volume regulation and modulation of Na^+/H^+ exchange. *Renal Physiol Biochem* 1990;13:164.
72. Baquet A, Meijer AJ, Hue L. Hepatocyte swelling increases inositol 1,4,5-trisphosphate, calcium

and cAMP concentration but antagonizes phosphorylase activation by calcium-dependent hormones. *FEBS Lett* 1991;278:103–106.

73. Graf J, Haddad P, Häussinger D, Lang F. Cell volume regulation in liver. *Renal Physiol Biochem* 1988;11:202–220.

74. Theodoropoulos PA, Stournaras C, Stoll B, et al. Hepatocyte swelling leads to rapid decrease of the G/total actin ratio and increases actin mRNA levels. *FEBS Lett* 1992;311:241–245.

74. Hesketh JE, Pryme IF. Interaction between mRNA, ribosomes and the cytoskeleton. *Biochem J* 1991;277:1–10.

75. Häussinger D, Stoll B, vom Dahl S et al. Microtubule stabilization and induction of tubulin mRNA by cell swelling in isolated rat hepatocytes. *Biochem Cell Biol* 1994;78: in press.

76. Hesketh JE, Pryme IF, Interaction between mRNA, ribosomes, and the cytoskeleton. *Biochem J* 1991;277:1–10.

77. Balavoine S, Feldmann G, Lardeux B. Rates of RNA degradation in isolated rat hepatocytes. Effects of amino acids and inhibitors of lysosomal function. *Eur J Biochem* 1990;189:617–623.

78. Lardeux BR, Mortimore GE. Amino acid and hormonal control of macromolecular turnover in perfused rat liver. *J Biol Chem* 1987;262:14514–14519.

79. Völkl H, Friedrich F, Häussinger D, Lang F. Effects of cell volume on acridine orange fluorescence in hepatocytes. *Biochem J* 1993;295:11–14.

80. Häussinger D, Newsome W, vom Dahl S et al. Control of liver function by the hydration state. *Biochem Soc Trans* 1994; in press.

81. Leake RE, Trench ME, Barry JM. Effect of cations on the condensation of hen erythrocate nuclei and its relation to gene activation. *Exp Cell Res* 1982;71:17–26.

82. Finkenzeller G, Newsome W, Lang F, Häussinger D. Increase of c-jun mRNA upon hypoosmotic cell swelling of rat hepatoma cells. FEBS Lett 1994;340:163–166.

83. Meijer AJ, Baquet A, Gustafson L et al. Mechanism of activation of glycogen synthase by swelling. *J Biol Chem* 192;267:5823–5828.

Organ Metabolism and Nutrition:
Ideas for Future Critical Care, edited by
J. M. Kinney and H. N. Tucker.
Raven Press, Ltd., New York © 1994.

16

Phosphatidylcholine: The Unappreciated Nutrient in Total Parenteral Nutrition

Steven H. Zeisel

Department of Nutrition, University of North Carolina at Chapel Hill,
Chapel Hill, North Carolina 27599-7400

Our understanding of the scientific bases for feeding humans parenterally is evolving continuously. Over several decades, the solutions administered have changed from blends of glucose and amino acids to complex mixtures of glucose, amino acids, lipids, trace minerals, vitamins, and other micronutrients. Most ingredients were added because of their perceived value as nutrients, but some were added because of food technology considerations. In this review, I discuss an ingredient, phosphatidylcholine, that was added because it stabilized parenteral lipid emulsions, but which now turns out to supply a needed nutrient. In addition, I review recent advances in our understanding of the molecular bases for intracellular signaling that suggest that commercial parenteral emulsions could be crafted so as to have important physiologic and pharmacologic effects that go well beyond their current use as sources of calories and essential fatty acids.

PHOSPHATIDYLCHOLINE, THE DETERGENT

Triacylglycerol is sufficiently hydrophobic that it will not stay in an aqueous solution. For this reason, food technologists have used phospholipids to stabilize lipid-water emulsions. Phospholipids have both hydrophobic and hydrophilic substituents, thus, they form an ideal interface between triacylglycerol and water. Phospholipids are major components of all membranes, and lecithin's designation as generally regarded as safe (GRAS) makes its use as a food additive more acceptable than other detergents. Huge quantities of phospholipids (usually in a mixture called lecithin) are used by the food industry each year. In the common chocolate bar, for instance, triglycerides are kept emulsified by the addition of lecithin. Without lecithin the candy bar turns white, as the lighter lipids rise to the surface.

Commercial parenteral emulsions (e.g., Intralipid), contain egg phospholipids (approximately 70% phosphatidylcholine) to stabilize the soybean triglyceride as an emulsion. These phospholipids have been included because of their detergent properties, not as a source of nutrients.

After intravenous infusions of lipid emulsions, there is an accumulation in liver and other tissues of abnormal lipids (i.e., lipoprotein-X). Lipoprotein-X appears to be a metabolite of one of the components of egg phospholipid rather than of the triglyceride in parenteral emulsions (1). For this reason, manufacturers are considering reducing the phospholipid content of parenteral emulsions. This might be accomplished by replacing egg phospholipid with an alternative detergent. However, before reformulation is attempted, it is important to realize that a component of egg phospholipid, phosphatidylcholine, is providing choline—an important nutrient.

CHOLINE

Choline is universally distributed in all cells, mostly in the form of choline esters such as phosphocholine, glycerophosphocholine, phosphatidylcholine, lysophosphatidylcholine, choline plasmalogen, platelet activating factor, and sphingomyelin (2). Choline is needed for acetylcholine biosynthesis, as a methyl donor, and for phosphatidylcholine biosynthesis. Phosphatidylcholine is the predominant phospholipid (>50%) in most mammalian membranes. Total body stores of choline in humans can be estimated based on measurement of choline pool concentrations in animal tissues; a 70-kg human should contain more than 5 mmol choline (500 mg) in unesterified form and more than 300 mmol choline (30 g) in esterified forms.

The importance of choline as a nutrient was accidentally discovered during the pioneering work on insulin (3,4). Depancreatized dogs developed fatty infiltration of the liver and died. Administration of raw pancreas prevented hepatic damage; the active component was the choline moiety of pancreatic phosphatidylcholine. The term *lipotropic* was coined to describe choline and other substances that prevented deposition of fat in the liver.

Several lines of evidence suggest that choline is indeed an essential nutrient for humans. Human cells grown in culture have an absolute requirement for choline (5). Healthy humans fed diets deficient in choline have decreased plasma choline concentrations (6), and malnourished humans have diminished plasma or serum choline concentrations (7,8). In most mammals, including the monkey, choline deficiency results in severe liver dysfunction (9,10). Humans fed parenterally with solutions containing little or no choline develop liver dysfunction, including fatty liver, that is similar to that seen in choline-deficient animals (7). Supplementation of these patients with a choline-containing phospholipid reverses the fatty liver (11).

DIETARY SOURCES OF CHOLINE

Choline chloride, choline bitartrate, and lecithin (phosphatidylcholine) are listed in the Code of Federal Regulations as nutrients and/or dietary supplements that are generally recognized as safe (12). More than 5,000 kg of choline chloride and more than 12,000 kg of choline bitartrate are used in the manufacture of foods in a single year (12).

Calculations of dietary choline intake are based only on estimates of the free choline and phosphatidylcholine content of foods (13–17). Our own measurements of the lysophosphatidylcholine, glycerophosphocholine, and phosphocholine contents of rat tissues (18) show that these choline-containing compounds are present in high concentrations in many tissues (e.g., muscle concentrations of these three esters were approximately 100 nmol/g each). Thus, the foods eaten by humans probably also contain significant amounts of these esters of choline. For these reasons, choline intake (especially unesterified choline intake) is probably underestimated by current tables. My best estimate of total choline intake in the adult human is >70 to 100 μmol/kg/d (700 to 1,000 mg/70 kg/d of choline moiety) (19,20). This estimate is substantiated by our observation that, when humans were switched from a diet of normal foods to a defined diet containing 500 mg choline (750 mg choline chloride), plasma choline and phosphatidylcholine concentrations decreased significantly in most subjects (6). This suggests that normal dietary intake of choline exceeds 500 mg (70 μmol/kg/d). The best estimate of the choline requirements for infants must be based on the assumption that they require the amount of choline present in breast milk. Colostrum and transitional milk contain approximately 1,400 μM choline moiety (500 μM free choline, 400 μM choline in phospholipids [17] and 400–500 μM choline as glycerophosphocholine and phosphocholine [22a]). Assuming a premature infant needs to ingest 100 kcal/kg/d, and that milk has a caloric density of 0.66 kcal/ml, the infant drinks 150 ml milk/kg/d. Thus, choline intake in a breast fed infant would be approximately 200 μmol/kg/d, two or three times that required by the adult human.

Normal fasting plasma choline concentrations in adults are between 8 and 12 μM; plasma phosphatidylcholine concentrations are approximately 1 to 1.5 mM (6,7, 21,22). In the adult human, serum choline concentrations fluctuate modestly (increase 1.5-fold) when common choline-containing foods are ingested (21).

The only source of choline other than diet is from the *de novo* biosynthesis of phosphatidylcholine catalyzed by phosphatidylethanolamine-N-methyltransferase (PeMT). This enzyme synthesizes phosphatidylcholine via sequential methylation of phosphatidylethanolamine using S-adenosylmethionine as a methyl donor (20,23–25). Most PeMT activity is found in the liver (26), but significant activity is present in brain (24,27) and mammary gland (28) and detectable activity is found in most other tissues (29–38). The presence of this pathway is the major reason that choline has been considered a dispensable nutrient for humans.

The demand for choline as a methyl donor is probably the major factor which determines how rapidly a diet deficient in choline will induce pathology. The pathways of choline and 1-carbon metabolism cross at the formation of methionine from homocysteine (39–41). Methionine is regenerated from homocysteine in a reaction catalyzed by betaine:homocysteine methyltransferase, in which betaine, a metabolite of choline, serves as the methyl donor (40). Betaine concentrations in livers of choline-deficient rats are markedly diminished (40–42). The only alternative mechanism for regeneration of methionine is via a reaction catalyzed by 5-methyltetrahydrofo-late:homocysteine methyltransferase, which uses a methyl group generated *de novo* from the 1-carbon pool (40,43). Methionine is converted to S-adenosylmethionine in a reaction catalyzed by methionine adenosyl transferase. S-adenosylmethionine is the active methylating agent for many enzymatic methylations.

A disturbance in folate or methionine metabolism results in changes in choline metabolism and visa versa. During choline deficiency, hepatic choline concentration decreases rapidly. At the same time, hepatic S-adenosylmethionine concentrations are decreased (44–47). It has been suggested that the availability of methionine limits S-adenosylmethionine synthesis during choline deficiency because the 5-methyltetra-hydrofolate homocysteine methyltransferase reaction alone cannot fulfill the total requirement for methionine, and the betaine-dependent remethylation of homocyste-ine is limited by the availability of betaine (40). Choline deficiency is also associated with inhibition of hepatic glycine-N-methyltransferase activity, which is believed to be important for the removal of excess S-adenosylmethionine from liver (48). Folate metabolism is also altered in choline deficiency (49,50), reflected by an immediate reduction in total folate pools, followed by a restoration of normal levels secondary to greater residence time of folate molecules within liver (50).

HEPATIC DYSFUNCTION AND CHOLINE DEFICIENCY

Hepatocyte turnover and leakage of hepatic cytosolic enzymes (alanine amino-transferase) are greatly increased during choline deficiency (51,52). In addition, ex-tremely large amounts of lipid (mainly triglycerides) accumulate in liver, eventually filling the entire hepatocyte (53–57). Fatty infiltration of the liver starts in the central area of the lobule and spreads peripherally (53). The accumulation of triacylglycerol within hepatocytes begins within hours after rats are started on a choline-deficient diet, peaks within the first 6 months (at >2,000 mg/liver; in control rats, 28 mg/liver), and then diminishes as liver becomes fibrotic (58,59). Triacylglycerol accumulation occurs because triglyceride must be packaged as very low density lipoprotein (VLDL) to be exported from liver. Phosphatidylcholine is an essential component of VLDL (55,56); other phospholipids cannot substitute (55,56). Hepatocytes isolated from choline-deficient rats were unable to export VLDL until choline or methionine was made available (55). High-density lipoprotein secretion was not effected.

HUMAN REQUIREMENTS FOR CHOLINE

We fed healthy humans a choline-deficient diet to determine whether they devel-oped symptoms consistent with choline deficiency (6). Subjects were admitted to the Clinical Research Center and were constantly observed for 5 weeks. During the first week all subjects consumed the same choline-containing diet. During the middle 3 weeks of the study the control group continued on the choline-containing diet while the choline-deficient group consumed the same diet without choline. During the fifth

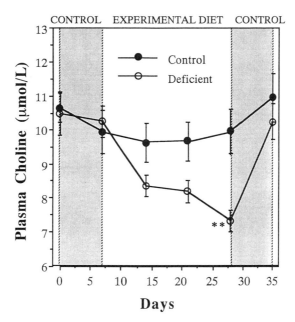

FIG. 1. Plasma choline in humans ingesting a control or choline-deficient diet. Healthy male subjects were hospitalized for 5 weeks. During the first and last weeks of the study, all subjects consumed the same choline-containing standard diet; during the middle 3 weeks of the study, subjects were divided into two groups, one that continued on the choline-containing diet and one that consumed the same diet without choline. During the fifth week of the study, all subjects consumed the choline-containing diet. Plasma choline was measured using a mass spectrometric method. Data are expressed as mean choline concentration (μmol/l) ± standard error of the mean. ** = $p < 0.01$ different from day-7 value. From Zeisel SH, daCosta K-A, Franklin PD, et al. Choline, an essential nutrient for humans. *FASEB J* 1991;5:2093–2098; with permission.

week all subjects consumed the choline-containing diet. We observed that humans ingesting a choline-deficient diet for 3 weeks had diminished plasma choline (Fig. 1) and phosphatidylcholine concentrations (Fig. 2), as well as diminished erythrocyte membrane phosphatidylcholine concentrations. Serum alanine transaminase (ALT) activity, a measure of hepatocyte damage, increased significantly when a choline-deficient diet was ingested (Fig. 3). The design of the study, as approved by our Institutional Review Board, was such that clinically significant changes in liver function (ALT>0.58 μkat/l) were not to be induced in the subjects. We suggest that choline deficiency of longer duration would have resulted in more prominent evidence of liver dysfunction. We also observed a significant decrease in serum cholesterol (derived from VLDL secreted by liver) in the choline-deficient subjects (6).

Patients Likely to Be Vulnerable to Choline Deficiency

Choline deficiency may be of clinical importance in several groups of patients. Bypass surgery involving large segments of the bowel (i.e., to produce weight loss

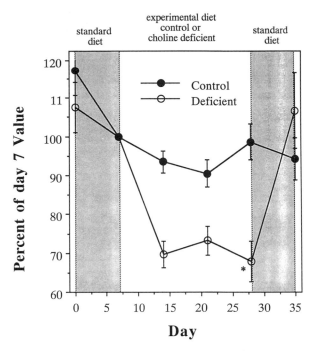

FIG. 2. Plasma phosphatidylcholine in humans ingesting a control or choline-deficient diet. Subjects were treated as described in Fig. 1. Plasma phosphatidylcholine was measured using thinlayer chromatography and phosphorus determination. Data are expressed as mean percent of day-7 phosphatidylcholine concentration ± standard error of the mean. ˙ = $p < 0.05$ different from day-7 value. From Zeisel SH, daCosta K-A, Franklin PD, et al. Choline, an essential nutrient for humans. *FASEB J* 1991;5:2093–2098; with permission.

in very obese humans) is associated with fatty liver. In obese rats that have had 90% of their small intestine bypassed, fatty liver develops. Choline supplementation prevented this, and choline-deficient diets in such animals exacerbated the accumulation of fat in the liver (60).

Malnourished humans, in whom stores of choline, methionine, and folate have been depleted (7,8), are also likely to need more dietary choline than did our healthy adult subjects. Malnourished humans, at the time they were referred for total parenteral nutrition (TPN) therapy, had significantly lower plasma choline concentrations than did well-fed control subjects (7,61).

Hepatic complications associated with TPN, which include fatty infiltration of the liver and hepatocellular damage, have been reported by many clinical groups (62). Frequently TPN must be terminated because of the severity of the associated liver disease. It is possible that some of the liver disease associated with TPN is related to choline deficiency. Amino acid–glucose solutions used in TPN contain no choline (7,61). Plasma choline concentrations declined, from their already subnormal levels, in patients intravenously fed with an amino acid–glucose solution lacking choline

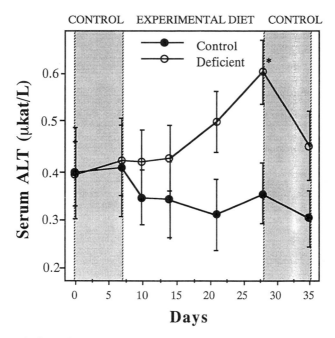

CONTROL   EXPERIMENTAL DIET   CONTROL

FIG. 3. Serum alanine aminotransferase activity in humans ingesting a control or choline-deficient diet. Subjects were treated as described in Fig. 1. Serum alanine aminotransferase was determined using an automated spectrophotometric assay. Data are expressed as mean activity (μkat/l) ± standard error of the mean. * = $p < 0.05$ different from day-7 value. From Zeisel SH, daCosta K-A, Franklin PD, et al. Choline, an essential nutrient for humans. *FASEB J* 1991;5:2093–2098; with permission.

during the first week of therapy (7). However, when patients were treated with lipid emulsion as well as an amino acid–glucose solution, their plasma choline concentrations rose slightly. Neither group received sufficient choline to restore plasma choline concentrations to normal.

Commercial parenteral emulsions (e.g., Intralipid) contain egg phospholipids (12 mg/ml, 70% to 75% of which is phosphatidylcholine) to stabilize 100 or 200 mg of soybean triglyceride. As discussed earlier, the healthy adult human requires approximately 100 μmol choline/kg/d. Healthy babies may require 200 μmol choline/kg/d. Given that a liter of 20% lipid emulsion contains approximately 10 mmol of choline as phosphatidylcholine, a patient treated with the recommended 3 g/kg/d of lipid receives approximately 150 μmol/kg/d choline. We observed that TPN patients required approximately this amount of lipid emulsion during the first week of TPN therapy to maintain plasma choline levels (7). Burt et al. (63) and Buchman et al. (11) reported that low plasma choline concentrations in TPN patients were associated with liver dysfunction (as measured by transaminase leakage). Conditions that enhance hepatic triglyceride synthesis (such as infusion of glucose) increase the requirement for the choline for export of triglyceride from liver (64). Thus, treatment of malnourished patients with high-calorie TPN solutions, at a time when choline stores are depleted, might enhance the likelihood of hepatic dysfunction. When rats were fed intravenously with choline-free TPN solutions (4.25% FreAmine II in 25% glucose), they developed fatty infiltration of the liver and had elevated serum levels of conjugated bilirubin and transaminases (65). In these animals, oral or intravenous supplements of choline were effective in reversing hepatic lipid accumulation. Others have not observed this effect (66). The definitive experiment, in which supplemental choline (in the form of lecithin) was administered during long-term TPN has recently been performed (11). Patients studied had been treated with TPN (average duration 7 years) including 4 kcal/kg/day as 20% Intralipid (delivering approximately 50 μmol/kg/d choline as phosphatidylcholine). These patients had low plasma choline concentrations (average 6.3 μM). In a double-blind protocol, 20 grams lecithin (30% phosphatidylcholine; delivering approximately 300 μmol choline moiety/kg/d) or placebo (soybean oil) were administered orally twice a day for 6 weeks. At the end of this experimental period, plasma choline had risen by more than 50% in the lecithin group, while in the placebo group it had decreased by 25%. Fatty liver was defined using computed tomography. In the treated group, liver density increased (fat decreased) by approximately 30% ($p < 0.05$); in the placebo group, liver density increased by only 8% (nonsignificant). This strongly suggests that choline is an essential nutrient during long-term TPN.

CHOLINE DEFICIENCY AND CARNITINE

Carnitine is a cofactor for long-chain acetyl-CoA carnitine transferase; human deficiency syndromes have been identified (67), and the carnitine content of optimal TPN solutions is being carefully considered. Rats fed a choline-deficient diet had reduced levels of carnitine in liver, heart, and skeletal muscle (68,69). This finding has been attributed to a methyl-group deficiency, i.e., carnitine is derived from trimethyllysine. However, a single injection of choline (but not of methionine, betaine, or sarcosine) was able to raise the concentration of hepatic carnitine in these animals to control values within 1.5 hours (69). This suggests that choline was capable of facilitating carnitine release from some storage pool, as de novo synthesis of carnitine would have taken much more time. Paradoxically, plasma carnitine was higher in choline-deficient rats (69), probably because transport into tissues was inhibited. It is likely that carnitine transport is linked to choline transport across cell membranes; perhaps a choline molecule must exit the cell in order to flip the carnitine carrier from the inside of the outside of the plasma membrane.

CHOLINE, SIGNAL TRANSDUCTION, AND CARCINOGENESIS

Choline is the only single nutrient for which dietary deficiency in experimental animals is associated with development of cancer (58,70). We have suggested that

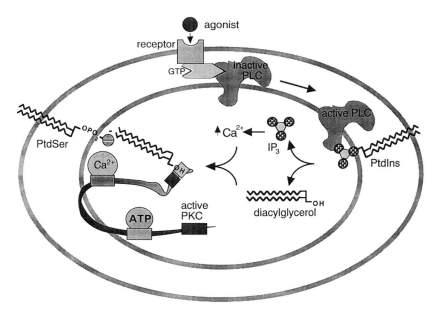

FIG. 4. Phosphoinositide-mediated signal transduction. When an appropriate receptor is stimulated by an agonist, there is a change in the conformation of a GTP binding protein (G-protein). This causes the activation of a phospholipase C (PLC) specific for phosphatidylinositide (PtdIns). Activated PLC hydrolyzes PtdIns bisphosphate to form inositol-1,4,5-trisphosphate (IP$_3$). IP$_3$ acts to release calcium from intracellular storage sites. PtdIns hydrolysis also forms diacylglycerol. Calcium, diacylglycerol (DAG), and phosphatidylserine (PtdSer) activate protein kinase C (PKC) by unmasking the catalytic site of the enzyme. Modified from Zeisel SH. Choline phospholipids: signal transduction and carcinogenesis. *FASEB J* 1993;7:551–557, with permission.

this effect of choline deficiency involves a "short-circuiting" of normal cellular signal transduction.

Our understanding of signal transduction has evolved rapidly, therefore, a brief review of current thinking is appropriate. Signals are transmitted across membranes via a highly interactive network of molecular events (Fig. 4). Basically, an extracellular sensor detects a signal and transmits this message into the interior of the cell via a protein phosphorylation cascade to a final component that acts as a regulator of gene transcription. Occupation of a surface receptor activates one of a series of phospholipases, which break down membrane phospholipid to generate second messengers. The activation of phospholipase C activity (PLC) hydrolyzes the glycerophosphate bond of intact phospholipids to generate 1,2-sn-diacylglycerol (DAG) and an aqueous soluble head group. Numerous phosphatidylinositide (PtdIns)-specific PLCs exist (71). It is believed that specific receptors couple to specific PtdIns-PLC isotypes (71). In a similar manner, specific receptors appear to be linked to activation of specific phosphatidylcholine-PLCs (72).

The products generated by PLC trigger the next event in the signal cascade, which is the activation of protein kinase C (PKC). The first step in PKC activation is the formation of a ternary enzyme + Ca^{2+} + phospholipid-membrane complex. Products generated by PtdIns-PLC include inositol-1,4,5-triphosphate (IP_3) and DAG. IP_3 is a water-soluble product that acts to release calcium from stores in the endoplasmic reticulum. This increase in cytosolic calcium makes more calcium available for binding to PKC isotypes that are Ca^{2+} dependent (73). Calcium increases the tightness of association of these PKCs with the membrane, thereby increasing membrane occupancy. This facilitates binding of DAG. The DAG-PKC complex approaches the membrane more closely, placing the kinase in a pocket of negatively charged phosphatidylserine head groups, into which Ca^{2+} is attracted. Thus, DAG increases the affinity of PKC for calcium. Normally PKC is folded so that an endogenous "pseudosubstrate" region on the protein is bound to the catalytic site, thereby inhibiting activity. The combination of DAG and Ca^{2+} causes a conformational change in PKC, causing flexing at a hinge region so as to withdraw the pseudosubstrate and unblock the PKC catalytic site. The appearance of diacylglycerol in membranes is usually transient, and therefore PKC is activated only for a short time after a receptor has been stimulated. The events that occur downstream from PKC are just beginning to be characterized. Clearly, PKC signals impinge on several known intracellular control circuits (73). The targets for phosphorylation by PKC include receptors for insulin, epidermal growth factor and many proteins involved in control of gene expression, cell division, and differentiation (74,75). Several lines of evidence indicate that cancers might develop secondary to abnormalities in PKC-mediated signal transduction (75). First, many mitogens activate PKC (76). Second, several known tumor promoters mimic activation of PKC. The phorbol esters (DAG analogs) are potent mitogens and tumor promoters (74) whose effects may be explained by their interactions with PKC. Okadaic acid (an inhibitor of protein phosphatases whose net effect is to increase protein phosphorylation of PKC targets) is also a potent tumor promoter (77).

A major line of reasoning that links carcinogenesis to perturbation of signal transduction is based on the study of genes that are overexpressed in cancers. Oncogenes can be divided into four classes: growth factors *(sis, hist)*, growth factor receptors *(erbB, fms, kit)*, transducers of growth factors *(src, abl, ras, raf)*, and transcription factors *(jun, fos, myc)*. Anti-oncogenes, such as the neurofibromatosis type 1 (NF1) locus, also can act to modulate signal transduction. NF1 encodes a protein that is a GTPase-activating protein which inhibits the activation of PLC (77). Thus, the pathways responsible for start-stop signals during cell division and growth use intermediary steps mediated by the protein products made by protooncogenes. The expression of oncogenes can perturb PKC-mediated signal transduction in a manner similar to that which we previously described for choline deficiency. In *erbB*-transformed fibroblasts, DAG accumulates because it is not removed as rapidly by DAG kinase activity (78). Transformation by *ras* or *src* oncogenes is associated with permanent translocation of PKC to the cytoplasmic membrane (79). DAG is elevated in vivo in *ras*-transformed liver of neonatal transgenic mice (80). NIH 3T3 cells transformed with Ha-*ras*, Ki-*ras*, v-*src*, or v-*fms* oncogenes have elevated DAG levels as well as tonic activation and partial down-regulation of PKC (81). These elevated DAG levels are produced by activation of degradation of phosphatidylcholine (79,82). Activated PKC, in turn, may induce expression of the *myc* oncogene (*myc* is thought to trigger hepatocytes to enter the cell division cycle) (83–85). Indeed, *myc* is overexpressed in liver and tumor tissue from choline-deficient rat liver (85,86). Thus, many observations suggest that chronically increased DAG concentration with subsequent sustained activation of PKC may be a perturbation of signal transduction which results in carcinogenesis.

CHOLINE AND CANCER

We have suggested that the mechanism responsible for the carcinogenic effect of choline deficiency involves a short-circuiting of normal cellular signal transduction when lipid-derived second messenger accumulates. The fatty liver of choline deficiency is associated with the accumulation of the second messenger—DAG (Fig. 5) (58). In plasma membrane, DAG reaches values higher than those occurring after stimulation of a receptor linked to PLC activation (e.g., vasopressin receptor), and choline deficiency is associated with significant increases in PKC activity in hepatic plasma membranes. There is a stable activation of PKC and/or an increase in the total PKC pool in the cell (58) with changes in several PKC isotypes (at 6 weeks of choline deficiency, amounts of PKC α and δ are increased twofold and tenfold, respectively). The accumulation of DAG and subsequent activation of PKC within liver during choline deficiency may be the critical abnormality that eventually contributes to the development of hepatic cancer in these animals (58).

There are several other mechanisms which have been suggested for the cancer-promoting effect of a choline devoid diet. In the choline deficient liver, there is a progressive increase in cell proliferation, related to regeneration after parenchymal cell death (59,87,88). Cell proliferation, with associated increased rate of DNA synthesis, could be the cause of greater sensitivity to chemical carcinogens (51). Activation of PKC activity would be expected to trigger cell proliferation. Other stimuli

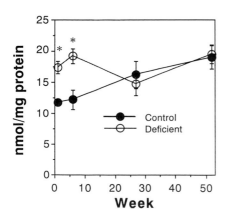

Week

FIG. 5. Elevated diradylglycerol in hepatic plasma membrane from choline-deficient rats. Rats were fed a defined diet containing choline (control) or devoid of choline (deficient) for 52 weeks. During this period, 23% of deficient rats developed hepatocarcinoma (all deficient rats had atypical hepatic foci), while none of the controls developed carcinoma or atypical foci. *sn*-1,2-Diradylglycerol was measured in hepatic plasma membrane using a radioenzymatic assay at indicated times. Data are expressed as mean $\pm$ SEM (n = 6/point). * = p <0.01 by one-way ANOVA and Scheffe's test. Data from daCosta KA, Cochary EF, Blusztajn JK, et al. Accumulation of 1,2-*sn*-diradylglycerol with increased membrane-associated protein kinase C may be the mechanism for spontaneous hepatocarcinogenesis in choline deficient rats. 1993; *J Biol Chem* 1993;268:2100–2105.

for increased DNA synthesis can be associated with carcinogenesis: Hepatectomy and necrogenic chemicals are examples. Shinozuka and Lombardi (89), however, found that the overall rate of liver cell proliferation could be dissociated from the rate at which preneoplastic lesions formed during choline deficiency, suggesting that cell proliferation is not the sole condition acting as a promoter of liver cancer. Methylation of DNA is important for the regulation of expression of genetic information. It has been suggested that the under-methylation of DNA, observed during choline deficiency (despite adequate dietary methionine), is responsible for carcinogenesis (90,91). Another proposed mechanism is based on the observation that, when rats are fed a choline deficient diet, increased lipid peroxidation occurs within liver (presence of diene conjugates in lipids isolated from purified hepatic nuclei; [92]). Lipid peroxides in the nucleus could be a source of free radicals, which could modify DNA, and cause carcinogenesis. It is likely that a combination of these mechanisms contributes to carcinogenesis during choline deficiency.

It is interesting that choline-deficient rats not only have a higher incidence of spontaneous hepatocarcinoma, but also are markedly sensitized to the effects of a variety of administered carcinogens (88). This has important implications, as choline status may modulate the threshold for sensitivity to environmental carcinogens. In addition, it has direct applicability to TPN therapy in humans because many of these patients are also being treated with chemotherapy. When choline-deficient male rats were treated with procarbazine, a chemotherapeutic agent, they had 50% higher mammary tumor incidence than did controls treated with procarbazine (93). This could be extremely important if choline deficiency has the same effect in humans. Cancer patients treated with chemotherapeutic agents have increased incidences of secondary and primary malignancies compared with patients not so treated (94). These patients are often on TPN therapy and might be choline deficient. Methotrexate, an inhibitor of folate metabolism, exacerbates choline deficiency (95). This occurs because folate-methyl groups are the only alternative source when choline is not available. The choline depletion secondary to TPN therapy in combination with methotrexate treatment might be a very toxic combination.

These observations are consistent with the hypothesis that, during a crucial period, choline deficiency can either initiate carcinogenesis, or promote endogenously initiated cells, or make hepatocytes susceptible to initiation. Perturbed PKC signal transduction may lower the threshold dose of carcinogen needed to initiate the development of cancers.

MIGHT PARENTERAL PHOSPHATIDYLCHOLINE HAVE IMPORTANT EFFECTS ON SIGNAL TRANSDUCTION?

While signal transduction is occupying our thoughts, it may be worthwhile to consider whether parenterally administered phosphatidylcholine might be used to modulate these messenger systems.

Phosphatidylcholine hydrolysis can be catalyzed by PLC and phospholipase D, and can act to sustain a message that was initially transmitted via inositide breakdown. Sustained activation of PKC is essential for triggering cell differentiation and proliferation (76). Phosphatidylcholine breakdown can generate second messengers independent of PtdIns breakdown. The fatty-acid species in phosphatidylcholine are different from those in PtdIns, therefore the DAGs generated from each will differ. Other products of phosphatidylcholine hydrolysis, such as phosphatidic acid, lysophosphatidylcholine, and free fatty acids also are second messengers (72,96). Phosphatidic acid can act as a mitogen (97). Lysophosphatidylcholine stimulates PKC activity (76), but it is a membrane-lytic detergent with potential toxic effects. Lysophosphatidylcholine generation is important in chemotaxis, relaxation of smooth muscle and activation of T-lymphocytes (76). Phospholipase A_2 (PLA_2) generates free fatty acids from phosphatidylcholine (76). Arachidonic acid, generated by PLA_2, can be a precursor for lipoxygenase or cyclooxygenase-generated products (73).

Thus, the phosphatidylcholine in parenteral fat emulsions might be used to modulate signal transduction. In addition, it would be useful to consider whether intravenously administered DAG might have important effects. It should be possible to substitute DAG for triglyceride in the emulsions; there may even be DAG in the emulsions as currently constituted. These questions need to be addressed in future research studies.

SPECIAL REQUIREMENTS FOR CHOLINE IN THE NEWBORN

Newborn infants are commonly fed parenterally. The demand for choline in children is likely to be higher than the demand for choline in adults, as large amounts of choline must be used to make phospholipids in growing organs (2). A reasonable estimate for dietary intake of choline in the infant can be derived from analyses of milk. As discussed earlier, milk contains approximately 1,400 μM choline moiety, delivering 200 μmol choline/kg/d to the healthy suckling baby. An infant treated with the recommended 3g/kg/d of parenteral lipid emulsion receives only approximately 150 μmol/kg/d choline.

CHOLINE AND BRAIN FUNCTION

The availability of choline to infants may be of special importance, as critical areas of brain are developing at around the time of birth. Choline supplementation during both pre- and postnatal development had long-term enhancing effects on spatial memory in rats, and this improvement was still detected in adults that had been treated as infants (98,99). Effects persist beyond 26 months of age (W. Meck, March, 1993, personal communication). Choline supplementation during the perinatal period led to a significant reduction in both the number of working memory errors and the number of reference memory errors made both during acquisition and at steady-state performance. The mechanism for this effect of choline on brain function has not been elucidated. Acetylcholine neurotransmission is important for memory in normal humans and rodents (100), and acetylcholine synthesis can be driven by increased availability of choline (101). Increased choline can enhance activity in the basal forebrain cholinergic system, thereby leading to improved memory function in a variety of species, including rats, mice, mollusks, and humans (102–106). Choline may also be influencing brain function via effects of phospholipid biosynthesis (107–109).

SUMMARY

Phosphatidylcholine was added to parental lipid emulsions as a stabilizing agent. It now turns out to supply a needed nutrient. Choline is required to make certain phospholipids, which are essential components of all membranes. It is a precursor for biosynthesis of the neurotransmitter acetylcholine and also is an important source of labile methyl groups. Healthy humans fed diets deficient in choline and humans fed parenterally have decreased plasma choline concentrations and develop liver dysfunction that is similar to that seen in choline-deficient animals. In experimental animals, fatty liver occurs in choline deficiency because phosphatidylcholine synthesis is required for VLDL secretion. This accumulation of lipids (especially the second-messenger DAG) in choline-deficient liver may explain why choline-deficient rats spontaneously develop hepatocarcinoma. Fatty liver is an important complication of parenteral nutrition therapy, and phosphatidylcholine supplementation may prevent it from developing. Phosphatidylcholine is parenteral emulsions may be especially important in the neonate, where demand for choline is higher and where critical areas of brain are developing. Choline supplements administered to rats *in utero* or shortly after birth permanently alter brain function.

ACKNOWLEDGMENT

The work described in this review was supported by a grant from the American Institute for Cancer Research.

REFERENCES

1. Hajri T, Ferezou J, Lutton C. Effects of intravenous infusions of commercial fat emulsions (Intralipid 10 or 20%) on rat plasma lipoproteins: phospholipids in excess are the main precursors of lipoprotein-X-like particles. *Biochim Biophys Acta* 1990;1047:121–130.
2. Zeisel SH. Choline deficiency. *J Nutr Biochem* 1970;1:332–349.
3. Best CH, Huntsman ME. The effects of the components of lecithin upon the deposition of fat in the liver. *J Physiol* 1932;75:405–412.
4. Best CH, Huntsman ME. Effect of choline on liver fat of rats in various states of nutrition. *J Physiol* 1935;83:255–274.
5. Eagle H. The minimum vitamin requirements of the L and Hela cells in tissue culture, the production of specific vitamin deficiencies, and their cure. *J Exp Med* 1955;102:595–600.
6. Zeisel SH, DaCosta K-A, Franklin PD, et al. Choline, an essential nutrient for humans. *FASEB J* 1991;5:2093–2098.
7. Sheard NF, Tayek JA, Bistrian BR, et al. Plasma choline concentration in humans fed parenterally. *Am J Clin Nutr* 1986;43:219–224.

8. Chawla RK, Wolf DC, Kutner MH, Bonkovsky HL. Choline may be an essential nutrient in malnourished patients with cirrhosis. *Gastroenterology* 1989;97:1514–1520.
9. Zeisel SH. "Vitamin-like" molecules: choline. In: Shils M, Young V, eds. *Modern Nutrition in Health and Disease*. Philadelphia: Lea & Febiger, 1988;440–452.
10. Hoffbauer FW, Zaki FG. Choline deficiency in the baboon and rat compared. *Arch Pathol* 1965; 79:364–369.
11. Buchman AL, Dubin M, Jenden D, et al. Lecithin increases plasma free choline and decreases hepatic steatosis in long-term total parenteral nutrition patients. *Gastroenterology* 1992;102: 1363–1370.
12. Federation of American Societies for Experimental Biology. *Evaluation of the Health Aspects of Choline Chloride and Choline Bitartrate as Food Ingredients*. National Technical Information Service, #PB262–654, 1975.
13. Engel RW. The choline content of animal and plant products. *J Nutr* 1943;25:441–446.
14. McIntire JM, Schweigert BS, Elvehjem CA. The choline and pyridoxine content of meats. *J Nutr* 1944;28:219–223.
15. Food and Nutrition Board. Comprehensive GRAS survey, usage levels reported for NAS appendix A substances (group 1) used in regular foods. In National Academy of Sciences USA. Washington, D.C., 1973.
16. Weihrauch JL, Son Y-S. The phospholipid content of foods. *J Am Oil Chem Soc* 1983;60:1971–1978.
17. Zeisel SH, Char D, Sheard NF. Choline, phosphatidylcholine and sphingomyelin in human and bovine milk and infant formulas. *J Nutr* 1986;116:50–58.
18. Pomfret EA, daCosta KA, Schurman LL, Zeisel SH. Measurement of choline and choline metabolite concentrations using high-pressure liquid chromatography and gas chromatography-mass spectrometry. *Anal Biochem* 1989;180:85–90.
19. Federation of American Societies for Experimental Biology. *Effect of Consumption of Choline and Lecithin on Neurological and Cardiovascular Systems*. Prepared for the Bureau of Foods, Food and Drug Administration, National Technical Information Service, #PB82-133257. Springfield, VA, 1981.
20. Zeisel SH. Dietary choline: biochemistry, physiology, and pharmacology. *Annu Rev Nutr* 1981;1: 95–121.
21. Zeisel SH, Growdon JH, Wurtman RJ, et al. Normal plasma choline responses to ingestion of lecithin. *Neurology* 1980;30:1226–1229.
22. Aquilonius SM, Ceder G, Lying TU, et al. The arteriovenous difference of choline across the brain of man. *Brain Res* 1975;99:430–433.
22a. Rohlfs EM, Garner SC, Mar MH, Zeisel SH. Glycerophosphocholine and phosphocholine are the major choline metabolites in rat milk. *J Nutr* 1993;123:1762–1768.
23. Blusztajn JK, Zeisel SH, Wurtman RJ. Developmental changes in the activity of phosphatidylethanolamine N-methytransferases in rat brain. *Biochem J* 1985;232:505–511.
24. Blusztajn JK, Zeisel SH, Wurtman RJ. Synthesis of lecithin (phosphatidylcholine) from phosphatidylethanolamine in bovine brain. *Brain Res* 1979;179:319–327.
25. Ridgway ND, Vance DE. Purification of phosphatidylethanolamine N-methyltransferase from rat liver. *J Biol Chem* 1987;262:17231–17239.
26. Bjornstad P, Bremer J. In vivo studies on pathways for the biosynthesis of lecithin in the rat. *J Lipid Res* 1966;7:38–45.
27. Crews FT, Calderini G, Battistella A, Toffano G. Age dependent changes in the methylation of rat brain phospholipids. *Brain Res* 1981;229:256–259.
28. Yang EK, Blusztajn JK, Pomfret EA, Zeisel SH. Rat and human mammary tissue can synthesize choline moiety via the methylation of phosphatdiyethanolamine. *Biochem J* 1988;256:821–828.
29. Davis PB. Lymphocyte and granulocyte phosphatidylethanolamine N-methyltransferase: properties and activity in cystic fibrosis. *Pediatr Res* 1986;20:1290–1296.
30. Fonlupt P, Dubois M, Gallet H, et al. Changes in leukocyte phospholipid-N-methyltransferase activity after chronic treatment of allergic patients with mequitazine. *Comptes Rendus* 1983;296: 1005–1007.
31. Harari Y, Castro GA. Phosphatidylethanolamine methylation in intestinal brush border membranes from rats resistant to *Trichinella spiralis*. *Mol Biochem Parasitol* 1985;15:317–326.
32. Laychock SG. Phosphatidylethanolamine N-methylation and insulin release in isolated pancreatic islets of the rat. *Mol Pharmacol* 1985;27:66–73.
33. Nieto A, Catt KJ. Hormonal activation of phospholipid methyltransferase in the Leydig cell. *Endocrinology* 1983;113:758–762.

34. Niwa Y, Sakane T, Taniguchi S. Phospholipid transmethylation in the membrane of human neutrophils and lymphocytes. *Arch Biochem Biophys* 1984;234:7–14.
35. Panagia V, Ganguly PK, Okumura K, Dhalla NS. Subcellular localization of phosphatidylethanolamine N-methylation activity in rat heart. *J Mol Cell Cardiol* 1985;17:1151–1159.
36. Hirata F, Tallman JF, Henneberry RC, et al. Phospholipid methylation: a possible mechanism of signal transduction across biomembranes. *Prog Clin Biol Res* 1981;63:383–388.
37. Saceda M, Garcia MP, Mato JM, et al. Phospholipid methylation in pancreatic islets. *Biochem Int* 1984;8:445–452.
38. Robinson BS, Snoswell AM, Runciman WB, Kuchel TR. Choline biosynthesis in sheep. Evidence for extrahepatic synthesis. *Biochem J* 1987;244:367–373.
39. Mudd SH, Poole JR. Labile methyl balances for normal humans on various dietary regimens. *Metab Clin Exp* 1975;24:721–735.
40. Finkelstein JD, Martin JJ, Harris BJ, Kyle WE. Regulation of the betaine content of rat liver. *Arch Biochem Biophys* 1982;218:169–173.
41. Wong ER, Thompson W. Choline oxidation and labile methyl groups in normal and choline-deficient rat liver. *Biochim Biophys Acta* 1972;260:259–271.
42. Barak AJ, Tuma DJ. Betaine, metabolic by-product or vital methylating agent? *Life Sci* 1983;32: 771–774.
43. Finkelstein JD, Martin JJ, Harris BJ. Methionine metabolism in mammals. The methionine-sparing effect of cystine. *J Biol Chem* 1988;263:11750–11754.
44. Shivapurkar N, Poirier LA. Tissue levels of S-adenosylmethionine and S-adenosylhomocysteine in rats fed methyl-deficient, amino acid-defined diets for one to five weeks. *Carcinogenesis* 1983;4: 1051–1057.
45. Poirier LA, Grantham PH, Rogers AE. The effects of a marginally lipotrope-deficient diet on the hepatic levels of S-adnosylmethionine and on the urinary metabolites of 2-acetylaminofluorene in rats. *Cancer Res* 1977;37:744–748.
46. Barak AJ, Beckenhauer HC, Tuma DJ. Use of S-adenosylmethionine as an index of methionine recycling in rat liver slices. *Anal Biochem* 1982;127:372–375.
47. Zeisel SH, Zola T, daCosta K, Pomfret EA. Effect of choline deficiency on S-adenosylmethionine and methionine concentrations in rat liver. *Biochem J* 1989;259:725–729.
48. Cook RJ, Horne DW, Wagner C. Effect of methyl group deficiency on one-carbon metabolism in rats. *J Nutr* 1989;119:612–617.
49. Horne DW, Cook RJ, Wagner C. Effect of dietary methyl group deficiency on folate metabolism in rats. *J Nutr* 1989;119:618–621.
50. Selhub J, Seyoum E, Pomfret EA, Zeisel SH. Effects of choline deficiency and methotrexate treatment upon liver folate content and distribution. *Cancer Res* 1991;51:16–21.
51. Ghoshal AK, Ahluwalia M, Farber E. The rapid induction of liver cell death in rats fed a choline-deficient methionine-low diet. *Am J Pathol* 1983;113:309–314.
52. Ghoshal AK, Farber E. The induction of liver cancer by dietary deficiency of choline and methionine without added carcinogens. *Carcinogenesis* 1984;5:1367–1370.
53. Lombardi B, Pani P, Schlunk FF. Choline-deficiency fatty liver: impaired release of hepatic triglycerides. *J Lipid Res* 1968;9:437–446.
54. Lombardi B. Effects of choline deficiency on rat hepatocytes. *Fed Proc* 1971;30:139–142.
55. Yao ZM, Vance DE. The active synthesis of phosphatidylcholine is required for very low density lipoprotein secretion from rat hepatocytes. *J Biol Chem* 1988;263:2998–3004.
56. Yao ZM, Vance DE. Head group specificity in the requirement of phosphatidylcholine biosynthesis for very low density lipoprotein secretion from cultured hepatocytes. *J Biol Chem* 1989;264: 11373–11380.
57. Blusztajn JK, Zeisel SH. 1,2-sn-diacylglycerol accumulates in choline-deficient liver. A possible mechanism of hepatic carcinogenesis via alteration in protein kinase C activity? *FEBS LETT* 1989; 243:267–270.
58. daCosta KA, Cochary EF, Blusztajn JK, et al. Accumulation of 1,2-*sn*-diradylglycerol with increased membrane-associated protein kinase C may be the mechanism for spontaneous hepatocarcinogenesis in choline deficient rats. *J Biol Chem* 1993;268:2100–2105.
59. Chandar N, Lombardi B. Liver cell proliferation and incidence of hepatocellular carcinomas in rats fed consecutively a choline-devoid and a choline-supplemented diet. *Carcinogenesis* 1988;9:259–263.
60. Kaminski DL, Mueller EJ, Jellinek M. Effect of small intestinal bypass on hepatic lipid accumulation in rats. *Am J Physiol* 1980;239:G358–G362.

61. Chawla RK, Berry CJ, Kutner MH, Rudman D. Plasma concentrations of transsulfuration pathway products during nasoenteral and intravenous hyperalimentation of malnourished patients. *Am J Clin Nutr* 1985;42:577–584.
62. Poley JR. Liver and nutrition: hepatic complications of total parenteral nutrition. In: Lebenthal E, ed. *Textbook of Gastroenterology and Nutrition in Infancy*. New York: Raven Press, 1981;743–763.
63. Burt ME, Hanin I, Brennan MF. Choline deficiency associated with total parenteral nutrition. *Lancet* 1980;2:638–639.
64. Carroll C, Williams L. Choline deficiency in rats as influenced by dietary energy somics. *Nutr Rep Int* 1982;25:773.
65. Kaminski DL, Adams A, Jellinek M. The effect of hyperalimentation on hepatic lipid content and lipogenic enzyme activity in rats and man. *Surgery* 1980;88:93–100.
66. Hall RI, Ross LH, Bozovic MG, Grant JP. The effect of choline supplementation on hepatic steatosis in the parenterally fed rat. *JPEN* 1985;9:597–599.
67. Borum PR. Carnitine. *Annu Rev Nutr* 1983;3:233–259.
68. Corredor C, Mansbach C, Bressler R. Carnitine depletion in the choline-deficient state. *Biochim Biophys Acta* 1967;144:366–374.
69. Carter AL, Frenkel R. The relationship of choline and carnitine in the choline deficient rat. *J Nutr* 1978;108:1748–1754.
70. Rogers AE, Newberne PM. Lipotrope deficiency in experimental carcinogenesis. *Nutr Cancer* 1980; 2:104–112.
71. Meldrum E, Parker PJ, Carozzi A. The Ptd-Ins-PLC superfamily and signal transduction. *Biochim Biophys Acta* 1991;1092:49–71.
72. Exton JH. Signaling through phosphatidylcholine breakdown. *J Biol Chem* 1990;265:1–4.
73. Stabel S, Parker PJ. Protein kinase C. *Pharmacol Ther* 1991;51:71–95.
74. Nishizuka Y. Studies and perspectives of protein kinase C. *Science* 1991;233:305–312.
75. Weinstein IB. The role of protein kinase C in growth control and the concept of carcinogenesis as a progressive disorder in signal transduction. *Adv Second Messenger Phosphoprotein Res* 1990;24: 307–316.
76. Nishizuka Y. Intracellular signaling by hydrolysis of phospholipids and activation of protein kinase C. *Science* 1992;258:607–614.
77. Hunter T. Cooperation between oncongenes. *Cell* 1991;64:249–270.
78. Kato M, Kawai S, Takenawa T. Defect in phorbol acetate-induced translocation of diacylglycerol kinase in erbB-transformed fibroblast cells. *FEBS Lett* 1989;247:247–250.
79. Diaz-Laviada I, Larrodera P, Diaz-Meco M, et al. Evidence for a role of phosphatidylcholine-hydrolysing phospholipase C in the regulation or protein kinase C by ras and src oncogenes. *Embo J* 1990;9:3907–3912.
80. Wilkison WO, Sandgren EP, Palmiter RD, et al. Elevation of 1,2-diacylglycerol in ras-transformed neonatal liver and pancreas of transgenic mice. *Oncogene* 1989;4:625–628.
81. Wolfman A, Wingrove TG, Blackshear PJ, Macara IG. Down-regulation of protein kinase C and of an endogenous 80-kDa substrate in transformed fibroblasts. *J Biol Chem* 1987;262:16546–16552.
82. Price BD, Morris JD, Marshall CJ, Hall A. Stimulation of phosphatidylcholine hydrolysis, diacylglyc-erol release, and arachidonic acid production by oncogenic ras is a consequence of protein kinase C activation. *J Biol Chem* 1989;264:16638–16643.
83. Rozengurt E. Early signals in the mitogenic response. *Science* 1986;234:161–166.
84. Kaibuchi K, Tsuda T, Kikuchi A, et al. Possible involvement of protein kinase C and calcium ion in growth factor-induced expression of c-myc oncogene in Swiss 3T3 fibroblasts. *J Biol Chem* 1986; 261:1187–1192.
85. Hsieh LL, Wainfan E, Hoshina S, et al. Altered expression of retrovirus-like sequences and cellular oncogenes in mice fed methyl-deficient diets. *Cancer Res* 1989;49:3795–3799.
86. Chandar N, Lombardi B, Locker J. c-myc gene amplification during hepatocarcinogenesis by a choline-devoid diet. *Proc Natl Acad Sci USA* 1989;86:2703–2707.
87. Chandar N, Amenta J, Kandala JC, Lombardi B. Liver cell turnover in rats fed a choline-devoid diet. *Carcinogenesis* 1987;8:669–673.
88. Newberne PM, Rogers AE. Labile methyl groups and the promotion of cancer. *Annu Rev Nutr* 1986;6:407–432.
89. Shinozuka H, Lombardi B. Synergistic effect of a choline-devoid diet and phenobarbital in promoting the emergence of foci of gamma-glutamyltranspeptidase-positive hepatocytes in the liver of carcino-gen-treated rats. *Cancer Res* 1980;40:3846–3849.

90. Locker J, Reddy TV, Lombardi B. DNA methylation and hepatocarcinogenesis in rats fed a choline devoid diet. *Carcinogenesis* 1986;7:1309–1312.
91. Dizik M, Christman JK, Wainfan E. Alterations in expression and methylation of specific genes in livers of rats fed a cancer promoting methyl-deficient diet. *Carcinogenesis* 1991;12:1307–1312.
92. Rushmore T, Lim Y, Farber E, Ghoshal A. Rapid lipid peroxidation in the nuclear fraction of rat liver induced by a diet deficient in choline and methionine. *Cancer Lett* 1984;24:251–255.
93. Rogers AE, Akhtar R, Zeisel SH. Procarbazine carcinogenicity in methotrexate-treated or lipotrope-deficient male rats. *Carcinogenesis* 1990;11:1491–1495.
94. Byrd R. Late effects of treatment of cancer in children. *Pediatr Clin North Am* 1985;32:835–856.
95. Pomfret EA, daCosta K-A, Zeisel SH. Effects of choline deficiency and methotrexate treatment upon rat liver. *J Nutr Biochem* 1990;1:533–541.
96. Besterman JM, Duronio V, Cuatrecasas P. Rapid formation of diacylglycerol from phosphatidylcholine: a pathway for generation of a second messenger. *Proc Natl Acad Sci USA* 1986;83:6785–6789.
97. Wakelam MJO, Cook SJ, Currie S, et al. Regulation of the hydrolysis of phosphatidylcholine in Swiss 3T3 cells. *Biochem Soc Trans* 1991;19:321–324.
98. Meck WH, Smith RA, Williams CL. Pre- and postnatal choline supplementation produces long-term facilitation of spatial memory. *Dev Psychobiol* 1988;21:339–353.
99. Meck WH, Smith RA, Williams CL. Organizational changes in cholinergic activity and enhanced visuospatial memory as a function of choline administered prenatally or postnatally or both. *Behav Neurosci* 1989;103:1234–1241.
100. Bartus RT, Dean R, Beer B, Lippa AS. The cholinergic hypothesis of geriatric memory dysfunction. *Science* 1982;217:408–414.
101. Blusztajn JK, Wurtman RJ. Choline and cholinergic neurons. *Science* 1983;221:614–620.
102. Barry SR, Gelperin A. Exogenous choline augments transmission at an identified cholinergic synapse in terrestrial mollusk *Limax maximus*. *J Neurophysiol* 1982;48:439–450.
103. Sahley CL, Barry SR, Gelperin A. Dietary choline augments associative memory function in *Limax maximus*. *Neurobiology* 1986;17:113–120.
104. Bartus RT, Dean RL, Goas JA, Lippa AS. Age-related changes in passive avoidance retention: modulation with dietary choline. *Science* 1980;209:301–303.
105. Sitaram N, Weingartner H, Gillin JC. Human serial learning: enhancement with arecoline and choline impairment with scopolamine. *Science* 1978;201:274–276.
106. Sitaram N, Weingartner H, Caine ED, Gillin JC. Choline: selective enhancement of serial learning and encoding of low imagery words in man. *Life Sci* 1978;22:1555–1560.
107. Schmidt DE, Wecker L. CNS effects of choline administration: evidence for temporal dependence. *Neuropharmacology* 1981;20:535–539.
108. Wecker L. Neurochemical effects of choline supplementation. *Can J Physiol Pharmacol* 1986;64:329–333.
109. Wecker L. Dietary choline: a limiting factor for the synthesis of acetylcholine by the brain. *Adv Neurol* 1990;51:139–145.

Organ Metabolism and Nutrition:
Ideas for Future Critical Care, edited by
J. M. Kinney and H. N. Tucker.
Raven Press, Ltd., New York © 1994.

17

Exogenous Lipids and Hepatic Function

Yvon A. Carpentier, D. Y. Dubois, V. S. Siderova,
and M. Richelle

*L. Deloyers Laboratory for Experimental Surgery, Université Libre de Bruxelles, B-1070
Brussels, Belgium*

THE ROLE OF THE LIVER IN LIPID METABOLISM

The liver is a central organ playing a major role in lipid and lipoprotein metabolism. It is involved in the assembly and secretion of some lipoproteins, in the transformation and remodelling of others, and also plays an essential role in the removal and endocytosis of specific particles. In addition, the liver is the exclusive or main site for the production of apoproteins (apos) B-100, A-II, C-I, C-II, and C-III, as well as serum amyloid (SAA) and H; it is also largely associated in the production of apo A-I, D, E, and J. Some enzymes involved in the intravascular metabolism of lipoproteins are also essentially produced in the liver, e.g., lecithin cholesterol acyltransferase (LCAT).

High-density lipoproteins (HDLs) mostly originate from the liver and the intestine. In patients fed parenterally, the liver represents the major source of HDL, but the possibility for HDL to be formed from surface components released during peripheral lipolysis of triglyceride (TG)-rich particles should be considered. High-density lipoproteins play a major role in the "reverse cholesterol transport," a process that results in the transfer of cholesterol from peripheral tissues to the liver (1). As detailed later, they are also involved in the exchange of neutral lipids with other lipoproteins (1,2) or emulsion particles (3). In addition to their contribution in cholesterol transport, there is increasing evidence to recognize antithrombogenic (4) and antiinflammatory (5,6) properties of HDL.

Very low density lipoproteins (VLDL) are mostly from hepatic origin (7,8). In fasting conditions, more than 90% of plasma TGs are transported by VLDL. Whereas chylomicron TGs are from dietary source, VLDL-TGs are derived from fatty acids (FAs) delivered to the liver from peripheral tissues or synthetized in situ (9). In contrast to a widespread opinion, VLDL secretion is predominant during the postprandial (vs. the fasting) period (10). The type of substrate delivered to the liver determines the secretion of two different types of VLDL (Fig. 1A). Carbohydrates stimulate the hepatic production of TG, but not of cholesteryl esters (CE) and apo B, which result in the secretion of large $VLDL_1$ with a high TG content (Fig. 1B).

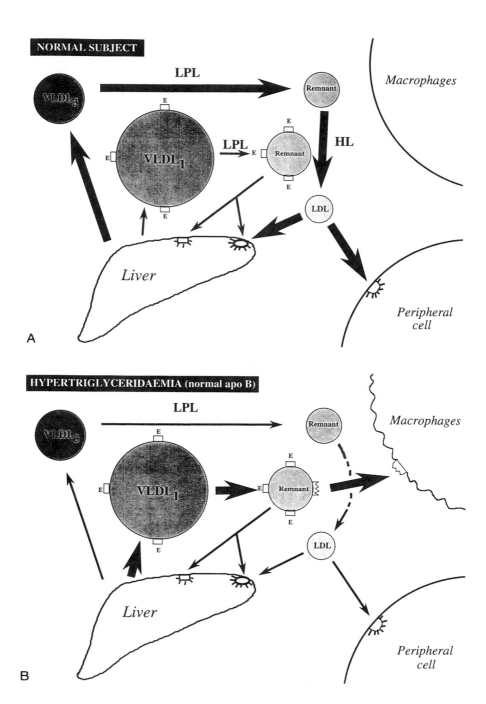

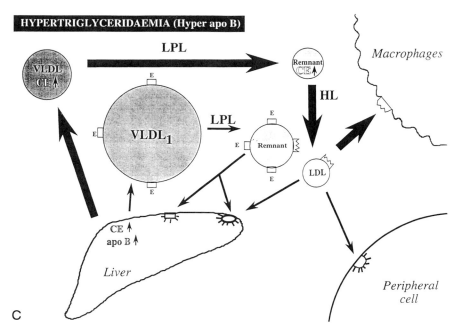

FIG. 1. C: Large delivery of long-chain fatty acids (LCFAs) to the liver stimulates cholesteryl ester (CE) and apo B production, which leads to the secretion of a large number of small CE-rich VLDLs. Lipolysis by LPL and by HL leads to the formation of small and dense LDLs, which are particularly sensitive to peroxidation. These modified LDLs may be removed (at a fast rate) by receptors present in macrophages.

Many long-chain fatty acids (LCFA) stimulate the production of not only TG but also CE and apo B, which results in the secretion of a large number of small VLDL$_3$ with a relatively high CE content (Fig. 1C). Lipoprotein lipase (LPL), a vascular endothelium-anchored enzyme, hydrolyzes a major part of VLDL-TG and releases FAs that are largely assimilated by extrahepatic (namely adipose) tissues (11). This lipolytic process and lipid exchanges between lipoproteins transform VLDL into CE-enriched remnants (2). Apart from their main function as lipid carrier, it has been

←

FIG. 1. Hepatic secretion of very low density lipoproteins (VLDL). **A:** In normal conditions, mainly one type of VLDL (VLDL$_3$) is produced by the liver, while secretion of large TG-rich and apo E–rich VLDL$_1$ is limited. Both VLDL$_1$ and VLDL$_3$ undergo lipolysis by lipoprotein lipase (LPL). This leads to the formation of remnant particles. Remnants from VLDL$_3$ are further lipolyzed by hepatic lipase (HL), which leads to the formation of low-density lipoproteins (LDLs). Low-density lipoproteins bind to specific B,E receptors present in the hepatocytes and in selected peripheral cells. Remnants from VLDL$_1$ are essentially removed in the liver; they can bind to both the LDL receptor and to a specific apo E receptor. **B:** Large carbohydrate supply stimulates the formation of large VLDL$_1$ and induces hypertriglyceridemia without raising apo B level. If these particles remain for a prolonged period in the circulation, plasma proteases can alter apos (mainly apo B). Remnants derived from these modified VLDLs may be removed (at fast rate) by receptors present in macrophages.

suggested that VLDLs (and other TG-rich particles) play a specific role in septic conditions by trapping and neutralizing endotoxins (12).

The vast majority of remnants derived from $VLDL_3$ are converted into low-density lipoproteins (LDLs) through further TG lipolysis by hepatic lipase (13,14). At the final stage of their intravascular stay, LDLs are removed by receptor-mediated endocytosis, mainly in the liver but also in other tissues (15). A substantial proportion of remnants derived from $VLDL_1$ are directly removed from the circulation by hepatocytes, via apo E binding receptors (16,17). HDL are also partially catabolized in the liver by the combination of hepatic lipase activity, cholesterol diffusion, and receptor-mediated processes (18,19).

Thus, while being a key-organ in the secretion and conversion of lipoproteins, the liver also plays an important role in the uptake of TG, CE, phospholipids (PLs), and, of special interest, liposoluble vitamins contained in circulating lipoproteins.

The hepatic metabolism of FA comprises different aspects and involves several pathways. The liver metabolizes FA from both endogenous and exogenous origin (20). Endogenous FAs include those synthesized *de novo* and those released upon lipolysis of hepatocellular TG stores. Exogenous FAs are derived from the plasma pool of nonesterified FA (Nefas) and the lipid components of circulating lipoproteins and emulsion particles. A number of regulatory mechanisms determine the balance between lipogenesis and FA oxidation in relation to the physiopathologic status.

Lipogenesis represents the formation of nonessential FA (mainly palmitate and myristate) from excess acetyl-CoA derived from carbohydrates. These FA may also be produced by elongation or chain reduction of nonessential or essential FA (21). Although at a much lower rate than observed in more specialized tissues (such as, e.g., the central nervous system), the liver is an active site for elongation and desaturation, leading to the formation of nonessential mono-unsaturated FA such as oleate (using the delta-9 desaturase), but also of essential long-chain polyunsaturated acids, such as arachidonate and eicosapentanoate or docosahexanoate (using the delta-6, delta-5, and delta-4 desaturases) (Table 1).

The regulation of FA oxidation in mammalian liver has been recently reviewed (20) and a summary is provided in Table 2. Beta-oxidation of FA takes place mainly in mitochondria, but also (and, to a substantial extent, for some very long chain FA) in peroxysomes. In the mitochondria, acetyl-CoA can then be oxidized by entering the tricarboxylic acid cycle (22) or be converted to ketone bodies (and, to a limited extent, to short-chain carnitine esters) (23). In the cytosol, acetyl-CoA can lead to the formation of FAs (using acetyl-CoA carboxylase) or of cholesterol using hydroxymethyl glutaryl (HMG) CoA synthase and reductase. Esterification of FA into diglycerides can further lead to the formation of TG, but also of PLs (with a selection of saturated FA in sn-1 and of unsaturated in sn-2 position) (24). Acylcholesterol acyltransferase (ACAT) preferentially uses oleate for the formation of CEs. Distribution of FA into these different pathways is largely regulated by the state of nutrition and the hormonal milieu, but also by the type of FA. Since lipid emulsions have been developed on the model of TG-rich chylomicron and show many similarities to this lipoprotein with respect to composition and size range (while providing FA pat-

TABLE 1. *Desaturase-elongase pathways for n-6 and n-3 essential fatty acids.* *

		n-6 series	n-3 series
		Linolenic C18:2n-6	Alpha-linolenic C18:3n-3
Δ6-Desaturase	→	↓	↓
		Gamma-linolenic C18:3n-6	Octadecatetraenoic C18:4n-3
Elongation	→	↓	↓
		Dihomo-gamma-linolenic C20:3n-6	Eicosatetraenoic C20:4n-3
Δ5-Desaturase	→	↓	↓
		Arachidonic C20:4n-6	Eicosapentaenoic C20:5n-3
Elongation	→	↓	↓
		Docosatetraenoic C22:4n-6	Docosapentaenoic C22:5n-3
Δ4-Desaturase	→	↓	↓
		Docosapentaenoic C22:5n-6	Docosahexaenoic C22:6n-3

The same enzymatic pathway is used for elongation and desaturation of C18 n-6 and n-3 fatty acids. Fatty acids playing a major role in humans (at the exception of those involved in brain metabolism) are presented in capital letters.

TABLE 2. *Fatty acid oxidation in the liver.*

Process	Main enzyme(s)	Rate-limiting	Control
Cell uptake	FABP ?	?	?
	Lipoprotein receptor	+ +	Cellular effectors
Cytosolic transport	L-FABP	?	?
Activation	acyl-CoA synthetases	±	?
Transport into mitochondria	CPT_o CPT_i	+ + + ?	Malonyl-CoA, diet, hormones ?
Transport into peroxisomes	CPT_p	+ + +	Malonyl-CoA, diet
Beta-oxidation	"Metabolon"	+ +	NADH/NAD$^+$, osmolarity cellular effectors?
Ketogenesis	HMG-CoA synthase	+ + +	Diet, hormones
Complete oxidation	TCA cycle	+ + +	Ca^{2+} (mobilization & distribution) diet, hormones

Adapted from Guzman and Geelen (20).
FABP, fatty acid binding protein; L-FABP, liver fatty acid binding protein; CPT_o, carnitine palmitoyltransferase activity in the mitochondrial outer membrane; CPT_i, carnitine palmitoyltransferase activity in the mitochondrial inner membrane; CPT_p, carnitine palmitoyltransferase activity in peroxisomes; "metabolon": the chain of mitochondrial enzymes involved in the beta-oxidation; HMG-CoA, 3 hydroxy–3 methylglutaryl-CoA; TCA, tricarboxylic acid (or Krebs) cycle.

tern substantially different from that of dietary FA) (25), several interactions may be expected between the metabolism of emulsion particles and hepatic function.

INTRAVASCULAR METABOLISM OF LIPID EMULSIONS

In emulsion particles, the TG core is stabilized by a PL surface. However, PLs are present in greater amounts in lipid emulsions than in chylomicrons, and the surplus of PLs can be isolated by ultracentrifugation as a separate fraction of vesicular or liposomal particles (26).

Metabolism of Triglyceride-rich Particles

Hydrolysis of triglycerides present in the core of emulsion particles takes place first at the endothelial site of extrahepatic tissues under the action of LPL. Immediately after their infusion into the circulation, emulsion particles acquire different apos transferred from the HDL pool (Fig. 2). Apo C-II plays an essential role in the recognition of emulsion particles by LPL receptor site and activation of its hydrolytic site (27). Transfer of apo C-II is very efficient (28) and only small amounts are required for activating LPL; thus, except for extreme conditions of altered protein synthesis or massive losses, apo C-II deficiency is unlikely to be rate limiting for extrahepatic lipolysis. Hydrolysis of exogenous TG is regulated by endogenous factors (such as the availability of active LPL and its distribution between various tissues), as well as by the lipid composition of the emulsion. Indeed, in order to become accessible to the hydrolytic action of the lipase, TG molecules have to partition from particle core into the PL surface (29). The amount of TG that can be dissolved into a PL layer is largely dependent on the chain length and degree of unsaturation of triglyceride FA, but also on PL composition. For example, medium-chain TG (MCT) are four to five times more soluble into the same phospholipid layer than soybean-derived long-chain TG (LCT). This factor probably plays an important role in the faster hydrolysis by LPL of MCT versus LCT and explains why MCTs disappear more rapidly than LCTs from a particle containing a mixture of both types of TG (30).

In normal postprandial conditions, it is generally believed that most FAs resulting from TG hydrolysis by LPL are taken up by adjacent tissues and that only a small fraction is released into the circulation to increase the plasma pool of Nefas largely associated to albumin. The situation can be quite different in parenteral nutrition since lipid emulsions are sometimes infused at a fast rate. The immediate effect of TG hydrolysis by LPL is to release large amounts of FA at the site of the endothelial wall. If they are not efficiently assimilated by the adjacent tissues, FAs accumulate and exert a feedback inhibition on LPL activity (31); this effect is more pronounced for LCFA than medium-chain FA. In addition, locally high concentrations of FA can disrupt the attachment of LPL to the endothelium and release the enzyme into the circulation. Lipoprotein lipase was recently suggested to act as a ligand promoting the binding to their receptors of TG-rich remnants (32) and other lipoproteins (33).

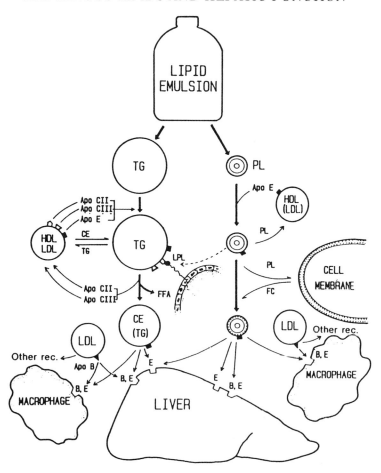

FIG. 2. Intravascular metabolism of both triglyceride (TG)-rich and phospholipid (PL)-rich particles present in a lipid emulsion. On the left side, four main steps are represented for the metabolism of TG-rich particles: (1) acquisition of apoproteins (apo) E, CII, and CIII by transfer from high-density lipoproteins (HDLs); (2) lipolysis by lipoprotein lipase (LPL) at the endothelial site of extrahepatic tissues releasing fatty acids (FAs); (3) exchanges of neutral lipids TG and cholesteryl esters (CEs) between emulsion particles and low-density lipoproteins (LDLs) and HDL; these exchanges are mediated by the CE transfer protein (CETP); (4) uptake of particle remnants by the liver, but potentially also by macrophages. On the right side, the formation of PL-free cholesterol complexes having acquired apo E is represented, as is the competitive effect of liposomes for LPL. In the lower part, we have speculated on the potential competition of exogenous remnants between themselves and with endogenous lipoproteins for binding to the LDL B,E receptor and the chylomicron remnant E receptor, at the site of different tissues. FFA, free fatty acids. From Carpentier, 26a.

One can speculate a similar role for LPL towards emulsion remnants. Thus, the infusion rate of lipid emulsions, together with the capacity of extrahepatic tissues for assimilating FA released from TG hydrolysis, may largely influence not only the release of Nefas and LPL in the plasma, but also the amount of TG remaining in remnant particles to be delivered to the liver. Indeed, recent work from Sniderman and his associates strongly suggests that assimilation of FA by peripheral tissues (and namely adipose tissues) is regulated by an acylation-stimulating protein (ASP) which is more potent than insulin in promoting reesterification of FA into TG (34). An impaired tissue response to ASP would lead to an increased content of TG in remnant particles, together with a higher release of Nefas into the circulation (Fig. 3). Although LPL is capable of hydrolyzing various lipid components contained into different lipoproteins, the enzyme appears to interact preferentially with large-sized particles such as chylomicrons and VLDL, and its activity on PLs represents only a few percent of that directed on TG. In addition, the enzyme shows a specificity for preferentially cleaving FA with a chain length not longer than 18 carbon atoms from the sn-1 and the sn-3 positions of TG molecules. It was recently suggested that the hepatic lipase (HL) could have a complementary role by hydrolyzing, from the particle surface, residual lipids (mono- and diglycerides, PLs, etc.) that have not been properly attacked by LPL (35). This would result in a preferential channeling of some FA to the periphery while others are mainly delivered to the liver.

Exchange of core components between TG-rich particles and cholesterol-rich lipoproteins represents another important step in the intravascular metabolism of lipid emulsions. This process is mediated by the cholesteryl ester transfer protein (CETP), which is actively present in humans and in only some animal species (2). These exchanges are regulated by the amount (and the composition) of TG-rich particles present in the circulation, but also by the concentration of PLs and Nefas. Transfer of TG to LDL (and HDL), in exchange of CE, results in a substantial core remodelling, which can affect particle recognition by specific receptors (13,36). At the same time, emulsion particles lose TG (both by hydrolysis and transfer) and acquire CE to form remnants that may play a substantial role in the reverse transport of cholesterol from peripheral tissues to liver. In vitro and in vivo data from our group support the concept that MCT-containing particles transfer more TG to LDL and HDL but accept much less CE from these lipoproteins than pure LCT emulsions, these effects being related to a higher concentration of MCT in surface PLs (30,37,38). Thus, higher peripheral lipolysis and low enrichment with CE result in a low concentration of TG and CE in remnants formed from MCT-containing particles.

Uptake of remnants by the liver is the last, but crucial, step in the intravascular metabolism of emulsion TG-rich particles. It has been long known that remnant removal could proceed not only through the B, E receptors, but also through a receptor recognizing only apo E. More recently, it was shown that infusion of recombinant apo E in rabbits largely accelerates the elimination of CE contained in remnants (39,40). Evidence is developing that the recently isolated low-density receptor-related protein (LRP) could be the long-sought chylomicron remnant (or apo E) receptor (41). Confirmation that LRP is this putative receptor would be extremely relevant

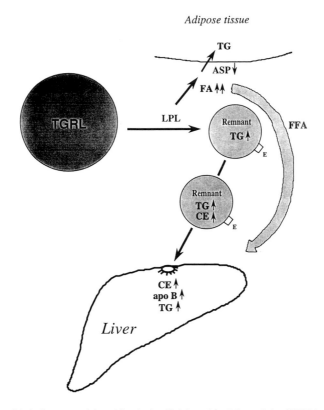

Adipose tissue

FIG. 3. Relationship between peripheral lipolysis of triglyceride-rich particles (TGRL) and delivery of fatty acids (FA) to the liver. In normal conditions, FAs released at the endothelial site by the action of lipoprotein lipase (LPL) are largely taken up by peripheral (namely adipose) tissues. Acylation stimulating protein (ASP) stimulates FA reesterification into triglycerides (TG) and increases FA assimilation by adipose tissue. When tissue response to ASP is reduced, high amounts of FA are present at the endothelial site. This leads to the release of abnormally TG-enriched remnants into the circulation which acquire substantial amounts of cholesteryl esters (CEs) by exchange from other lipoproteins. In addition, a large proportion of FAs are released into the circulation and increase the plasma pool of nonesterified FA (FFA). Massive delivery to the liver of FA (as FFA and as TGFA in remnants) stimulates the production of CE, apoprotein (apo) B and TG.

for the care of patients because (a) LRP has been isolated not only in hepatocytes, but also in other tissues such as bone marrow; and (b) LRP also binds some proteins, such as alpha-2 macroglobulin and plasminogen activator inhibitor (PAI-1). If there was a competition between these proteins and remnants for the same receptor sites, this could not only delay the catabolism of tumor necrosis factor (TNF) (and other cytokines linked with alpha-2 macroglobulin), but also enhance the tendency to thrombosis by impairing the fibrinolytic process.

In the case of impaired hepatic uptake or prolonged stay in the circulation, remnants may be diverted to other tissues (e.g., macrophages) where they can be removed by receptor-mediated (or possibly non–receptor-mediated) pathway(s).

Although some aspects of this integrated view on the intravascular metabolism of TG-rich particles are still speculative, the concept that emulsion FA partitioning between peripheral tissues and the liver may be affected by TG composition and by different mediators is gaining support.

Metabolism of Phospholipid-rich Particles

The proportion of PLs present in the liposomal fraction is much higher in the classical 10% emulsions with a PL:TG (wt:wt) ratio of 0.12 than in 20% emulsions with a PL:TG ratio of 0.06 (42).

Because the plasma elimination of liposomal particles is relatively slow, infusion of PL-rich emulsions at a high rate induces their prolonged accumulation (43,44). In the circulation, these particles may interfere with other lipoproteins and emulsion particles at several steps of their metabolism (Fig. 2) (10). For example, they compete with TG-rich particles for binding to LPL, which may impede peripheral hydrolysis of TG (26). They acquire apoproteins (e.g., apo E) from the HDL reservoir and are capable of competing with other particles for binding to apo E and B,E receptors (45). In addition, liposomal PL can substantially modify the composition of cell membranes by attracting free cholesterol, as demonstrated for erythrocytes (46). Phospholipid-free cholesterol complexes bind to albumin and form particles similar to lipoprotein X (LpX), which was primarily isolated from the plasma of cholestatic patients. LipoproteinX is expected to be eliminated in the liver; hepatic accumulation of PL has been reported to occur in patients on long-term total parenteral nutrition (TPN) with lipids (47).

Because of these effects, at several steps of lipid metabolism, attention has recently been paid to reduce the liposomal content of lipid emulsions (42). In addition to the 20% preparations, PL-reduced 10% emulsions as well as 30% emulsions with a PL:TG ratio of 0.06 and 0.04, respectively) have now become available. Of interest is that not only the amount of PLs, but also their composition, may affect emulsion metabolism. For instance, we found differences of TG elimination and FA release into the circulation between two preparations differing only in the phosphatidylcholine:phosphatidylethanolamine ratio of egg PLs.

HEPATIC COMPLICATIONS DURING LONG-TERM PARENTERAL NUTRITION

Elevated plasma values of hepatic enzymes and bilirubin are commonly observed in patients receiving nutrients exclusively by the intravenous route (48–50). Such alterations have long been recognized in infants (51–53) and subsequently in adult patients on long-term TPN (54,55).

In clinical practice, the incidence of such alterations was particularly high with use of hypercaloric parenteral regimens based predominantly on carbohydrates as an energy source (56–60). Occurrence of abnormal liver function tests has also been

TABLE 3. *Triglyceride fatty acid composition of the soy-derived LCT and the mixed MCT/LCT emulsion.*

Emulsions	LCT	MCT/LCT
C8–C12	0	53
C14–C16	13	5
C18:1n9	19	10
C18:2n6	55	26
C18:3n3	8	3
C20:4n6	0	0
C20:5n3	0	0
C22:6n3	0	0

attributed to fat emulsions (61). Nevertheless, reduction of total caloric intake and partial isocaloric substitution of glucose with lipids are associated with normal values of liver enzymes in a majority of adult patients receiving parenteral nutrition for average periods of about 1 month (62–65). Still, abnormal hepatic function tests remain a matter of serious concern in some patients requiring long-term parenteral nutrition, particularly those with inflammatory bowel disease or short bowel syndrome (55,66–68). Although uncommon, cases of progression to irreversible liver damage have been reported (66,69,70).

Studies from our group and others demonstrated substantial differences in the metabolism of MCT-containing emulsion by comparison to conventional soy-derived emulsions, consisting mainly of, (a) a faster and more complete TG hydrolysis at peripheral sites leading to the formation of remnants poorly loaded with TG and CE, (b) a marked enlargement of plasma Nefa pool with a substantial contribution of medium-chain FA, and (c) higher levels of ketone bodies. These properties made us hypothesize that use of a mixed emulsion may offer a better protection of liver function, particularly in patients requiring long-term TPN.

In a prospective crossover study (71), eight patients with inflammatory bowel disease on home parenteral nutrition (HPN) were randomized to receive 50% of nonprotein calories as exclusively long-chain TG (provided with a 20% soy-derived emulsion Endolipid [B. Braun, Melsungen, Germany]) or a 50:50 (wt:wt) mixture of long-chain TG and MCT (provided with a 20% emulsion Medialipide [B. Braun]) for 3 months and then switched to the other emulsion during a second period of 3 months (Table 3). The other HPN components remained unchanged. Three patients with inflammatory bowel disease showed an increase in plasma levels of liver transaminases, gamma glutamyltranspeptidase, and alkaline phosphatase while receiving HPN with Endolipid. After a second measurement (at a week interval) confirming the alteration, these three patients were switched to the mixed emulsion and the abnormalities resolved within 2 to 8 weeks. A slower elimination of emulsion TG was observed during the period of abnormal hepatic tests. For example, in two patients with high plasma bilirubin levels, a twofold increase in plasma TG, free cholesterol, and PLs was observed in samples taken at 6 hours postinfusion. This occurred almost exclusively in the 1.006 < d < 1.063 g/l or LDL fraction, which contains not only endogenous LDL, but also remnants formed from emulsion (TG-rich) particles and LpX-like material. No alteration of liver tests occurred during nutritional support with the mixed emulsion. If one assumes the average incidence for altered hepatic tests to be 25% in patients on long-term HPN with standard soy-derived emulsions (68,72), the probability calculated by binomial distribution that none of the eight patients would have developed liver dysfunction during 3 months of HPN is 0.023.

In a subsequent longitudinal study, 24 HPN patients receiving the mixed emulsion (contributing up to 50% of nonprotein calories) were prospectively followed for periods of 3 to more than 60 months (Fig. 4). Six patients started with altered hepatic parameters. In five of them, liver function tests progressively improved and remained normal after 12 and 24 months. In one patient who was treated with phenytoin, hepatic enzymes remained elevated, but the levels did not exceed 50% above the upper normal range. This latter patient and two others developed biliary microlithiases after periods of 6, 30, and 60 months, respectively, and two patients underwent a cholecystectomy. Among the 18 patients who entered the study with normal liver function tests, only two showed a transitory elevation of alkaline phosphatase level (at 3 and 6 months), with subsequent normalization.

These results suggest that the use of a mixed lipid emulsion has the potential to substantially reduce the incidence of liver complications in the growing population of patients requiring prolonged HPN but, because the etiology of TPN-associated liver dysfunction is multifactorial (73), the mechanisms through which this beneficial effect is exerted remain speculative.

Pathologic changes observed in the liver of animals and patients during TPN include steatosis, intra- and extrahepatic cholestasis, but also inflammatory foci, namely in the periportal areas (58,59). In some instances, evolution toward fibrosis or cirrhosis is observed.

Hepatic fatty infiltration, the most common and earliest alteration noted (74), has been thought to result from excessive infusion of macronutrients (and particularly of carbohydrates) (56,63,75,76), unbalanced calorie-protein intake, unbalanced amino acid intake (77), delivery to the liver of exogenous or endogenous toxic products (72), or deficiencies in essential FA (78,79), choline (80,81) or carnitine. Lipid supplementation can reduce steatosis by correcting essential FA deficiency (78) and by lowering the portal insulin:glucagon ratio, an effect that can also be obtained by l-glutamine addition (82). Medium-chain TGs appear to protect better than long-chain TGs against fatty infiltration (83). It is difficult to evaluate FA delivery to the liver during TPN with a mixed versus a soy-derived emulsion. On the one hand, low contents of TG (and CE) in emulsion remnants probably indicate efficient peripheral lipolysis; on the other, large amounts of Nefas are available for all tissues, including the liver. Medium-chain FA can readily cross hepatic mitochondrial membrane to undergo beta-oxidation (without previous coupling to carnitine) and stimulate ketogenesis (20). Hence, they are probably less prone to elongation and reesterification than long-chain FA (84). In vitro, octanoate stimulates TG production and formation of CE much less than long-chain FAs such as oleate (85).

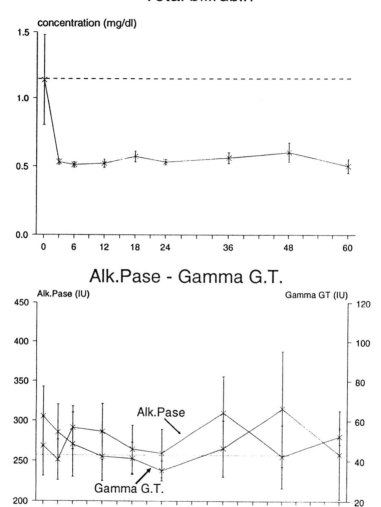

FIG. 4. Evolution of liver tests in 24 patients receiving home parenteral nutrition with MCT/LCT for 6 to 60 months. Shown are average values for plasma total bilirubin, alkaline phosphatase (Alk. Pase) and gamma glutamyltranspeptidase (Gamma G.T.) over the 60-month follow-up. Upper normal range is indicated by a dotted line.

Higher concentrations of ketones (86) and short-chain carnitine esters (87) during TPN with MCTs may at least partly obviate the failure of parenteral solutions to provide adequate nutrients to the gut and immune cells. Whether this may have a protective effect against increased permeability of intestinal barrier and delivery of toxins or bacteria to the liver remains to be determined.

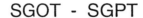

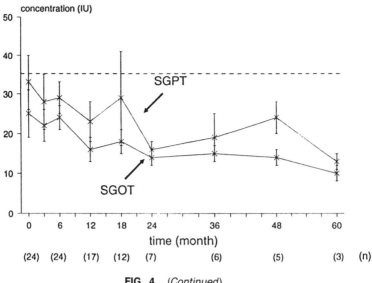

FIG. 4. (*Continued*)

It was recently shown that infusion of soy-derived emulsions in rats increases the toxic effects of TNF-alpha on hepatocytes (88). This could be due to an effect of remnants delaying TNF catabolism (see previous section) or to an increased inflammatory reaction resulting from large provision of n-6 FA. One may speculate that the different metabolism of remnants as well as the lower n-6 FA supply with the mixed emulsion could influence this reaction.

The pattern of essential FA in extra- and intracellular membrane PLs is known to regulate cell metabolic functions by influencing membrane physical properties as well as the expression and activity of receptors and enzymes. In patients on long-term HPN, our group showed that alterations of erythrocyte FA composition induced by soy-derived emulsions could be largely reduced by using the mixed emulsion (89). Whether this applies to other cells and to what extent it is associated with functional consequences is not known.

Polyunsaturated FAs, which contribute to 63% of soy TGFA, are very sensitive to free radicals. Peroxidative injury to hepatic mitochondrial lipids, produced by dietary copper overload in rats, is related to vitamin E deficiency (90). It is well recognized that TPN with conventional lipids is associated with the formation of peroxyl radicals (91–93) and that current supply of antioxidants is insufficient in long-term HPN patients (94,95). At the same time, infusion of alpha-tocopherol-enriched emulsion in humans maintains a normal vitamin E distribution among plasma lipoproteins (96). It is tempting to speculate that the use of a mixed emulsion may reduce the need for vitamin E supplementation.

Lipid composition of remnants suggests that reverse cholesterol transport to the liver is much lower with mixed than long-chain emulsions. Whether this influences bile composition and lithogenicity remains to be elucidated. Observations of biliary sludge and gallstones in some of our long-term patients emphasize the fact that bile stasis is a major factor in the development of cholestasis (97) and suggests the need for appropriate therapy (98).

CONCLUSIONS

The liver plays a key role in the metabolism of lipids and lipoproteins in humans. This is also true in patients receiving parenteral nutrition with lipids. In such conditions, peripheral metabolism of emulsion particles at the endothelial site of extrahepatic tissues regulates the delivery of various lipid components to the liver.

Alterations of hepatic function tests are not uncommon during long-term parenteral nutrition. The etiology is multifactorial and several morphopathologic changes are observed. Although rare, an irreversible evolution toward cirrhosis can occur. We report a study suggesting that the use of a lipid emulsion containing MCTs can substantially reduce the incidence of HPN-associated liver complications and speculate on potential factors contributing to this beneficial effect. Both a direct role for MCTs and the influence of decreasing soy long-chain TGFA intake are considered.

ACKNOWLEDGMENTS

The studies summarized in this chapter were performed with the support of Grants nr 9.4585.90 and 9.4511.91 from the Belgian "Fonds de la Recherche Scientifique Medicale." The emulsions were kindly provided by B. Braun (Melsungen, Germany). I wish to thank R. J. Deckelbaum, T. Olivecrona, P. Fürst, and D. Haumont for a long-standing scientific collaboration and many friendly discussions, and my secretary N. Van Laer for her tremendous help in organizing and typing this manuscript.

REFERENCES

1. Tall AR. Plasma high density lipoproteins. Metabolism and relationship to atherogenesis. *J Clin Invest* 1990;86:379–384.
2. Tall AR. Plasma lipid transfer protein. *J Lipid Res* 1986;27:361–368.
3. Granot E, Deckelbaum RJ, Eisenberg S, et al. Core modification of human low density lipoprotein by artificial triacylglycerol emulsion. *Biochim Biophys Acta* 1985;833:308–315.
4. Aoyama T, Yui Y, Morishita H, Kawai C: Prostaglandin I₂ half-life regulated by high density lipoprotein is decreased in acute myocardial infarction and unstable angina pectoris. *Circulation* 1990;81:1784–1791.
5. Blackburn WD Jr, Dohlman JC, Venkatachalapathi YV, et al. Apolipoprotein A-I decreases neutrophil degranulation and superoxide production. *J Lipid Res* 1991;32:1911–1918.
6. Packman CH, Rosenfeld SI, Leddy JP. High-density lipoproteins and its apolipoproteins inhibit cytolytic activity of complement. Studies of the nature of the inhibitory moieties. *Biochim Biophys Acta* 1985;812:107–115.

7. Alexander CA, Hamilton RL, Havel RJ. Subcellular localization of B apoprotein of plasma lipoproteins in rat liver. *J Cell Biol* 1976;69:241–263.
8. Chao F-F, Stiers DL, Ontko JA. Hepatocellular triglyceride synthesis and transfer to lipid droplets and nascent very low density lipoproteins. *J Lipid Res* 1986;27:1174–1181.
9. Gotto AM Jr, Pownall HJ, Havel RJ. Introduction to the plasma lipoproteins. *Methods Enzymol* 1986;128:3–41.
10. Sniderman AD, Cianflone K. Substrate delivery as a determinant of hepatic apo B secretion. *Arterioscler Thromb* 1993;13:629–636.
11. Olivecrona T, Bengtsson-Olivecrona G. Lipoprotein lipase from milk—the model enzyme in lipoprotein lipase research. In: Borensztajn J, ed. *Lipoprotein Lipase*. Chicago: Evener Publishers, 1987; 15–58.
12. Harris HW, Grunfeld C, Feingold KR, Rapp JH. Human very low density lipoproteins and chylomicrons can protect against endotoxin-induced death in mice. *J Clin Invest* 1990;86:696–702.
13. Packard CJ, Munro A, Lorimer AR, et al. Metabolism of apolipoprotein B in large triglyceride-rich hypertriglyceridemic subjects. *J Clin Invest* 1984;74:2178–2192.
14. Havel RJ. The formation of LDL: mechanisms and regulation. *J Lipid Res* 1984;25:1570–1576.
15. Goldstein JL, Brown MS. Progress in understanding of the LDL receptor and HMG-CoA reductase, two membrane proteins that regulate plasma cholesterol. *J Lipid Res* 1984;25:1450–1461.
16. Mahley RW, Innerarity TL. Lipoprotein receptors and cholesterol homeostasis. *Biochim Biophys Acta* 1983;737:197–222.
17. Mahley RW, Hussain MM. Chylomicron and chylomicron remnant catabolism. *Curr Opin Lipidol* 1991;2:170–176.
18. Collet X, Perret B-P, Simar G, et al. Behaviour of phospholipase-modified HDL towards cultured hepatocytes. I. Enhanced transfers of HDL sterols and apoproteins. *Biochim Biophys Acta* 1990; 1043:301–310.
19. Hidaka H, Fidge NH. Affinity purification of the hepatic high-density lipoprotein receptor identifies two acidic glycoproteins and enables further characterization of their binding properties. *Biochem J* 1992;284:161–167.
20. Guzman M, Geelen JH. Regulation of fatty acid oxidation in mammalian liver. *Biochim Biophys Acta* 1993;1167:227–241.
21. Wakil SJ, Stoops JK, Joshi V. Fatty acid synthesis and its regulation. *Annu Rev Biochem* 1983;52: 537–579.
22. Krebs HA. The history of the tricarboxylate cycle. *Perspect Biol Med* 1970;14:154–170.
23. McGarry JD, Foster DW. Regulation of hepatic fatty acid oxydation and ketone body production. *Annu Rev Biochem* 1980;49:395–420.
24. Bell RM, Coleman RA. Enzymes in glycerolipids synthesis in eucaryotes. *Annu Rev Biochem* 1980; 49:459–487.
25. Wretlind A. Development of fat emulsions. *JPEN* 1981;5:230–235.
26. Haumont D, Deckelbaum RJ, Richelle M et al. Plasma lipid and plasma lipoprotein concentrations in low birth weight infants given parenteral nutrition with twenty or ten percent lipid emulsion. *J Pediatr* 1989;115:787–793.
26a.Carpentier VA. Intravascular metabolism of fat emulsions. *Clin Nutr* 1989;8:115–125.
27. Olivecrona T, Bengtsson-Olivecrona G. Lipases involved in lipoprotein metabolism. *Curr Opin Lipidol* 1990;1:116–121.
28. Tonouchi H, Iriyama K, Carpentier YA. Transfer of apolipoproteins between plasma lipoproteins and exogenous lipid particles after repeated bolus injections or during a continuous infusion of fat emulsion. *JPEN* 1990;14:381–385.
29. Deckelbaum RJ, Hamilton JA, Moser A, et al. Medium-chain versus long-chain triacylglycerol emulsion hydrolysis by lipoprotein lipase and hepatic lipase: implications for the mechanisms of lipase action. *Biochemistry* 1990;29:1136–1142.
30. Richelle M. Influence of intravenous lipid emulsions on cholesterol homeostasis. *Clin Nutr* 1992;11: 48–52.
31. Peterson J, Bihain BE, Bengtsson-Olivecrona G, et al. Fatty acid control of lipoprotein lipase: a link between energy metabolism and lipid transport. *Proc Natl Acad Sci* 1990;87:909–913.
32. Beisegel U, Weber W, Bengtsson-Olivecrona G. Lipoprotein lipase enhances the binding of chylomicrons to low density lipoprotein receptor-related protein. *Proc Natl Acad Sci USA* 1991;88:8342–8346.
33. Rumsey SC, Obunike JC, Arad Y, et al. Lipoprotein lipase-mediated uptake and degradation of low density lipoproteins by fibroblasts and macrophages. *J Clin Invest* 1992;90:1504–1512.

34. Sniderman AD, Baldo A, Cianflone K. The potential role of acylation stimulating protein as a determinant of plasma triglyceride clearance and intracellular triglyceride synthesis. *Curr Opin Lipidol* 1992; 3:202–207.
35. Melin T, Qi C, Bengtsson-Olivecrona G, et al. Hydrolysis of chylomicron polyenoic fatty acid esters with lipoprotein lipase and hepatic lipase. *Biochim Biophys Acta* 1991;1075:259–266.
36. Kleinman Y, Schonfeld G, Gavish D, et al. Hypolipidemic therapy modulates expression of apolipoprotein B epitopes on low density lipoproteins. Studies in mild to moderate hypertriglyceridemic patients. *J Lipid Res* 1987;28:540–548.
37. Richelle M, Carpentier YA, Deckelbaum RJ. Long-chain and medium-chain triacylglycerols in neutral lipid exchange processes with human low density lipoproteins. *Biochemistry*, in press.
38. Hamilton JA, Vural J, Carpentier YA, Deckelbaum RJ. Competition between LCT and MCT at phospholipid surfaces. A NMR spectroscopy approach. *Clin Nutr* 1991;10(Suppl):39.
39. Mahley RW, Weisgraber KH, Hussain MM, et al. Intravenous infusion of apolipoprotein E accelerates clearance of plasma lipoproteins in rabbits. *J Clin Invest* 1989;83:2125–2130.
40. Yamada N, Shimano H, Mokuno H, et al. Increased clearance of plasma cholesterol after injection of apolipoprotein E into Watanabe heritable hyperlipidemic rabbits. *Proc Natl Acad Sci* 1989;86: 665–669.
41. Brown MS, Herz J, Kowal RC, Goldstein JL. The low-density lipoprotein receptor-related protein: double agent or decoy? *Curr Opin Lipidol* 1991;2:65–72.
42. Haumont D, Richelle M, Deckelbaum RJ, et al. Effect of liposomal content of lipid emulsions on plasma lipids in low birth weight infants receiving parenteral nutrition. *J Pediatr* 1992;121:759–763.
43. Griffin E, Breckenridge WC, Kuksis A, et al. Appearance and characterization of lipoprotein X during continuous Intralipid infusions in the neonate. *J Clin Invest* 1979;64:1703–1712.
44. Untracht S. Alterations of serum lipoproteins resulting from total parenteral nutrition with Intralipid. *Biochim Biophys Acta* 1982;711:176–192.
45. Williams KJ, Scanu AM. Uptake of endogenous cholesterol by a synthetic lipoprotein. *Biochim Biophys Acta* 1986;875:183–194.
46. Dahlan W, Richelle M, Kulapongse S, et al. Modification of erythrocyte membrane lipid composition induced by a single intravenous infusion of phospholipid-triacylglycerol emulsions in man. *Clin Nutr* 1992;11:255–261.
47. Degott C, Messing B, Moreau D, et al. Liver phospholipidosis induced by parenteral nutrition: histologic, histochemical, and ultrastructural investigations. *Gastroenterology* 1988;95:183–191.
48. Sheldon GF, Petersen SR, Sanders R. Hepatic dysfunction during hyperalimentation. *Arch Surg* 1978;113:504–508.
49. Lindor KD, Fleming CR, Abrams A, Hirschkorn MA. Liver function values in adults receiving total parenteral nutrition. *JAMA* 1979;241:2398–2400.
50. Robertson JF, Garden DJ, Shenkin A. Intravenous nutrition and hepatic dysfunction. *JPEN* 1986; 10:172–176.
51. Peden VH, Witzleben CL, Skelton MA. Total parenteral nutrition. *J Pediatr* 1971;78:180–181.
52. Dahms BB, Halpin TC. Serial liver biopsies in parenteral nutrition associated cholestasis of early infancy. *Gastroenterology* 1981;81:136–144.
53. Bell RL, Ferry GD, Smith EO, et al. Total parenteral nutrition—Related cholestasis in infants. *JPEN* 1986;10:366–359.
54. Touloukian RJ, Downing SE. Cholestasis associated with long-term parenteral hyperalimentation. *Arch Sug* 1973;106:58–62.
55. Bowyer BA, Fleming CR, Ludwig J, et al. Does long-term home parenteral nutrition in adult patients cause chronic liver disease? *JPEN* 1985;9:11–17.
56. Lowry SF, Brennan MF. Abnormal liver function during parenteral nutrition: relation to infusion excess. *J Surg Res* 1979;26:300–307.
57. Robin AP, Carpentier YA, Askanazi J, et al. Metabolic consequences of hypercaloric glucose infusion: a review. *Acta Chir Belg* 1981;2–3:133–140.
58. Fisher RL. Hepatobiliary abnormalities associated with total parenteral nutrition. *Gastroenterol Clin North Am* 1989;18:645–666.
59. Campos AC, Oler A, Meguid MM, Chen T-Y. Liver biochemical and histological changes with graded amounts of total parenteral nutrition. *Arch Surg* 1990;125:447–450.
60. Messing B, Colombel JF, Heresbach D, et al. Chronic cholestasis and macronutrient excess in patients treated with prolonged parenteral nutrition. *Nutrition* 1992;8:30–36.
61. Allardyce DB. Cholestasis caused by lipid emulsions. *Surg Gynecol Obstet* 1982;154:641–647.

62. Messing B, Latrive JP, Bitoun A, et al. La stéatose hépatique au cours de la nutrition parentérale totale dépend-elle de l'apport calorique lipidique? *Gastroenterol Clin Biol* 1979;3:719–725.
63. Buzby GP, Mullen J, Stein TP, Rosato EF. Manipulation of TPN calorie substrate and fatty infiltrations of the liver. *J Surg Res* 1981;31:46–54.
64. Carpentier YA, Van Brandt M. Effect of total parenteral nutrition on liver function. *Acta Chir Belg* 1981;2:141–143.
65. Meguid MM, Schimmel E, Johnson WC, et al. Reduced metabolic complications in total parenteral nutrition: pilot study using fat to replace one-third of glucose calories. *JPEN* 1986;6:304–307.
66. Craig RM, Neumann T, Jeejeebhoy KN, Yokoo H. Severe hepatocellular reaction resembling alcoholic hepatitis with cirrhosis after massive small bowel resection and prolonged total parenteral nutrition. *Gastroenterology* 1980;79:131–137.
67. Baker AL, Rosenberg IH. Hepatic complications of total parenteral nutrition. *Am J Med* 1987;82:489–497.
68. Stanko RT, Nathan G, Mendelow H, Adibi SA. Development of hepatic cholestasis and fibrosis in patients with massive loss of intestine supported by prolonged parenteral nutrition. *Gastroenterology* 1987;92:197–202.
69. Rabenek L, Freeman H, Owen D. Death due to TPN-related liver failure (abstr). *Gastroenterology* 1984;86:1215.
70. Williams JW, Sankary HN, Foster PF. Splanchnic transplantation. An approach to the infant dependent on parenteral nutrition who develops irreversible liver disease. *JAMA* 1989;261:1458–1462.
71. Carpentier YA, Richelle M, Haumont D, Deckelbaum RJ. New developments in fat emulsions. *Proc Nutr Soc* 1990;49:375–380.
72. Fouin-Fortunet H, Le Quernec L, Erlinger S, et al. Hepatic alterations during total parenteral nutrition in patients with inflammatory bowel disease; A possible consequence of lithocholate toxicity. *Gastroenterology* 1982;82:932–937.
73. Jeejeebhoy KN. Hepatic manifestations of total parenteral nutrition: need for prospective investigation. *Hepatology* 1988;8:428–429.
74. Tulikoura I, Huikuri K. Morphological fatty acid changes and function of the liver, serum free fatty acids and triglycerides during parenteral nutrition. *Scand J Gastroenterol* 1982;17:177–185.
75. Hall RI, Grant JP, Ross LH, et al. Pathogenesis of hepatic steatosis in the parenterally fed rat. *J Clin Invest* 1984;74:1658–1668.
76. Keim NL. Nutritional effectors of hepatic steatosis induced by parenteral nutrition in the rat. *JPEN* 1987;11:18–22.
77. Belli DC, Fournier LA, Lepage G, et al. Total parenteral nurition-associated cholestasis in rats: comparison of different amino acid mixtures. *JPEN* 1987;11:67–73.
78. Jeejeebhoy KN, Langer B, Tsallas G, et al. Total parenteral nutrition at home. Studies in patients surviving four months to five years. *Gastroenterology* 1976;71:943–953.
79. Keim NL, Mares-Perlman JA. Development of hepatic steatosis and essential fatty acid deficiency in rats with hypercaloric, fat free parenteral nutrition. *J Nutr* 1984;114:1807–1815.
80. Buchman AL, Dubin M, Jenden D, et al. Lecithin increases plasma free choline and decreases hepatic steatosis in long-term total parenteral nutrition patients. *Gastroenterology* 1992;102:1363–1370.
81. Buchman AL, Moukarzel A, Jenden DJ, et al. Low plasma free choline is prevalent in patients receiving long term parenteral nutrition and is associated with hepatic aminotransferase abnormalities. *Clin Nutr* 1993;12:33–37.
82. Li S, Nussbaum MS, McFadden DW, et al. Addition of L-glutamine to total parenteral nutrition and its effects on portal insulin and glucagon and the development of hepatic steatosis in rats. *J Surg Res* 1990;48:421–426.
83. Baldermann H, Wicklmayr M, Rett K, et al. Changes of hepatic morphology during parenteral nutrition with lipid emulsions containing LCT or MCT/LCT quantified by ultrasound. *JPEN* 1991;15:601–603.
84. Sarda P, Lepage G, Roy CC, Chessex P. Storage of medium-chain triglycerides in adipose tissue of orally fed infants. *Am J Clin Nutr* 1987;45:399–405.
85. Deckelbaum RJ, Carpentier YA, Arad Y, et al. Effects of free fatty acids of varying chain length on cell cholesterol metabolism. In: Stein O, Eisenberg S, Stein Y, eds. *Atherosclerosis IX.* Tel Aviv, Israël, R & L Creative Communication Ltd, 1992;33–37.
86. Ball MJ. Hematological and biochemical effects of parenteral nutrition with medium-chain triglycerides: comparison with long-chain triglycerides. *Am J Clin Nutr* 1991;53:916–922.
87. Rössle C, Carpentier YA, Richelle M, et al. Medium-chain triglycerides induce alterations in carnitine metabolism. *Am J Physiol* 1990;258:E944–E947.

88. Matsui J, Cameron RG, Kuo GC, Jeejeebhoy KN. Nutritional, hepatic and metabolic effects of cachectin/TNF in rats receiving TPN. *Gastroenterology* 1993;104:235–243.
89. Dahlan W, Richelle M, Kulapongse S, et al. Effects of essential fatty acid contents of lipid emulsions on erythrocyte polyunsaturated fatty acid composition in patients on long-term parenteral nutrition. *Clin Nutr* 1992;11:262–268.
90. Sokol RJ, Devereaux M, Mierau GW, et al. Oxidant injury to hepatic mitochondrial lipids in rats with dietary copper overload. Modification by vitamin E deficiency. *Gastroenterology* 1990;99:1061–1071.
91. Van Gossum A, Lemoyne M, Sharriff R, et al. Increased lipid peroxidation after lipid emulsion as measured by breath pentane output. *Am J Clin Nutr* 1988;48:1394–1399.
92. Lemoyne M, Van Gossum A, Kurian R, Jeejeebhoy KN. Plasma vitamin E and selenium and breath pentane in home parenteral nutrition patients. *Am J Clin Nutr* 1988;48:1310–1315.
93. Pitkänen O, Hallman O, Andersson S. Generation of free radicals in lipid emulsion used in parenteral nutrition. *Pediatr Res* 1991;29:56–59.
94. Steephen AC, Traber MG, Ito Y, et al. Vitamin E status of patients receiving long term parenteral nutrition: is vitamin E supplementation adequate? *JPEN* 1991;15:647–652.
95. Kayden HJ, Traber MG. Absorption, lipoprotein transport, and regulation of plasma concentrations of vitamin E in humans. *J Lipid Res* 1993;34:343–358.
96. Traber M, Carpentier YA, Kayden HJ, et al. Alteration in plasma alpha- and gamma-tocopherol concentrations in response to intravenous infusion of lipid emulsions in humans. *Metabolism* 1993; 42:701–709.
97. De Boer SY, Masclee AAM, Jebbink MCW, et al. Effect of intravenous fat on cholecystokinin secretion and gallbladder motility in man. *JPEN* 1992;16:16–19.
98. Sitzmann JV, Pitt HA, Steinborn PA, et al. Cholecystokinin prevents parenteral nutrition induced biliary sludge in humans. *Surg Gynecol Obstet* 1990;170:25–31.

Organ Metabolism and Nutrition:
Ideas for Future Critical Care, edited by
J. M. Kinney ∠nd H. N. Tucker.
Raven Press, Ltd., New York © 1994.

18

Sepsis and Human Splanchnic Metabolism

Jukka Takala

Critical Care Research Program, Department of Intensive Care, Kuopio University Hospital,
FIN-70211 Kuopio, Finland

The systemic inflammatory response to severe infection, sepsis, is a common cause of morbidity and mortality in intensive care patients (1–3). A similar systemic inflammatory response can also be associated with a number of clinical conditions without infection, e.g., acute pancreatitis, major trauma, severe hypovolemic shock, visceral ischemia, and the adult respiratory distress syndrome. These conditions are characterized by hypermetabolism and increased substrate requirements, once circulation has been stabilized (4,5). The phrase "systemic inflammatory response syndrome (SIRS)" has recently been introduced to describe the systemic inflammatory process, regardless of its cause (6). According to this rationale, the term *sepsis* is used when the SIRS is the result of a confirmed infection. For the purpose of this review, *sepsis* is used interchangeably with SIRS.

Sepsis induces marked changes in energy and substrate metabolism, which reflect a complex interaction between peripheral tissues and the splanchnic organs (7). The splanchnic region appears to have a central role in the pathogenesis of organ dysfunction, which is characteristic to sepsis. Intestinal mucosal injury due to tissue hypoxia may promote the translocation of intraluminal bacteria and toxins and thereby trigger the cascade of mediators, which causes further tissue injury and perfusion defects. The splanchnic organs contain large numbers of tissue macrophages, which by producing cytokines may modify both the local metabolic response to sepsis and the function of extrasplanchnic tissues and organs (6,7).

The metabolic changes may be further modified by the cardiovascular and respiratory effects of sepsis. Myocardial depression may limit the response of cardiac output to the increased metabolic demands, abnormal vasoregulation alter the blood flow distribution and cause oxygen supply/demand mismatch, the concomitant respiratory failure reduce the oxygen delivery to the tissues (8,9).

Abnormal tissue oxygen utilization is a major metabolic defect in severe sepsis. Oxygen consumption can be supply dependent at high levels of oxygen delivery, and the ability of the tissues to increase oxygen extraction in response to the increased metabolic demand is impaired in sepsis. Oxygen uptake is enhanced in response to increased oxygen delivery, and increased blood levels of lactate are common, both suggesting the presence of tissue hypoxia (10–12). Maldistribution of blood flow due to abnormal vasoregulation (9,13), interstitial edema due to capillary leakage (14), and direct cellular damage as the result of cell-mediated and humoral inflammatory response (15) all contribute to the abnormal oxygen utilization and tissue hypoxia in sepsis. Because the metabolic demand for oxygen is increased and the utilization of available oxygen impaired, it is conceivable that an elevated oxygen delivery is necessary to prevent tissue hypoxia. Indeed, recent studies indicate that supranormal oxygen delivery, whether achieved spontaneously or by therapy aimed at increasing oxygen delivery, is associated with improved outcome after major surgery and in septic shock (16–18).

Splanchnic tissue hypoxia, demonstrated as gastric intramucosal acidosis, is associated with increased morbidity and mortality in intensive care patients (19–21). Reversal of the splanchnic tissue hypoxia by administration of fluids and vasoactive drugs improves the outcome (21,22). It is evident that the splanchnic region can be both a target and a source of the inflammatory response in sepsis.

Only very limited data are available on the effects of sepsis on splanchnic metabolism in humans. The reasons for this are obvious: Access to the splanchnic organs, tissues, and vascular beds requires invasive methods and the inherent instability of the patient with severe sepsis presents severe limitations for most traditional metabolic research techniques; the new sophisticated imaging techniques may offer less invasive alternatives in the future. Extrapolation of data obtained from experimental models of sepsis is difficult due to the major differences between models in the overall circulatory and blood volume status (23–25). For example, endotoxin shock models demonstrate normal or reduced splanchnic blood flow (23,24), whereas models based on intraabdominal infection tend to have increased splanchnic blood flow (25), which is consistent with observations in hemodynamically stable clinical sepsis (26–30). In contrast, endotoxin injection in healthy human volunteers reproduces many of the hemodynamic and metabolic changes of clinical sepsis (31,32).

The available data on splanchnic metabolism in clinical sepsis and septic shock largely focus on splanchnic oxygen transport (26–30,33,34). Splanchnic substrate metabolism has been studied only following endotoxin injection (31) and in hemodynamically stable sepsis (28,29).

METABOLIC RESPONSE TO ENDOTOXIN

The hemodynamic and metabolic alterations associated with severe sepsis due to invasive infection by gram-negative bacteria have traditionally been attributed to endotoxin (31,35). Experimental studies have demonstrated that although endotoxin alone is sufficient to produce the typical cardiovascular and metabolic pattern of septic shock, an identical pattern results from sepsis due to gram-positive bacteria with no endotoxemia (35). In human septic shock, endotoxemia has been observed in approximately half of the patients, and gram-negative infection is not a prerequisite for endotoxemia (31,35). It has now been well established that endotoxin is not the universal mediator of sepsis. Nevertheless, administration of small doses of endotoxin to healthy human subjects has been shown to produce a hyperdynamic cardiovascular state with myocardial depression and left ventricular dilatation, impaired pulmonary gas exchange and alveolar permeability, and activation of the fibrinolytic system, all changes qualitatively similar to those observed in clinical sepsis (6,35). Accordingly, changes in splanchnic metabolism following endotoxin administration can give an insight to the changes in splanchnic metabolism likely to occur in clinical sepsis.

Fong et al. (31) injected endotoxin (20 U/kg) to healthy volunteers and followed the splanchnic and peripheral metabolic changes and cytokine responses for 6 hours. Total splanchnic blood flow and arterial-venous concentration differences of oxygen and substrates were obtained by regional catheterization techniques. The injection of endotoxin produced a characteristic acute hypermetabolic response (up to 40%) that persisted throughout the study. In the beginning of the whole-body hypermetabolism, leg oxygen uptake remained unchanged and then decreased by 36%. Both splanchnic oxygen uptake and blood flow increased after endotoxin injection, reached the maximum by 2 to 3 hours, and then gradually declined. In the early phase of the experiment, the increase in splanchnic oxygen consumption could explain approximately 75% of the increase in whole-body oxygen consumption; by the end of the

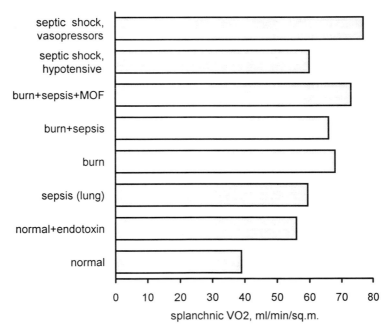

FIG. 1. Increasing severity of sepsis or systemic inflammatory response increases splanchnic oxygen consumption. Injection of endotoxin induces similar splanchnic hypermetabolism as hemodynamically stable sepsis. In septic shock, marked splanchnic hypermetabolism is present even during the hypotension. Adapted from Wilmore et al. (28), Dahn et al. (29,30), Fong et al. (31), and Ruokonen et al. (33).

study, approximately 15% of the whole-body hypermetabolism could be attributed to splanchnic hypermetabolism. At the peak of splanchnic metabolic activity, the splanchnic oxygen consumption represented 43% of the whole-body oxygen consumption (Fig. 1). The hypermetabolism was accompanied by increased splanchnic glucose release (Fig. 2), hyperglycemia, and increased peripheral glucose uptake. An increase in the splanchnic uptake and peripheral release of lactate and free fatty acids and a transient increase in splanchnic release of triglycerides were also observed. Changes in amino acid metabolism were characterized by reduced circulating amino acid levels and increased splanchnic uptake of amino acids, especially alanine and glutamine. The overall changes in splanchnic substrate metabolism were in favor for increased splanchnic glucose production.

The metabolic changes following endotoxin administration were clearly more distinct in the splanchnic region than in the periphery. The observed changes support the concept that the alterations in the peripheral substrate fluxes served to provide substrates for the increased splanchnic metabolic activity, presumably hepatic synthesis of glucose, protein, and lipids.

The administration of endotoxin to the systemic circulation was followed rapidly by splanchnic release of tumor necrosis factor (TNF) and a later increase in the blood

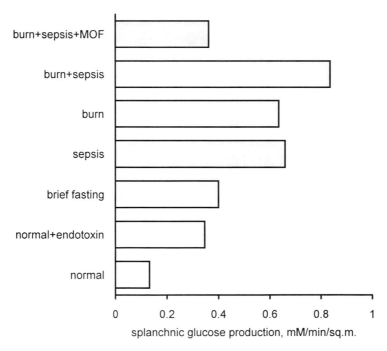

FIG. 2. Splanchnic glucose production initially increases, when the septic condition becomes more severe; in multiple organ failure (MOF), an abrupt reduction in glucose production occurs despite continuing splanchnic hypermetabolism. Adapted from Wilmore et al. (28), Dahn et al. (30), and Fong et al. (31).

levels of interleukin-6. The time course of the metabolic changes and the splanchnic release of TNF, and the very similar splanchnic metabolic effects of TNF in experimental models, all support the concept that the splanchnic metabolic effects of endotoxin are mediated via a complex cascade of endogenous mediators. These mediators include cytokines, especially TNF, and the traditional counterregulatory hormones. It is noteworthy that the administration of endotoxin in the study of Fong et al. was associated with a persistent increase in arterial cortisol level, whereas epinephrine increased only transiently, and glucagon and insulin remained unchanged.

SPLANCHNIC METABOLISM AND OXYGEN TRANSPORT IN CLINICAL SEPSIS

The pioneer studies on splanchnic oxygen and substrate transport in septic patients were published in the early 1970s by Gump et al. (26,27) and in the early 1980s by Wilmore et al. (28). These studies in burn patients and patients with intraperitoneal infections demonstrated the changes in blood flow distribution and splanchnic oxygen consumption that have later been confirmed to be characteristic of hemodynamically stable sepsis in general (29,30).

Whole-body and splanchnic blood flow and oxygen consumption were measured in hemodynamically stable, febrile patients with intraperitoneal infections and without respiratory failure (26). Splanchnic blood flow was normal in patients without whole-body hypermetabolism, but its fraction of cardiac output was slightly reduced and represented 17% of whole-body blood flow. The splanchnic oxygen consumption was within the normal range and corresponded to 20% of whole-body oxygen consumption. In contrast, patients with whole-body hypermetabolism had increased splanchnic blood flow and splanchnic hypermetabolism. The splanchnic blood flow represented 24% of cardiac output and the splanchnic oxygen consumption 26% of whole-body oxygen consumption. The increase in splanchnic oxygen consumption could explain half of the increase in whole-body oxygen consumption. An increase in splanchnic blood flow appeared to be the primary mechanism to compensate for the increased splanchnic metabolic demand. The results clearly demonstrated the importance of the splanchnic region to the hypermetabolic response to infection. Gump et al. also studied splanchnic blood flow in three patients with severe burns and observed that the splanchnic blood flow was only slightly increased despite hyperdynamic circulation. If the splanchnic metabolic demands were elevated in these circumstances, the lack of increase in splanchnic blood flow represented maldistribution of the increased cardiac output (27). The study of Wilmore et al. (28) on the effects of burn injury with and without infection on splanchnic metabolism and circulation still provides the most detailed, available information on the impact of sepsis on splanchnic metabolism and the dynamic changes that occur when sepsis progresses to multiple organ failure.

Splanchnic blood flow, oxygen consumption, and substrate exchange were studied in three groups of patients with major burns: noninfected patients with stable vital functions, patients with bacteremia and a systemic septic response, and patients with bacteremia and multiple organ failure. All patients were grossly hypermetabolic. Splanchnic blood flow was higher than normal in all three groups and tended to be lowest in the group with bacteremia and multiple organ failure. Splanchnic oxygen consumption was increased by 50% to 100% and accounted for 25% to 30% of whole-body oxygen consumption (Fig. 1). The highest splanchnic oxygen extraction was observed in patients with sepsis and organ failures. The high splanchnic oxygen extraction (48%) and splanchnic hypermetabolism were combined with reduced hepatic extraction of indocyanine green, suggesting functional deterioration of the liver.

The splanchnic glucose output was increased by approximately 50% above normal in the noninfected patients (Fig. 2). In patients with sepsis without multiple organ failure, the splanchnic glucose output increased further to approximately twice the normal rate. In contrast, when sepsis was associated with multiple organ failure, the splanchnic glucose output sharply decreased to the low normal range, despite the persistent splanchnic hypermetabolism.

The splanchnic uptake of amino acids was increased in the noninfected patients and increased further by two- to threefold in patients with sepsis, due to increased fractional extraction of amino acids in the splanchnic bed. In patients with sepsis and multiple organ failure, the splanchnic uptake and fractional extraction of amino acids decreased. Specifically, the uptake of gluconeogenetic precursors alanine and serine was reduced to approximately one fifth of that observed in patients with sepsis but without organ failures.

These results provide a basis for a dynamic model of interaction between increased splanchnic metabolic demand, oxygen transport, and the pathogenesis of splanchnic organ failures. The following sequence of events can be hypothesized: In patients with burn injury without infection, the increase in splanchnic metabolic demand is increased as compared to the overall hypermetabolic response to the injury, but the increased demand is well matched with the increase in splanchnic blood flow and oxygen delivery. The distinct increase in splanchnic oxygen consumption in excess of the whole-body metabolic response is probably related to the systemic inflammatory response that is typically observed in major burns even without infection, and which is most likely mediated by cytokines.

Once the inflammatory response is further magnified as the result of infection, the metabolic activity, especially gluconeogenesis, is further increased, without a concomitant increase in oxygen consumption. This shift in the splanchnic metabolic activity precedes the deterioration of liver function and the rather dramatic reduction of gluconeogenesis and amino acid uptake that occurs in the next stage of sepsis. It is possible that the marked increase in gluconeogenesis occurs at the expense of other oxygen-consuming processes within the liver or in other splanchnic organs, e.g., the gut. It is also possible that the lack of further increase in oxygen consumption and the relatively normal total splanchnic oxygen extraction are the result of blood flow redistribution within the splanchnic region, in order to favor the metabolic demand of increased hepatic gluconeogenesis.

Once sepsis progresses further and signs of multiple organ failure develop, the splanchnic glucose output is abruptly shut down, suggesting failure of the gluconeogenetic processes. At this point, the persistently high splanchnic oxygen consumption is accompanied by very high splanchnic oxygen extraction, close to 50%, strongly suggesting that the splanchnic metabolic activity may be limited because of insufficient oxygen delivery, and tissue hypoxia in the gut and the liver is likely to occur.

Burn injury per se may have altered the regulation of blood flow and metabolism due to the extensive and specific tissue injury. The similar findings in burns patients and in patients with intraperitoneal infection support the concept that splanchnic hypermetabolism is characteristic to sepsis in general. This was confirmed by Dahn et al. (29,30) in intensive care patients with sepsis and, in most cases, concomittant acute respiratory failure. As such, the patients in Dahn's studies represent a more severely ill group of patients than the previously studied patients with intraperitoneal infections.

Splanchnic oxygen transport and metabolism was studied in patients with sepsis due to gram-negative infection of various locations. A control group of patients considered as stressed but nonseptic (most with respiratory failure following trauma or major surgery) was included. Both groups of patients were moderately hypermetabolic and the whole-body oxygen consumption was similar in the two groups. Both patient groups had a hyperdynamic circulation, but as can be expected, the cardiac index was higher in patients with sepsis. Accordingly, the septic patients had a lower systemic oxygen extraction fraction than the patients without infection. Splanchnic blood flow was higher than normal in both groups and tended to be higher in patients with sepsis. Splanchnic oxygen consumption was substantially increased in the patients with sepsis, and accounted for 44% of the whole-body oxygen consumption. In the patients without infection, the splanchnic oxygen consumption represented 30% of the whole-body oxygen consumption. This is still higher than normal and probably reflects some degree of inflammatory response also in the noninfected patients, who had acute respiratory failure of various severity, including the adult respiratory distress syndrome. In sepsis, the splanchnic hypermetabolism was clearly disproportionate to the moderately increased splanchnic blood flow and resulted in a high splanchnic oxygen extraction fraction (0.39 vs. 0.23 for systemic oxygen extraction). While sepsis has been associated traditionally with impaired oxygen extraction, the extraction capability seems to be well preserved regionally. The results demonstrate a dissociation between the distribution of blood flow and metabolic demand in sepsis. Furthermore, the marked splanchnic hypermetabolism and increased oxygen extraction occurred despite normal or high mixed venous oxygen saturation and normal arterial lactate levels, both often regarded as indications of sufficient oxygen delivery. Even minor changes in cardiac output and splanchnic blood flow may, under these circumstances, lead to precipitation of tissue hypoxia in the splanchnic region.

Splanchnic glucose production was higher than normal in both groups and higher in the septic patients when compared with patients without infection. When compared with the findings of Wilmore et al., the septic patients in Dahn's study had a glucose production comparable or slightly higher than noninfected burns patients, clearly higher than burns patients with multiple organ failure, but lower than burn patients with culture-positive sepsis (Fig. 2). In contrast, the splanchnic lactate uptake in the septic patients was roughly twofold compared with the highest values observed in patients with burns (the bacteremic group without multiple organ failure).

A crude estimation, based on the available data on lactate flux across the splanchnic bed, suggests that the splanchnic fractional extraction of lactate was markedly higher in the study of Dahn et al. compared with the burns patients in the study of Wilmore et al., possibly due to differences in liver function or splanchnic blood flow distribution.

The disproportionate increase in splanchnic oxygen consumption, compared with the increase in splanchnic blood flow in hemodynamically stable sepsis, was confirmed in another study by Dahn et al. (30) in patients whose sepsis was, in most cases, because of pneumonia. In this study, splanchnic oxygen consumption and blood flow in sepsis was compared with measurements obtained in healthy subjects. The splanchnic fractional extraction of indocyanine green and galactose were both reduced in sepsis, suggesting impaired hepatocellular function.

The traditional perception of hypoxia-induced tissue injury is that tissue hypoxia develops as a result of reduced oxygen delivery, which is the case, e.g., in splanchnic tissue hypoxia secondary to hypovolemic shock. These studies clearly demonstrate that in hemodynamically stable sepsis, the splanchnic region is at risk of tissue hypoxia because of increased metabolic activity and oxygen demand. The subtle changes in liver function that occur early in sepsis, even in the absence of major hemodynamic alterations, may well be related to transient episodes of tissue hypoxia due to the high metabolic activity of the splanchnic tissues in sepsis.

SPLANCHNIC OXYGEN TRANSPORT IN SEPTIC SHOCK

Septic shock can be characterized as a distributive shock, because after correction of hypovolemia, hyperdynamic circulation with high cardiac output and low peripheral resistance usually prevails. Despite high cardiac output, signs of insufficient tissue perfusion, e.g., metabolic acidosis with increased blood levels of lactate, are common. Multiple organ dysfunction is observed so early in shock that the hypotension alone does not explain the pathogenesis of organ failures (36). It is likely that the various mediator cascades, at least in part, explain the pathogenesis of organ damage (7,15). The possibility that the metabolic changes in the splanchnic region preceding the shock might contribute to organ dysfunction has largely been overlooked. Assuming that the splanchnic hypermetabolism is present before the clinical manifestation of septic shock, it seems evident that the prerequisites for splanchnic tissue hypoxia exist in septic shock. The myocardial dysfunction and hypovolemia that are common early in septic shock (35) may indeed precipitate tissue hypoxia in the hypermetabolic splanchnic region. Ruokonen et al. have recently demonstrated that once the hypovolemia has been corrected in septic shock, the splanchnic region is grossly hypermetabolic (Fig. 1) and the blood flow to the splanchnic region is normal or increased (33). When the hypotension was corrected with vasopressor drugs, the splanchnic oxygen consumption tended to be increased further (Fig. 1), and parallel changes in splanchnic oxygen delivery and consumption were observed in most patients. Splanchnic oxygen extraction was relatively well preserved, even during hypotension, supporting the hypothesis that the increased metabolic demand in the splanchnic region contributed to tissue hypoxia. The parallel changes in splanchnic oxygen delivery and consumption may have been related to a tissue oxygen debt or, alternatively, reflect changes in splanchnic metabolism induced by the sympathomimetic amines.

The splanchnic metabolic effects of sympathomimetic amines have not been well documented in humans and no data on their splanchnic effects in sepsis are available. Because the catecholamines may markedly modify the activity of various metabolic pathways in the liver and simultaneously alter the splanchnic blood flow and its distribution, their effects on splanchnic oxygen transport and substrate metabolism in clinical sepsis should be evaluated.

SPLANCHNIC HYPERMETABOLISM, ENDOTOXIN, AND CYTOKINES

As discussed previously, injection of endotoxin induces splanchnic hypermetabolism and release of TNF in healthy volunteers. It would be tempting to speculate that

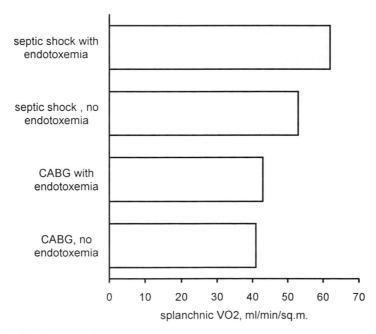

FIG. 3. In clinical sepsis and after coronary artery bypass surgery (CABG), the pattern of splanchnic metabolism is not acutely influenced by the presence of endotoxin. Adapted from Takala (34).

the splanchnic hypermetabolism observed in clinical sepsis is also related to endo-toxin and TNF. We (Takala and Ruokonen) have recently compared the splanchnic oxygen consumption in endotoxemic patients with that in patients without endotoxe-mia (34). We studied patients with septic shock and postoperative patients after coronary artery by-pass surgery. In the latter group, transient peri- and postoperative endotoxemia is known to occur in approximately 30% to 40% of patients. Splanchnic oxygen consumption was higher in patients with septic shock than in the postopera-tive patients. In both diagnostic groups, no differences between patients with and without endotoxemia were observed (Fig. 3). Levels of TFN were increased in pa-tients with endotoxemia and not detectable in patients without endotoxemia. Accord-ingly, no relationship between splanchnic oxygen consumption and endotoxin or TNF-levels were observed. These findings emphasize that the splanchnic metabolic response in clinical sepsis may differ substantially from responses seen following endotoxin injection. The possible role of endotoxin and TNF as mediators of the splanchnic metabolic changes in sepsis is not excluded, but the causal relationship is not as straightforward as suggested by endotoxin challenge studies.

REFERENCES

1. Tran DD, Groenveld ABJ, van der Meulen J, et al. Age, chronic disease, sepsis, organ system failure, and mortality in a medical intensive care unit. *Crit Care Med* 1990;18:474–479.
2. Goris PJA, te Boekhorst TPA, Nuytinck JKS, Gimbère JSF. Multiple-organ failure. Generalized autodestructive inflammation? *Arch Surg* 1985;120:1109–1115.
3. Danner RL, Elin RJ, Hosseini JM, et al. Endotoxemia in human septic shock. *Chest* 1991;99:169–175.
4. Barton R, Cerra FB. The hypermetabolism multiple organ failure syndome. *Chest* 1989;96:1153–1160.
5. Pitkänen O, Takala J, Pöyhönen M, Kari A. Nitrogen and energy balance in septic and injured intensive care patients: response to parenteral nutrition. *Clin Nutr* 1991;10:258–265.
6. American College of Chest Physicians/Society of Critical Care Medicine Consensus Conference: Definitions for sepsis and multiple organ failure and guidelines for the use of innovative therapies in sepsis. *Crit Care Med* 1992;20:864–874.
7. Tracey KJ. TNF and other cytokines in the metabolism of septic shock and cachexia. *Clin Nutr* 1992;11:1–11.
8. Vincent J-L, Roman A, Kahn RJ. Dobutamine administration in septic shock: addition to a standard protocol. *Crit Care Med* 1990;18:689–693.
9. Ruffolo RR Jr, Fondacaro JD, Levitt B, et al. Pharmacologic manipulation of regional blood flow. In: Snyder JV, Pinsky MR, eds. *Oxygen Transport in Critically Ill*. 1st ed. Chicago: Year Book Medical Publishers, 1987;450–474.
10. Haupt MT, Gilbert EM, Carlson RW. Fluid loading increases oxygen consumption in septic patients with lactic acidosis. *Am Rev Respir Dis* 1985;131:912–916.
11. Vincent J-L, Roman A, DeBacker D, Kahn RJ. Oxygen uptake/supply dependency: effects of short-term dobutamine infusion. *Am Rev Respir Dis* 1990;142:2–8.
12. Bihari D, Smithies M, Gimson A, Tinker J. The effects of vasodilation with prostacyclin on oxygen delivery and uptake in critically ill patients. *N Engl J Med* 1987;317:397–403.
13. Schumacker PT, Cain SM. The concept of a critical oxygen delivery. *Intensive Care Med* 1987;13:223–229.
14. Fleck A, Raines G, Hawker F, et al. Increased vascular permeability: a major cause of hypoalbuminae-mia in disease and injury. *Lancet* 1985;1(8432):781–784.
15. Colten HR. Tissue-specific regulation of inflammation. *J Appl Physiol* 1992;72:1–7.
16. Shoemaker WC, Appel P, Kram HB, et al. Prospective trial of supranormal values of survivors as therapeutic goals in high-risk surgical patients. *Chest* 1988;94:1176–1186.
17. Tuchschmidt J, Fried J, Astiz M, Rackow E. Elevation of cardiac output and oxygen delivery improves outcome in septic shock. *Chest* 1992;102:216–220.

18. Boyd O, Grounds RM, Bennet ED. The beneficial effect of supranormalisation of oxygen delivery with dopexamine hydrochloride on perioperative mortality. *Intensive Care Med* 1992;18(Suppl 2):72.
19. Fiddian-Green RG, Baker S. Predictive value of the stomach wall pH for complications after cardiac operations: comparison with other monitoring. *Crit Care Med* 1987;15:153–156.
20. Fiddian-Green RG, Gantz NM. Transient episodes of sigmoid ischemia and their relation to infection from intestinal organisms after abdominal aortic operations. *Crit Care Med* 1987;15:835–839.
21. Gutierrez G, Palizas F, Doglio G, et al. Gastric intramucosal pH as a therapeutic index of tissue oxygenation in critically ill patients. *Lancet* 1992;339:195–199.
22. Doglio GR, Pusajo JF, Egurrola MA, et al. Gastric mucosal pH as a prognostic index of mortality in critically ill patients. *Crit Care Med* 1991;19:1037–1040.
23. Breslow MJ, Miller CF, Parker SD, et al. Effect of vasopressors on organ blood flow during endotoxin shock in pigs. *Am J Physiol* 1987;252:H291–H300.
24. Hussain SNA, Rutledge F, Roussos C, Magder S. Effects of norepinephrine and fluid administration on the selective blood flow distribution in endotoxic shock. *J Crit Care* 1988;3:32–42.
25. Fink MP, Heard SO. Laboratory models of sepsis and septic shock. *J Surg Res* 1990;49:186–196.
26. Gump FE, Price JB Jr, Kinney JM. Whole body and splanchnic blood flow and oxygen consumption measurements in patients with intraperitoneal infection. *Ann Surg* 1970;171:321–328.
27. Gump FE, Price JB, Kinney JM. Blood flow and oxygen consumption in patients with severe burns. *Surg Gynecol Obstet* 1970;130:23–28.
28. Wilmore DW, Goodwin CW, Aulick LH, et al. Effect of injury and infection on visceral metabolism and circulation. *Ann Surg* 1980;192:491–500.
29. Dahn MS, Lange P, Lobdell K, et al. Splanchnic and total body oxygen consumption differences in septic and injured patients. *Surgery* 1987;101:69–80.
30. Dahn MS, Lange P, Wilson RF, et al. Hepatic blood flow and splanchnic oxygen consumption measurements in clinical sepsis. *Surgery* 1990;107:295–301.
31. Fong Y, Marano MA, Moldaver LL, et al. The acute splanchnic and peripheral tissue metabolic response to endotoxin in humans. *J Clin Invest* 1990;85:1896–1904.
32. Suffredini AF, Shelhamer JH, Neumann RD, et al. Pulmonary and oxygen transport effects of intravenously administered endotoxin in normal humans. *Am Rev Respir Dis* 1992;145:1398–1403.
33. Ruokonen E, Takala J, Kari A, et al. Regional blood flow and oxygen transport in septic shock. *Crit Care Med* 1993;21:1296–1303.
34. Takala J, Ruokonen E. Regoinal oxygen consumption in sepsis and after surgery: effects of endotoxemia and increased blood levels of TNF. *Clin Nutr* 1992;11(Special suppl):36.
35. Parrillo JE, Parker MM, Natanson C, et al. Septic shock in humans. *Ann Intern Med* 1990;113; 227–242.
36. Ruokonen E, Takala J, Kari A, Alhava E. Septic shock and multiple organ failure. *Crit Care Med* 1991;19:1146–1151.

Organ Metabolism and Nutrition:
Ideas for Future Critical Care, edited by
J. M. Kinney and H. N. Tucker.
Raven Press, Ltd., New York © 1994.

19

AIDS versus Acute Septic States: Similarities and Dissimilarities

Hans P. Sauerwein

Department of Endocrinology and Internal Medicine, Academic Medical Center,
1105 AZ Amsterdam, The Netherlands

Rapid weight loss, associated with the loss of body fat and skeletal muscle mass, frequently accompanies short-term self-limiting disease processes such as infection and injury. The loss of body tissue may be minimal and of little consequence in a patient with a brief self-limiting short-lasting illness, but when the disease is prolonged, a variety of clinical events occur in association with the catabolic state. These alterations include immunosuppression characterized by an increase in the frequency of nosocomial infections, loss of muscle strength and diminished activity (1). These clinical events are accompanied by metabolic changes: net protein loss, increased lipolysis, and glucose intolerance due to insulin resistance (2,3). Although increased lipolysis can be suppressed and glucose intolerance can be overcome by the administration of insulin (3), maintenance or replenishment of body protein has been proven to be extremely difficult or even impossible in critically ill patients (4).

One of the most striking symptoms of acquired immunodeficiency syndrome (AIDS) is extreme and progressive weight loss with debilitation (5). Weight loss is due to loss of fat and body cell mass (6). Maintenance or replenishment of body cell mass has been proven to be extremely difficult or even impossible in major subgroups of patients with AIDS (7). These similarities in the clinical picture and reaction to treatment in critically ill patients and patients with AIDS would suggest similarities in metabolic and hormonal changes in critical illness, e.g., sepsis, and AIDS. However, the first studies show some similarities but also highly remarkable differences between critically illness (sepsis) and AIDS. In this review, those similarities and dissimilarities are discussed.

Because AIDS is a disease predominantly found in humans, only data obtained in this species are considered. In all of the articles on metabolic changes in AIDS, control groups are included. For this reason, only those publications on the metabolic changes in sepsis are considered for this review when control groups are included.

ENERGY METABOLISM

No studies on total daily expenditure or diet-induced thermogenesis in HIV infection have been published, therefore the discussion concentrates on resting energy expenditure (REE).

It is stated that there is a graded rise in metabolic rate following injury in proportion to the severity of trauma. In invasive sepsis, rises in metabolic rate up to twice the normal levels in hospitalized patients have been reported (2). Those values obtained in patients were frequently compared to calculated estimations of REE. When the data are compared to those obtained from matched healthy controls, many fewer impressive increases in REE in sepsis or acute infection are found, with, in general, values for REE around 20% higher than in control subjects (3,8–10; Godfried MH, personal communication). Fever is frequently found in sepsis. The presence of fever has been found to increase REE approximately 13% for each degree Celsius (11). Many of the studies of the past decade have shown that fever is not an obligatory component for the induction of an increase in REE. Normal body temperature does not exclude the possibility of hypermetabolism, and human immunodeficiency virus (HIV) infection is no exception to this finding. In four full papers, data on REE in HIV infection have been published (12–15). They show that hypermetabolism is a frequent but not obligatory finding in HIV infection. Hommes et al. (12) studied 18 consecutive outpatients with stable AIDS, defined as free of clinically active infections for a period of at least 2 months before participation, and compared them with the data from 11 healthy matched controls. They found an increase in REE by 9%, quite similar to the data by Melchior et al. in a comparable group of AIDS patients (REE + 12%) (13). The data by Grünfeld et al. show slightly higher increases in REE in stable AIDS patients (REE + 25%) (14). In their patients with AIDS, during secondary infection (AIDS-SI), REE was increased by 29% (14). Resting energy expenditure is already increased in the early asymptomatic stage of HIV infection, as shown by Hommes et al. (15) (REE + 8%) and Grünfeld et al. (14) (REE + 14%).

HIV infection and sepsis both induce an increase in REE. This increase is not very impressive. It is a little more evident in sepsis than in HIV infection, unless the latter is complicated by an opportunistic infection (AIDS-SI).

LIPID METABOLISM

Lipolysis

Reliance on fat as a major source of energy in the injured human was already recognized in the early studies by Moore (16) on the metabolic response to injury. It is therefore not unexpected that lipolysis is increased in sepsis. In vitro studies from adipose tissue specimens obtained from septic patients have shown that adipocyte adrenergic-stimulated lipolysis was increased when the patients were septic for more than 24 hours (17), and in vivo studies have confirmed this finding. Both glycerol turnover and free fatty acid (FFA) turnover were doubled in these patients compared with healthy controls after an overnight fast (18,19). During glucose administration, the differences were even more striking (3,19). During a euglycemic clamp, with insulin concentrations around 100 μU/ml, FFA turnover was still five times higher in septic patients compared with the controls (3).

Lipolysis is not thoroughly studied in HIV infection. Hommes et al. studied basal lipid metabolism in stable AIDS patients (20). They found that FFA concentration and FFA turnover after an overnight fast did not differ from the values obtained in healthy subjects matched for body composition. Grünfeld et al. reported a small but significant increase in FFA concentrations (+25%) (21). (FFA turnover was not measured in this study). When the fasting period is prolonged for an additional 6 hours, FFA turnover is significantly higher (+23%) in the patients than in the control subjects (20). This increase in FFA turnover in stable AIDS patients may be called accelerated lipolysis. Remarkably, FFA concentrations were comparable in patients and controls, despite the difference in FFA turnover, indicating that the relationship between FFA concentrations and FFA turnover is changed in the HIV-infected patients, as can be observed in healthy subjects (22). Such alterations in lipid metabolism have been described before in a wide variety of acute bacterial and viral infections (2,23). Despite the accelerated lipolysis, FFA concentrations are suppressable by glucose in AIDS to very low values, contrary to sepsis (3,24). In asymptomatic HIV infection, serum FFA levels are normal (21; M. J. T. Hommes, personal communication).

Triglycerides

The concentrations of triglycerides in plasma are elevated fourfold in gram-negative sepsis in humans (23). The rise in triglyceride concentration is due to an elevation of very low density lipoprotein (VLDL), explained at least in part by concomitant reductions of lipoprotein lipase activity (25). Studies in septic dogs have shown that the increase in the production of VLDL is presumably more important as a factor contributing a hypertriglyceridemia in sepsis than a decreased rate of clearance (26).

Plasma triglyceride concentrations are strikingly elevated in patients with AIDS. The concentration in stable AIDS patients is approximately doubled when compared with controls, with possibly a small additional increase during opportunistic infections (20,21,27). In asymptomatic HIV-positive subjects, values between those found in AIDS patients and healthy control subjects are reported (21,28). As in sepsis, triglyceride clearance time and postheparin lipase activity are significantly decreased in AIDS and asymptomatic HIV-positive subjects (21). Recent data suggest that hepatic synthesis of FFA is also increased in AIDS (5). Increased VLDL production can therefore contribute to the high triglyceride in AIDS.

AIDS and sepsis both induce, in a qualitative sense, comparable changes in lipid metabolism. Sepsis is characterized by marked hypertriglyceridemia due to increased production and decreased clearance of VLDL and an impressive stimulation of lipolysis. The increases in triglyceride concentration in AIDS is much less marked, with about 50% of the increase found in sepsis. The mechanisms by which this increase is induced are probably the same in sepsis and AIDS. Lipolysis in AIDS can be better defined as accelerated lipolysis than as increased lipolysis.

Thus far, the data suggest that the metabolic changes induced by AIDS or sepsis are comparable and in relation to the severity of the clinical picture. This is true for REE and lipid metabolism. The differences in glucose and protein metabolism between both diseases are quite remarkable, however.

GLUCOSE METABOLISM

Basal and Insulin-stimulated Glucose Metabolism in Sepsis

It has been known since the time of Claude Bernard that injury causes hyperglycemia, and hyperglycemia is a frequent but not invariable finding in sepsis and other acute infections under basal circumstances (2,9–11,29–33). Hyperglycemia can be caused by an increase in glucose production, a decrease in glucose clearance, or a combination of both; the latter is usually found (10,29,31). In sepsis, total glucose production is approximately twice the basal rate in normal volunteers (30–32). Despite this increase, endogenous glucose production is easily suppressable with only slightly higher insulin concentrations than those necessary for suppression in healthy subjects (3,31,32), suggesting, at most, moderate insulin resistance at the hepatic level. This has been confirmed in other acute infections (10,33). An increase in glucose production does not invariably lead to hyperglycemia. This is well illustrated by the frequently normal plasma glucose concentrations in sepsis despite an increase in basal hepatic glucose production or the dissociation between the degree of increase in glucose production and increase in plasma glucose concentration (30–32). This suggests that basal glucose utilization is, in general, increased in septic states. In the basal state, glucose utilization is mainly insulin independent (34). In insulin-stimulated circumstances, major defects in glucose utilization are found in sepsis and other acute infections (3,10,32,33). With the euglycemic clamp technique, it can be shown that infectious patients require about 50% less glucose than control subjects to maintain euglycemia even when endogenous glucose production is completely suppressed (3,10,32). Glucose is either oxidized or stored after uptake. In acute infections, including sepsis, glucose oxidation is, in general, not different from that of healthy subjects during an euglycemic clamp as long as plasma insulin concentration is above 30 μU/ml (10,29,31–33,35). A defect in nonoxidative glucose disposal in insulin-dependent tissues seems, therefore, a characteristic finding in sepsis and other acute infections. The possible etiology of this apparent blockade in glucose storage can result from diminished glycogen synthesis, accelerated glycogenolysis, or both (10). These possibilities have not been formally tested in septic humans, but studies in patients with other predominant acute infections have been published (10,33). Virkamäki et al.

studied mechanisms of hepatic and peripheral insulin resistance during acute infections in humans (33). Their data indicate that insulin resistance is predominantly localized to skeletal muscle and to a lesser extent to the liver. The defect in insulin action in skeletal muscle is localized to glycogen synthesis rather than glycolysis.

Glucose Metabolism in AIDS

The data on changes in glucose metabolism in HIV infection are scarce. Only three full papers on the influence of stable AIDS on glucose metabolism have been published (20,24,36). Data about the changes in asymptomatic HIV infection are lacking.

Plasma glucose concentrations after an overnight fast are consistently, although not always, significantly lower in stable AIDS patients compared with healthy controls (20,24,36). This (tendency to a) lower plasma glucose concentration cannot simply be ascribed to lower endogenous glucose production, as in two of the three studies, the rate of appearance of glucose tended to be higher than in the control subjects (Table 1). This combination of a decrease in glucose concentration despite an increase in production rate is contrary to the findings in other infectious diseases in which both (tend to) increase. Although glucose uptake is mainly noninsulin-mediated in the basal state (34), these changes in basal glucose metabolism in acute infections are ascribed to an increase in insulin resistance. It could therefore be possible that the peculiar changes in basal glucose metabolism in stable AIDS were caused by an increase in insulin sensitivity, which would be a highly remarkable finding, considering all the published data on acute infections and glucose metabolism. The suggestion of an increase in insulin sensitivity was confirmed by a two-step euglycemic hyperinsulinemic clamp study (24). This study showed that insulin clearance was increased in stable AIDS, a usual finding also in injury and sepsis (37). This increase in clearance resulted in significantly lower insulin concentrations in the patients, compared with the control subjects, in both steps of the clamp (42 ± 2 vs. 52 ± 4 µU/ml, $p < 0.05$ and 255 ± 17 vs. 392 ± 14 µU/ml, $p < 0.001$). Total glucose uptake increased similarly

TABLE 1. *Basal glucose metabolism in stable AIDS.*

Reference	Group	Plasma-glucose (mmol/l)	Endog-glucose production (µmol/kg/min)
Hommes et al. (20)	Patients	5.02 ± 0.15*	14.0 ± 0.39
	Controls	5.46 ± 0.14	12.44 ± 0.95
Hommes et al. (24)	Patients	4.6 ± 0.1	12.62 ± 0.78
	Controls	5.0 ± 0.1	12.75 ± 0.72
Heyligenberg et al. (36)	Patients	5.2 ± 0.1	15.9 ± 0.5
	Controls	5.3 ± 0.1	15.2 ± 0.4

* $p < 0.05$ versus control.

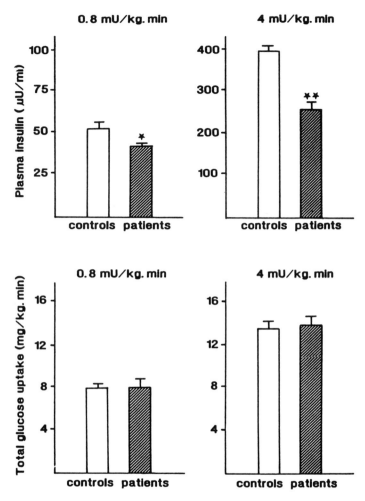

FIG. 1. Plasma insulin concentrations in relation to total glucose uptake during the clamp periods in healthy controls and stable AIDS patients *P <0.05, **<0.001 patients compared with controls. From Hommes et al. (24). Reproduced with permission from the editor.

in patients and controls despite the significant difference in plasma insulin concentration (44.4 ± 5 μmol/kg/min vs. 44.0 ± 3 μmol/kg/min and 77.8 ± 4 μmol/kg/min vs. 75.9 ± 4 μmol/kg/min) (Fig. 1). Because 19% and 35% lower insulin concentrations were sufficient to metabolize the same amount of glucose, it can be argued that the sensitivity to insulin of peripheral tissue in stable AIDS patients is increased. No definite conclusions regarding the insulin sensitivity of the liver could be drawn from that study because the lowest insulin infusion rate was already too high to assess its sensitivity. Rates of oxidative and nonoxidative glucose disposal were similar in the patients and the control subjects in the basal state and during the two-step euglycemic clamp (Table 2), suggesting that both pathways are undisturbed in stable AIDS.

TABLE 2. *Glucose disposal in the basal state and during an euglymic hyperinsulinemic clamp in stable AIDS patients.*

	Group	Basal	Insulin ($\pm$ 50 μU/ml)	Insulin ($\pm$ 300 μU/ml)
Glucose oxidation	Patients	1.44 $\pm$ 0.5	10.35 $\pm$ 0.8	19.5 $\pm$ 1.7
(μmol/kg/min)	Controls	1.46 $\pm$ 1.0	10.96 $\pm$ 1.5	15.00 $\pm$ 0.8
Nonoxidative glucose disposal	Patients	12.56 $\pm$ 0.3	34.04 $\pm$ 2.7	58.73 $\pm$ 3.2
(μmol/l/kg/min)	Controls	10.98 $\pm$ 0.9	33.04 $\pm$ 2.0	59.17 $\pm$ 2.3

Two mechanisms of glucose uptake are present in vivo: insulin-mediated glucose uptake (IMGU) and noninsulin-mediated glucose uptake (NIMGU). The suggestion of increased insulin sensitivity from whole-body glucose tissue uptake will only be true if the size of NIMGU and IMGU is comparable in patients and controls. In rats, it has been shown that gram-negative sepsis increased substantially the rate of whole-body glucose disposal. Most of the sepsis-induced increment in glucose disposal could be accounted for by increased rates of glucose uptake by macrophage-rich tissues (38). These data indicate that the degree of whole-body glucose disposal will also be influenced by the activity (i.e., the rate of glucose uptake) in the insulin-insensitive and relatively insulin-nonsensitive tissues, and two components in which NIMGU occurs. An increase in NIMGU in stable AIDS can be an alternative explanation for the finding of similar glucose tissue uptake rates in the presence of lower insulin concentrations. If NIMGU is considerably increased in stable AIDS, compared with controls, the contribution of IMGU will be overestimated. Consequently, an increase in insulin sensitivity in HIV infection will be erroneously presumed. The possibility of an increase in NIMGU in stable AIDS is a real one. One of the tissues

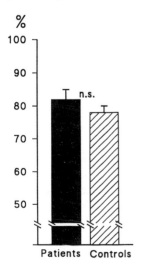

FIG. 2. Noninsulin-mediated glucose uptake (NIMGU), expressed as percentage of basal glucose uptake in AIDS patients *(solid bars)* and controls *(open bars)*. From Heyligenberg et al. (36). Reproduced with permission from the editor.

TABLE 3. *Basal glucose metabolism in asymptomatic HIV-positive subjects.*

Group	Glucose concentration (mmol/L/n)	Endogenous glucose production (μmol/kg/min)	Glucose oxidation (μmol/kg/min)	Nonoxidative glucose disposal (μmol/kg/min)
Patients (n = 11)	5.27 ± 0.14	13.0 ± 0.67	0.89 ± 0.4	12.11 ± 0.54
Controls (n = 11)	5.31 ± 0.12	12.5 ± 0.84	3.90 ± 1.6	8.6 ± 1.2

in which glucose can be taken up without the intervention of insulin is the monocyte-macrophage system, the major harbor of the HIV virus. As in gram-negative septic rats, this system is also stimulated in AIDS (39,40). The effect of HIV infection/stable AIDS on NIMGU and IMGU was studied in stable AIDS patients and controls, using intravenous somatostatin to block endogenous insulin production and induce temporary insulin deficiency (34,36). The study indicated that in stable AIDS, glucose tissue uptake during somatostatin-induced insulinopenia, representing NIMGU, was not different from the value obtained in the control subjects. In the patients, the euglycemic glucose uptake during somatostatin was 82% ± 3% of the basal glucose uptake. In the control subjects, this value was 78% ± 2% (Fig. 2), in good accordance with findings in the literature (34). HIV infection in humans does not seem to influence NIMGU, a finding clearly different from the influence of sepsis, at least in rodents.

No data on glucose metabolism in asymptomatic HIV-positive subjects have been published. Our group has studied only basal glucose metabolism (Hommes et al., unpublished results). No significant differences in the plasma glucose concentration, endogenous glucose production, glucose oxidation, and nonoxidative glucose disposal were found (Table 3).

Sepsis is like all other types of injury characterized by insulin resistance at hepatic and, especially, peripheral level. The latter is due to a defect in nonoxidative glucose disposal. This defect seems to be a defect in glycogen synthesis. AIDS is, unlike all other types of injury, characterized by increased insulin sensitivity with undisturbed oxidative and nonoxidative glucose disposal.

PROTEIN METABOLISM

Acute wasting of lean body mass is a well-known feature of sepsis. The protein content of the lean body mass is the result of the processes of synthesis and breakdown. It is evident that in sepsis those processes must be out of balance, resulting in an increased rate of urea appearance (31). During starvation and in lesser illnesses this imbalance is mainly due to a decrease in the protein synthesis rate (41), while in sepsis an increase in the protein breakdown rate is the most impressive finding (4,42,43). Nutrition is only able to diminish net protein catabolism, not bring the rates of synthesis and breakdown of protein into balance (4,31,44).

Cross-sectional studies in AIDS patients, with and without opportunistic infections, have indicated that body cell mass, estimated from measurements of total body potassium, was significantly diminished in these patients, compared with HIV-negative homosexual males and heterosexuals (6). This finding is not unexpected in patients with active opportunistic infections. Comparable results, however, have been obtained in stable AIDS patients despite seemingly normal caloric intake (45). It can always be argued that malabsorption with subsequent semistarvation is the cause of these abnormalities, but even in patients without any clinical sign of malabsorption, fat free mass is almost always less than in control groups (M. J. T. Hommes, personal communication). These clinical data would suggest abnormalities in protein metabolism in AIDS patients. Published studies are scarce, one full article (46) and one abstract (47,48). Stein et al. (46) studied nine male subjects with AIDS who were free of disease and without evidence of malabsorption or diarrhea and with normal nutritional intake. Whole-body protein kinetics were measured with ^{15}N-glycine. It was documented that only one of them was slowly losing weight; the others were weight-stable or had increasing weight. The protein synthetic rate was 28% lower in the AIDS patients than in control subjects (4.38 ± 0.34 vs. 3.16 ± 0.29 g protein/kg/d), while the breakdown rate differed by 23% (4.66 ± 0.29 in controls) vs. 3.57 ± 0.33 g protein/kg/d (in AIDS patients). The authors considered their findings consistent with malnutrition rather than a hypermetabolic type of response. A different picture was found by Macallan et al. (47,48). They measured protein turnover, using ^{13}C-labeled leucine as a tracer, in 14 unspecified HIV-infected patients in stage IV and three patients in stage II. Whole-body protein turnover was 29% higher in the subjects with AIDS compared with healthy controls. The values of the subjects in stage II were intermediate between those of the subjects with stage-IV infection and those of the controls. The elevation of protein turnover was seen in persons with HIV infection who were well and had stable weight as well in those who were losing weight. Data on rates of protein synthesis and breakdown were not given. The measurements were repeated during short-term total parenteral nutrition (TPN) (0.2 g N/kg/d and 31.9 kcal/kg/d). Remarkably, individuals with HIV infection made an anabolic response to feeding of similar magnitude as did controls.

No statement can be made about similarities or dissimilarities in protein metabolism in septic versus HIV-infected patients, as the results obtained thus far in AIDS patients are quite confusing. Increased and decreased protein turnover is reported in seemingly comparable patient groups. The elevation of protein turnover, consistent with a catabolic pattern, is seen in persons with HIV infection and stable weight as well in those who are losing weight. The normal anabolic response to feeding in these patients is dissimilar to the response of patients with sepsis and does not explain the gradual weight loss in some of them, unless the study group is quite variable concerning absorptive capacity of the gut.

THYROID HORMONE METABOLISM

Nonthyroidal Illness

Several characteristics make hormones such as insulin, glucagon, and catecholamines ideal short-term regulators of metabolism. They can be secreted briskly, are water-soluble, have short half-lives, and act through binding at membrane receptors to elicit intracellular effects. As demonstrated by the clinical features of hyper- and hypothyroidism, thyroid hormones are also powerful metabolic regulators. They differ greatly, however, with respect to metabolism and action compared with the above-mentioned hormones. Thyroid hormone secretion increases rather slowly upon stimulation by thyroid-stimulating hormone (TSH). Thyroid hormones are hydrophobic and are transported in blood predominantly bound to plasma proteins. They have long half-lives (T3: $\pm$ 1 day; T4 $\pm$ 7 days) and act primarily through binding to nuclear receptors. Their metabolic effects are caused by modulations of gene transcription, which eventually result in changes in protein metabolism. It is evident that thyroid hormones are slow metabolic regulators. The circulating concentrations of the thyroid hormones are profoundly influenced by a wide variety of clinical syndromes without intrinsic thyroid disease (nonthyroidal illness, NTI). As the subjects are nevertheless considered to be euthyroid, the alterations in thyroid functions in NTI are referred to as the "euthyroid sick syndrome" (49,50).

Under normal circumstances, plasma triiodothyronine (T3) is derived predominantly (approximately 80%) from extrathyroidal conversion from thyroxine (T4) (only secreted by the thyroid gland), whereas the remainder of T3 is secreted by the thyroid. The remainder of T4, not converted to T3, is converted to reverse-T3 (r-T3), an inactive metabolite. Type II 5'-deiodinase catalyzes the conversion from T4 to T3 and from rT3 to other metabolites (51). Inhibition of this enzyme will induce low T3 and high rT3 levels. Multiple alterations of T4 distribution and metabolism occur in patients with NTI disorders, such as infectious diseases, myocardial infarction, surgery, and renal failure. These include increased or decreased total T4 and free T4 concentrations, a low T3 and an increased rT3 concentration, and TSH values usually in the normal range. Inhibition of 5'-deiodinase type II, altered concentrations and binding kinetics of thyroid hormones to the thyroid hormone-transporting proteins, and changes in the regulation of thyroid hormone secretion are therefore involved in the pathogenesis of NTI. The severity of the underlying disease (e.g., the infection) is correlated with thyroidal abnormalities with a reciprocal relationship between severity and serum T3 levels (50). A direct relationship is found between the magnitude of the decrease in serum T4 and patient outcome, with a high mortality in patients with very low T4 values (52). As can be expected, the typical findings of NTI with decreased total T4 and T3, increased rT3, and normal TSH are also found in bacterial sepsis (53) and other infections (52).

Nonthyroidal Illness and HIV Infection

The single best prognostic indicator of acute mortality due to *Pneumocystis carinii* pneumonia in AIDS appeared to be a very low T3 concentration (54). This would suggest that the impact of HIV infection on thyroid hormone metabolism would be not different from other infectious diseases. Reality proved to be otherwise, as patients with an HIV infection have a unique pattern of alterations in their serum thyroid hormone indices, even in the initial asymptomatic seropositive phase of the disease. These changes become more pronounced with progression of the disease into more advanced stages. These unique changes include a significant increase in serum T4 associated with a paradoxical decrease in rT3 and maintenance of a normal T3. Decreases in serum T3 develop only in critically ill patients with HIV and *Pneumocystis carinii* pneumonia. However, even in these cases, the changes are modest compared with those observed in patients in a medical intensive care unit with similar mortality rates (54). These findings have been confirmed by others (55–57).

Several observations indicate that the hypothalamo-pituitary-thyroid relations are altered in NTI. Despite profound depression in circulatory T3 and T4, TSH concentration is usually in the normal range (50,58,59), and pharmacologically induced decrements in serum T4 and T3 by administration of stable iodine do not result in the expected rise of serum TSH in about half of the patients with NTI (50). The nocturnal TSH surge found in healthy subjects is blunted, or even absent, in NTI, which is probably related to altered hypothalamic regulation because this phenomenon was not related to ambient plasma T4 of T3 concentration or pituitary TSH responsiveness to thyroid-regulating hormone (TRH) (54).

From the studies published on thyroid hormone concentrations in HIV infection, it is not clear how HIV infection influences regulation of thyroid hormone secretion. Our group therefore studied thyroid hormone secretion in relation to pulsatile characteristics of TSH secretion (Fig. 3) and pituitary TRH responsiveness in asymptomatic HIV positive patients and patients with stable AIDS (56). The data clearly showed

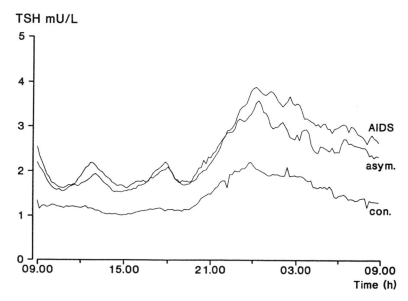

FIG. 3. Twenty-four hour plasma thyroid-stimulating hormone (TSH) concentrations. Curves represent the mean in eight healthy controls (con), eight asymptomatic HIV-positives (asym), and six stable AIDS patients (AIDS). From Hommes et al. (56). Reproduced with permission from the editor.

that, compared with carefully matched controls, the HIV-infected patients (both the asymptomatics and the stable patients) had significantly increased TSH secretion, albeit still in the normal range, suggesting a primary hypothyroid-like regulation of the pituitary-thyroid axis. This suggestion was supported by the TRH study showing an exaggerated TSH response after TRH.

The changes in thyroid hormone metabolism in regular NTI are induced by influencing peripheral hormone metabolism and altering hypothalamic regulation. In HIV infection, the thyroid gland seems to be the primary goal of regulation. Because HIV infection and its consequences are not known to cause thyroid disease (60), this change in thyroid hormone regulation can not simply be ascribed to subclinical thyroid gland destruction.

PATHOPHYSIOLOGIC CONSIDERATIONS

The pathogenetic mechanisms that induce NTI is unknown, but the altered hormonal environment has long been held responsible for the characteristic metabolic changes in sepsis. Septicemia is associated with a profound neuroendocrine response initiated by the hypothalamus and the sympathetic nervous system (2,61,62). This response is characterized by increases in the plasma concentrations of catecholamines, growth hormone, corticosteroids, and glucagon, and a variable response of insulin. The degree of these increases is generally not very impressive, and sometimes no difference in plasma values between patients and healthy controls is found. By example, in the previously cited studies on the influence of acute infection on glucose metabolism, no increase in the plasma concentrations of these hormones was found despite impressive disturbances in glucose metabolism (10,33). In the cited studies on the influence of sepsis on metabolism, plasma catabolic hormone concentrations were variable, differing between no change up to a fourfold increase of one of these hormones in some studies. On the average, a twofold increase was reported (3,4,8, 9,19,29,31,61).

Attempts to stimulate the metabolic response to injury by the combined infusion of catecholamines, cortisol, and glucagon showed that much higher concentrations are needed to produce metabolic changes of a comparable magnitude to those found in sepsis (61,63,64). Other factors must therefore be also involved in the induction of the metabolic changes of sepsis. In AIDS, it is even more clear that other factors must be involved, as the plasma concentrations of insulin and the catabolic hormones are not different between patients with stable AIDS and healthy controls (Table 4) (65).

Recent work convincingly shows that cytokines, especially TNF, interleukin-1 (IL-1), and interleukin-6 (IL-6), are among these mediators, with a prominent role for TNF (1,2,66–68). Short-lasting intravenous administration of TNF to non–weight-losing adult subjects with disseminated cancer induced a dose-related maximal increase in energy expenditure of 30%. Whole-body protein turnover, measured by primed-constant infusion of ^{15}N-glycine for 42 hours during a metabolically defined

TABLE 4. *Plasma concentrations of catabolic hormones in patients with stable AIDS and healthy controls (mean ± SE).*

	AIDS	Controls
Cortisol (μmol/l)	0.32 ± 0.05	0.28 ± 0.03
Glucagon (ng/l)	130 ± 23	84 ± 10
Epinephrine (ng/l)	47 ± 11	68 ± 9
Norepinephrine (ng/l)	253 ± 28	351 ± 38
Growth hormone (mU/l)	6 ± 2*	<2.0 (all)

Data from Hommes (65).
* $p < 0.005$ versus controls.

diet, increased by 14%, and whole-body protein synthesis rate increased by 25%; whole-body protein catabolism also increased but this change did not reach statistical significance. Closer inspection of the data suggests that the average protein catabolic rate was a higher-than-average synthesis rate before TNF administration, while the reverse was found afterward. This apparently mitigated effect of TNF on protein metabolism during a balanced diet is supported by the data on nitrogen balance. This balance became negative (or more negative) after TNF in only four of the nine patients. Changes in lipid metabolism were very obvious, with a >80% turnover in glycerol, a >60% increase in FFA turnover, and an increase in triglyceride concentration. Glucose metabolism was not studied. Levels of insulin were not significantly altered by TNF. An increase in plasma cortisol was the only statistically significant change in the concentrations of the catabolic hormones induced by TNF in these studies (69,70). Cancer itself affects metabolism (71). There are reports that suggest that cancer patients are chronically exposed to increased endogenous TNF levels, and prolonged exposure of TNF may lead to increased tolerance (72,73). As it was uncertain if these data would influence the metabolic response to TNF injection and the study was done during feeding, our group performed a crossover saline-controlled study in healthy males during short-term starvation (<24 hours) (68,74). Tumor necrosis factor induced an impressive but transient stress hormone response lasting between 2 hours (catecholamines) and 8 hours (cortisol and glucagon), with an intermediate growth hormone response. Insulin levels were not influenced. Resting energy expenditure showed an increase (34 ± 2% at 4 hours) and was still raised at the end of the study (9 hours after the TNF injection). Plasma glucose concentration increased early and was sustained, with no tendency to decline before the end of the study. This increase must be ascribed to the combined effects of increased production and decreased disposal because the increase in plasma concentration was double the increase in production rate (+23% ± 7% for concentration vs. 10% ± 3% for glucose production). Glucose oxidation was completely inhibited, as in the control period. The effect on parameters of lipid metabolism was transient, with peak values of plasma FFA and glycerol at four hours and a decline to control values at 8 hours after injection. The increase in FFA concentration was due to an increase in FFA turnover. This stimulation of lipolysis was followed by a marked increase in ketogenesis, different from the data obtained in sepsis. Data on protein metabolism were not obtained (62). During the aforementioned study, thyroid hormone concentrations were measured at regular intervals. A significant decrease in plasma T3 and TSH and a significant increase in plasma rT3 were found with no change in plasma T4, with the hormonal picture typical for NTI at the end of the observation period (10 hours after TNF injection) (75). These changes were already apparent within the first few hours after injection, and the rapidity of these changes suggest that NTI is not merely a secondary adaptation to the catabolic state as has been proposed (50).

These data together suggest a prominent role for TNF as mediator in sepsis. The contribution of IL-1 and IL-6 to the metabolic picture of sepsis is not known, as no data on the changes in metabolic parameters induced by these cytokines in healthy humans have been published. Preliminary and unpublished results by our group suggest that IL-6, except for its well-known induction of the acute-phase response, has other metabolic influences as well, but these seem to be less impressive than those induced by TNF, except for its influence on REE (J. M. C. Stouthard, personal communication).

The role of TNF, IL-6, and IL-1 as mediators of the metabolic changes found in HIV infection is unconvincing, with publications showing increased cytokine production and others vehemently denying this. Even the data on in vitro studies on modulation of cytokine production by cell lines infected by HIV virus are inconclusive, showing or denying increased expression of cytokine in RNA in cell lines infected by the HIV virus (76–78). The interest in TNF as a possible mediator of metabolic disturbances in HIV infection surged with a publication showing high levels in serum (79). This was confirmed by some (80,81) although others failed to find a significant increase in TNF levels (5,21,82). In the positive studies, the occurrence of secondary infection was either apparent or not stated, and secondary infection is, among others, a likely explanation for these differences (5). The controversy is not resolved when ex vivo basal and lipopolysaccharide (LPS)-induced TNF production by circulating monocytes is measured; some authors find increased production while others do not. This existence of concomitant opportunistic infection is no explanation for these differences, as increased production is also sometimes reported in asymptomatic seropositives (83–85). Unpublished results from our group suggest that unstimulated peripheral monocytes from HIV-infected subjects do not produce cytokines. Lipopolysaccharide-stimulated TNF production in our patients with stable AIDS was about 70% higher than in the matched control group. No increase in stimulated IL-1 and IL-6 production in these patients was found. Very preliminary data in asymptomatic HIV-infected subjects showed normal LPS-stimulated production (Godfried MH, personal communication). The dilemma is not resolved, but there is some suggestion that TNF production may be increased in stable AIDS.

The metabolic alterations induced by sepsis and AIDS are summarized and are related to those induced by TNF injection in Table 5. When these data are compared, the similar changes found in sepsis and AIDS, as increases in REE, lipolytic rate, and triglyceride concentrations, can also be induced by TNF administration. When

TABLE 5. *Metabolic alterations induced by sepsis, TNF administration to healthy subjects, and stable AIDS.*

	Sepsis	AIDS	TNF
REE	↑↑	↑	↑↑
Protein turnover	↑↑	↑/↓	↑
Synthesis	↑	↑	↑
Breakdown	↑↑		↑/−
Lipolysis	↑↑	↑	↑↑
Triglyceride concentration	↑↑	↑	↑
Ketone body concentration	N/↓	N	↑
Glucose concentration	↑	−/↓	↑
Turnover	↑	N	↑
Oxidation	N	−	NA
Nonoxidative disposal	↓	−	NA
Insulin resistance	↑	↓	↑
Plasma insulin	N/↑	N	N
Plasma catabolic hormones	↑	N	↑
NTI	+	+	+
tissue of regulation	Peripheral/CNS	Thyroid gland	Peripheral/CNS

↑, increase; ↓, decrease; N, normal; NA, not available; REE, resting energy expenditure; NTI, nonthyroid illness, TNF, tumor necrosis factor; CNS, central nervous system;

our data on increased TNF production in AIDS are confirmed, it is a real possibility that TNF is involved in the induction of these changes, directly or indirectly.

The differences between sepsis and AIDS in regard to glucose metabolism are remarkable and relate mainly to a difference in peripheral glucose handling. In the basal state, TNF administration to healthy subjects induces changes comparable to those found in sepsis. This would suggest that TNF is not involved in the metabolic alterations in glucose metabolism as is found in AIDS. This is not necessarily so, however, as a major increase in the concentration of the catabolic hormones by TNF is also found. Combined hormone infusions have shown that these hormones can easily induce an insulin-resistant state (63,64). In vitro and in vivo data in animals suggest that TNF may have a stimulating influence on glucose uptake (for a review, see ref. 66). When these data are combined, it is a possibility that increased insulin sensitivity is a feature of increased TNF production in humans when catabolic hormone secretion is not influenced. Future studies will explore this possibility.

The data on protein metabolism in AIDS are too scarce and too contradictory to make any useful concluding remarks. Nonthyroid illness is induced by sepsis, TNF administration, and HIV infection. The similarity between the tissues of regulation in sepsis and after TNF and the dissimilarity between these two situations and AIDS suggest a major role for TNF in the induction of NTI in sepsis, but not in AIDS.

The possibility of a major role for TNF in the induction of the metabolic changes by sepsis is more apparent than its role in the induction of the metabolic changes in AIDS, but enough pieces of evidence have been sampled to make it worthwhile to explore further this possibility in HIV infection.

REFERENCES

1. Wilmore DW. Catabolic illness. Strategics for enhancing recovery. *N Engl J Med* 1991;325:695–702.
2. Watters JM, Wilmore DW. The metabolic response to trauma and sepsis. In: LJ DeGroot, ed. *Endocrinology*. Philadelphia: WB Saunders, 1989;2367–2393.
3. Sauerwein HP, Pesola GR, Godfried MH, et al. Insulin sensitivity in septic cancer-bearing patients. *JPEN* 1991;15:653–658.
4. Shaw JHF, Wildbore M, Wolfe RR. Whole body protein kinetics in severely septic patients. The response to glucose infusions and total parenteral nutrition. *Ann Surg* 1987;205:288–294.
5. Grünfeld C, Feingold KR. Metabolic disturbances and wasting in the acquired immunodeficiency syndrome. *N Engl J Med* 1992;327:329–337.
6. Kotler DP, Wang J, Pierson RN. Body composition studies in patients with the acquired immunodeficiency syndrome. *Am J Clin Nutr* 1985;42:1255–1265.
7. Kotler DP, Tierney AR, Culpepper-Morgan JA,et al. Effect of home total parenteral nutrition on body composition in patients with acquired immunodeficiency syndrome. *JPEN* 1990;14:454–458.
8. Arnold J, Shipley KA, Scott NA, et al. Thermic effect of parenteral nutrition in septic and nonseptic individuals. *Am J Clin Nutr* 1989;50:853–860.
9. Arnold J, Leinhardt D, Carlson G, et al. Thermogenic and hormonal responses to amino acid infusion in septic humans. *Am J Physiol* 1992;263:E129–E135.
10. Yki-Järvinen H, Sammalkorpi K, Koivisto VA, Nikkilä EA. Severity, duration and mechanisms of insulin resistance during acute infections. *Clin Endocrinol Metab* 1989;69:317–323.
11. Kinney JM, Fürst P, Elwyn DH, Carpentier YA. The intensive care patient. In: Kinney JM, Jeejeebhoy KN, Hill GL, Owen VE, eds. *Nutrition and Metabolism in Patient Care*. Philadelphia: WB Saunders, 1988;656–671.
12. Hommes MJT, Romijn JA, Godfried MH, et al. Increased resting energy expenditure in HIV-infected men. *Metabolism* 1990;39:1186–1190.
13. Melchior JC, Salmon D, Rigand D, et al. Resting energy expenditure is increased in stable malnourished HIV-infected patients. *Am J Clin Nutr* 1991;53:437–441.
14. Grünfeld C, Pang M, Shimizu L, et al. Resting energy expenditure, caloric intake and short-term weight change in human immunodeficiency virus infection and the acquired immunodeficiency syndrome. *Am J Clin Nutr* 1992;55:455–460.
15. Hommes MJT, Romijn JA, Endert E, Sauerwein HP. Resting energy expenditure and substrate oxidation in human immunodeficiency virus (HIV)-infected asymptomatic men. HIV affects host metabolism in the early asymptomatic stage. *Am J Clin Nutr* 1991;54:311–315.
16. Moore FD. *Metabolic care of the surgical patients*. Philadelphia: WB Saunders, 1959;35–36.
17. Forse RA, Leibel R, Askanazi J, et al. Adrenergic control of adipocyte lipolysis in trauma and sepsis. *Ann Surg* 1987;206:744–751.
18. Carpentier YA, Askanazi J, Elwyn DH, et al. Effects of hypercaloric glucose infusion on lipid metabolism in injury and sepsis. *J Trauma* 1979;19:649–654.
19. Shaw JHF, Wolfe RR. Fatty acid and glycerol kinetics in septic patients and in patients with gastrointestinal cancer. The response to glucose infusion and parenteral feeding. *Ann Surg* 1987;205:368–376.
20. Hommes MJT, Romijn JA, Endert E, et al. Basal fuel homeostasis in symptomatic immunodeficiency virus (HIV) infection. *Clin Sci* 1991;80:359–365.
21. Grünfeld C, Pang M, Doerrler W, et al. Lipids, lipoproteins, triglyceride clearance and cytokines in human immunodeficiency virus infection and the acquired immunodeficiency syndrome. *J Clin Endocrinol Metab* 1992;74:1045–1052.
22. Issekutz B, Bortz WM, Miller HI, Paul P. Turnover rate of plasma FFA in humans and dogs. *Metabolism* 1967;16:1001–1009.
23. Gallin JI, Kaye D, O'Leary WM. Serum lipids in infection. *N Engl J Med* 1969;281:1081–1086.
24. Hommes MJT, Romijn JA, Endert E, et al. Insulin sensitivity and insulin clearance in HIV infected men. *Metabolism* 1991;40:651–656.
25. Sammalkorpi K, Valtonen V, Kerttula Y, et al. Changes in serum lipoprotein pattern induced by acute infections. *Metabolism* 1988;37:859–865.
26. Wolfe RR, Shaw JHF, Durkot MJ. Effect of sepsis on VLDL kinetics: responses in basal state and during glucose infusion. *Am J Physiol* 1985;248:E732–E740.
27. Grünfeld C, Kotler DP, Hamadek R, et al. Hypertriglyceridemia in the aquired immunodeficiency syndrome. *Am J Med* 1989;86:27–31.

28. Grünfeld C, Kotler DP, Shigenaga JK, et al. Circulating interferon-α levels and hypertriglyceridemia in the acquired immunodeficiency syndrome. *Am J Med* 1991;90:154–162.
29. White RN, Frayn KN, Little RA, et al. Hormonal and metabolic responses to glucose infusion in sepsis studied by the hyperglycemic glucose clamp technique. *JPEN* 1987;11:345–353.
30. Long CL, Spencer L, Kinney JM, Geiger JW. Carbohydrate metabolism in man: effect of elective operations and major injury. *J Appl Physiol* 1971;31:110–116.
31. Shaw JHF, Klein S, Wolfe RR. Assessment of alanine, urea and glucose interrelationships in normal subjects and in patients with stable isotopic tracers. *Surgery* 1985;97:557–567.
32. Shangraw RE, Jahoor F, Mihyoshi H, et al. Differentiation between septic and postburn insulin resistance. *Metabolism* 1989;38:983–989.
33. Virkamäki A, Puhakainen I, Koivisto VA, et al. Mechanisms of hepatic and peripheral insulin resistance during acute infections in humans. *J Clin Endocrinol Metab* 1992;74:673–679.
34. Baron AD, Kolterman OG, Mandarino LJ, Olefski JM. Rates of non-insulin mediated glucose uptake in type II diabetic subjects. *J Clin Invest* 1985;76:1782–1788.
35. Sauerwein HP, Pesola GR, Groeger JS, et al. Relationship between glucose oxidation and FFA concentration in septic cancer-bearing patients. *Metabolism* 1988;37:1045–1050.
36. Heyligenberg R, Romijn JA, Hommes MJT, et al. Insulin mediated and non-insulin mediated glucose uptake in HIV-infected men. *Clin Sci* 1993;84:209–216.
37. Dahn MS, Lange MP, Mitchell RA, et al. Insulin production following injury and sepsis. *J. Trauma* 1987;27:1031–1038.
38. Lang CH, Dobrescu C. Sepsis-induced increases in glucose uptake by macrophage rich tissues persist during hypoglycemia. *Metabolism* 1991;40:585–593.
39. Pantales C, Graziosi C, Butini L, et al. Lymphoid organs function as major reservoirs for human immunodeficiency virus. *Proc Natl Acad Sci* 1991;88:9838–9842.
40. Fauci AJ. Immunopathogenic mechanims in human immunodeficiency virus (HIV) infection. *Ann Intern Med* 1991;114:678–693.
41. Claque MB,Keir MJ, Wright PD, Johnston IDA. The effects of nutrition and trauma on whole-body protein metabolism in man. *Clin Sci* 1983;65:165–175.
42. Long CL, Jeevanandam M, Kim BM, Kinney JM. Whole body protein synthesis and catabolism in septic man. *Am J Clin Nutr* 1977;30:1340–1344.
43. Jahoor F, Shangraw RE, Miyoshi H, et al. Role of insulin and glucose oxidation in mediating the protein catabolism of burns and sepsis. *Am J Physiol* 1989;257:E323–E331.
44. Streat SJ, Beddoe AH, Hill GL. Aggressive nutritional support does not prevent protein loss despite fat gain in septic intensive care patients. *J Trauma* 1987;27:262–266.
45. Kotler DP, Tierney AR, Brenner SK, et al. Preservation of short-term energy balance in clinically stable patients with AIDS. *Am J Clin Nutr* 1990;51:7–13.
46. Stein TP, Nutinsky C, Condoluci D, et al. Protein and energy substrate metabolism in AIDS patients. *Metabolism* 1990;39:876–881.
47. Macallan DC, McNurlan NA, Garlick PJ, Griffin GE. Infection with human immunodeficiency virus increases whole body protein turnover but does not prevent the acute anabolic response to nutrition. *Clin Nutr* 1992;11(Suppl): 14.
48. Macallan DC, Griffin GE. Metabolic disturbances in AIDS. *N Engl J Med* 1992;327:1530–1531.
49. Romijn JA. *On metabolic modulation by starvation and disease* [Thesis]. University of Amsterdam, 1990.
50. Wartofsky L, Burman K. Alterations in thyroid function in patients with systemic illnesses: the euthyroid sick syndrome. *Endocr Rev* 1982;3:164–217.
51. Pangaro LN. Physiology of the thyroid gland. In: Becker KL, ed. *Principles and Practice of Endocrinology and Metabolism*. Philadelphia: JB Lippincot, 1990;271–275.
52. Kaptein EM, Weiner JM, Robinson WJ, et al. Relationship of altered thyroid hormone indices to survival in nonthyroidal illnesses. *Clin Endocrinol* 1982;16:565–574.
53. Richmond DA, Molitch ME, O'Donnell TF. Altered thyroid hormone levels in bacterial sepsis: the role of nutritional adequacy. *Metabolism* 1980;29:936–942.
54. Fried JC, LoPresti JS, Micon M, et al. Serum triiodothyronine values. Prognostic indicators of acute mortality due to *Pneumocystis carinii* pneumonia associated with the acquired immuno-deficiency syndrome. *Arch Intern Med* 1990;150:406–409.
55. Feldt-Rasmussen U, Sestoft L, Berg H. Thyroid function tests in patients with acquired immune deficiency syndrome and healthy HIV1-positive out-patients. *Eur J Clin Invest* 1991;21:59–63.
56. Hommes MJT, Romijn JA, Brabant G, et al. Hypothyroid-like regulation of the pituitary-thyroid axis in stable HIV-infection. *Metabolism* (in press).

57. Grünfeld C, Pang M, Doerrler W, et al. Indices of thyroid function and weight loss in human immuno-deficiency virus and the acquired immunodeficiency syndrome (submitted).
58. Brent GA, Hershman JM. Thyroxine therapy in patients with severe nonthyroidal illnesses and low serum thyroxine concentrations. *J Clin Endocrinol Metab* 1986;63:1–8.
59. Romijn JA, Wiersinga WM. Decreased nocturnal surge of thyrotropin in non-thyroidal illness. *J Clin Endocrinol Metab* 1990;70:35–42.
60. Grinspoon SK, Bilezikian JP. HIV disease and the endocrine system. *N Engl J Med* 1992;327: 1360–1365.
61. Frayn KN. Hormonal control of metabolism in trauma and sepsis. *Clin Endocrinol* 1986;24:577–599.
62. Douglas RG, Shaw JHF. Metabolic response to sepsis and trauma. *Br J Sug*1989;76:115–122.
63. Bessey PQ, Watters JM, Aoki TT, Wilmore DW. Combined hormonal infusion stimulates the metabolic response to injury. *Ann Surg* 1984;200:264–281.
64. Gelfand RA, Matthews DE, Bier DM, Sherwin RS. Role of counter regulatory hormones in the catabolic response to stress. *J Clin Invest* 1984;74:2238–2248.
65. Hommes MJT. *Host metabolism in chronic HIV infection* [Thesis]. University of Amsterdam, 1990.
66. vd Poll T, Sauerwein HP. Tumor necrosis factor α: its role in the metabolic response to sepsis. *Clin Sci* 1993;84:247–256.
67. Tracey KJ. TNF and other cytokines in the metabolism of septic shock and cachexia. *Clin Nutr* 1992;11:1–11.
68. vd Poll T. *Tumor necrosis factor: biological responses in humans* [Thesis]. University of Amsterdam, 1991.
69. Warren RS, Starnes HF, Gabrilove JL, et al. The acute metabolic effects of tumor necrosis administration in humans. *Arch Surg* 1987;122:1396–1400.
70. Starnes HF, Warren RS, Jeevanandam M, et al. Tumor necrosis factor and the acute metabolic response to tissue injury in man. *J Clin Invest* 1988;82:1321–1325.
71. Brennan MF. Total parenteral nutrition in the cancer patient. *N Engl J Med* 1981;305:375–382.
72. Balkwill F, Osborne R, Burke F, et al. Evidence for tumor necrosis factor/cachectin production in cancer. *Lancet* 1987;ii:1229–1232.
73. Tracey KJ, Wei H, Manogue KR, et al. Cachectin/tumor necrosis factor induces cachexia, anemia and inflammation. *J Exp Med* 1988;167:1211–1227.
74. vd Poll T, Romijn JA, Endert E,et al. Tumor necrosis factor mimics the metabolic response to acute infection in healthy humans. *Am J Physiol* 1991;261:E457–E466.
75. vd Poll T, Romijn JA, Wiersinga WM, Sauerwein HP. Tumor necrosis factor: a putative mediator of the sick euthyroid sick syndrome in man. *J Clin Endocrinol Metab* 1990;71:1567–1572.
76. Molina JM, Scadden DT, Bryn R, et al. Production of tumor necrosis factor α and interleukin 1β by monocytic cells infected with human immunodeficiency virus. *J Clin Invest* 1989;84:733–737.
77. Munis JR, Richman DD, Kornbluth RS. Human immunodeficiency virus-1 infection of macrophages in vitro neither induces tumor necrosis factor (TNF)/cachectin gene expression nor alters TNF/cachectin induction by lipopolysaccharide. *J Clin Invest* 1990;85:591–596.
78. Yamato K, Hajjaoui Z, Simon K, Koeffler HP. Modulation of interleukin-1β RNA by monocytic cells infected with human immunodeficiency virus-1. *J Clin Invest* 1990;86:1109–1114.
79. Lahdevirta J, Maury CPJ, Teppo AM, Repo H. Elevated levels of circulating cachectin/tumor necrosis factor in patients with acquired immunodeficiency syndrome. *Am J Med* 1988;85:289–291.
80. Rautonen J, Rautonen N, Martin NL, et al. Serum interleukin-6 concentrations are elevated and associated with elevated tumor necrosis factor-α and immunoglobulin G and A concentrations in children with HIV infection. *AIDS* 1991;5:1319–1325.
81. Noronka IL, Daniel V, Schimpf K,Opelz G. Soluble IL-2 receptor and tumor necrosis factor-α in plasma of haemophilia patients infected with HIV. *Clin Exp Immunol* 1992;87:287–292.
82. Kalinkovich A, Engelmann H, Harpaz N, et al. Elevated serum levels of soluble tumor necrosis factor receptors (s TNF-R) in patients with HIV infection. *Clin Exp Immunol* 1992;89:351–355.
83. Lau AS, Livesey JF. Endotoxin induction of tumor necrosis factor is enhanced by acid-labile interferon α in acquired immunodeficiency syndrome. *J Clin Invest* 1989;84:738–743.
84. Vyarkarnam A, Matear P, Meager A, et al. Altered production of tumor necrosis factor alpha and beta and interferon gamma by HIV infected individuals. *Clin Exp Immunol* 1991;84:109–115.
85. Peters AMJ, Jäger FS, Warneke A, et al. Cytokine secretion by peripheral blood monocytes from human immunodeficiency virus-infected patients is normal. *Clin Immunol Immunopathol* 1991;61: 343–352.

Organ Metabolism and Nutrition:
Ideas for Future Critical Care, edited by
J. M. Kinney and H. N. Tucker.
Raven Press, Ltd., New York © 1994.

Overview:
Splanchnic Organ Function, Metabolism, and Nutrition

Jukka Takala

Critical Care Research Program, Department of Intensive Care, Kuopio University Hospital, PSF-70211 Kuopio, Finland

Severe infection and other conditions that acutely and severely disturb the homeostasis induce a systemic inflammatory response, which is characterized by hypermetabolism and increased substrate turnover and requirements (1). The inflammatory response induces a remarkably consistent clinical picture, which is not dependent on the triggering cause or the presence of infection (2). In this overview, the term *sepsis* is used to refer to the systemic inflammatory response, regardless of the presence of infection.

Accumulating data from several lines of research suggest that the splanchnic region has a central role not only in the metabolic response, but also in the pathogenesis of organ dysfunction and failure in sepsis (2–6).

SPLANCHNIC TISSUE OXYGENATION (see Chapter 18)

Adequate balance between splanchnic tissue oxygen supply and demand is the prerequisite for normal function and metabolism in the splanchnic region. Modern intensive care has facilitated rapid restoration of vital functions and reduced the duration of overt shock and tissue hypoperfusion in various categories of acutely ill patients. Recent studies have demonstrated that signs of splanchnic tissue hypoxia may persist despite stabilization of vital signs and normalization of systemic hemodynamics (5,7–10). Assessment of gastric intramucosal pH using gastrointestinal tonometry has facilitated clinical monitoring of the adequacy of splanchnic tissue oxygenation (5,7–9). Transient splanchnic tissue hypoxia, demonstrated as gastric intramucosal acidosis, is relatively common in various groups of intensive care patients: Up to 80% of patients with multiple organ failure, 50% of patients undergoing elective cardiac surgery, and 18% of patients undergoing abdominal aortic surgery have episodes of gastric intramucosal acidosis (5,7–9). Gastric intramucosal acidosis is also associated with higher occurrence rate of multiple organ failure and increased mortality (7–9). Furthermore, treatment of gastric mucosal acidosis by administration of fluids and vasoactive drugs improves the outcome (5,9).

It has been suggested that intestinal mucosal injury due to tissue hypoxia promotes translocation of intraluminal bacteria and toxins and thereby triggers the cascade of mediators, which may cause further tissue injury and perfusion defects (11). Increased intestinal permeability, but not the bacterial or endotoxin translocation, has been demonstrated in infected burn patients (12). In contrast to experimental models, where bacterial translocation has been shown to occur, the relevance of translocation in clinical sepsis has not been demonstrated. Although the association between splanchnic tissue hypoxia and increased morbidity and mortality seems evident, the actual mechanisms appear much more complex than the translocation hypothesis assumes.

The pathogenesis of splanchnic tissue hypoxia in intensive care patients is multifactorial. In hypovolemia, perfusion of the heart and the central nervous system is maintained at the expense of the peripheral tissues and the splanchnic region. Prolonged hypovolemia will inevitably lead to severe splanchnic tissue hypoxia and increase the risk of multiple organ failure. In sepsis, the metabolic demand for oxygen in the splanchnic region appears to be markedly increased (3,10,13–16). While the total splanchnic blood flow is also higher than normal, the increase in oxygen consumption is disproportionate to the increase in blood flow and necessitates high oxygen extraction. Endothelial injury is common in sepsis and contributes to abnormal vascular tone, blood flow maldistribution, and development of hypovolemia (2). In addition, severe sepsis is almost invariably accompanied by acute respiratory failure (17), which limits the systemic oxygen delivery. Myocardial depression is also common in sepsis and may limit the response of systemic blood flow to the increased oxygen demand (18). Under these circumstances, the splanchnic hypermetabolism increases the risk of splanchnic oxygen delivery/demand mismatch, and even subtle changes in blood volume, cardiac output, arterial oxygenation, or oxygen demand in other tissues may precipitate splanchnic tissue hypoxia. It is evident that severe tissue hypoxia is present in septic shock (10); in contrast, the role and presence of tissue hypoxia in hemodynamically stable sepsis have not been well established. Because the metabolic demand for oxygen is increased and the utilization of available oxygen may be impaired, it is conceivable that an elevated oxygen delivery may be necessary to prevent splanchnic tissue hypoxia.

SPLANCHNIC REGION AND THE INFLAMMATORY RESPONSE
(see Chapters 6 and 18)

The splanchnic region can be both the target and the source of the inflammatory response in sepsis (6,11,19). For example, circulatory shock or a source of sepsis outside the splanchnic region may, via changes in circulation and oxygen transport cause splanchnic tissue injury, activate tissue macrophages in the splanchnic organs, and thereby trigger the release of cytokines in the splanchnic region. On the other hand, sepsis from the splanchnic region may modify both the local metabolic responses and the function of extrasplanchnic tissues and organs.

The pathogenesis of splanchnic organ damage is certainly multifactorial (6,11). Local tissue injury and perfusion defects due to excessive activation of cell-mediated inflammatory reaction cascades and humoral mediators, and disturbance of oxidative metabolism in the tissues, are likely to contribute. Regardless of the primary mechanism, tissue hypoxia increases the risk of organ failure and may contribute to the progression of tissue injury caused by other factors.

The hemodynamic and metabolic alterations associated with severe sepsis due to invasive infection by gram-negative bacteria have traditionally been attributed to endotoxin (4,6,18,20). Experimental studies have demonstrated that although endotoxin alone is sufficient to produce the typical cardiovascular and metabolic pattern of septic shock, an identical pattern results from sepsis due to gram-positive bacteria with no endotoxemia. In human septic shock, endotoxemia has been observed in approximately half of the patients, the gram-negative infection is not a prerequisite for endotoxemia (10,20). It has now been well established that endotoxin is not the universal mediator of sepsis, but rather one trigger of the complex cascade of endogenous mediators that includes cytokines, especially tumor necrosis factor (TNF) and the traditional counterregulatory hormones (2,4,6).

SPLANCHNIC ORGAN FUNCTION AND NUTRITION
(see Chapters 10 and 13)

While lack of sufficient oxygen inevitably leads to tissue injury, recent studies strongly suggest that insufficient supply of other substrates may rapidly lead to altered splanchnic organ function. The importance of intraluminal nutrients in the gut for maintaining the gut mucosal integrity has been known for several years. The enhanced metabolic and cytokine response to endotoxin in parenterally fed normal subjects, compared with enterally fed subjects, suggested that either the lack of intraluminal nutrients or the lack or insufficient supply of some nutrients in the parenteral nutrition contributed to the altered response (21). Soeters and Deutz have now demonstrated that the lack of glutamine from the parenteral nutrition regimens contributes to increased mucosal permeability in the gut in surgical patients (see Chapter 13). Glutamine supplementation effectively prevented the increase in permeability. Although the importance of the increased mucosal permeability in the development of splanchnic organ dysfunction and in the activation of inflammatory reaction cascades has not been confirmed, modification of the permeability changes by nutrient supply certainly opens up new possibilities to explore the basic pathophysiology of the response of the splanchnic region to injury and sepsis.

The clinical relevance of the increased intestinal permeability is unclear. Intestinal permeability is increased in a variety of conditions, e.g., in response to endotoxin injection, in burn patients, and after major vascular surgery, major trauma, and hemorrhagic shock (22–25).However, the increase in intestinal permeability correlates poorly with infectious postraumatic complications. If the changes in permeability can be manipulated by administration of glutamine, as suggested by Soeters and Deutz, the clinical relevance of the permeability changes can hopefully be better evaluated in the near future.

Several studies support the concept that enteral nutrition may reduce the risk of postoperative and posttraumatic infectious complications (26–28). Since the hypothesis of bacterial translocation as a major cause of infectious complications in surgical and intensive care patients is not supported by available data, the possible protective effect of enteral nutrition is most likely based on other mechanisms. Once again, one possible explanation is that parenteral nutrition regimens lack some substrates that are necessary for optimum host defense; glutamine has been proposed as a candidate.

GLUTAMINE AND REGULATION OF HEPATIC METABOLISM
(see Chapter 15)

Glutamine appears to have functions that go far beyond acting as a nutritional compound. Experimental studies have demonstrated that the hepatocellular hydration state, i.e., cell volume, is an important determinant of hepatocellular function (29). The following discussion of these regulatory mechanisms is based entirely on experimental studies in vitro, and their potential clinical relevance has not been assessed.

Nevertheless, rapid changes in extracellular water and osmolality, and consequently also in cell volume, are common in the intensive care patient. If cell volume is an important determinant of hepatocellular function also in vivo, the interaction between hepatic metabolism and body fluid and osmolality shifts may be clinically important.

Amino acids, especially glutamine, and hormones, such as insulin and glucagon, can induce changes in the intracellular hydration state in the liver, which are accompanied by changes in hepatic metabolism (30,31). Many of the glutamine-induced metabolic responses in the liver can be reproduced by such hypoosmotic cell swelling as corresponds to the increase in cell volume induced by glutamine. Representative examples include glycogen synthesis, inhibition of proteolysis, and stimulation of amino acid uptake. Experimental data suggest that cell swelling acts like an anabolic proliferative signal for the cell, whereas cellular dehydration is catabolic and antiproliferative (29–31). The sodium-dependent glutamine transporter in the plasma membrane can be viewed as a transmembrane signaling system, which triggers hepatocellular function changes via alterations of the hepatocellular hydration state.

If the cell volume indeed acts as a major signal for protein metabolism, changes similar to those described for glutamine should occur following changes in cell volume induced by any mechanism. Clinically relevant examples of conditions that induce acute changes in cell volume include hypo- and hypernatremia, hyperglycemia, hypo- and hypertonic dehydration, and the acute changes in body water content and its distribution that accompany severe injury, shock, and sepsis.

SPLANCHNIC METABOLISM IN SEPSIS (see Chapter 18)

Sepsis induces marked changes in energy and substrate metabolism, which reflect a complex interaction between peripheral tissues and the splanchnic organs. Based on available data in various groups of septic patients (burns, intraabdominal sepsis, sepsis from extraabdominal focus, septic shock) and the response to endotoxin administration in humans, the general features of splanchnic metabolism in sepsis can be summarized as follows (3,4,10,13–16).

Splanchnic oxygen consumption is increased and the splanchnic region is hypermetabolic. Despite normal or low whole-body oxygen extraction, the splanchnic oxygen extraction is markedly increased because the increase in splanchnic blood flow does not match the increase in splanchnic oxygen demand. Consequently, the splanchnic region is at risk of tissue hypoxia. The subtle changes in splanchnic organ function that are common in sepsis may well be related to transient episodes of tissue hypoxia. The splanchnic hypermetabolism persists even during multiple organ failure.

Splanchnic glucose output is markedly increased in sepsis, but may abruptly decrease, when multiple organ failure develops. The splanchnic uptake of amino acids is also markedly increased and provides substrates for increased gluconeogenesis. In multiple organ failure, the uptake of amino acids may decrease in parallel with the reduction of splanchnic glucose production. The distribution of the metabolic activity and blood flow within the splanchnic region is unclear. It is possible that during marginal oxygen supply, the increased hepatic gluconeogenesis is maintained at the expense of other metabolic processes within the splanchnic region, e.g., in the gut.

EXOGENOUS LIPIDS AND HEPATIC FUNCTION (see Chapter 17)

Recent studies have revealed important new aspects of the intravascular metabolism of lipid emulsions. Several interactions may be expected between the metabolism of emulsion particles, the composition of triglycerides, and hepatic function. In addition to acting as lipid carriers, it seems possible that triglyceride-rich particles or their remnants may interact with endotoxin, various mediators, and cytokines.

The extrahepatic lipolysis of the exogenous triglycerides by lipoprotein lipase is regulated by both endogenous factors and the lipid composition of the emulsion. The phospholipid composition of the surface layer of an emulsion particle and the chain length and degree of unsaturation of triglyceride fatty acids both influence the rate of hydrolysis of emulsion triglycerides. The faster hydrolysis of medium-chain triglycerides in a mixed emulsion is probably related to their greater solubility in the surface phospholipid layer of the emulsion particle, as compared with long-chain triglycerides (32). The infusion rate of the emulsion may influence the release of nonesterified fatty acids and lipoprotein lipase in the plasma and the amount of triglycerides in the emulsion remnant particles taken up by the liver. In addition to hydrolysis, the triglyceride-rich emulsion particles lose triglycerides and acquire cholesteryl esters in the exchange of core components with lipoproteins.

The last step of the intravascular metabolism of emulsion particles is the hepatic uptake of the remnants through receptor-mediated pathways. It is possible, but not confirmed, that the uptake of the remnants may compete for the same receptor sites with proteins that are linked with TNF and other cytokines.

The phospholipid-rich particles of the emulsions may interfere with the metabolism of other lipoproteins and emulsion particles and also modify the composition of cell membranes (33,34). In addition to the amount of phospholipids, their composition may influence the metabolism of the emulsion.

The clinical applications of the new information on the intravascular metabolism of fat emulsions have not yet been established. Promising results have been obtained in avoiding liver dysfunction in the specific subgroup of patients receiving long-term home parenteral nutrition (35). The etiology of altered liver function during total parenteral nutrition is multifactorial and of varying severity. In rare cases, an irreversible progress toward liver cirrhosis may occur. The use of a mixed, medium-chain triglyceride containing lipid emulsion can substantially reduce the incidence of liver function abnormalities during long-term parenteral nutrition. It is also possible that choline deficiency may contribute to liver function abnormalities during long-term parenteral nutrition (see Chapter 16).

The studies by Carpentier et al. (35) have clearly demonstrated that the complex intravascular metabolism of lipid emulsions is dramatically influenced by a delicate interaction of the various components of the emulsion, the rate of administration, the interaction between the peripheral and hepatic lipid metabolism, and probably also by different mediators. It is possible in the future that the exchange between exogenous and endogenous lipids, and the receptor-binding characteristics of lipid particles may enable the use of exogenous lipids as pharmacologic tools.

REFERENCES

1. Barton R, Cerra FB. The hypermetabolism multiple organ failure syndrome. *Chest* 1989;96:1153–1160.
2. American College of Chest Physicians/Society of Critical Care Medicine Consensus Conference. Definitions for sepsis and multiple organ failure and guidelines for the use of innovative therapies in sepsis. *Crit Care Med* 1992;20:864–874.
3. Wilmore DW, Goodwin CW, Aulick LH, et al. Effect of injury and infection on visceral metabolism and circulation. *Ann Surg* 1980;192:491–500.
4. Fong Y, Marano MA, Moldawer LL, et al. The acute splanchnic and peripheral tissue metabolic response to endotoxin in humans. *J Clin Invest* 1990;85:1896–1904.
5. Gutierrez G, Palizas F, Doglio G, et al. Gastric intramucosal pH as a therapeutic index of tissue oxygenation in critically ill patients. *Lancet* 1992;339:195–199.
6. Tracey KJ. TNF and other cytokines in the metabolism of septic shock and cachexia. *Clin Nutr* 1992;11:1–11.
7. Fiddian-Green RG, Baker S. Predictive value of the stomach wall pH for complications after cardiac operations: comparison with other monitoring. *Crit Care Med* 1987;15:153–156.
8. Fiddian-Green RG, Gantz NM. Transient episodes of sigmoid ischemia and their relation to infection from intestinal organisms after abdominal aortic operations. *Crit Care Med* 1987;15:835–839.
9. Doglio GR, Pusajo JF, Egurrola MA, et al. Gastric mucosal pH as a prognostic index of mortality in critically ill patients. *Crit Care Med* 1991;19:1037–1040.

10. Ruokonen E, Takala J, Kari A, et al. Regional blood flow and oxygen transport in septic shock. *Crit Care Med* 1993;21:1296–1303.
11. Meakins JL, Marshall JC. The gastrointestinal tract: the "motor" of multiple organ failure. *Arch Surg* 1986;121:197–201.
12. Ziegler TR, Snith RJ, O'Dwyer ST, et al. Increased intestinal permeability associated with infection in burn patients. *Arch Surg* 1988;123:1313–1319.
13. Gump FE, Price JB Jr, Kinney JM. Whole body and splanchnic blood flow and oxygen consumption measurements in patients with intraperitoneal infection. *Ann Surg* 1970;171:321–328.
14. Gump FE, Price JB, Kinney JM. Blood flow and oxygen consumption in patients with severe burns. *Surg Gynecol Obstet* 1970;130:23–28.
15. Dahn MS, Lange P, Lobdell K, et al. Splanchnic and total body oxygen consumption differences in septic and injured patients. *Surgery* 1987;101:69–80.
16. Dahn MS, Lange P, Wilson RF, et al. Hepatic blood flow and splanchnic oxygen consumption measurements in clinical sepsis. *Surgery* 1990;107:295–301.
17. Ruokonen E, Takala J, Kari A, Alhava E. Septic shock and multiple organ failure. *Crit Care Med* 1991;19:1146–1151.
18. Parrillo JE, Parker MM, Natanson C, et al. Septic shock in humans. *Ann Intern Med* 1990;113:227–242.
19. Goris PJA, te Boekhorst TPA, Nuytinck JKS, Gimbère JSF. Multiple-organ failure. Generalized autodestructive inflammation? *Arch Surg* 1985;120:1109–1115.
20. Danner RL, Elin RJ, Hosseini JM, et al. Endotoxemia in human septic shock. *Chest* 1991;99:169–175.
21. Fong Y, Marano MA, Barber A, et al. Total parenteral nutrition and bowel rest modify the metabolic response to endotoxin in humans. *Ann Surg* 1989;210:449–457.
22. O'Dwyer ST, Michie HR, Ziegler TR, et al. A single dose of endotoxin increases intestinal permeability in healthy humans. *Arch Surg* 1988;231:1459–1464.
23. Deitch EA. Intestinal permeability is increased in burn patients shortly after injury. *Surgery* 1990;107:411–416.
24. Harris CE, Griffiths RD, Freestone N, et al. Intestinal permeability in the critically ill. *Intensive Care Med* 1992;18:38–41.
25. Roumen RMH, Hendricks T, Wevers RA, Goris RJA. Intestinal permeability after severe trauma and hemorrhagic shock is increased, without relation to septic complications. *Arch Surg* 1993;128:453–457.
26. Moore FA, Moore EE, Jones TN, et al. TEN versus TPN following major abdominal trauma—Reduced septic morbidity. *J Trauma* 1989;29:916–922.
27. Kudsk KA, Croce MA, Fabian TC, et al. Enteral versus parenteral feeding. Effects on septic morbidity after blunt and penetrating abdominal trauma. *Ann Surg* 1992;215:503–513.
28. Moore FA, Feliciano DV, Andrassy RJ, et al. Early enteral feeding, compared with parenteral, reduces postoperative septic complications. The results of a meta-analysis. *Ann Surg* 1992;216:172–183.
29. Häussinger D, Lang F. Cell volume in the regulation of hepatic function: a mechanism for metabolic control. *Biochim Biophys Acta* 1991;1071:331–350.
30. Stoll B, Gerok W, Lang F, Häussinger D. Liver cell volume and protein synthesis. *Biochem J* 1992;287:217–222.
31. Häussinger D, Lang F. Cell volume and hormone action. *Trends Pharmacol Sci* 1992;13:371–373.
32. Richelle M. Influence of intravenous lipid emulsions on cholesterol homeostasis. *Clin Nur* 1992;11:48–52.
33. Sniderman AD, Cianflone K. Substrate delivery as a determinant of hepatic apo-B secretion. *Arterioscler Thromb* 1993;13:629–636.
34. Dahlan W, Richelle M, Kulapongse S, et al. Modification of erythrocyte membrane lipid composition induced by a single intravenous infusion of phospholipid-triacylglycerol emulsions in man. *Clin Nutr* 1992;11:255–261.
35. Carpentier YA, Richelle M, Haumont D, Deckelbaum RJ. New developments in fat emulsions. *Proc Nutr Soc* 1990;49:375–380.

Organ Metabolism and Nutrition:
Ideas for Future Critical Care, edited by
J. M. Kinney and H. N. Tucker.
Raven Press, Ltd., New York © 1994.

20

Neutrophil and Lung Endothelial Interactions

Ruth Simpson, *Raphael Alon, **C. R. Valeri, †David Shepro, and
‡Herbert B. Hechtman

*University Hospital of South Manchester, Didsbury, United Kingdom; *Department of
Surgery, Ichilov Hospital, Tel Aviv Medical Center, Tel Aviv, Israel 64239; **Naval Blood
Research Laboratory, Boston University School of Medicine, Boston, Massachusetts 02118;
†Biology Department, Boston University, Boston, Massachusetts 02215; ‡Department of
Surgical Oncology, Brigham and Women's Hospital, Boston, Massachusetts 02115.*

Lung injury is a common clinical problem, varying from minor changes in pulmonary function associated with most viral infections to major respiratory failure with increase in microvascular permeability, pulmonary edema, and an impaired ability to oxygenate blood—hallmarks of the adult respiratory distress syndrome (ARDS). Injury may be by both local and systemic inflammatory fibers. All these factors, particularly the neutrophil, have been implicated as a cause of lung injury while at the same time being considered a major component of the body's defense. The circulating neutrophil has an assortment of weapons at its disposal to fight off invasion by infecting organisms. If not regulated, however, the neutrophil may easily damage host tissues. Following infection or injury, circulating neutrophils are recruited to that site. These neutrophils interact with the endothelium, diapedese, and release their toxic substances. Inappropriate adhesion of activated neutrophils in organs such as the lungs, remote to the site of injury due to the systemic release of endothelial cell activators, may lead to multisystem organ failure.

POLYMORPHONUCLEAR NEUTROPHIL AND ENDOTHELIAL CELL INTERACTIONS

An inappropriate interaction of polymorphonuclear neutrophils (PMN) and pulmonary endothelial cells (EC) results in pulmonary injury. Polymorphonuclear neutrophil sequestration may be due to a local extravascular stimulus such as acid aspiration

Supported in part by The National Institute of Health, Grants GM24891-14, GM35141-06, HL43875-02; The Brigham Surgical Group Inc., and The Trauma Research Foundation; and the U.S. Navy (Office of Naval Research Contract No. N00014-88-C-0018, with the funds provided by the Naval Medical Research and Development Command). The opinions or assertions contained herein are those of the authors and are not to be construed as official or reflecting the views of the Navy Department or Naval Service at large.

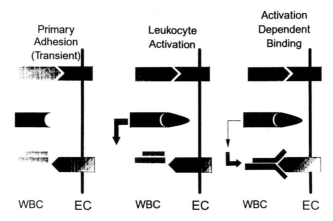

FIG. 1. Leukocyte-endothelial interaction. On the left, initial adhesion is transient and is mediated via selectins. In the center panel, a soluble factor (e.g., C5a) or cell surface factor (e.g., platelet activating) signals the leukocyte to functionally up-regulated the integrins, which leads to more secure binding. Adapted from Butcher EC. Leukocyte-endothelial cell recognition: three (or more) steps to specificity and diversity. *Cell* 1991;67:1033–1036.

or secondary to a remote insult such as ischemia-reperfusion of a systemic organ. With severe inflammation remote from the lungs, mediators gain access to the circulation, thereby activating circulating PMN as well as pulmonary and systemic organ EC. In general there are three steps in PMN-EC interactions (Fig. 1).

1. Binding of constitutively functional leukocyte adhesion receptors to EC counterreceptors.
2. Activation of the leukocyte by locally generated chemoattractants.
3. Interaction of the activation-dependent adhesion receptor on the PMN with its EC counterreceptor.

Within minutes of tissue injury, neutrophils begin to interact loosely with the walls of postcapillary venules, "rolling" along affected segments. In the lungs this likely occurs in capillaries. This reversible adhesion is mediated by the selectins, a family of three integral membrane proteins (2). Each member of the family consists of an amino terminal domain similar to mammalian C-type lectins, an epidermal growth factor–like sequence, a variable number of repeats similar to the short consensus units in complement regulatory proteins, a transmembrane domain, and a short cytoplasmic tail (3). The lectin domain and Ca^{2+} are required for adhesion (4).

The inflammatory response involves a complex chain of events culminating in the adhesion and migration of neutrophils from the circulation into inflamed tissue where they release free radicals and proteolytic enzymes. It is important that release occurs only in areas of inflammation because these agents are capable of injuring healthy tissue. Thus, in such situations as reperfusion injury, autoimmune disease, and organ transplantation, the inflammatory response can have deleterious effects.

The selectins play an important role in the initial localization of neutrophils to inflamed tissue. They comprise three members, all of which can mediate PMN-EC adhesion. The genes for the three selectins have been sequenced and cloned.

1. *L-selectin.* This was the first defined as the homing receptor for lymphocytes to enable them to escape from the circulation into lymph nodes (5). L-selectin is constitutively present on the neutrophil as well as other leukocytes and participates in the adherence of unstimulated PMN to cytokine-stimulated EC under conditions of flow (1). It is then lost from the neutrophil surface, coincident with the engagement of CD 18–dependent mechanisms, which in turn lead to firm adhesion and transendothelial migration. One counterreceptor for L-selectin has been sequenced and cloned and is called GlyCAM; another is P-selectin.

2. *E-selectin.* This adhesion molecule is not basally expressed and is only found on activated EC (6). It is up-regulated by cytokines such as interleukin-1 (IL-1) and tumor necrosis factor (TNF), a process occurring at the level of transcription. E-selectin is upregulated in 1 hour. Levels are maximal at 4 to 8 hours and have returned to baseline by 24 to 48 hours (6).

3. *P-selectin.* This is found on both activated platelets and EC. In the former, P-selectin is a component of the alpha granules and in the latter, the Weibel-Palade bodies. Within seconds of stimulation by thrombin, it is translocated to the plasma membrane and then rapidly reinternalized (7). P-selectin mediates unstimulated PMN adherence to EC without involvement of the beta-2 integrins (8). Further, the time course of P-selectin expression provides a mechanism that regulates a transient adhesive interaction. Coexpression of endothelial P-selectin and platelet activating factor (PAF) is required for maximum PMN adhesion (8).

Initial cell adhesion occurs via the interaction of circulation PMN with activated EC by selectin receptors. Sialic acid is required as L-selectin mediated binding is abolished in vitro and in vivo by treatment with broad spectrum sialidases (9). Two molecules of 50 kd and 90 kd are precipitated from EC by a specific monoclonal antibody (10). These components have been termed GlyCAMs, which represent biological ligands for L-selectin (11). This initial interaction brings the PMN within the microenvironment of EC-derived PMN-activating cytokines or chemoattractants. These soluble or cell-bound factors could then act on the EC-associated PMN to upregulate integrins (e.g., CD11/CD18) and lead to firm PMN-EC bonding. Further, it is thought that these chemoactivators then lead to the shedding of L-selectin (12). This may function as a regulatory stimulus to prevent PMN from rolling and subsequently adhering at a site remote from the inflammation. L-selectin mediates the initial adherence but not migration. When L-selectin is blocked by monoclonal antibodies, adhesion is reduced. Polymorphonuclear neutrophil diapedesis of adherent cells is not altered. However, the number of migrating cells per unit surface area of the vessel is reduced because of the reduced number of rolling PMNs.

Since L-selectin is shed soon after the PMNs are activated, it is unlikely that L-selectin is involved in adhesion of PMNs exposed to chemoactivators. Thus, in the presence of monoclonal antibodies to the integrins or in patients with leukocyte adhesion deficiency, chemotactic stimulation of PMN results in complete loss of adherence, as L-selectin is shed (13,14).

Counter receptors for the selectins are not fully characterized. There is evidence that both P-selectin and E-selectin recognize sialyl-Lewis X (sLex), a terminal carbohydrate containing sialic acid and fucose, found in leukocyte glycolipids and glycoproteins. L-selectin accounts for a maximum of about 5% of protein-associated sLex and an even smaller fraction of the total PMN cell surface sLex. It is thought that L-selectin acts as a presenter of sLex for P- and E-selectin, partly due to its unique topographical location on microvillous processes of the PMN surface (15). This area of the PMN initially interacts with the EC. The preferential localization of L-selectin on microvillous processes, is certainly consistent with the proposed role of this molecule in initiating PMN-EC interactions. Its exposure may explain the functional dominance of the oligosaccharides located here rather than in other sites on the PMN surface. The characterization of sLex does not exclude the role of other carbohydrates. Indeed, it is likely that others will be found to be of functional importance (16).

In vitro, L-selectin shedding is induced by chemoattractants and low-dose chymotrypsin, but surprisingly not by elastase, trypsin, or collagenase. Chymotrypsin leads to a rapid activation-independent loss of greater than 90% of L-selectin. This treatment prevents the homing of PMNs to inflamed tissue but has no effect on integrin mediated events.

LEUKOCYTE ACTIVATION

PMN may be activated by cytokines produced locally or systemically, such as TNF or IL-1. Infusion of such cytokines leads to rapid shedding of L-selectin from the PMN. Within 15 to 30 minutes there is a profound neutropenia with PMN trapping within the pulmonary circulation (17). CD 18, a member of an integrin family of adhesion receptors (4) is up-regulated, quantitatively and qualitatively (18). The latter is an interesting event and is illustrated by infusion of another PMN activator, PAF. This causes CD 18–dependent binding to EC before new copies of the integrin can be translocated to the cell surface membrane. Further, inhibition of quantitative upregulation of CD 18 does not prevent PMN-EC adhesion (19).

All integrins are heterodimeric cell surface proteins composed of two noncovalently linked polypeptide chains, alpha and beta. The latter subunit distinguishes three subfamilies: beta-1 (CD29), beta-2 (CD18) an beta-3 (CD61). The alpha and beta chains comprise transmembrane and cytoplasmic segments. The extracellular domain of the two chains binds to various ligands, which include complement components, extracellular matrix glycoproteins, and proteins on the surface of other cells. The cytoplasmic tail of the integrin interacts with cytoskeletal components. Integrins coordinate the binding of cells to extracellular proteins with a resultant alteration in the cell's cytoskeleton. For PMN, this leads to changes in cell shape, motility, and

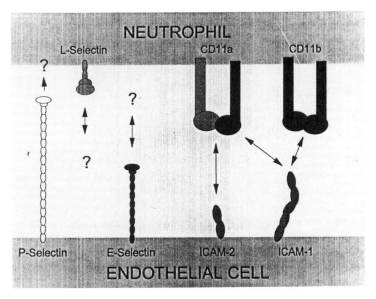

FIG. 2. Selectin and integrin receptors and counterreceptors. Adapted from Springer TA. Adhesion receptors of the immune system. *Nature* 1991;346:425–434.

phagocytic response. It is hypothesized that the PMN integrins coupled with a counterreceptor signal the cell to alter F-actin, thereby affecting motion and shape (20).

The beta-1 integrins include receptors that bind to extracellular matrix components, fibronectin, laminin, and collagen. These proteins are expressed on leukocytes and nonhemopoietic cells (4). The beta-1 integrins are involved in the interaction of lymphocytes with extracellular matrix during extravascular tissue migration. They are not expressed on PMNs, which are destined to die once they reach a site of extravascular inflammation.

The beta-2 family are also known as the leukocyte integrins because they are confined to white blood cells. There are two beta-2 members that are involved in PMN-EC interactions (Fig. 2). The first, CD11a/CD18 (LFA-1), is constitutively expressed on PMN plasma membranes and can also be up-regulated. The second, CD11b/CD18 (MAC-1), binds to the complement component C3bi, as well as to the intercellular-adhesion molecule-1 (ICAM-1) and other as yet undetermined ligands. CD11b/CD18 is present on the cell surface and in subcellular granules that are rapidly fused with the plasma membrane which permits receptor translocation upon activation (21). A third molecule CD11c/CD18 is poorly described.

In addition to cytokines, other methods of leukocyte activation are by contact with complement fragments fixed on the EC (22) or contact with the eicosanoids, leukotriene B_4 or thromboxane A_2. All activate the CD11/CD18 complex (23). In addition, the soluble anaphylatoxin C5a activates EC, which in turn will rapidly express PAF on its surface. This in turn up-regulates CD11a/CD18 and CD11b/CD18

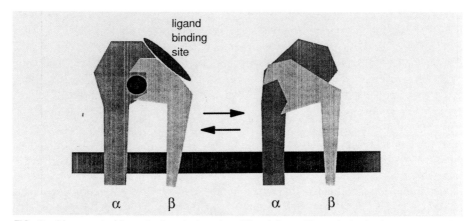

FIG. 3. Movement of the cytoplasmic domains of the alpha and beta chains leads to an extracellular realignment with expression of a receptor. Adapted from Dransfield I, Buckle AM, Hogg N. Early events of the immune response mediated by leukocyte integrins. *Immunol Rev* 1990;114;29–44.

(24). Endothelial cell–associated PAF will also prime the granulocyte for an enhanced response to other chemotactic factors, a so-called juxtacrine activity (8). Chemoactivators such as C5a cause a surprisingly rapid PMN-EC adhesion. Within 1 minute of intravenous injection, neutropenia is noted due to transient EC adhesion. The PMNs soon detach and normal levels of circulating PMNs are restored in 15 to 20 minutes (25,26). As observed with an infusion of PAF, this increased adherence does not correlate with temporal changes in the number of integrin molecules expressed on the PMN cell surface, but is inhibited by monoclonal antibodies to CD 18 (18). Increased integrin expression occurs in 15 minutes, due to translocation from subcellular granules, but lasts for over 1 hour, by which time the PMNs are detached. Further, the increase in expression is only two- to threefold, whereas the increase in binding is three- to tenfold (18). Therefore, there must be a qualitative change in the avidity of the constitutively present CD11b/CD18 adhesion molecule. This is a "functional" up-regulation (23). The mechanism is likely by way of movement of the cytoplasmic portion of the alpha and beta chains leading to positioning of the extracellular domains such that a receptor becomes expressed (Fig. 3). Inhibition of quantitative up-regulation of CD11b/CD18 does not reduce PMN adhesion to EC (26,27).

OXYGEN FREE RADICALS

The integrins modulate firm adhesion, which is a prerequisite for the establishment of a microenvironment favoring the localized action of neutrophil-derived oxygen-free radicals and proteases. In addition, integrin-mediated adhesion is needed for diapedesis. Activation of PMN triggers the enzyme NADPH oxidase on the PMN plasma membrane to generate oxygen free radicals, which include superoxide anion, hydrogen peroxide, and free hydroxyl ions (28,29). The unpaired electron in the outer shell renders these agents highly reactive (30). Myeloperoxidase, a granular enzyme, is also released and generates hypohalus acids from the free radicals (31). The most common product is hypochlorous acid, due to the abundance of chloride ions the extracellular fluid. This acid is sufficiently reactive to exert its toxic effect by directly attacking membrane-associated targets, whereas less reactive chloramines, especially those with lipophilic characteristics, diffuse across the plasma membrane to attack cytosolic components (29).

Endothelial cells, independently of PMNs, are capable of generating oxygen free radicals (32). During ischemia, cellular levels of adenosine triphosphate can be depleted to 40% of baseline values. This is associated with a tenfold increase in hypoxanthine. Normally, hypoxanthine is oxidized by the enzyme xanthine dehydrogenase to xanthine using nicotinamide adenine dinucleotide (NAD) in a reaction converting NAD to NADH. However, during ischemia, xanthine dehydrogenase is converted to xanthine oxidase. This enzymatic conversion is central to the thesis of oxygen radical–mediated reperfusion injury (Fig. 4).

During ischemia, hypoxanthine accumulates in the tissue because xanthine dehydrogenase is no longer present and because there is no oxygen available as a substrate for xanthine oxidase to catalyze the conversion of hypoxanthine to xanthine. When oxygen is reintroduced during reperfusion, xanthine oxidase converts hypoxanthine to xanthine, with the generation of large amounts of superoxide anion. This burst of superoxide production starts a cascade of reactions with the release of other oxygen radicals within the EC.

In addition to direct cell injury, oxygen free radicals may act indirectly to promote

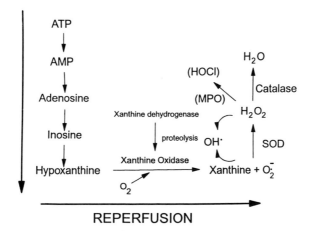

FIG. 4. Proposed mechanism for the development of oxygen free radical–dependent injury due to xanthine oxidase and neutrophils. Ischemia leads to a build-up of hypoxanthine and xanthine oxidase in the EC. The reintroduction of O_2 with reperfusion leads to the generation of superoxide ions (O_2^-), hydrogen peroxide (H_2O_2), and hydroxyl ions (OH^-). Adapted from Granger DN. Role of xanthine oxidase and granulocytes in ischemia-reperfusion injury. *Am J Physiol* 1988;255: H1269–1275.

proteolytic injury from PMN enzymes. This occurs by destruction of naturally occurring antiproteases such as alpha$_2$-macroglobulin. In addition, oxygen free radicals may act as chemoattractants, thereby promoting further neutrophil-dependent injury. Finally, oxygen radicals will activate the complement system producing additional chemoattractants as well as the C5b-C9 membrane attack complex, which can cause osmotic lysis of cells.

Oxygen free radicals can be produced by stimulation with exogenous agents. Thus, the breathing of enriched oxygen mixtures and the parenteral administration of paraquat or bleomycin will cause acute pulmonary toxicity secondary to oxygen radicals. Doxorubicin leads to a cardiomyopathy via a similar mechanism (30).

PROTEOLYTIC ENZYMES OF THE NEUTROPHIL

Apart from free radicals, PMNs contain enzymes that are capable of injuring tissue (33). These proteolytic enzymes, serine protease, elastase, and two metallo-proteinases, collagenase and gelatinase, are active for longer periods than oxygen free radicals. The enzymes are held in check from damaging normal tissue by antiproteinases: alpha-1-proteinase inhibitor, alpha-2-macroglobulin, and secretory leukoproteinase inhibitor (34). If not inhibited, the proteinase can break down extracellular matrix components. In overwhelming sepsis and reperfusion injuries, it is thought that the oxidants may not independently mediate injurious effects but may destroy the antiproteinase shield, which then allows the up-regulated proteinases to attack and degrade host tissues (35).

CYTOKINES

Cytokines are a diverse group of proteins, produced by a variety of cells, including mononuclear phagocytes and lymphocytes. Cytokines are produced during the effector phase of natural and specific immunity and function to mediate and regulate immune and inflammatory responses. Some cytokines induce the synthesis of other cytokines. Most are pleiotropic. The cytokines include cell division and mediate some of the effector functions of mononuclear phagocytes. Cytokines will also activate both PMN and EC by binding to specific receptors on the cell surface, which results in transcriptional and translational events. Two of the important cytokines known to cause pulmonary injury are TNF and IL-1.

Tumor necrosis factor is thought to mediate lung injury and multisystem organ dysfunction following endotoxemia (36), acid aspiration (37), and intestinal (38) and hindlimb ischemia-reperfusion (39). Intravenous injection of TNF results in PMN sequestration in the lungs, pulmonary permeability, and edema (40). In moderate dose, TNF will cause death. Blocking TNF, using antisera or a binding protein (TNF$_{bp}$), reduces the lung leukosequestration, permeability, and edema that follow intestinal ischemia (40a). The TNF-mediated injury is dependent on EC-PMN adhesion via the CD18 integrin. Tumor necrosis factor is a potent activator of PMN, inducing generation of leukotriene B_4, superoxide ion, hydrogen peroxide, and release of granular enzymes, especially elastase (41). Tumor necrosis factor is also known to up-regulate CD18 and ICAM-1 (40). The latter is the EC counterreceptor for CD18. However, the CD18-mediated binding of PMN to EC is not wholly due to ICAM-1 because blocking this adhesion molecule only partially prevents PMN-EC adhesion. Further, CD18–independent mechanisms are involved with certain inducers of lung injury, such as *Streptococcus pneumoniae* or hydrochloric acid aspiration.

Interleukin-1 exists as one of two polypeptides, IL-1 alpha and IL-1 beta (42). Both produce a wide range of inflammatory changes. Many nucleated cells synthesize IL-1, including phagocytes, EC, and smooth muscle cells (43). Low levels of IL-1 result in fever, drowsiness, anorexia, malaise, and arthralgias. Higher levels cause hypotension, leukopenia, pulmonary congestion, tissue neutrophil infiltration, and necrosis.

In contrast to TNF, high levels of IL-1 are not lethal. Blockade of the IL-1 receptor with IL-1 receptor antagonist attenuates hypotension, leukopenia, and pulmonary neutrophil infiltration in rabbit endotoxemia (45). Tumor necrosis factor potentiates the effect of IL-1. Even though TNF and IL-1 have specific and distinct receptors, it is likely that TNF and IL-1 stimulate similar intracellular messages and lead to similar alterations in cell metabolism (43). Cyclooxygenase inhibitors block many but not all the effects of TNF (44). Thus, they will inhibit the febrile response but not the pulmonary leukosequestration, permeability, or edema.

ENDOTHELIAL CELL ACTIVATION

Endothelial cell activation means a quantitative change in the level of expression of specific gene products that endow ECs with new capacities and functions (46). Thus, cytokines secreted by mononuclear blood cells may activate EC. Several are involved in PMN-lung EC interactions. They can cause selective induction of E-selectin on postcapillary venules, a receptor that is not present in unstimulated EC. Expression of E-selectin allows PMN to loosely adhere and "roll" along endothelium. A second receptor, ICAM-1, is constitutively expressed on EC, but is markedly up-regulated by cytokines. As a counter-ligand for leukocyte CD18 integrins, this coupling results in firm PMN adhesion and subsequent migration. ICAM-1 is a member of the immunoglobulin superfamily of adhesion receptors. These receptors comprise five extracellular immunoglobulin domains formed in two sheets of antiparallel beta-strands stabilized by a disulphide bond, a transmembrane domain, and a short cytoplasmic tail. Up-regulation is largely controlled at the mRNA level and therefore is seen after 4 hours and is usually maximal by 24 hours. However, up-regulation of ICAM-1 does not itself increase PMN adhesion. Functional up-regulation of the beta-2 integrins is also required (48). Polymorphonuclear neutrophil transendothelial migration requires the presence of two distinct EC adhesion molecules, E-selectin and ICAM-1, as monoclonal antibodies to block over 90% of PMN transmigration

(47). There must, therefore, be a complex interplay of PMN and EC-dependent adhesion mechanisms for transmigration to occur across activated EC.

Modulation of adhesion receptors as a result of activation of EC by cytokines leads to an alteration of EC morphology. There is a reorganization of the cytoskeleton, cell membrane, and matrix (46). The normally confluent monolayer of EC loses its epithelioid organization and develops a fibroblastoid character with overlapping, elongated, spindle-shaped cells (49). There is a loss of fibronectin from the basement membrane and the actin fibers are rearranged from dense peripheral bands to longitudinal arrays of stress fibers. With increased activation, the ECs become plump and retract, leaving dentritic processes and intracellular gaps, resulting in increased microvascular permeability.

COMPLEMENT

The complement system consists of serum and membrane protein that interact in a highly regulated fashion to produce biologically active protein products. Complement activation is organized into two convergent proteolytic pathways: the classical and the alternative (50). The classical pathway is activated principally by antibody-antigen complexes and is the major effector mechanism for antibody-mediated immune responses. The alternate pathway is activated in the absence of antibody and promotes the destruction of infecting organisms. It has a primitive capacity to discriminate between autologous cells and foreign microbes.

Factors C3a and C5a are anaphylotoxins and bind to specific receptors on leukocytes and smooth muscle cells. C5a binding results in PMN activation, adhesion, chemotaxis, diapedesis, release of PMN granular enzymes, the production of eicosanoids, and reactive oxygen metabolites. Activation of the complement system leads to PMN adhesion to EC, in part mediated by CD11/CD18 (21), whereas others have noted the importance of P-selectins (51). Within 1 minute of complement activation, PMN adhere, a phenomenon that is maximum at 20 minutes and lasts for 8 hours. This event can be modified by monoclonal antibodies to CD11b/CD18 as well as P-selectin. This is in contrast to cytokine activation of EC, which is slow and requires protein synthesis (52). Generalized complement activation from septicemia or reperfusion can therefore result in neutrophil sequestration and pulmonary injury. Following hindlimb ischemia, there is a local deposition of complement fragments as early as 10 minutes after reperfusion. Subsequently large numbers of complement fragments can be identified in the muscle interstitium (unpublished observations). It is postulated that free radicals, generated during reperfusion, activate the alternative pathway leading to this complement deposition.

LOCAL LUNG INJURY

Local lung injury can result from conditions such as acid aspiration or pneumonia. In the former there is a delayed local injury associated with the adhesion of PMN

(52). Thromboxane A_2 (TxA_2) and TNF are synthesized causing PMN infiltration into the alveolae and pulmonary microvascular permeability. Inhibition of TxA_2 with a synthetase inhibitor (54) and TNF with antisera (37) reduces but does not eliminate the leukosequestration and permeability. However, unlike remote lung injury secondary to acid aspiration, CD 18 is not involved. A monoclonal antibody to CD 18 failed to prevent the local leukosequestration or local injury. Further, CD 18 is not involved in the PMN infiltration and pulmonary edema caused by instillation of *S. pneumoniae* into rabbit lung (55). In contrast, when *Escherichia coli* endotoxin is instilled into rabbit lungs under the same conditions, pretreatment with an anti–CD 18 antibody prevents PMN infiltration and the injury (55). CD 18–independent lung leukosequestration is also found in the infected lungs of people suffering from leukocyte adhesion deficiency that results from a congenital defect in CD 18. Therefore, several adhesion mechanisms appear to be significant.

Atelectasis is a common postoperative complication arising from retention of bronchial secretions or hypoventilation. Reexpansion of an atelectatic area can cause pulmonary permeability and edema. Although the exact mechanism of atelectasis-induced microvascular barrier dysfunction has not yet been determined, it is believed that tissue ischemia is created due to hypoxic pulmonary vasoconstriction or mechanical deformation of the pulmonary capillary bed. Reexpansion with reperfusion then leads to the generation of eicosanoid chemoattractants, PMN activation with sequestration in the pulmonary capillary bed. In a rabbit model of lobar atelectasis, monoclonal antibody inhibition of CD 18 or ICAM-1 prevents to an equal degree the reexpansion induced systemic leukopenia, PMN lung sequestration, microvascular protein leak, and lung weight gain (56). Rendering these rabbit neutropenic with nitrogen mustard is also effective in reducing all parameters of injury. In this model of atelectasis there is also PMN sequestration in the nonatelectic lung. This can be reduced by treatment with monoclonal antibodies to CD 18 or ICAM-1.

REMOTE PULMONARY INJURY

Pulmonary injury remote from a stimulus occurs in a variety of clinical settings, including hindlimb and intestinal ischemia-reperfusion, acute pancreatitis, and endotoxemia. The injury most commonly presents as ARDS, in which there is tachypnea, hypoxia, pulmonary hypertension, a rise in physiological shunting, and noncardiogenic pulmonary edema. These changes are largely due to increased pulmonary vascular permeability causing a flux of protein-rich fluid across the endothelial barrier.

In the setting of abdominal aortic aneurysm repair, the lower torso is rendered ischemic during the period of aortic cross-clamping (57). On release of the clamp there is a transient leukopenia and after several hours, pulmonary edema by chest X-ray. In animal experiments it can be shown that following hindlimb ischemia there is an increase in both lung lymph flow and the lymph/plasma protein ratio confirming increased permeability. Polymorphonuclear neutrophils play a role in this injury because there is a marked accumulation of these cells in the pulmonary capillary bed

(58). Injury can be prevented by inducing neutropenia. Further, these PMNs are known to be activated because PMN-derived proteolytic enzymes have been recovered from alveolar lavage fluid. Circulating PMNs also produce increased H_2O_2.

Polymorphonuclear neutrophils are usually, but not always, involved in lung injury. In the setting of endotoxemia there are documented cases of ARDS occurring in leukopenic patients. Presumably, in these settings, a vasotoxin, such as the complement attack complex, acts directly on the EC to damage the microvascular barrier.

The use of monoclonal antibodies against EC and PMN adhesion molecules can help define the role of PMN in remote pulmonary injury. Within 10 minutes following hindlimb ischemia, there is a rise in plasma leukotriene B_4 (59) and TxA_2 (60), likely originating from activated PMN. This is coincident with a transient circulating neutropenia. Subsequently, over the course of hours, neutrophils become sequestered within the pulmonary vasculature. There is pulmonary edema and protein loss into the alveolar spaces. Although TNF is not detected during reperfusion, TNF antisera reduces the PMN sequestration and the pulmonary microvascular leak (38). The use of a monoclonal antibody to CD 18 completely prevents the systemic neutropenia, PMN lung sequestration, and lung injury, showing that these remote events are CD18–dependent. Involvement of PMN and their products can also be shown in experiments where inhibition of elastase by methylsuccinyl-L-Ala-L-ALA-L-Pro-L-Val-chloromethylketone (MAAPV) or oxygen free radicals by superoxide dismutase and catalase reduce pulmonary permeability after bilateral hindlimb ischemia and reperfusion (61).

When plasma taken from rabbits after 3 hours of hindlimb ischemia and 10 minutes of reperfusion (the time of peak plasma LTB_4 levels) is incubated with PMN from a normal rabbit, surprisingly there is no change in CD 18 expression. The same plasma induces diapedesis when introduced into a dermabrasion chamber on normal rabbits. This event is prevented by a monoclonal antibody to CD 18. Therefore, hindlimb ischemia-reperfusion results in CD 18–dependent lung injury and CD 18–dependent lung PMN sequestration, which does not require increased expression of CD 18 on the surface of the PMN, but likely a conformational change in the CD 18 molecule (Fig. 2).

Complement is involved in both the local and the remote organ injury following bilateral hindlimb ischemia and reperfusion. Thus, soluble complement receptor type 1 (sCR1), a genetically engineered segment of the receptor present on erythrocytes and PMN, which inhibits the alternate and the classical pathways, reduces hindlimb skeletal muscle permeability, neutrophil sequestration, and weight gain. Further, lung injury is attenuated, as determined by pulmonary permeability (62).

Intestinal ischemia-reperfusion also results in both local and remote organ injury. The intestinal mucosa loses its barrier function, leading to the translocation of endotoxin from the intestinal lumen to the lymphatic circulation (63), which can be detected after 30 minutes of ischemia. Tumor necrosis factor levels in plasma rise after 15 minutes of reperfusion. The levels peak at 30 minutes and remain elevated throughout 3 hours of reperfusion. Polymorphonuclear neutrophil sequestration within the pulmonary microvessels and pulmonary permeability develop after 60 minutes of reperfusion. After 3 hours of reperfusion there is also a significant liver PMN sequestration and injury, as determined by the rise of serum glutamine-pyruvate transaminase (SGPT).

Treatment of rats subjected to 1 hour of superior mesenteric artery occlusion with TNF antisera reduces the rise in SGPT and the pulmonary permeability (38). These observations suggest that endotoxin stimulates the Kupffer cells in the liver to synthesize TNF, which in turn mediates the leukosequestration and the changes in the liver function and pulmonary permeability. These postulates, however, are tentative. Indeed, because endotoxin levels are highest in intestinal lymphatics which empty into the chest, it is possible that TNF is synthesized by many sites in addition to the liver. Although IL-1 is not detectable in the serum of rats undergoing intestinal ischemia-reperfusion, the IL-1 receptor antagonist, given prior to reperfusion, reduces the leukosequestration as well as the increase in SGPT and lung microvascular permeability (40a). Therefore, cytokines are strongly implicated in the lung injury following intestinal ischemia-reperfusion. They likely stimulate the EC to up-regulate the expression of ICAM, because lung leukosequestration can be prevented with a monoclonal antibody to CD 18 (40). That the cytokine-mediated increase in lung permeability is neutrophil dependent can be shown by prior depletion of circulating PMN.

Finally, the lung injury after gut ischemia is also mediated by integrins. Interestingly, an anti–CD 11b antibody reduces to baseline the pulmonary permeability, but not the leukosequestration (64). Therefore, although adhesion is a prerequisite for injury, the injury can be abolished without preventing adhesion. Antibodies to CD 11b have been shown to prevent the PMN respiratory burst without influencing adhesion. Similarly, inhibition of oxygen free radicals by scavengers or the inhibition of PMN elastase prevents lung injury but not adhesion following hindlimb ischemia-reperfusion (60).

In the rat model of intestinal ischemia, inhibition of the complement cascade has also been shown to prevent lung injury. Similar to the monoclonal antibody against CD 11b, sCR1 effectively reduces pulmonary permeability without reducing leukosequestration. Further, this is the only agent that has been found to reduce the local gut injury and improve survival in our model of complete intestinal ischemia and reperfusion (65). It seems, therefore, that complement is a major mediator of local and lung injury, but not pulmonary leukosequestration. It appears that the PMN adhesion in the lung is dependent on cytokines and integrins, but that a complement component, likely C3bi, is a key factor in signaling adherent PMN to produce products leading to tissue injury.

Complement inhibition by sCR1 reduces pulmonary injury induced by intravascular activation of complement by cobra venom factor and by immune complex alveolitis (66). In these two models, antibodies to CD 18 are equally effective. Blocking CD 11b reduces the injury to cobra venom factor but not immune complexes if the anti-CD 11b monoclonal antibody is given intravenously. However, if the antibody is instilled directly into the lungs, the injury is abrogated. This suggests that both CD 11b and CD 18 are required for full expression of the injury.

SHEAR STRESS

The importance of shear stress has only recently come to light (67–69). Blood flow–induced shear forces in the circulation act to limit PMN adhesion to EC. Shear will also promote detachment of PMN once they have loosely adhered. In vitro tests of PMN-EC adhesion is often carried out under static conditions. However, recent studies with flow show the importance of shear in that CD 18 and ICAM-dependent adhesion is not observed if the shear rate is above 2.0 dynes/cm^2 (66). Diapedesis is also shown to be dependent upon the interaction of these two adhesion molecules in non-static conditions. Thus, antibodies to CD 18 and ICAM-1 significantly inhibit transmigration under all flow conditions (66).

The selectin family is found to mediate adhesion in both shear and non-shear states. At shear rates of 1.85 dynes/cm^2 L-selectin is responsible for adhesion to stimulated EC. Activation of the PMN then results in firm adhesion via CD 18 with subsequent migration and/or release of free radicals and proteolytic enzymes. In the lungs the shear forces are low, facilitating the adhesion process. Indeed, in the pulmonary bed, stimulated PMNs that have shed their L-selectin can adhere via integrin mechanisms. This is perhaps the reason that the lungs are so vulnerable to PMN-mediated injury. We hypothesize that only when systemic hypotension develops will shear forces in systemic organs be sufficiently low to allow leukosequestration of activated PMN and thereby multisystemic organ dysfunction.

MECHANICAL ENTRAPMENT OF POLYMORPHONUCLEAR NEUTROPHILS

Lung injury may be exacerbated by the entrapment of PMNs in capillary beds. PMNs are large, stiff viscoelastic cells that have to deform to pass through most capillaries. PMNs take a thousand times as long as erythrocytes to pass through the precapillary sphincter (58). Therefore, in areas of low shear stress such as the lungs, and particularly in the presence of inflammatory mediators, the PMN cytoskeleton may be altered to make them stiff and thereby lodge within the capillaries. Even in the systemic microvasculature, once the perfusion pressure returns to normal, PMNs may not be washed from the capillary due to firm adhesion. This is the theory underlying the "no reflow" phenomenon, which aggravates an initial injury by perpetuating ischemia. While lodged in the capillary, the PMN may release its oxidants and proteases, further exacerbating the trauma (68).

CONCLUSION

Lung injury is a common clinical event arising from local and systemic causes. Both the PMN and the EC play important roles. Their activation and interaction leads to the generation of toxic oxidants and enzymes that directly injure the pulmonary tissue. If treatment is aimed at the underlying pathologic process sufficiently early in the course of the disease, inflammatory events can be modified. However, even after the initial cascade of PMN and adhesion has occurred, inhibition of these chemoactivators and the adhesion molecules themselves may be of benefit in limiting injury from subsequent waves of ischemia or endotoxemia.

REFERENCES

1. Butcher EC. Leukocyte-endothelial cell recognition: three (or more) steps to specificity and diversity. *Cell* 1991;67:1033–1036.
2. Ley K, Gaehtgens P, Fennie C, et al. Lectin-like cell adhesion molecule 1 mediates leukocyte rolling in mesenteric venules in vivo. *Blood* 1991;124:117–123.
3. Stoolman LM. Adhesion molecules controlling lymphocyte migration. *Cell* 1989;56:907–910.
4. Springer TA. Adhesion receptors of the immune system. *Nature* 1990;346:425–434.
5. Lasky LA, Signer MS, Yednock TA, et al. Cloning of a lymphocyte homing receptor reveals a lectin domain. *Cell* 1989;56:1045–1055.
6. Luscinskas FW, Brock AF, Arnaout MA, Gimbrone MA. Endothelial-leukocyte adhesion molecule-1–dependent and leukocyte (CD11/CD18)–dependent mechanisms contribute to polymorphonuclear leukocyte adhesion to cytokine-activated human vascular endothelium. *J Immunol* 1989;142: 2257–2263.
7. Hattori R, Hamilton KK, Fugate RD, et al. Stimulated secretion of endothelial von Willibrand factor is accompanied by rapid redistribution of the cell surface of the intracellular granule membrane protein GMP-140. *J Biol Chem* 1989;264:7768–7771.
8. Lorant DE, Patel KD, McIntyre TM, et al. Coexpression of GMP-140 and PAF by endothelium stimulated by histamine or thrombin: a juxtacrine system for adhesion or activation of neutrophils. *J Cell Biol* 1991;115:223–234.
9. Rosen SD, Chi S-I, True DD, et al. Intravenously injected sialidase inactivates attachment sites for lymphocytes on human endothelial venules. *J Immunol* 1989;142:1895–1902.
10. Streeter PR, Rouse BTN, Butcher EC. Immunohistologic and functional characterization of a vascular adressin involved in lymphocyte homing to peripheral lymph nodes. *J Cell Biol* 1988;107:1853–1862.
11. Lasky LA, Rosen SD. The selectins: carbohydrate-binding adhesion molecules of the immune system. In: Gallin JI, Goldstein IM, Snyderman R, eds. *Inflammation: Basic Principles and Clinical Correlates.* New York: Raven Press, 1992;407–412.
12. Kishimoto TK, Jutila MA, Berg EL, Butcher EC. Neutrophil Mac-1 and MEL-14 adhesion proteins inversely regulated by chemotactic factors. *Science* 1989;245:1238–1241.
13. Anderson DC, Springer TA. Leukocyte adhesion deficiency: an inherited defect in the Mac-1, LFA-1 and p150,95 glycoproteins. *Annu Rev Med* 1987;38:175–194.
14. Hallman R, Jutila MA, Smith CW, et al. The peripheral lymph node homing receptor, LECAM-1, is involvd in CD 18–independent adhesion of human neutrophils to endothelium. *Biochem Biophys Res Commun* 1991;174:236–243.
15. Picker LJ, Warnock A, Burns AR, et al. The neutrophil selectin LECAM-1 presents carbohydrate ligands to the vascular selectins ELAM-1 and GMP140. *Cell* 1991;66:921–933.
16. Kishimoto TK, Warnock RA, Jutila MA, et al. Antibodies against human LECAM-1 (LAN-1/Leu-8/DREG 56 antigen) and endothelial cell ELAM-1 inhibit a common CD 18–independent adhesion pathway in vitro. *Blood* 1991;78:805–811.
17. Stephens K, Ishizara A, Wu Z, et al. Granulocyte depletion prevents TNF-mediated acute lung injury in guinea pigs. *Am Rev Respir Dis* 1988;138:1300–1307.
18. Nathan C, Srimal S, Farber G, et al. Cytokine-induced respiratory burst of human neutrophils: dependence on extracellular matrix proteins and CD 11/CD 18 integrins. *J Cell Biol* 1989;109: 1341–1349.
19. Lo SK, Detmers PA, Levin SM, Wright SD. Transient adhesion of neutrophils to endothelium. *J Exp Med* 1989;169:1779–1793.
20. Tamkyn JW, DeSimone DW, Fonda D, et al. Structure of integrin, a glycoprotein involved in the transmembrane linkage between fibronectin and actin. *Cell* 1986;46:271–282.
21. Carlos TM, Harlan JM. Membrane proteins involved in phagocytic adherence to endothelium. *Immunol Rev* 1990;114:5–28.

22. Marks RM, Todd RF III, Ward PA. Rapid induction of neutrophil-endothelial adhesion by endothelial complement fixation. *Nature* 1989;339:314–317.
23. Wiles ME, Welbourn R, Goldman G, et al. Thromboxane-induced neutrophil adhesion to pulmonary microvascular and aortic endothelium is regulated by CD18. *Inflammation* 1991;15:181–199.
24. Zimmermann GA, Prescott SM, McIntyre TM. Endothelial cell interactions with granulocytes: tethering and signaling molecules. *Immunol Today* 1992;13:93–100.
25. Lundberg C, Marceau F, Hugli TE. C5a-induced hemodynamic and hematologic changes in the rabbit. Role of cyclooxygenase products and polymorphonuclear leukocytes. *Am J Physiol* 1987;128:471.
26. O'Flaherty JT, Showell HJ, Ward PA. Neutropenia induced by systemic infusion of chemotactic factors. *J Immunol* 1977;118:1586–1589.
27. Vedder NB, Harlan JM. Increased surface expression of CD 11b/CD 18 (Mac-1) is not required for stimulated neutrophil adherence to cultured endothelium. *J Clin Invest* 1988;81:676–682.
28. Granger DN. Role of xanthin oxidase and granulocytes in ischemia-reperfusion injury. *Am J Physiol* 1988;255:H1269–1275.
29. Weiss SJ. Tissue destruction by neutrophils. *N Engl J Med* 1989;320:365–376.
30. Reilly PM, Schiller HJ, Bulkley GB. Pharmacologic approach to tissue injury mediated by free radicals and other reactive oxygen metabolites. *Am J Surg* 1991;161:488–501.
31. Klebanoff SJ. Phagocytic cells: products of oxygen metabolism. In: Gallin JI, Goldstein IM, Snyderman R, eds. *Inflammation: Basic Principles and Clinical Correlates*. New York: Raven Press, 1988;391–441.
32. Welbourn R, Goldman G, Paterson IS, et al. Ischemia-reperfusion injury: pathophysiology and treatment. *Br J Sug* 1991;78:651–655.
33. Henson PM, Henson JE, Fittschen C, et al. Phagocytic cells: degranulation and secretion. In: Gallin JI, Goldstein IM, Snyderman R, eds. *Inflammation: Basic Principles and Clinical Correlates*. New York: Raven Press, 1988;391–441.
34. Travis J, Salveson GS. Human plasma protease inhibitors. *Annu Rev Biochem* 1983;52:655–709.
35. Albrich JM, Gilbaugh JH III, Calahan KB, Hurst JK. Effects of the putative neutrophil-generated toxin, hypochorous acid on membrane permeability and transport systems of *Escherichia coli*. *J. Clin Invest* 1986;78:177–184.
36. Michie HR, Manogue KR, Spriggs DR, et al. Detection of circulating TNF after endotoxin administration. *N Engl J Med* 1988;318:1481–1486.
37. Goldman G, Welbourn R, Kobzik L, et al. Tumor necrosis factor-α mediates acid aspiration-induced systemic organ injury. *Ann Surg* 1990;212:513–520.
38. Caty MG, Guice KS, Oldham KT, et al. Evidence for tumor necrosis factor–induced pulmonary injury after intestinal ischemia–reperfusion injury. *Ann Sug* 1990;212:694–700.
39. Welbourn R, Goldman G, O'Riordain M, et al. Role of tumor necrosis factor as mediator of lung injury following lower torso ischemia. *J Appl Physiol* 1991;70:2645–2649.
40. Lo SK, Everitt J, Gu J, Malik AB. Tumor necrosis factor mediates experimental pulmonary edema by ICAM-1 and CD 18-dependent mechanisms. *J Clin Invest* 1992;89:981–988.
40a.Simpson R, Alon R, Kobzik L, et al. Neutrophil and nonneutrophil-mediated injury in intestinal ischemia-reperfusion. *Ann Surg* 1993;218:444–454.
41. Movat HZ, Cybulsky M, Colditz IG, et al. Acute inflammation in gram-negative infection: endotoxin, interleukin 1, tumor necrosis factor and neutrophils. *Fed Proc* 1987;46:97–104.
42. Dinarello CA. Interleukin-1 and interleukin-1 antagonism. *Blood* 1991;77:1627–1652.
43. Dinarello CA. Cytokines: interleukin-1 and tumor necrosis factor (cachetin). In: Gallin JI, Goldstein IM, Snyderman R, eds. *Inflammation: Basic Principles and Clinical Correlates*. New York: Raven Press, 1987;195–208.
44. Kettelhut IC, Fiers W, Goldberg AL. The toxic effects of tumor necrosis factor in vivo and their prevention by cyclooxygenase inhibitors. *Proc Natl Acad Sci USA* 1987;84:4273–4277.
45. Wakabayashi G, Gelfand JA, Burke JF, et al. A specific receptor antagonist for interleukin 1 prevents *Escherichia coli*–induced shock in rabbits. *FASEB* 1991;340:338–343.
46. Pober JS. Cytokine-mediated activation of vascular endothelium. *Am J Physiol* 1988;133:426–433.
47. Luscinskas FW, Cybulsky MI, Kiley J-M, et al. Cytokine-activated human endothelial monolayers support enhanced neutrophil transmigration via a mechanism involving both endothelial-leukocyte adhesion molecule-1 and intercellular adhesion molecule-1. *J Immunol* 1991;146:1617–1625.
48. Hibbs ML, Jakes S, Stacker SA, et al. The cytoplasmic domain of the integrin lymphocyte function-associated antigen 1 beta subunit: sites required for binding to intercellular adhesion molecule 1 and the phorbol ester-stimulated phosphorylation site. *J Exp Med* 1991;174:1227–1238.

49. Stolpen AH, Golan DE, Pober JS. TNF and immune IFN act singly and in combination to reorganize human vascular endothelial cell monolayers. *Am J Pathol* 1986;123:16–24.
50. Frank MM. Complement in the pathophysiology of human disease. *N Engl J Med* 1987;316:1525–1530.
51. Mulligan MS, Polley MJ, Bayer RJ, et al. Neutrophil-dependent acute lung injury. *J Clin Invest* 1992; 90:1600–1607.
52. Gamble JR, Harlan JM, Klebanoff SJ, Vades MA. Stimulation of the adherence of neutrophils to umbilical Ven endothelium by human recombinant tumor necrosis factor. *Proc Natl Acad Sci USA* 1985;82:8667–8671.
53. Goldman G, Welbourn R, Klausner JM, et al. Leukocytes mediate acid aspiration induced multi-organ injury. *Surgery* 1993;114:13–20.
54. Goldman G, Welbourn R, Klausner JM, et al. Local acid aspiration leads to thromboxane-dependent generalized pulmonary edema. *Surg Forum* 1989;40:258–261.
55. Doerschuk CM, Winn RK, Coxson HO, Harlan JM. CD 18–dependent and –independent mechanisms of neutrophil emigration in the pulmonary and systemic microcirculation of rabbits. *J Immunol* 1990; 144:2327–2333.
56. Goldman G, Welbourn R, Rothlien R, et al. Adherent neutrophils mediate permeability after atelectasis. *Ann Surg* 1992;216:372–380.
57. Paterson IS, Klausner JM, Pugatch R, et al. Non-cardiogenic pulmonary edema after abdominal aortic aneurysm surgery. *Ann Surg* 1989;209:231–236.
58. Klausner JM, Paterson IS, Mannick JA, et al. Reperfusion pulmonary edema. *JAMA* 1989;261: 1030–1035.
59. Welbourn R, Goldman G, Kobzik L, et al. Neutrophil adherence receptors (CD 18) in ischemia: dissociation between quantitative cell surface expression and diapedesis mediated by leukotriene B_4. *J Immunol* 1990;145:1906–1911.
60. Anner H, Kaufman RP, Valeri CR, et al. Reperfusion of ischemic lower limbs increases pulmonary microvascular permeability. *J Trauma* 1988;28:607–610.
61. Welbourn CRB, Goldman G, Paterson IS, et al. Neutrophil elastase and oxygen radicals: synergism in lung injury after hindlimb ischemia. *Am J Physiol* 1991;269:H1852–H1856.
62. Lindsay TF, Hill J, Ortiz F, et al. Blockade of complement activation prevents local and pulmonary leak following lower torso ischemia-reperfusion. *Ann Surg* 1992;216:677–683.
63. Simpson R, Hill J, Lindsay TF, et al. Importance of bacterial and endotoxin translocation via mesenteric lymph following ischemia. *Surg Forum* 1992;112:163–165.
64. Hill J, Lindsay T, Rusche J, e al. A Mac-1 antibody reduces liver and lung injury but not neutrophil sequestration following intestinal ischemia-reperfusion. *Surgery* 1992;112:166–172.
65. Hill J, Lindsay TF, Ortiz F, et al. Soluble complement receptor type 1 ameliorates the local and remote organ injury following intestinal ischemia-reperfusion in the rat. *J Immunol* 1992;149:1723–1728.
66. Mulligan MS, Yeh CG, Rudolph AR, Ward PA. Protective effects of soluble CR1 in complement- and neutrophil-mediated tissue injury. *J Immunol* 1992;148:1479–1485.
67. Lawrence MB, Smith CW, Eskin SG, McIntyre LV. Effect of venous shear stress on CD 18–mediated neutrophil adhesion to cultured endothelium. *Blood* 1990;75:227–237.
68. Schmid-Schonbein GW. Capillary plugging by granulocytes and the no-reflow phenomenon in the microcirculation. *Fed Proc* 1987;46:2397–2401.
69. Lawrence MB, Eskin SG, McIntyre LV. Effect of flow on polymorphonuclear leukocyte/endothelial cell adhesion. *Blood* 1987;70:1284–1292.

*Organ Metabolism and Nutrition:
Ideas for Future Critical Care,* edited by
J. M. Kinney and H. N. Tucker.
Raven Press, Ltd., New York © 1994.

21

Free Radicals, Tissue Injury, and Human Disease: A Potential for Therapeutic Use of Antioxidants?

Barry Halliwell, Patricia J. Evans, Harparkash Kaur, and
Okezie I. Aruoma

*Pharmacology Group, University of London, Kings College, London SW3 6LX,
United Kingdom*

It is difficult these days to open a medical journal without seeing some paper on the role of "reactive oxygen species" or "free radicals" in human disease. These species have been implicated in more than 100 conditions, from arthritis and hemorrhagic shock to AIDS (1,2). This wide range implies that free radicals are not something esoteric, but are involved as a general mechanism of tissue injury in most, if not all, human diseases. Sometimes they make a significant contribution to the disease pathology; at other times they may not (3). Telling the difference requires accurate assays of free radical activity that are applicable to humans: the lack of such assays has greatly impeded progress in our understanding of the role played by free radicals in disease pathology, but the recent development of assays applicable to humans should lead to rapid progress (3).

WHAT IS A FREE RADICAL?

Electrons in atoms occupy regions of space known as *orbitals*. Each orbital can hold a maximum of two electrons. A free radical is simply defined as *any species capable of independent existence that contains one or more unpaired electrons,* an unpaired electron being one that is alone in an orbital. Most biological molecules are nonradicals, containing only paired electrons. A superscript dot is used to denote free radical species.

Radicals can react with other molecules in a number of ways (reviewed in refs. 3,4). Thus, if two radicals meet, they can combine their unpaired electrons and join to form a covalent bond (a shared pair of electrons).

$$A^{\cdot} + A^{\cdot} \rightarrow A—A \qquad [1]$$

An example is the reaction of superoxide radical ($O_2^{\cdot-}$) with nitric oxide radical (NO$^{\cdot}$) to form the nonradical peroxynitrite (5).

$$O_2^{\cdot-} + NO^{\cdot} \rightarrow ONOO^-$$ [2]

A radical might donate its unpaired electron to another molecule. Thus $O_2^{\cdot-}$ reduces ferric (Fe^{3+}) cytochrome c to ferrous (Fe^{2+}) cytochrome c. A radical might take an electron from another molecule in order to pair. Thus, $O_2^{\cdot-}$ oxidizes ascorbic acid and is itself simultaneously reduced to hydrogen peroxide, H_2O_2. Finally, a radical might join up with another molecule in an addition reaction.

When a radical gives one electron to, takes one electron from, or simply adds on to a nonradical, that nonradical becomes a radical. Thus, a feature of the reaction of free radicals with nonradicals is that they tend to proceed as *chain reactions:* One radical begets another. Free radicals generated in vivo are likely to set off chain reactions, simply because most molecules found in vivo are nonradicals.

The Reactivity of Free Radicals

The chemical reactivity of free radicals varies enormously, depending on their chemical structure. The most reactive radical known to chemistry is hydroxyl radical, OH$^{\cdot}$. This species can attack and damage almost every molecule found in living cells (4,6). Because it is so reactive, OH$^{\cdot}$ does not persist for even a microsecond in vivo before combining with whatever molecule is in its immediate vicinity. Because it is a radical, however, the reactions of OH$^{\cdot}$ leave behind a legacy in the cell in the form of chain reactions. For example, if OH$^{\cdot}$ attacks DNA, free radical chain reactions produce chemical alterations in the purine and pyrimidine bases (that can lead to mutations) as well as strand breakage. Indeed, the pattern of chemical change that results is so characteristic that it can be used as a diagnostic for OH$^{\cdot}$ radical attack on DNA (7). Imperfect repair of oxidative DNA damage can result in cancer (8). It has recently been shown that DNA from human cancerous tissues shows elevated levels of damage products characteristic of attack by OH$^{\cdot}$ (9,10).

Another type of biological damage caused by OH$^{\cdot}$ is its ability to stimulate the destruction of membranes by setting off a free radical chain reaction known as *lipid peroxidation* (11). This occurs when the OH$^{\cdot}$ is generated close to membranes and attacks the fatty-acid side-chains of the membrane phospholipids. It preferentially attacks fatty acid side-chains with several double bonds, such as arachidonic acid. The OH$^{\cdot}$ abstracts an atom of hydrogen from one of the carbon atoms in the side-chain and combines with it to form water. This reaction removes the OH$^{\cdot}$, but leaves behind a carbon-centered radical ($-\overset{\cdot}{C}-$) in the membrane. Carbon-centered radicals formed from polyunsaturated fatty-acid side-chains usually undergo molecular rearrangement to give conjugated diene radicals, which can have various fates. Thus, if two such radicals collide in the membrane, crosslinking of fatty-acid side-chains can occur as the two electrons join to form a covalent bond. Reaction with membrane proteins is also a possibility. However, under physiologic conditions, the most likely fate of carbon-centered radicals is to combine with oxygen, creating yet another type of radical, the *peroxyl radical* (sometimes abbreviated to peroxy radical).

$$-\overset{.}{\underset{}{C}}- \; + \; O_2 \; \rightarrow \; -\overset{\overset{\textstyle O_2^{.}}{|}}{\underset{}{C}}- \tag{3}$$

Peroxyl radicals are reactive enough to attack adjacent unsaturated fatty-acid side-chains, abstracting hydrogen.

$$-\overset{\overset{\textstyle H}{|}}{\underset{}{C}}- \; + \; -\overset{\overset{\textstyle O_2^{.}}{|}}{\underset{}{C}}- \; \rightarrow \; -\overset{.}{\underset{}{C}}- \; + \; -\overset{\overset{\textstyle O_2H}{|}}{\underset{}{C}}- \tag{4}$$

Another carbon-centered radical is generated, and so the chain reaction continues. Hence one OH˙ can result in the conversion of many fatty-acid side-chains into *lipid hydroperoxides* (Eq. 4). Accumulation of lipid hydroperoxides in a membrane alters its fluidity and may eventually lead to membrane breakdown. In addition, lipid hydroperoxides can decompose to yield a range of highly cytotoxic products, perhaps the most unpleasant of which are aldehydes (12) such as malondialdehyde and hydroxynonenal. Peroxyl radicals and cytotoxic aldehydes can also cause severe damage to membrane proteins, inactivating receptors, signal transduction mechanisms, transport proteins, and membrane-bound enzymes (e.g., refs. 12,13).

Other Oxygen-Containing Free Radicals

Several oxygen-containing radicals are known that are much less reactive than OH˙. One of these is *superoxide radical*. Despite its impressive name, superoxide radical does not attack most biological molecules.

Superoxide is made by adding one electron to the diatomic oxygen molecule.

$$O_2 \; + \; e^- \; \rightarrow \; O_2^{.-} \tag{5}$$

Between 1% and 3% (14) of the oxygen we inhale may be used to make superoxide radical (almost all of the rest, of course, is used in the process of oxidative phosphorylation in mitochondria). Some of the $O_2^{.-}$ formation in vivo is a chemical accident. For example, when mitochondria are functioning, some of the electrons passing through the respiratory chain leak from the electron carriers and combine directly with oxygen, reducing it to $O_2^{.-}$ (14,15). Many molecules oxidize on contact with oxygen, e.g., an epinephrine solution left on the bench "goes off" and eventually forms a pink product. The first stage in this oxidation is transfer of an electron from the hormone onto oxygen, giving $O_2^{.-}$. The $O_2^{.-}$ then oxidizes more adrenalin in a chain reaction (14). Such oxidations presumably proceed in vivo as well.

Oxidants and Phagocyte Action

Some of the $O_2^{\cdot-}$ production in vivo may be accidental, but much is functional. Thus activated phagocytic cells generate $O_2^{\cdot-}$, as has been shown for monocytes, neutrophils, eosinophils, and many types of macrophage (16,17). Radical production is important in allowing phagocytes to kill some of the bacterial strains that they can engulf. This importance is simply illustrated by examining patients with chronic granulomatous disease, a collective name for inborn conditions in which the membrane-bound NADPH oxidase system in phagocytes that makes the $O_2^{\cdot-}$ does not work (16). Such patients have phagocytes that engulf and process bacteria normally, but several bacterial strains are not killed and are released in viable form when the phagocytes die. Thus, patients suffer severe, persistent, and multiple infections by such common organisms as *Staphylococcus aureus.* Another killing mechanism used by neutrophils (but not by macrophages) is the enzyme myeloperoxidase (18). It uses H_2O_2 produced from $O_2^{\cdot-}$ to oxidize chloride ions into hypochlorous acid, HOCl, a powerful antibacterial agent (many household bleaches are solutions of the sodium salt of hypochlorous acid, NaOCl).

$$H_2O_2 + Cl^- \rightarrow HOCl + OH^- \qquad [6]$$

Free Radicals and the Vascular Endothelium

Another example of a useful role for $O_2^{\cdot-}$ may be provided by vascular endothelium. It is known that endothelium-derived relaxing factor (EDRF), a humoral agent that is produced by endothelium and is an important mediator of vasodilator responses induced by several pharmacologic agents, including acetylcholine and bradykinin, is closely related to or identical with nitric oxide (19). Several papers (e.g., refs. 20,21) have claimed that the endothelium also produces small amounts of $O_2^{\cdot-}$. Superoxide can react with $NO^{\cdot}$ (Eq. 1). Both $NO^{\cdot}$ and $O_2^{\cdot-}$ are free radicals (each with one unpaired electron) and so they can combine to give a nonradical product, peroxynitrite.

One possibility is that controlled variations in the production of $NO^{\cdot}$ and $O_2^{\cdot-}$ by endothelium provide a mechanism for regulation of vascular tone (22). Another possibility is that increased $O_2^{\cdot-}$ formation in vivo could antagonize $NO^{\cdot}$ and contribute to the impaired endothelium-mediated vasodilation in diabetic patients (23), to the pathogenesis of hypertension (24), and to pathologic vasoconstriction (25). Indeed, the interaction of $O_2^{\cdot-}$ and $NO^{\cdot}$ could be a dangerous event (26). Peroxynitrite may be directly toxic to cells (26,27). It may also decompose, after protonation, to form several reactive species, such as $OH^{\cdot}$ and NO_2^+ (26–28), e.g.,

$$ONOO^- + H^+ \rightarrow ONOOH \rightarrow NO_2^{\cdot} + OH^{\cdot} \qquad [7]$$

Thus, excessive production of $NO^{\cdot}$ and $O_2^{\cdot-}$, as may happen in, for example, septic shock (17,29), might lead to severe oxidative damage by producing highly reactive hydroxyl radicals. However, another view is that NO˙ could be protective, by removing $O_2^{˙-}$ and preventing metal-ion–dependent OH˙ generation (22,29a).

Transition Metals

Many transition metals have variable oxidation numbers, e.g., iron as Fe^{2+} or Fe^{3+} and copper as Cu^+ or Cu^{2+}. Changing between oxidation states involves accepting and donating single electrons, e.g.,

$$Fe^{3+} + e^- \rightleftarrows Fe^{2+} \qquad [8]$$

$$Cu^{2+} + e^- \rightleftarrows Cu^+ \qquad [9]$$

Thus transition metal ions are remarkably good promoters of free radical reactions (4). For example, they react with hydrogen peroxide (H_2O_2) to form OH˙ radicals (4,30).

$$Cu^+ + H_2O_2 \rightarrow Cu^{2+} + OH˙ + OH^- \qquad [10]$$

$$Fe^{2+} + H_2O_2 \rightarrow Fe^{3+} + OH˙ + OH^- \qquad [11]$$

They also accelerate the decomposition of lipid hydroperoxides into cytotoxic products such as aldehydes, alkoxyl radicals, and peroxyl radicals (4,12).

ANTIOXIDANT DEFENSES

Much of the $O_2^{˙-}$ generated in vivo is removed by superoxide dismutase (SOD) enzymes, which catalyze the reaction

$$O_2^{˙-} + O_2^{˙-} + 2H^+ \rightarrow H_2O_2 + O_2 \qquad [12]$$

In the absence of SOD, reaction (Eq. 12) occurs nonenzymically but at a rate approximately four orders of magnitude less at pH 7.4 (14). Because the SOD enzymes produce H_2O_2, they work in conjunction with two other types of enzyme that remove H_2O_2: catalases and glutathione peroxidases (15). It is widely thought that glutathione peroxidase is more important than catalase in removing H_2O_2 in humans, probably because it is located in the same subcellular compartments as SOD (mitochrondria and cytosol), whereas catalase is restricted to the peroxisomes in most tissues (4). The H_2O_2-removing glutathione peroxidase enzymes have the distinction of being among the few known enzymes that require the element selenium for activity: a selenocysteine residue (side-chain $-SeH$ instead of $-SH$, as in normal cysteine) is present at their active sites (31). It is unlikely, however, that the sole function of selenium in humans is to act as a cofactor for glutathione peroxidase (31). Glutathione peroxidases remove H_2O_2 by using it to oxidize reduced glutathione (GSH) into oxidized glutathione (GSSG).

$$2GSH + H_2O_2 \rightarrow GSSG + 2H_2O \qquad [13]$$

It is important to remove both $O_2^{\cdot-}$ and H_2O_2 in vivo, one reason being that $O_2^{\cdot-}$ can accelerate the production of $OH^{\cdot}$ from H_2O_2 in the presence of transition metal ions (Eqs. 10 and 11), reducing Fe^{3+} and Cu^{2+} back to Fe^{2+} and Cu^+, respectively, and allowing further reaction with H_2O_2 to make more $OH^{\cdot}$ (4,30). Superoxide might also generate $OH^{\cdot}$ from $NO^{\cdot}$ (eqs. 2 and 7).

Because of the "catalytic" effect of transition metal ions on free radical reactions, the human body has evolved to keep as many iron and copper ions as possible safely bound in storage or transport proteins (32,33). Thus there is three times as much transferrin iron-binding capacity in human blood plasma as iron needing to be transported, so that there are essentially no catalytic iron ions in plasma from healthy adults. Iron ions bound to transferrin cannot stimulate lipid peroxidation or generation of $OH^{\cdot}$ (32,33). The same is true of copper ions bound to the plasma protein ceruloplasmin (32,33). Hence copper catalytic for free radical reactions is similarly absent from the plasma of healthy humans (34), which is particularly fortunate in view of the ability of "free" copper to stimulate peroxidation of low-density lipoproteins (LDLs) (35), an event that facilitates the development of atherosclerosis (36). The value of this sequestration of metal ions is illustrated by an inspection of the severe pathology suffered by patients with iron or copper overload diseases. For example, in patients with idiopathic hemochromatosis, iron ions catalytic for free radical reactions circulate in the blood (37), and these patients can suffer liver damage, diabetes, joint inflammation, cardiac malfunction, and hepatoma (38).

As well as the primary antioxidant defenses (scavenger enzymes and metal-ion sequestration), there are secondary defenses. Thus, cell membranes and plasma lipoproteins contain α-tocopherol, which functions as a chain-breaking antioxidant (39). It is a lipid-soluble molecule located inside biological membranes and lipoprotein particles. Attached to the hydrophobic structure of α-tocopherol is an $-OH$ group whose hydrogen atom is very easy to remove. Thus when peroxyl radicals are generated during lipid peroxidation, they abstract hydrogen preferentially from the tocopherol.

$$CO_2^{\cdot} + TOH \rightarrow CO_2H + TO^{\cdot} \qquad [14]$$

This stops the peroxyl radical from attacking an adjacent fatty-acid side-chain or protein and terminates the chain reaction, hence the name *chain-breaking antioxidant*. It also converts the α-tocopherol into a radical, tocopherol-$O^{\cdot}$. This radical is poorly reactive, being unable to attack adjacent fatty-acid side-chains at a significant rate, so that the chain reaction is stopped. It is widely thought, on the basis of experiments in vitro, that the tocopherol radical can migrate to the membrane surface and be converted back to α-tocopherol by reaction with ascorbic acid (vitamin C). Thus, both vitamin C and α-tocopherol may cooperate to minimize the consequences of lipid peroxidation in membranes and lipoproteins (35,39). It is important to inhibit peroxidation in plasma lipoproteins, particularly LDLs, since peroxidized LDLs play a role in the development of atherosclerosis (36). α-Tocopherol is the most important antioxidant in LDL, but carotenoids such as beta-carotene also contribute (35) and part of the antioxidant capacity of human LDL is unaccounted for (40). Many other compounds may also sometimes function as antioxidants in vivo; suggestions include ubiquinol, carnosine, and bilirubin. However, the experimentation needed to prove that these compounds actually exert antioxidant actions in vivo has not yet been performed (discussed in ref. 41).

The antioxidant defenses of the human body are not 100% efficient. Thus, cells contain systems that can repair DNA after attack by radicals (8), degrade proteins damaged by radicals (42), and metabolize lipid hydroperoxides in membranes (43). It may be that antioxidant defense is not perfect because some free radical formation is useful, as already explained. As with most things, whether free radicals are good or bad is largely a question of amount, time, and location. The antioxidant defense enzymes operate as a balanced, coordinated system (44). Thus, too much SOD, in relation to the activities of H_2O_2-destroying enzymes, may be harmful rather than beneficial (44,45). For example, the gene for the copper, zinc-containing SOD is located on chromosome 21 in humans. Trisomy 21 results in a 50% elevation of this enzyme in human tissues, and experiments with transgenic mice are consistent with the view that this increased SOD may contribute to the symptoms of Down's syndrome (45).

Oxidative stress (46) is said to result when oxygen free radicals are generated in excess in the human body. This can occur if antioxidant levels are too low. For example, malnutrition can cause low body levels of α-tocopherol, vitamin C, beta-carotene, and glutathione. Oxidative stress can also be caused by increased free radical formation, which can happen by a number of mechanisms. Thus several toxins are metabolized so as to increase free radical formation in vivo (reviewed in ref. 4). They include the herbicide paraquat, the anthracycline antitumor antibiotic adriamycin, the hepatotoxin carbon tetrachloride, and cigarette smoke (47). Inhaling air polluted with O_3 or with the free radical nitrogen dioxide ($NO_2^{\cdot}$) may also cause oxidative stress (48–50).

Cells can tolerate mild oxidative stress and often respond to it by increased synthesis of antioxidant defense enzymes (51,52). Severe oxidative stress, however, can lead to cell injury or death. Depending on the cell-type used and the means by which oxidative stress is imposed, injury and death can result from damage to DNA, proteins, and/or lipids. Thus, several molecular targets must be considered when attempting to measure, or to explain the consequences of, oxidative stress in vivo (1,3,7,53–56).

FREE RADICALS AND HUMAN DISEASE

What is the exact role played by free radicals in human disease? Limitations in methodology have, until very recently, precluded precise answers to this question (3). Some human diseases may be *caused* by oxidative stress. Thus ionizing radiation generates $OH^{\cdot}$ directly by splitting water molecules (6).

$$H_2O \rightarrow H^{\cdot} + OH^{\cdot} \qquad [15]$$

Many of the biological consequences of excess radiation exposure may be due to free radical damage to lipids, proteins, and DNA (6). The signs produced by chronic dietary deficiencies of selenium (the cardiomyopathy known as Keshan disease) or of α-tocopherol (neurologic disorders seen in patients with inborn errors in the mechanism of intestinal fat absorption) might also be mediated by oxidative stress (31,57). In the premature infant, exposure of the incompletely vascularized retina to elevated concentrations of oxygen can lead to retinopathy of prematurity, which in its most severe forms can result in blindness. Several controlled clinical trials have documented the efficiency of α-tocopherol in minimizing the severity of the retinopathy, consistent with some role of lipid peroxidation (discussed in ref. 58).

Secondary Production of Radicals in Human Disease

For most human diseases, however, the oxidative stress is *secondary* to the primary disease process (Fig. 1). For example, activated neutrophils produce $O_2^{\cdot -}$, H_2O_2, and HOCl in order to kill bacteria. However, if a large number of phagocytes becomes activated in a localized area, they can produce tissue damage. For example, the synovial fluid in the swollen knee joints of rheumatoid patients swarms with activated neutrophils. There is good evidence that free radicals and other products derived from neutrophils are contributing to the joint injury. Indeed, the ease of access to the inflamed rheumatoid joint makes this a good system in which to develop assays of free radical formation that are applicable to humans (3). Figure 1 summarizes the various mechanisms by which tissue injury (whatever the means by which it is caused) can result in oxidative stress.

Ischemia-Reoxygenation Injury

One of the most exciting research areas in recent years has been that of the role of free radicals in ischemia-reperfusion injury (59). When tissues are deprived of oxygen, they are injured and, after a period, the injury becomes irreversible and the tissue will die. The length of this critical period depends on the extent of O_2 deprivation (whether it is ischemia or merely hypoxia) and the tissue in question: Skeletal muscle can be rendered bloodless for hours without much injury, whereas in the brain the period is in minutes. For heart, up to about 60 minutes of ischemia seems to be tolerable. Thus ischemia injures cells and will eventually kill them, and the aim should be to restore blood flow as soon as possible, hence the use of thrombolytic agents in the treatment of myocardial infarction (60).

Studies on isolated organs and in animals, however, have shown that, provided the period of ischemia does not itself do irreversible damage, tissue function is better preserved if antioxidants are included in the reoxygenation medium (59–61). Hence restoration of O_2, although obviously beneficial overall, causes increased free radical formation in the damaged tissue and temporarily worsens the injury (59), and inclusion of antioxidants when blood flow is restored offers improved recovery of tissue function upon reoxygenation. Antioxidants that have been used include recombinant

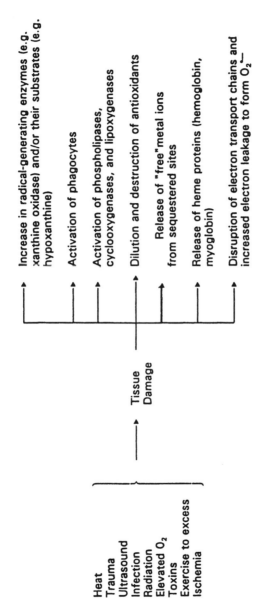

FIG. 1. Some of the mechanisms by which tissue damage can cause oxidative stress.

human superoxide dismutase, thiol compounds, and desferrioxamine (59–63). Desferrioxamine is a chelating agent that binds iron ions and usually stops them from accelerating free radical reactions (63–65). The use of antioxidants in the treatment of septic or hemorrhagic shock and in the preservation of organs for transplantation is an area receiving increasing attention (61,66–69). Although most clinical testing of antioxidants in cardiac reperfusion injury has been carried out with SOD (59), this may be one of the least promising antioxidants to use (discussed in refs. 64,68,69). As originally proposed by Gutteridge et al. (64), the use of iron chelators that inhibit free radical damage may be a more promising approach for short-term treatment (63).

Why should ischemia lead to more free radical generation when tissues are reoxygenated? Possibilities, summarized in Fig. 1, include release of iron ions, catalytic for free radical reactions, from their normal storage sites within the cell (1,22,63,66,67), disruption of mitochondrial respiratory chains so that more electrons leak to oxygen to form $O_2^{\cdot-}$ (70), activation of Kupffer cells in the liver (17,71,72), and increases in the activities of enzymes that generate $O_2^{\cdot-}$ and H_2O_2. Particular attention has centered on xanthine oxidase (59,73). Although this enzyme may be of importance in some aspects of human reperfusion injury (74–76), it probably plays little, if any, role in human myocardial injury, simply because no convincing evidence has been published to show that this enzyme is present in significant amounts in human hearts (discussed in ref. 76a).

Traumatic Injury

There are many examples in which tissue injury by a nonradical mechanism appears to lead to increased free radical reactions. Thus, not only ischemic but also mechanical (e.g., crushing) or chemical injury to tissues can cause cells to rupture and release their contents into the surrounding area. These contents will include transition metal ions and heme proteins (Fig. 1). Cell injury can also activate phospholipases, lipoxygenases, and cycloxygenases. For example, administration of cytotoxic drugs to patients with acute myeloid leukemia has been shown to create a temporary "iron overload" state, presumably due to extensive drug-induced lysis of the leukemic cells (77,78). This increased iron availability could contribute to the side effects of cytotoxic cancer chemotherapy (77,78) because certain anthracycline anti-tumor drugs are known to increase $O_2^{\cdot-}$ and H_2O_2 production in vivo (79). Thus, the extra $O_2^{\cdot-}$ and H_2O_2 could interact with iron to generate damaging $OH^{\cdot}$ radicals (77).

Another area of related interest lies in the sequelae of traumatic or ischemic injury to the brain. Some areas of the human brain are rich in iron, and cerebrospinal fluid has no significant iron-binding capacity because its content of transferrin is very low (reviewed in ref. 80). Thus it has been proposed (80) that injury to the brain by mechanical means (trauma) or by oxygen deprivation (stroke) can result in release of iron ions into the surrounding area. These ions can help to spread damage by accelerating free radical reactions (Fig. 1). This proposal has been given support from animal studies using antioxidants, including chelating agents that bind iron ions and prevent them from catalyzing free radical reactions. Promising results have been obtained with aminosteroid-based antioxidants (the "lazaroids") (81), although the clinical usefulness of these compounds has yet to be evaluated.

Fulminant Hepatic Failure and "Shock" Syndromes

Fulminant hepatic failure (FHF) is the most severe form of acute liver disease, with widespread defects in bodily function (e.g., encephalopathy, coagulation defects) and a high mortality rate. Causes of FHF include overdoses of paracetamol, viral hepatitis, halothane hepatitis, and idiosyncratic reactions to drugs. Treatment of FHF requires high-intensity clinical management, but the prognosis is poor. Liver transplantation is an effective therapeutic option, but only if a suitable organ is available.

The liver plays a central role in the metabolism of transition metals in the human body. For example, it takes up transferrin-bound iron from the circulation and unloads iron from it for use in the synthesis of iron proteins, releasing the apotransferrin into the circulation (reviewed in ref. 4). It has been shown in animals that the liver also possesses an efficient system for the uptake of "low molecular mass" iron ions catalytic for free radical reactions (82–84). Iron ions released from disrupted cells (Fig. 1) may eventually be removed from the circulation by this mechanism. The liver also takes up copper ions bound to albumin and incorporates the resulting copper into ceruloplasmin (reviewed in ref. 85). Presumably because of this efficient uptake system, concentrations of nonceruloplasmin copper in the plasma of healthy people are very low, and may even be zero (34,85). Concentrations of catalytic iron are also zero (reviewed in ref. 86).

Research in our laboratory has shown, however, that plasma from patients with FHF often contains "free" iron ions and sometimes "free" copper ions (Table 1). In patients who received liver transplantation, ions of both metals disappeared after receipt of the new liver, suggesting that the newly transplanted organ had taken them up (Table 2). Thus FHF, and perhaps other conditions in which there is multiorgan dysfunction, may cause oxidative stress in other body tissues by making catalytic transition metal ions more available. For example, Sanan et al. (66) found that desferrioxamine protects dogs against the lethal effects of severe hemorrhagic shock. Low blood pressure due to septic or hemorrhagic shock may lead to ischemia-reperfusion injury in many body tissues, and activated phagocytes contribute an oxidant load during sepsis (61,72). During septic shock, increases in the circulating tumor necrosis factor alpha (TNFα) may also contribute to oxidative stress in tissues (87–92).

Adult Respiratory Distress Syndrome

Adult respiratory distress syndrome (ARDS) is a form of acute lung injury that is estimated to affect up to 150,000 patients per year in the United States. In the original description of the syndrome (93), 12 patients developed clinical features similar to infantile respiratory distress syndrome within 96 hours of the associated injury or

TABLE 1. *"Catalytic" iron and copper in the plasma of patients with fulminant hepatic failure.*

Patient code	Cause of FHF	Bleomycin-detectable iron ($\mu mol/dm^3$)	Phenanthroline-detectable copper ($\mu mol/dm^3$)
A	Paracetamol O/D	4.9	0
B	Paracetamol O/D	0	0.25
C	Paracetamol O/D	0.85	0
D	Non (A or B) hepatitis	0	0
E	Paracetamol O/D	2.05	0
F	Paracetamol O/D	6.0	0
G	Paracetamol O/D	6.2	0
H	Budd-Chiari syndrome	0	0
I	Paracetamol O/D	>5	0
J	Paracetamol O/D	1.1	0.5
K	Non (A or B) hepatitis	1.3	0.7
L	Non (A or B) hepatitis	1.0	2.3
M	Paracetamol O/D	2.7	0
N	Paracetamol O/D	1.1	0
Normal Values	—	Always Zero	Always Zero

O/D, overdose.

illness (e.g., sepsis, aspiration of gastric contents, or severe trauma). The mortality rate of ARDS is high and does not appear to be decreasing as a result of "advances" in patient management.

It is widely thought that ARDS caused by sepsis results from bacterial lipopolysaccharide triggering the sequential expression of a number of cytokines (e.g., TNFα and interleukins 1, 2, and 8) and activation of complement and coagulation cascades

TABLE 2. *Effects of liver transplantation on "catalytic" iron and copper in the plasma of patients with fulminant hepatic failure.*

Patient code	Cause of FHF	Days after transplant[a]	Bleomycin-detectable iron ($\mu mol/dm^3$)	Phenanthroline-detectable copper ($\mu mol/dm^3$)
X	Wilson's disease	−1	6.1	5.1
		7	0	0.7
		14	0	0
		35	0	0
Y	Paracetamol O/D	−1	3.5	0
		1	2.8	0.7
		2	0.9	0
Z	Wilson's disease	−1	ND	5.1
		1	ND	0.7
		2	ND	0

[a] A negative value is days *before* transplantation
FHF, fulminant hepatic failure; O/D, overdose; ND, not done.

that have important activation and priming effects on several cellular systems, including circulating neutrophils, and macrophages normally resident in the lung (94–97). This is accompanied by the entrapment within the lung of neutrophils, where they become activated to release $O_2^{\cdot-}$, H_2O_2, HOCl, eicosanoids, proteases, and other damaging agents (94). The effects of TNFα may also involve oxidative stress to some extent (87–91,98). However, ARDS can develop in patients with neutropenia (e.g., ref. 99). Thus neutrophils are not always essential, but it must not be forgotten that alveolar macrophages are also capable of being primed and activated with subsequent release of proteases, oxygen-derived species, and other potentially toxic species.

Evidence for increased oxidative stress in patients with ARDS includes the recovery of myeloperoxidase and oxidized α_1-antiproteinase in bronchoalveolar lavage fluids (99–101), the exhalation of excess H_2O_2 in the breath (102,103), and the depletion of ascorbic acid and glutathione in body fluids (104,105). Some evidence for increased rates of lipid peroxidation has also been obtained (104). Oxidative stress may be potentiated in ARDS, as an unavoidable complication of treatment, by O_2 administration.

However, none of this evidence *proves* that oxidative stress is a clinically significant mediator of lung injury in ARDS. Much current research activity is focused on strategies designed to prevent or to ameliorate the early activator processes, such as infusing antibodies directed at bacterial lipopolysaccharide, TNFα, or at vascular endothelial or leukocyte adhesion molecules that play a role in the sequestration of activated neutrophils in the lung. However, given the multiplicity of the initiating stimuli and subsequent tissue-injury mechanisms, and the fact that the relative importance of such mechanisms may differ from patient to patient, the authors suggest that antioxidants not be tested alone, but *in combination* with other putative protective agents. We doubt that any single therapeutic approach will be strikingly successful after the onset of ARDS.

DISTINGUISHING SIGNIFICANCE FROM TRIVIALITY: THE IMPORTANCE OF ASSAY METHODOLOGY

Tissue destruction and degeneration can result in increased free radical damage (Fig. 1) by such processes as metal ion release, phagocyte activation, and disruption of mitochondrial electron transport chains (so that more electrons "escape" to oxygen to form $O_2^{\cdot-}$). It follows that almost any disease is likely to be accompanied by increased oxidative stress (1,3,106). It is not therefore surprising that the list of diseases in which free radical formation has been implicated is long and is growing longer. For atherosclerosis (36), rheumatoid arthritis (107), possibly some forms of ARDS (see previous section), reoxygenation injury (see previous section), and traumatic or ischemic damage to the central nervous system (80,81), there is reasonable evidence consistent with the view that free radical reactions make a significant contribution to the disease pathology. As has been stressed previously, however (1,3,106), it is equally likely that in some (perhaps most) diseases, the increased free radical formation makes no significant contribution to the progression of the disease. Each proposal for a role of free radicals in a particular disease must be subjected to stringent examination. Attention must be paid to the molecular targets of injury by oxidative stress and to whether or not any antioxidants administered actually succeed in diminishing oxidative stress. To do the latter requires good assay methodology.

ASSAYS FOR OXYGEN-DERIVED SPECIES: "TRAPPING" ASSAYS

The only technique that can "see" free radicals directly is electron spin resonance (ESR) spectroscopy, which measures the energy changes that occur as unpaired electrons align in response to an external magnetic field. Biologically relevant oxygen radicals ($O_2^{\cdot -}$, $OH^{\cdot}$), however, do not accumulate to high enough concentrations to be directly observable by ESR. Identifying these radicals in vivo can be achieved by two general approaches, the first of which is *trapping*. The radical is allowed to react with a trap molecule to give one or more stable products, which are then measured. Mention of trapping usually brings to mind the technique of *spin trapping*, in which the radical reacts with a spin trap to form a more stable radical, which is detectable by ESR (108). Spin traps such as phenyl-*t*-butyl nitrone have been useful in detecting certain free radicals in whole animals (108,109), but currently available spin traps have not yet succeeded in detecting $O_2^{\cdot -}$ or $OH^{\cdot}$ in vivo, nor are they approved for administration to humans. The metabolic fate of the traps themselves and of trap-free radical adducts must be carefully considered (109).

Aromatic Hydroxylation

There are many trapping methods other than spin trapping. For example, Babbs and Griffin (110) used dimethylsulfoxide to trap $OH^{\cdot}$ in animals, measuring the end-products produced. The authors developed the technique of aromatic hydroxylation as an assay for $OH^{\cdot}$ in humans (reviewed in ref. 111). The principle behind aromatic hydroxylation assays is that $OH^{\cdot}$ generated under physiologic conditions reacts with aromatic compounds to give predominantly hydroxylated end-products (111). An aromatic hydroxylation assay was first applied to humans with the use of salicylate (2-hydroxybenzoate) as a trap for $OH^{\cdot}$. The high doses of aspirin (acetylsalicylate) sometimes given to rheumatoid patients result in concentrations of salicylate in synovial fluid that could conceivably trap some $OH^{\cdot}$ (112). Attack of $OH^{\cdot}$ upon salicylate produces two major hydroxylated products: 2,3-dihydroxybenzoate and 2,5-dihydroxybenzoate. The latter product can also be generated by the action of cytochromes P-450 upon salicylate, whereas 2,3-dihydroxybenzoate apparently cannot (113). Hence, the formation of the latter product may be an index of $OH^{\cdot}$ production in vivo (112,113). Higher levels of 2,3-dihydroxybenzoate have been observed in rheumatoid patients than in normal controls after aspirin administration (112).

Another aromatic trap for $OH^{\cdot}$ is the amino acid phenylalanine (114). In vivo, the L-isomer of this amino acid is hydroxylated by phenylalanine hydroxylase at position

4 on the ring to give L-*p*-tyrosine. D-phenylalanine is not recognized by this enzyme. By contrast, OH˙ cannot distinguish between the two isomers: It acts on both L- and D-phenylalanine to produce a mixture of *o*-, *m*-, and *p*-tyrosines (ref. 114 and 114a). Formation of these tyrosines has already been used to measure OH˙ production by cells (114) and in reperfused heart (115). Similarly, we have found that plasma or synovial fluid from patients with rheumatoid arthritis contain little or no *o*- or *m*- tyrosines. However, if synovial fluid is aspirated from the knee joints of patients with active inflammation and added immediately to a solution of phenylalanine, these products often appear, suggesting that the joint contents are in the process of generating OH˙.

Uric Acid Degradation

In primates (including humans), uric acid is an end-product of purine metabolism because an active urate oxidase enzyme is not present (116). Ames et al. (117) proposed that uric acid acts as an antioxidant in vivo. We reasoned that, if this is the case, measuring the products of attack of oxygen-derived species on uric acid might be a potential marker of oxidative damage uniquely applicable to humans and to other primates (118). Uric acid is degraded upon exposure to OH˙, HOCl, and mixtures of hemoglobin (or myoglobin) with H_2O_2, but it appears unaffected by H_2O_2 alone or by O_2˙⁻. The major product of uric acid oxidation by these first three species is allantoin, but others include oxonic acid, oxaluric acid, cyanuric acid, and parabanic acid (119). The concentrations of all these products are increased in synovial fluid and serum from many rheumatoid patients (118) and in serum from patients with iron overload arising as a consequence of idiopathic hemochromatosis (unpublished results). These data are consistent with the occurrence of oxidative stress in vivo in both these conditions.

ASSAYS FOR OXYGEN-DERIVED SPECIES: "FINGERPRINT" ASSAYS

Instead of attempting to trap oxygen-derived species, one can sometimes implicate them as agents of tissue injury by examining the pattern of chemical change that they produce when they react with certain biological molecules. For example, attack of OH˙ upon DNA produces a pattern of chemical changes to all four of the DNA bases that seems characteristic of OH˙. Other oxygen-derived species either do not attack the DNA bases at all or they modify only guanine (7). For example, examination of this pattern of base changes has been used to show that damage to isolated DNA by copper ions plus H_2O_2, or by copper-phenanthroline chelates, involves OH˙, whereas DNA strand-breakage by the antibiotic bleomycin does not (7). Similarly, this "DNA fingerprinting" has been used to show that at least some of the DNA base damage that occurs when cells are subjected to oxidative stress involves OH˙ formation in the nucleus (7,120) and that the DNA of human cancerous tumors shows increased levels of damage, apparently mediated by OH˙ (9,10).

Measurement of end-products of lipid peroxidation can also be regarded as a finger-print assay. However, there is no simple foolproof method of measuring lipid peroxidation (121). Specific and accurate assays for lipid hydroperoxides and for certain aldehydes exist (reviewed in refs. 12,121). For example, erythrocytes obtained from patients suffering circulatory shock showed increases in bound aldehyde end-products of lipid peroxidation (122). However, measurement of these products reveals only part of the overall peroxidation process. Thus, lipid hydroperoxides may break down to other products, and a huge number of different aldehydes, other carbonyls, and other compounds are produced by peroxide decomposition (12). The "classical" thiobarbituric acid (TBA) test, although frequently applied to human body fluids, has an enormous false-positive rate: Most, if not all, of the TBA-reactive material in human body fluids is not lipid-derived (121,123). Some increase in specificity can be achieved by applying double-derivative spectroscopy (124) to the TBA test (125) or by separating the TBA-malondialdehyde (MDA) adduct from the body fluid after heating with TBA to remove different chromogens that are produced by the reaction of TBA with amino acids, carbohydrates, and aldehydes other than MDA (e.g., see refs. 121,123,126).

ANTIOXIDANT THERAPY: WHAT CAN BE ACHIEVED?

Free radical generation occurs normally in the human body, and rates of free radical generation are probably increased in most diseases (Fig. 1). Their importance as a mechanism of tissue injury is still uncertain, largely because the assays used to measure them have, until recently, been primitive. The development of new assays applicable to humans should allow rapid evaluation of the role of free radicals in disease pathology and provide a logical basis for the therapeutic use of antioxidants. Attempts to use antioxidants in the treatment of human disease can be divided into 3 main areas:

1. Administration of antioxidants that occur naturally in the human body, such as α-tocopherol, glutathione, or SOD.
2. Administration of synthetic antioxidants, such as probucol (36), or chelating agents that suppress iron ion-dependent free radical reactions, or xanthine oxidase inhibitors.
3. The possibility that drugs developed to protect against other mechanisms of tissue injury might have additional physiologic action because they have antioxidant properties.

It must not be forgotten, however, that tissue injury mechanisms in human disease are complex. Taking ischemia-reperfusion injury as an example, the extent of protection by antioxidants in different animal model systems can vary enormously. Just by slight changes in experimental conditions, a mechanism of tissue injury that is largely free radical–dependent can be easily changed to something that is scarcely affected by antioxidants. For example, patients with myocardial infarction are all different.

They have had different periods of ischemia. Some of them may have been treated with thrombolytic agents, some not, and so on. Thus, free radical scavengers alone may not afford satisfactory protection against ischemia-reperfusion. To overcome this problem, we might attempt to protect against all potential mechanisms of cell injury simultaneously. Polypharmacy is not encouraged, but in fact quite often a single drug may act by multiple mechanisms. Many of the drugs in clinical use may well be acting in several different ways. Drugs with multiple mechanisms of protective action, including antioxidant properties, may be one way forward in minimizing tissue injury in human disease.

ACKNOWLEDGMENTS

We are very grateful for research support from the Arthritis and Rheumatism Council, Ministry of Agriculture, Fisheries, and Food (MAFF), Science and Engineering Research Council (SERC), British Heart Foundation, Cancer Research Campaign, and the National Institutes of Health.

REFERENCES

1. Halliwell B. Oxidants and human disease: some new concepts. *FASEB J* 1987;1:358–364.
2. Halliwell B, Cross CE. Reactive oxygen species, antioxidants, and acquired immunodeficiency syndrome, *Arch Intern Med* 1991;151:29–31.
3. Halliwell B, Gutteridge JMC, Cross CE. Free radicals and human disease—where are we now? *J Lab Clin Med* 1992;6:598–620.
4. Halliwell B, Gutteridge JMC. *Free Radicals in Biology and Medicine.* 2nd ed. Oxford: Clarendon Press, 1989.
5. Saran M, Michel C, Bors W. Reactions of NO with $O_2{}^-$. Implications for the action of endothelium-derived relaxing factor. *Free Rad Res Comms* 1989;10:221–226.
6. Von Sonntag C. *The Chemical Basis of Radiation Biology.* London: Taylor and Francis, 1987.
7. Halliwell B, Aruoma OI. DNA damage by oxygen-derived species. Its mechanism and measurement in mammalian systems. *FEBS Lett* 1991;281:9–19.
8. Breimer LH. Repair of DNA damage induced by reactive oxygen species. *Free Rad Res Comms* 1991;14:159–171.
9. Olinski R, Zastawny T, Budzbon J, et al. DNA base modifications in chromatin of human cancerous tissue. *FEBS Lett* 1992;309:193–198.
10. Malins DC, Haimanot R. Major alterations in the nucleotide structure of DNA in cancer of the female breast. *Cancer Res* 1991;51:5430–5432.
11. Stark G. The effect of ionizing radiation on lipid membranes. *Biochim Biophys Acta* 1991;1071:103–122.
12. Esterbauer H, Zollner H, Schaur RJ. Hydroxyalkenals: cytotoxic products of lipid peroxidation. *ISI Atlas Sci Biochem* 1988;1:311–315.
13. Dean RT, Thomas SM, Garner A. Free-radical–mediated fragmentation of monoamine oxidase in the mitochondrial membrane. Role of lipid radicals. *Biochem J* 1986;240:489–494.
14. Fridovich I. Superoxide radical: an endogenous toxicant. *Annu Rev Pharmacol Toxicol* 1983;23:239–257.
15. Chance B, Sies H, Boveris A. Hydroperoxide metabolism in mammalian organs. *Physiol Rev* 1979;59:527–605.
16. Curnutte JT, Babior BM. Chronic granulomatous disease. *Adv Hum Genet* 1987;16:229–245.
17. Bautista AP, Schuler A, Spolarico Z, Spitzer JJ. Tumor necrosis factor-α stimulates superoxide anion generation by perfused rat liver and Kupffer cells. *Am J Physiol* 1991;261:G891–G895.
18. Weiss SJ. Tissue destruction by neutrophils. *N Engl J Med* 1989;320:365–376.

19. Knowles RG, Moncada S. Nitric oxide as a signal in blood vessels. *Trends Pharmacol Sci* 1992; 17:399–402.
20. Arroyo CM, Carmichael AJ, Bouscarel B, et al. Endothelial cells as a source of oxygen-free radicals. An ESR study. *Free Rad Res Comms* 1990;9:287–296.
21. Babbs CF, Creger MD, Turek JJ, Badylak SF. Endothelial superoxide production in the isolated rat heart during early reperfusion after ischemia. A histochemical study. *Am J Pathol* 1991;139: 1069–1080.
22. Halliwell B. Superoxide, iron, vascular endothelium and reperfusion injury. *Free Rad Res Comms* 1989;5:315–318.
23. DeTejada IS, Goldstein I, Azadzoi K, et al. Impaired neurogenic and endothelium-mediated relaxation of penile smooth muscle from diabetic men with impotence. *N Engl J Med* 1989;320:1025–1030.
24. Nakazano K, Watanabe N, Matsuno K, et al. Does superoxide underly the pathogenesis of hypertension: *Proc Natl Acad Sci USA* 1991;88:10045–10048.
25. Laurindo FRM, da Luz PL, Uint L, et al. Evidence for superoxide radical-dependent coronary vasospasm after angioplasty in intact dogs. *Circulation* 1991;83:1705–1715.
26. Beckman JS, Beckman TW, Chen J, et al. Apparent hydroxyl radical production by peroxynitrite: implications for endothelial injury from nitric oxide and superoxide. *Proc Natl Acad Sci USA* 1990; 87:1620–1624.
27. Radi R, Beckman JS, Bush KM, et al. Peroxynitrite oxidation of sulfhydryls. The cytotoxic potential of superoxide and nitric oxide. *J Biol Chem* 1990;266:4244–4250.
28. Hogg N, Darley-Usmar VM, Wilson MT, Moncada S. Production of hydroxyl radicals from the simultaneous generation of superoxide and nitric oxide. *Biochem J* 1992;281:419–424.
29. Nava E, Palmer RMJ, Moncada S. Inhibition of nitric oxide synthesis in septic shock—how much is beneficial? *Lancet* 1991;338:1555–1557.
29a. Harbrecht BG, Billiar TR, Stadler J, et al. Inhibition of nitric oxide synthesis during endotoxemia promotes intrahepatic thrombosis and an oxygen radical–mediated hepatic injury. *J Leukocyte Biol* 1992;52:390–394.
30. Halliwell B, Gutteridge JMC. Biologically relevant metal ion–dependent hydroxyl radical generation—an update. *FEBS Lett* 1992;307:108–112.
31. Levander OA. A global view of human selenium nutrition. *Annu Rev Nutr* 1987;7:227–250.
32. Halliwell B, Gutteridge JMC. Oxygen free radicals and iron in relation to biology and medicine; some problems and concepts. *Arch Biochem Biophys* 1986;246:501–514.
33. Halliwell B, Gutteridge JMC. The antioxidants of human extracellular fluids. *Arch Biochem Biophys* 1990;280:1–8.
34. Evans PJ, Bomford A, Halliwell B. Non-ceruloplasmin copper and ferroxidase activity in mammalian serum. Ferroxidase activity and phenanthroline-detectable copper in human serum in Wilson's disease. *Free Rad Res Comms* 1989;7:55–62.
35. Esterbauer H, Striegl G, Puhl H, Rotheneder M. Continuous monitoring of in vitro oxidation of human low density lipoprotein. *Free Rad Res Comms* 1989;6:67–75.
36. Steinberg D, Parthasarathy S, Carew TE, et al. Beyond cholesterol. Modifications of low-density lipoprotein that increase its atherogenicity. *N Engl J Med* 1989;320:915–924.
37. Grootveld M, Bell JD, Halliwell B, et al. Non–transferrin-bound iron in plasma or serum from patients with idiopathic hemochromatosis. *J Biol Chem* 1989;264:4417–4422.
38. McLaren GD, Muir WA, Kellermeyer RW. Iron overload disorders: natural history, pathogenesis, diagnosis and therapy. *CRC Crit Rev Clin Lab Sci* 1983;19:205–266.
39. Burton GW, Traber MG. Vitamin E: antioxidant activity, biokinetics and bioavailability. *Annu Rev Nutr* 1990;10:357–382.
40. Esterbauer H, Puhl H, Dieber-Rotheneder M, et al. Effect of antioxidants on oxidative modification of LDL. *Ann Med* 1991;23:573–581.
41. Halliwell B. How to characterize a biological antioxidant. *Free Rad Res Comms* 1990;9:1–32.
42. Marcillat O, Zhang Y, Lin SW, Davies KJA. Mitochondria contain a proteolytic system which can recognize and degrade oxidatively-denatured proteins. *Biochem J* 1988;254:677–683.
43. Maiorino M, Chu FF, Ursini F, et al. Phospholipid hydroperoxide glutathione peroxidase is the 18KDa selenoprotein expressed in human tumor cell lines. *J Biol Chem* 1991;266:7728–7732.
44. Amstad P, Peskin A, Shah G, et al. The balance between Cu, Zn-superoxide dismutase and catalase affects the sensitivity of mouse epidermal cells to oxidative stress. *Biochemistry* 1991;30:9305–9313.
45. Groner Y, Elroy-Stein O, Avraham KB, et al. Down syndrome clinical symptoms are manifested in transfected cells and transgenic mice overexpressing the human Cu/Zn-superoxide dismutase gene. *J Physiol (Paris)* 1990;84:53–77.
46. Sies H. *Oxidative Stress, Oxidants and Antioxidants.* New York, London: Academic Press, 1991.

47. Pryor WA. Cigarette smoke and the involvement of free radical reactions in chemical carcinogenesis. *Br J Cancer* 1987;55(Suppl VIII):19–23.
48. Pryor WA. Can vitamin E protect humans against the pathological effects of ozone in smog? *Am J Clin Nutr* 1991;53:702–722.
49. Halliwell B, Hu ML, Louie S, et al. Interaction of nitrogen dioxide with human plasma-antioxidant depletion and oxidative damage. *FEBS Lett* 1992;313:62–66.
50. Cross CE, Motchnik PA, Bruener BA, et al. Oxidative damage to plasma constituents by ozone. *FEBS Lett* 1992;298:269–272.
51. Storz G, Tartaglia LA. Oxy R—a regulator of antioxidant genes. *J Nutr* 1992;122:627–630.
52. Frank L. Developmental aspects of experimental pulmonary oxygen toxicity. *Free Rad Biol Med* 1991;11:463–494.
53. Hyslop PA, Hinshaw DB, Halsey WR Jr, et al. Mechanisms of oxidant-mediated cell injury. The glycolytic and mitochondrial pathways of ADP phosphorylation are major intracellular targets inactivated by hydrogen peroxide. *J Biol Chem* 1988;263:1665–1675.
54. Stadtman ER, Oliver CN. Metal-catalyzed oxidation of proteins—physiological consequences. *J Biol Chem* 1991;266:2005–2008.
55. Orrenius S, McConkey DJ, Bellomo G, Nicotera P. Role of Ca^{2+} in toxic cell killing. *Trends Pharmacol Sci* 1989;10:281–285.
56. Schreck R, Albermann K, Baeuerle PA. Nuclear factor kappa B: an oxidative stress-responsive transcription factor of eukaryotic cells (a review). *Free Rad Res Comms* 1992;17:221–237.
57. Muller DPR, Goss-Sampson MA. Neurochemical neurophysiological and neuropathological studies in vitamin E deficiency. *Crit Rev Neurobiol* 1990;5:239–265.
58. Ehrenkranz RA. Vitamin E and retinopathy of prematurity: still controversial. *J Pediatr* 1989;114:801–803.
59. McCord JM. Oxygen-derived free radicals in post ischemic tissue injury. *N Engl J Med* 1985;312:159–163.
60. Bolli R. Oxygen-derived free radicals and postischemic myocardial dysfunction ('stunned myocardium'). *J Am Coll Cardiol* 1988;12:239–249.
61. Youn YK, LaLonde C, Demling R. Use of antioxidant therapy in shock and trauma. *Circ Shock* 1991;35:245–249.
62. Bolli R, Jeroudi MO, Patel BS, et al. Marked reduction of free radical generation and contractile dysfunction by antioxidant therapy begun at the time of reperfusion: evidence that myocardial "stunning" is a form of reperfusion injury. *Circ Res* 1989;65:607–622.
63. Halliwell B. Drug antioxidant effects: a basis for drug selection? *Drugs* 1991;42:569–605.
64. Gutteridge JMC, Richmond R, Halliwell B. Inhibition of the iron-catalyzed formation of hydroxyl radicals from superoxide and of lipid peroxidation by desferrioxamine. *Biochem J* 1979;184:469–474.
65. Halliwell B. Protection against tissue damage in vivo by desferrioxamine. What is its mechanism of action? *Free Rad Biol Med* 1989;7:645–651.
66. Sanan S, Sharma G, Malhotra R, et al. Protection by desferrioxamine against histopathological changes of the liver in the post-oligemic phase of clinical hemorrhagic shock in dogs: correlation with improved survival rate and recovery. *Free Rad Res Comms* 1989;6:29–38.
67. Gower J, Healing G, Green C. Measurement by HPLC of desferrioxamine-available iron in rabbit kidneys to assess the effect of ischaemia on the distribution of iron within the total pool. *Free Rad Res Comms* 1989;5:291–299.
68. Bolli R. Superoxide dismutase ten years later: a drug in search of a function. *J Am Coll Cardiol* 1991;18:231–233.
69. Omar BA, McCord JM. The cardioprotective effect of Mn-superoxide dismutase is lost at high doses in the postischemic isolated rabbit heart. *Free Rad Biol Med* 1990;9:473–478.
70. Marklund SL. Role of toxic effects of oxygen in reperfusion damage. *J Mol Cell Cardiol* 1988;20(Suppl II):23–30.
71. Rymsa B, Wang JF, De Groot H. O_2^- release by activated Kupffer cells upon hypoxia reoxygenation. *Am J Physiol* 1991;24:G602–G607.
72. Bautista AP, Spitzer JJ. Superoxide anion generation by in situ perfused rat liver; effect of in vivo endotoxin. *Am J Physiol* 1990;259:G907–G912.
73. Anderson BO, Moore EE, Moore FA, et al. Hypovolemic shock promotes neutrophil sequestration in lungs by a xanthine oxidase-related mechanism. *J Appl Physiol* 1991;71:1862–1865.
74. Murrell GAC, Francis MJO, Bromley L. Free radicals and Dupuytren's contracture. *Br Med J* 1987;295:1373–1375.
75. Friedl HP, Smith DJ, Till GO, et al. Ischemia-reperfusion in humans. Appearance of xanthine oxidase activity. *Am J Pathol* 1990;136:491–495.

76. Merry P, Winyard PG, Morris CJ, et al. Oxygen free radicals, inflammation and synovitis: the current status. *Ann Rheum Dis* 1989;48:864–870.

76a.Podzuweit T, Beck H, Müller A, et al. Absence of xanthine oxidoreductase activity in human myocardium. *Cardiovasc Res* 1991;25:820–830.

77. Halliwell B, Aruoma OI, Mufti G, Bomford A. Bleomycin-detectable iron in serum from leukaemic patients before and after chemotherapy. Therapeutic implications for treatment with oxidant-generating drugs. *FEBS Lett* 1988;241:202–204.

78. Gordeuk VR, Brittenham GM. Bleomycin-reactive iron in patients with acute non-lymphocytic leukemia. *FEBS Lett* 1992;308:4–6.

79. Doroshow JH. Doxorubicin-induced cardiac toxicity. *N Engl J Med* 1991;324:843–845.

80. Halliwell B. Reactive oxygen species and the central nervous system. *J Neurochem* 1992;59: 1609–1623.

81. Hall ED, Braughler JM. Central nervous system trauma and stroke. *Free Rad Biol Med* 1989;6: 303–313.

82. Brissot P, Wright TL, Ma WA, Weisiger RA. Efficient clearance of non-transferrin-bound iron by rat liver *J Clin Invest* 1985;76:1463–1470.

83. Craven CM, Alexander J, Eldridge M, et al. Tissue distribution and clearance kinetics of non–transferrin-bound iron in the hypotransferrinemic mouse: a rodent model for hemochromatosis. *Proc Natl Acad Sci USA* 1987;84:3457–3461.

84. Kaplan J, Jordan I, Sturrock A. Regulation of the transferrin-independent iron transport system in cultured cells. *J Biol Chem* 1991;266:2997–3004.

85. Gutteridge JMC, Stocks J. Ceruloplasmin: physiological and pathological perspectives. *CRC Crit Rev Clin Lab Sci* 1981;14:257–329.

86. Gutteridge JMC, Halliwell B. Radical-promoting loosely-bound iron in biological fluids and the bleomycin assay. *Life Chem Rep* 1987;4:113–142.

87. Baud L, Fouqueray B, Philippe C, Affres H. Modulation of tumor necrosis factor by reactive oxygen metabolites. *News Physiol Sci* 1992;7:34–37.

88. Zimmerman RJ, Chan A, Leadon SC. Oxidative damage in murine tumor cells treated *in vitro* by recombinant human tumor necrosis factor. *Cancer Res* 1989;49:1644–1648.

89. Schulze-Osthoff K, Bakker AC, Vanhaesebroeck B, et al. Cytotoxic activity of tumor necrosis factor is mediated by early damage of mitochondrial functions. Evidence for the involvement of mitochondrial radical generation. *J Biol Chem* 1992;267:5317–5323.

90. Pogrebniak H, Matthews W, Mitchell J, et al. Spin-trap protection from tumor necrosis factor cytotoxicity. *J Surg Res* 1991;50:469–474.

91. Bautista AP, Schuler A, Spolarics Z, Spitzer JJ. Tumor necrosis factor-α stimulates superoxide anion generation by perfused rat liver and Kupffer cells. *Am J Physiol* 1991;261:G891–G895.

92. Jaeschke H, Farhood A. Neutrophil and Kupffer-cell induced oxidant stress and ischemia-reperfusion injury in rat liver. *Am J Physiol* 1991;260:G355–G362.

93. Asbaugh DG, Bigelow DB, Petty TL, Levine BE. Acute respiratory distress in adults. *Lancet* 1967; 2:19–23.

94. Tate RM, Repine JE. Neutrophils and the adult respiratory distress syndrome. *Am Rev Respir Dis* 1983;125:552–559.

95. Christman JW, Wheeler AP, Bernard GR. Cytokines and sepsis: what are the therapeutic implications? *J Crit Care* 1991;6:177–182.

96. Kunkel SL, Standiford T, Kasahara K, Strieter RM. Interleukin-8 (IL-8): the major neutophil chemotactic factor in the lung. *Exp Lung Res* 1991;17:17–23.

97. Fantone JC, Feltner DE, Brieland JK. Phagocytic cell-derived inflammatory mediators and lung disease. *Chest* 1987;91:428–434.

98. Ishii Y, Partridge CA, Del Vecchio PJ, Malik AB. Tumor necrosis factor-α-mediated decrease in glutathione increases the sensitivity of pulmonary vascular endothelial cells to H_2O_2. *J Clin Invest* 1992;89:794–802.

99. Maunder RJ, Hackman RC, Ritt E, et al. Occurrence of the adult respiratory distress syndrome in neutropenic patients. *Am Rev Respir Dis* 1986;133:313–316.

100. Cochrane CG, Spragg RG, Revak SD. The presence of neutrophil elastase and evidence of oxidation activity in bronchoalveolar lavage fluid of patients with adult respiratory distress syndrome. *Am Rev Respir Dis* 1983;127:525–527.

101. Weiland JE, Davis WB, Holter JF. Lung neutrophils in the adult respiratory distress syndrome: clinical and pathophysiological significance. *Am Rev Respir Dis* 1986;133:218–225.

102. Baldwin SR, Simon RH, Grum CM, et al. Oxidant activity in expired breath of patients with adult respiratory distress syndrome. *Lancet* 1986;i:11–14.
103. Sznajder JI, Fraiman A, Hall JB, et al. Increased hydrogen peroxide in the expired breath of patients with acute hypoxemic respiratory failure. *Chest* 1989;96:606–612.
104. Cross CE, Forte T, Stocker R, et al. Oxidative stress and abnormal cholesterol metabolism in patients with adult respiratory distress syndrome. *J Lab Clin Med* 1990;115:396–404.
105. Pacht ER, Timerman AP, Lykens MG, Merola AJ. Deficiency of alveolar fluid glutathione in patients with sepsis and the adult respiratory distress syndrome. *Chest* 1991;100:1397–1403.
106. Halliwell B, Gutteridge JMC. Lipid peroxidation, oxygen radicals, cell damage and antioxidant therapy. *Lancet* 1984;i:1396–1398.
107. Halliwell B, Hoult JRS, Blake DR. Oxidants, inflammation and anti-inflammatory drugs. *FASEB J* 1988;2:501–514.
108. Janzen EG. Spin trapping and associated vocabulary. *Free Rad Res Comms* 1990;10:63–68.
109. Chen GM, Bray TM, Janzen EG, McCay PB. Excretion, metabolism and tissue distribution of a spin-trapping agent alpha-phenyl-N-tert-butyl-nitrone (PBN) in rats. *Free Rad Res Comms* 1990;9: 317–323.
110. Babbs CF, Griffin DW. Scatchard analysis of methane sulfinic acid production from dimethyl sulfoxide. A method to quantify hydroxyl radical formation in physiologic systems. *Free Rad Biol Med* 1989;6:493–503.
111. Halliwell B, Grootveld M, Gutteridge JMC. Methods for the measurement of hydroxyl radicals in biochemical systems. Deoxyribose degradation and aromatic hydroxylation. *Methods Biochem Anal* 1988;33:59–90.
112. Grootveld M, Halliwell B. Aromatic hydroxylation of salicylate as a potential measure of hydroxyl radical formation *in vivo*. *Biochem J* 1986;232:699–504.
113. Ingelman-Sundberg M, Kaur H, Terelius Y, et al. Hydroxylation of salicylate by microsomal fractions and cytochrome P-450. Lack of production of 2,3-dihydroxybenzoate unless hydroxyl radical formation is permitted. *Biochem J* 1991;276:753–757.
114. Kaur H, Fagerheim I, Grootveld M, et al. Aromatic hydroxylation of phenylalanine as an assay for hydroxyl radicals. *Anal Biochem* 1988;172:360–367.
114a. Kaur H., Halliwell B. Aromatic hydroxylation of phenylalinine as an assay for hydroxyl radicals: measurement of hydroxyl radical formation from ozone and in blood from premature babies using improvised HPLC methodology. *Anal Biochem* (In press).
115. Bolli R, Kaur H, Li XY, et al. Demonstration of hydroxyl radical generation in "stunned" myocardium of intact dogs using aromatic hydroxylation of phenylalanine, *FASEB J* 1991;5:A704.
116. Yeldani AV, Wang X, Alvares K, et al. Human urate oxidase gene: cloning and partial sequence analysis reveal a stop codon within the fifth exon. *Biochem Biophys Res Commun* 1990;171:641–646.
117. Ames BN, Cathcart R, Schwiers E, Hochstein P. Uric acid provides an antioxidant defense in humans against oxidant and radical-caused aging and cancer: a hypothesis, *Proc Natl Acad Sci USA* 1981;78:6858–6862.
118. Grootveld M, Halliwell B. Measurement of allantoin and uric acid in human body fluids. A potential index of free radical reactions *in vivo*? *Biochem J* 1987;243:803–808.
119. Kaur H, Halliwell B. Action of biologically-relevant oxidizing species upon uric acid. Identification of uric acid oxidation products. *Chem Biol Interact* 1990;73:235–267.
120. Dizdaroglu M, Nackerdien Z, Chao BC, et al. Chemical nature of in vivo DNA base damage in hydrogen peroxide-treated mammalian cells. *Arch Biochem Biophys* 1991;285:388–390.
121. Gutteridge JMC, Halliwell B. The measurement and mechanism of lipid peroxidation in biological systems. *Trends Biochem Sci* 1990;15:129–135.
122. Poli G, Biasi F, Chiarpolto E, et al. Lipid peroxidation in human diseases: evidence of red cell oxidative stress after circulatory shock. *Free Rad Biol Med* 1989;6:167–170.
123. Largilliere C, Melancon SB. Free malondialdehyde determination in human plasma by high performance liquid chromatography. *Anal Biochem* 1988;170:123–126.
124. Corongiu FP, Poli G, Dianzani MU, et al. Lipid peroxidation and molecular damage to polyunsaturated fatty acids in rat liver. Recognition of two classes of hydroperoxides formed under conditions *in vivo*. *Chem Biol Interact* 1986;59:147–155.
125. Merry P, Grootveld M, Lunec J, Blake DR. Oxidative damage to lipids within the inflamed human joint provides evidence of radical-mediated hypoxic-reperfusion injury. *Am J Clin Nutr* 1991;56: 362S–369S.
126. Bird RP, Hung SSO, Hadley M, Draper HM. Determination of malonaldehyde in biological materials by high-pressure liquid chromatography. *Anal Biochem* 1983;128:240–244.

Organ Metabolism and Nutrition:
Ideas for Future Critical Care, edited by
J. M. Kinney and H. N. Tucker.
Raven Press, Ltd., New York © 1994.

22

Gas Exchange and Pulmonary Compromise

Simon Bursztein

Department of General Intensive Care, Israel Institute of Technology,
Rambam Medical Center, 31 096 Haifa, Israel

Being challenged by "Ideas for Future Critical Care" in relation to *Organ Metabolism and Nutrition,* and especially in a session on pulmonary function and gas exchange, it would be appropriate to recall that gas exchange, namely, oxygen consumption (VO_2) and carbon dioxide production (VCO_2), is in major part a function of energy expenditure and fuel utilization. To this end we review the basic principles of gas exchange and fuel utilization evaluated by indirect calorimetry to analyze if and how pulmonary compromise interacts with gas exchange.

GAS EXCHANGE

VO_2 and VCO_2 are values that may be easily obtained by noninvasive measurements of inspired and expired gases. However, it has to be emphasized that once the oxygen is taken into the lungs, it is carried by the blood to each single cell; only then, and mainly in the mitochondria, does the oxygen consumption actually take place. In the same way, the CO_2 is produced at cellular level, carried through the blood to the lungs, and exhaled.

Assuming that a human breathes at a frequency (F) of about 20 times per minute, inhaling and exhaling a tidal volume (VT) of about 500 ml of air each time, the minute volume (V) is then

$$V = VT \times F = 500 \times 20 = 10,000 \text{ ml/min} \qquad [1]$$

In room air, the concentrations of inspired oxygen (FIO_2) and of inspired carbon dioxide ($FICO_2$) remain at the constant values of about 21% and 0%, respectively. During expiration, the oxygen concentration (FEO_2) decreases from approximately 21% to a minimum of approximately 15%, and the carbon dioxide concentration ($FECO_2$) increases, from close to 0% to a maximum value of about 6%.

Breath-by-breath values of O_2 and CO_2 exchange may be obtained (1), but the methods are difficult to perform and the data not quite relevant to the evaluation of O_2 consumption and CO_2 production. The more usual technique to obtain these rates is to average the values of FEO_2 and $FECO_2$. When the expired air is mixed in a

Douglas bag or another mixing chamber, the concentration of O_2 and CO_2 in expired gases becomes homogeneous, and when respiratory volumes are obtained simultaneously, on-line measurements of VO_2 and VCO_2 can be obtained.

The only case in which the inspiratory minute volume (VI), equals the expiratory volume (VE) is when VO_2 is equal to VCO_2, and the ratio VCO_2/VO_2, or the respiratory quotient (RQ), equals 1. Therefore, for a more precise calculation of VO_2 and VCO_2, it is necessary to use the different values of VI and VE, instead of V. But to illustrate the VO_2 and VCO_2 determination, we may assume that VI = VE = 10,000 ml; that FIO_2 is 21% (0.21); that $FICO_2$ is 0%; and that FEO_2 and $FECO_2$, as measured by O_2 and CO_2 analyzers, are 18% (0.18) and 2.5% (0.025), respectively. Then:

$$VO_2 \text{ (ml/min)} = VI \times FIO_2 - VE \times FEO_2$$

$$= 10,000 \times 0.21 - 10,000 \times 0.18 \qquad [2]$$

$$= 300 \text{ ml/min}$$

and

$$VCO_2 \text{ (ml/min)} = VE \times FECO_2 - VI \times FICO_2$$

$$= 10,000 \times 0.025 - 10,000 \times 0.00 \qquad [3]$$

$$= 250 \text{ ml/min}$$

Measurements should be made between at least 20 and 30 minutes and the total volume divided by the time of measurement to express the values per minute. This is required because gas concentrations in O_2 and in CO_2, the respiratory rate, and respiratory volumes may vary from minute to minute, and sampling over a longer period improves accuracy. To calculate VO_2 and VCO_2, as shown in Eqs. 2 and 3, the values for VI, VE, FIO_2 and FEO_2, and $FECO_2$ have to be determined. It is not necessary, however, to make separate measurements for VI and VE because they are interrelated and the measurement of only one of them is necessary. Since nitrogen gas (N_2) is not metabolized in the body, the amount of N_2 exhaled is equal to the amount inhaled. If FIN_2 is the concentration of inspired nitrogen and FEN_2 is the concentration of expired nitrogen, we may write

$$VI \times FIN_2 = VE \times FEN_2 \qquad [4]$$

From Eq. 4, VI and VE can be derived:

$$VI = VE \times \frac{FEN_2}{FIN_2} \qquad [5]$$

$$VE = VI \times \frac{FIN_2}{FEN_2} \qquad [6]$$

Nitrogen analyzers are not commonly used in the clinical setting, but N_2 can be determined indirectly. Indeed, inspiratory gas and expiratory gas contain the full

composition of the air. If we assume that the air is dry (without water vapor) and if we neglect $FICO_2$, we may write the following equations.
For inspiratory gas:

$$FIO_2 + FIN_2 = 1 \ (100\%) \tag{7}$$

or

$$FIN_2 = 1 - FIO_2 \tag{8}$$

For expiratory gas:

$$FEO_2 + FECO2 + FEN_2 = 1 \ (100\%) \tag{9}$$

or

$$FEN2 = 1 - FEO_2 - FECO_2 \tag{10}$$

By replacing FIN_2 and FEN_2 in Eqs. 5 and 6 by their values in Eqs. 8 and 10, VI and VE can be obtained by measuring one volume instead of two, and by measuring the concentrations of O_2 in inspired gas and O_2 and CO_2 in expired gas. Then Eqs. 5 and 6 then become

$$VI = VE \times \frac{1 - FEO_2 - FECO_2}{1 - FIO2} \tag{11}$$

and

$$VE = VI \times \frac{1 - FIO_2}{1 - FEO_2 - FECO_2} \tag{12}$$

Because the difference between VI and VE is small, it may be negligible for clinical purposes, and the measurement of VE alone may be used for both VI and VE. In this way the values of VO_2 and VCO_2, calculated by Eqs. 2 and 3, become 300 and 250, respectively, and RQ becomes 0.83.

The value of RQ is normally less than 1, indicating that VO_2 is greater than VCO_2, and VI is greater than VE. One may thus wonder how is it that the subject is not inflated with air. This does not occur because the difference between the higher amount of oxygen inhaled, as compared with the amount of carbon dioxide exhaled, is utilized to form metabolic water, urea, uric acid, and other oxygen-containing compounds that will eventually be eliminated by the urine or by evaporation.

If for any reason there is an increase in the energy demand, because of exercise or because of acute disease associated with hypermetabolism, the only way to meet this increased energy need is to burn more substrate. This requires a higher oxygen uptake and brings about a simultaneous increase in CO_2 production. The way in which the body normally adjusts to higher oxygen demands is by increasing minute ventilation. Because FIO_2 is always constant in the equation $VO_2 = VI \times FIO_2 - VE \times FEO_2$, there are only two possibilities for increasing the VO_2: (a) by decreasing FEO_2, a way that is economical for the body because it requires no change in the work of breathing, yet is quantitatively of no great importance; or (b) by increasing VI and VE, which is the main adaptative mechanism to the increased metabolic demand, but causing also an increase in the work of breathing. The work of breathing requires about 3% to 5% of the total VO_2 at rest in normal subjects and increases exponentially with minute ventilation, as it is the case in the different types of respiratory impairments (2,3).

An alternative to the measuring of VO_2 in the respiratory gases is to measure the difference in O_2 content in arterial and mixed venous blood (a-vDO_2) and multiply it by blood flow or cardiac output. This requires samples of arterial blood and mixed venous blood taken from the right heart or the pulmonary artery. This method is never used to merely measure VO_2 for it is much more invasive and involves an unreasonable risk, especially when compared with measuring respiratory gas volumes and concentrations of O_2 and CO_2. However, for patients in whom a Swan Ganz catheter and arterial catheters have already been set for hemodynamic monitoring, drawing additional small blood samples to measure VO_2 represents a very minor risk. In such patients cardiac output is usually measured as part of the follow up, and VO_2 can then be calculated by the following equation:

$$VO_2(ml/min) = CO\ (ml/min) \times [a\text{-}vDO_2]\ ml/100\ ml \qquad [13]$$

where [a-vDO_2] is the arteriovenous difference of O_2 in ml per hundred ml of blood. With this method, the accuracy of VO_2 depends on the accuracy of the measurements of cardiac output and of arterial and venous O_2 contents. If, for instance, cardiac output is equal to 5,000 ml/min and the arterial (CaO_2) and venous content (CvO_2) of oxygen are, respectively, 21 and 15 ml/100 ml, we obtain

$$300\ ml/min = 5,000\ ml/min \times (21\text{--}15)\ ml/100\ ml \qquad [14]$$

CaO_2 and CvO_2 are readily available in the intensive care unit; most of the automatic blood gas analyzers calculate and display these values as a part of the regular analysis, and it is thus easily possible to obtain the value of VO_2 as part of the routine monitoring in these patients.

Theoretically, VCO_2 could be determined in a similar method by using the following formula:

$$VCO_2\ (ml/min) = CO\ (ml/min) \times [v\text{-}aDCO_2]\ ml/100\ ml \qquad [15]$$

Although this way of evaluating VCO_2 was proven to be acceptable for clinical use and some computer programs were even developed to this end, it was never used as a routine to determine carbon dioxide production (4,5).

ENERGY EXPENDITURE AND FUEL UTILIZATION EVALUATED BY INDIRECT CALORIMETRY

Energy expenditure (EE) can be accurately assessed via direct calorimetry by measuring heat loss. However, the method of choice for most patients is indirect calorimetry, which evaluates energy production by measuring VO_2, VCO_2, and nitrogen excretion (NM). Indirect calorimetry is based on two principles: The first is the law of conservation of energy; the second is that the energy produced by foodstuff oxidation in the body is equivalent to the energy produced by the combustion of this foodstuff in a bomb calorimeter.

For fat and carbohydrates, if the end-products (H_2O and CO_2) in the bomb calorimeter and in the body are the same, producing, respectively, 9.3 kcal and 4.17 kcal (3.75 for glucose), it is not true for protein. In the body, the end-products for protein are mainly urea and some other constituents such as creatinine, uric acid, ammonia, 3-methylhistidine, and about 4.4 kcal. In the bomb calorimeter, proteins are totally oxidized to form CO_2, H_2O, SO_4, and nitrogen and to produce about 5.7 kcal. From these measurements, equations can be derived for carbohydrate (dCH), protein (dP), and fat (dF) (6).

Carbohydrate:

$$1 \text{ g dCH} + 0.829 \text{ l } O_2 \rightarrow 0.829 \text{ l } CO_2 + 0.67 \text{ g } H_2O + 4.17 \text{ kcal} \qquad [16]$$

Protein:

$$1 \text{ g dP} + 0.966 \text{ l } O_2 \rightarrow 0.782 \text{ l } CO_2 + 0.41 \text{ g } H_2O + 4.4 \text{ kcal} \qquad [17]$$

Fat:

$$1 \text{ g dF} + 2.019 \text{ l } O_2 \rightarrow 1.427 \text{ l } CO_2 + 1.07 \text{ g } H_2O + 9.3 \text{ kcal} \qquad [18]$$

Equations 16, 17, and 18 represent fuel oxidation in the body, and the three nutrients are probably metabolized simultaneously in different proportions in relation with the patient's condition and other factors, most of which are not well known. The oxygen consumed in a given period of time is the amount of oxygen used to oxidate given quantities of carbohydrate, protein, and fat. Each of these nutrients uses 0.829, 0.966, and 2.019 l of oxygen per gram of metabolized substance, respectively. During the same period, carbon dioxide is produced in the amounts of 0.829, 0.782, and 1.427 l/g of carbohydrate, protein, and fat, respectively. When the three nutrients are being metabolized, there is also a heat production of 4.17 kcal for each gram of carbohydrate, 4.4 kcal for each gram of protein, and 9.3 kcal for each gram of fat. These relationships can be expressed by Eqs. 19, 20, and 21, representing simultaneously occurring processes and can therefore be considered a system of three equations with four unknowns. For solving these equations for dCH, dP, dF, and EE, the classical method is to derive the value of dP from the urea excretion in the 24-hour urinary output. Because 30 g of muscle are considered to contain 6.25 g of protein and 1 g of metabolized nitrogen (NM) is considered to be produced by 6.25 g of protein, the system of three equations with four unknowns becomes a system of four equations with four unknowns that can be solved.

$$VO_2 \text{ (l)} = 0.829 \text{ dCH} + 0.966 \text{ dP} + 2.019 \text{ dF} \qquad [19]$$

$$VCO_2 \text{ (l)} = 0.829 \text{ dCH} + 0.782 \text{ dP} + 1.427 \text{ dF} \qquad [20]$$

$$\text{EE (kcal)} = 4.17 \text{ dCH} + 4.4 \text{ dP} + 9.3 \text{ dF} \qquad [21]$$

$$\text{dP (g)} = 6.25 \text{ NM} \qquad [22]$$

Once the amount of metabolized proteins (dP) is known from the measured urea or nitrogen in the urine, as shown in Eq. 22, the resolution of this system of equations allows the calculation of EE, dCH, and dF as a function of VO_2, VCO_2, and NM, as shown by Eqs. 23, 24, and 25.

$$\text{EE (kcal)} = 3.586 \text{ } VO_2 + 1.443 \text{ } VCO_2 - 1.180 \text{ NM} \qquad [23]$$

$$\text{dCH (g)} = 4.113 \text{ } VCO_2 - 2.907 \text{ } VO_2 - 2.544 \text{ NM} \qquad [24]$$

$$\text{dF (g)} = 1.689 \text{ } (VCO_2 - VO_2) - 1.943 \text{ NM} \qquad [25]$$

Equations 16, 17, and 18 give the amounts of endogenic water produced by each foodstuff, and the total endogenic water production can be derived as a function of VO_2, VCO_2, and NM, by Eq. 26:

$$H_2OM \text{ (g)} = 0.949 \text{ } VCO_2 - 0.141 \text{ } VO_2 - 1.220 \text{ NM} \qquad [26]$$

NM can be derived from the measurements of urea in the 24-hour urinary excretion.

Although VO_2 and VCO_2 correspond directly to the O_2 consumed and the CO_2 produced by the oxidation of nutrients during the measurement, the nitrogen measured in the urine (NM) does not correspond to the protein breakdown during the same period. There are indeed great variations of hourly urea excretions in a single day, and therefore the determination of protein breakdown from nitrogen excretion has to be performed over a 24-hour period. It has to be emphasized, however, that for energy expenditure measurements, the factor NM is negligible. If we look at Eq. 27:

$$\text{EE (kcal/min)} = 3.586 \text{ } VO_2 + 1.443 \text{ } VCO_2 - 1.180 \text{ NM} \qquad [27]$$

and assuming a VO_2 of 0.250 l/min, a VCO_2 of 0.225 l/min, and an NM of 0.01 g/min (values that are within normal range), the calculated value of EE will be 1,775.52 kcal/d. A 10% error in VO_2 would cause a 7% error in EE; a 10% error in VCO_2 would cause a 3% error in EE, whereas a 100% error in NM would only be responsible for a 1% error in EE. For acutely ill patients presenting a hypercatabolic state with large and variable levels of protein breakdown, EE can be calculated from VO_2 and VCO_2 only (without taking into account NM), with a maximum error of no more than 2% (7).

Although, it is obvious that energy expenditure can be accurately measured without measuring nitrogen excretion, when looking at Eqs. 24 and 25, the numerical factors of NM are relatively greater because the two first terms of the equation are substracted one from the other; therefore, when calculating the amounts of metabolized carbohydrates (ΔCH) and fat (ΔF), while neglecting NM, the errors become much greater than in the calculation of EE (7).

DOES PULMONARY COMPROMISE INTERACT WITH GAS EXCHANGE?

Gas exchange, or VO_2 and VCO_2, is *in fine* what is needed for and resulting from fuel utilization for energy production at the cellular level, whereas pulmonary compromise, by reducing the elimination of CO_2 and/or the absorption of O_2, modifies blood gases without altering VO_2 and VCO_2. This process is maintained up to the point that the actual transport of oxygen, its delivery to the tissues, or its utilization at the mitochondrial level is jeoparized. Such a critical state may occur in several pathologic cases, but in respiratory failure, the reduction in VO_2 ensues only at the endstage of severe adult respiratory distress syndrome (ARDS) and will in most instances precede fatality.

The effect of oxygen delivery (DO_2) on VO_2 is broadly discussed in the literature and it is well proved that increased DO_2 affects VO_2 only beyond the point at which there is a lack in oxygen delivery to the tissues and an induction of anaerobic metabolism is evidenced by an increase in lactic acid (8–12).

When measurements of VO_2 and of VCO_2 are performed in chronic obstructive pulmonary disease (COPD) patients with major reduction in lung function, there will be an increase in VO_2 and in VCO_2 indicating an increased work of breathing (2,13). These patients undergo substantial and progressive weight loss that can be attributed to both the increase in resting energy expenditure (REE) secondary to the increased work of breathing and to a reduced caloric intake secondary to the efforts required by food intake. Studies on COPD patients show that a mean body weight loss of 13% is associated with a 10% increase in metabolic rate, a poor prognosis and an increased morbidity and mortality (16,17). Gas exchange is also affected by the type of nutrients supplied to patients with pulmonary compromise. The administration of carbohydrates, fat, or amino acids in different proportions has a serious effect on gas exchange and may considerably alter respiratory function (18,19).

Malnutrition, which is a frequent state found not only in hospitalized patients but also among a large population all over the world, is by itself affecting the respiratory system. The specific effects of denutrition on the respiratory muscles were first described in 1916, by Fromme (20). In a large necropsy study, a linear relationship was shown between mean body weight loss and diaphragm weight loss. For a mean body weight loss of 23%, there was a corresponding loss of 22% in mean diaphragm weight (20). In a more recent study, Arora and Rochester (21) observed that for a mean body weight loss of 31%, the corresponding weight loss of the diaphragm reached 43%. Both studies demonstrated a relationship between respiratory muscle mass and body weight, suggesting that changes in nutritional status have direct consequences on diaphragm muscle mass. Respiratory muscle weight loss, had, of course, an immediate effect on respiratory muscle strength, which decreased from 96% of normal in a control group to 37% in malnourished patients, while the vital capacity in underweight patients decreased to 63% of the normal value. In the same group of patients, the maximum voluntary ventilation decreased from 80% in the control group to 41% in the underweight patients (22).

The specific effects of nutritional deprivation on respiratory physiology, however, was first described by Keys et al. (23). In that study, normal subjects were put on a semistarvation diet for 24 weeks. During this period, subjects lost 24% of their body weight and presented a simultaneous progressive decline in respiratory function measured by vital capacity (VC) and resting minute ventilation (VE). Both VC and VE returned to normal after 12 weeks of refeeding (23). The authors concluded that the reduction in respiratory function was probably due to respiratory muscle weakness. In relation to the aforementioned studies, although gas exchange was not measured, it may be assumed that if there were an alteration in gas exchange, it was mainly an increase in VO_2 and VCO_2 because a major manifestation of pulmonary compromise was proven to be related to an increase in work of breathing (3).

The oxygen cost of the work of breathing, which in normal individuals at rest is below 5% of the total oxygen consumption (VO_2), increases with minute ventilation, as well as in different states of respiratory disfunction and during weaning from artificial ventilation. In a study performed more than 15 years ago, a mean increase of 24% in VO_2 was shown in intensive care patients when disconnected from artificial ventilation (2). This increase in VO_2 in itself renders the weaning procedure more difficult. A reduction in VO_2 with a simultaneous reduction in VCO_2 should therefore be termed *metabolic defect* or *defect in energy expenditure,* being often the endpoint of what has been recently called "systemic inflammatory response syndrome" (SIRS), which may be considered an aspect of multiple organ failure (24). Gas exchange alteration, namely a reduction in VO_2, is generally a manifestation of a life-threatening condition and is in most instances independent of pulmonary compromise; this can be evinced in the following states:

1. In cardiogenic, septic, hypovolemic or other kinds of shock, where the reduction in gas exchange is due to a lack of oxygen delivery to the tissues (e.g., because of hemodynamic compromise and reduced oxygen transport), the lack in oxygen delivery will induce anaerobic metabolism and lactate production.

2. In injury or burn, the healing tissue uses glucose for glycolysis rather than for oxidation. Wound requirements have been measured by Wilmore et al. (25) in severely burned patients in whom one leg was either severely burned (50% of the leg) or lightly burned (10% of the leg). Blood flow, O_2 consumption, as well as glucose utilization and lactate production, were measured both in the whole body and in the single leg. No significant differences in whole-body blood flow or in VO_2 were observed between the patients with the large or the small leg burns. However, blood flow, glucose utilization, and lactate production were much higher in the legs with large burns than in the legs with small burns, although there was only a small difference in VO_2. Almost all of the glucose utilized was converted to lactate. Thus the major difference between the legs with large and small burns was due to a difference in the amount of glucose used for glycolysis, not for oxidation. The energy derived from glucose by glycolysis is about one twentieth of that obtained by oxidation, or 0.2 kcal/g of glucose.

3. A serious alteration in VO_2 and VCO_2 can be induced by severe CO intoxications. The great affinity of hemoglobin for CO shifts to the left the oxihemoglobin dissociation curve and induces a reduction in oxygen delivery to the tissues.

4. Cyanide intoxication inhibits cytochrome oxidase, thereby reducing oxygen uptake at the cellular level. This becomes evident by the increase in oxihemoglobin saturation, a reduced arteriovenous oxygen concentration difference, and also a reduction in VO_2. Because cyanide also severely reduces cardiac output, VO_2 is even more compomised in this type of intoxication. The combination of both CO and cyanide intoxication was reported in experimental studies to reduce VO_2 and VCO_2 by 70% (26).

5. Other toxic agents, such as H_2S (hydrogen sulfide) (27), reduce oxygen uptake and CO production by inhibiting cytochrome oxidase, or as fluoroacetate (28) by blocking the Kreb's cycle.

In conclusion, it may be suggested that it would be more appropriate to relate the terminology of gas exchange to the defining of the alteration in oxygen consumption and CO production rather than to the qualification of the pulmonary function. If there is agreement that respiratory exchange is related to VO_2 and VCO_2, pulmonary compromise will alter these parameters only in specific conditions. Emphysema and COPD, for instance, increase VO_2 and VCO_2 by increasing the work of breathing, whereas severe ARDS reduces VO_2 and VCO_2 only in extreme cases in which oxygen delivery decreases to the point that anaerobic metabolism and lactate production ensue. Other alterations in gas exchange occur in severe intoxications and in hemodynamic disorders.

REFERENCES

1. Osborn JJ, Elliot SE, Segger FJ, Gerbode F. Continuous measurement of lung mechanics and gas exchange in the critically ill. *Med Res Eng* 1969;8:19–23.
2. Bursztein S, Taitelman U, De Myttenaere S, et al. Reduced oxygen consumption in catabolic states with mechanical ventilation. *Crit Care Med* 1978;6:162–164.
3. Cherniak RM, Cheniak L, Naimark A. Work of breathing. In: *Respiration in Health and Disease*. Philadelphia: Saunders, 1972;44–52.
4. Bar Joseph G, Taitelman U, Saphar P, et al. Proceedings of the 1st Pan American Congress of Critical Care Medicine, Mexico, *Excerpta Medica,* September, 1979.
5. Kelman GR. Digital computer procedure for the conversion of PCO2 into blood CO2 content. *Respir Physiol* 1967;3:111–115.
6. Bursztein S, Elwyn DH, Askanazi J, et al. The theoretical framework of indirect calorimetry and energy balance. In: *Energy Metabolism, Indirect Calorimetry and Nutrition.* Baltimore: Williams and Wilkins, 1989;47–70.
7. Bursztein S, Elwyn DH, Saphar P, Singer P. Critical analysis of indirect calorimetry measurements. *Am J Clin Nutr* 1989;50:227–230.
8. Moshenifar Z, Goldbach P, Tashkind D, Campisi DJ. Relationship between O2 delivery and O2 consumption in the adult respiratory distress syndrome. *Chest* 1983;81:267–271.
9. Cain SM. Supply dependency of oxygen uptake in ARDS: myth or reality? *Am J Med Sci* 1984;288: 119–124.
10. Haup MT, Gilbert EM, Carlson RW. Fluid loading increases oxygen consumption in septic patients with lactic acidosis. *Am Rev Respir Dis* 1985;131:912–916.
11. Annat G, Viale JP, Percival C, et al. Oxygen delivery and uptake in the adult respiratory distress

syndrome. Lack of relationship when measured independently in patients with normal blood lactate concentrations. *Am Rev Respir Dis* 1986;133:999–1001.

12. Kruse JA, Haup MT, Puri VK, Carlson RW. Lactate levels between oxygen delivery and consumption in ARDS. *Chest* 1990;98:959–962.

13. Annat GJ, Viale JP, De Reymez CP, et al. Oxygen cost of breathing and diaphragmatic pressure-time index. Measurement in patients with COPD during weaning with pressure support ventilation. *Chest* 1990;98(2):412–414.

14. Vandenbergh E, Van de Woestijne KP, Gyselen A. Weight changes in the terminal stages of chronic obstructive pulmonary disease: relation to respiratory function and prognosis. *Am Rev Respir Dis* 1967;95:557–566.

15. Openbrier DR, Irwin MM, Dauber JH, et al. Factors affecting nutritional status and the impact of nutritional support in patients with emphysema. *Chest* 1984;85:675–695.

16. Goldstein MS, Askanazi J, Weissman C, et al. Energy expenditure in patients with chronic obstructive pulmonary disease. *Chest* 1987;91:222–224.

17. Elwyn DH, Kinney JM, Gump EE, et al. Some metabolic effects of fat infusions in depleted patients. *Metabolism* 1980;29:125–132.

18. Askanazi JF, Nordenstrom J, Rosenbaum SH, et al. Nutrition for the patients with respiratory failure: glucose versus fat. *Anesthesiology* 1980;54:373–377.

19. Askanazi JF, Weissman, Lasala P, et al. Effects of increasing protein intake on ventilatory drive. *Anesthesiology* 1984;60:106–110.

20. Fromme H. Systematische untersuchungen uber die Gewichtsverhaltnisse des Zwerchfells. *Virchows Arch* 1916;221:117–155.

21. Arora NS, Rochester DF. Effect of body weight and muscularity on human diaphragam muscle mass, thickness and area. *J Appl Physiol* 1982;52:63–70.

22. Arora NS, Rochester DF. Respiratory muscle strength and maximal voluntary ventilation in under-nourished patients. *Am Rev Respir Dis* 1982;126:5–8.

23. Keys A, Brozek J, Henschel A, et al. *Biology of Human Starvation.* Minneapolis: University of Minnesota Press, 1950;601–606.

24. Deby-Dupont G, Lamy M, Dby C, et al. Adult respiratory distress syndrome: local system disease. In: Cerra FB, ed. *Perspectives in Critical Care.* Quality Medical Publishing, 1991;57–83.

25. Wilmore DW, Aulick LH, Mason AD Jr, et al. The influence of the burn wound on local and systemic responses to injury. *Ann Surg* 1977;186:444–458.

26. Isserles SA, Taitelman U, Westely J, et al. The effect of normobaric oxygen and thiosulfate on physiological and analytical variables in a canine model of combined CO-CN poisoning. (Abstract). AACT/AAPCC/ABMT/CAPCC Scientific Meeting, Toronto, 1991.

27. Nichols P. The effect of sulphide on cytochrome a_3: isoteric and allosteric shifts of the reduced peak. *Biochim Biophys Acta* 1976;396:188–196.

28. Peters RA. Lethal synthesis (Croonian lecture). *Proc R Soc Lond [Biol]* 1952;143–170.

Organ Metabolism and Nutrition:
Ideas for Future Critical Care, edited by
J. M. Kinney and H. N. Tucker.
Raven Press, Ltd., New York © 1994.

23

Evolving Concepts in Multiple Organ Failure Syndrome

Frank B. Cerra

Department of Surgery, University of Minnesota Hospital and Clinic, Minneapolis, Minnesota 55455

The current concepts of multiple organ dysfunction and failure as a response to tissue injury have evolved over a number of years. In large part, the syndrome was recognized as the knowledge base and technology of critical care evolved and the process of death after serious injury was retarded. This clinical problem is now the major cause of morbidity, mortality, length of stay, and resource utilization in intensive care units treating surgical patients (1).

The host response to tissue injury appears to be a spectrum within which one can identify several basic patterns (2). With a single uncomplicated injury, the response peaks on days 3 to 5 postinjury and abates by days 7 to 10 (Fig. 1). With a severe injury, death can result rapidly either during or following resuscitation. In between these extremes, two other patterns emerge. In one, the response persists and a complication is present; the response abates when the complication is treated. In the second, the response continues unabated, even when a treatable problem is discovered and treated, multiple organs fail, and the patient expires.

This last response pattern is called multiple organ failure syndrome (MOFS). This response pathway of organ failure can be entered from the etiologies of infection, inadequate perfusion, soft tissue and bone injury, and persistent inflammatory processes such as pancreatitis and adult respiratory distress syndrome (ARDS) (2–6). Once response occurs, the clinical alterations in vital signs, physiology, and metabolism are not discriminated by the etiology, or, in the case of infection, by the kind of microorganisms involved. Hence, the concept of the systemic inflammatory response syndrome (SIRS) has evolved, with the term *sepsis* reserved for SIRS where there is evidence for an infection as the etiologic protagonist (7).

Typically, there is an episode of identifiable microcirculatory compromise followed by a resuscitation intervention. Organ dysfunction associated with the injury, shock, and resuscitation become manifest, as in pulmonary failure with ARDS or renal failure from acute tubular necrosis. The organ dysfunction that occurs at this time is referred to as primary organ dysfunction. The SIRS response then is manifest and pathways of late postinjury (secondary) organ dysfunction occur (1,8). In one pattern, frequently seen after a pulmonary initiating event such as aspiration, the secondary

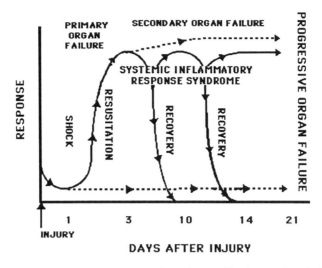

FIG. 1. Direct tissue injury from trauma or sepsis, or that resulting from reduced microcirculatory perfusion, induce responses described as shock-resuscitation and the systemic inflammatory response. Uncontrolled, these responses are associated with the development of multiple organ dysfunction and progressive organ failure and death.

organ dysfunction occurs very late (14 to 21 days). In another, commonly seen in septic shock with ARDS, multiple organ dysfunction is present from the time of injury. In both cases, the organ dysfunction can proceed to progressive organ failure and death (Fig. 2).

Several clinical settings are associated with the development of progressive organ failure (3–6,9). These include a persistent perfusion deficit, a persistent focus of infection, the combination of a perfusion deficit and a persistent septic focus, and a persistent inflammatory focus such as acute fulminant pancreatitis. There is increasing recognition, however, that a subgroup of patients is destined to develop MOFS irrespective of their management, and that there is another subgroup within which current therapy can successfully influence outcome (10).

The patients who develop the progressive form of the disease manifest increasing jaundice, biliary stasis, reduced hepatic amino acid extraction, and reduced hepatic and total body protein synthesis in the presence of nutrition support; increased hepatic triglyceride production (predominantly very low density lipoprotein [VLDL]) with reduced peripheral triglyceride clearance, increased ureagenesis with prerenal azotemia, reduced hepatic redox potential as reflected in the betahydroxybutyrate/ acetoacetate ratio, and, terminally, a failure of glucose release and hypoglycemia (10–12).

The transition to MOFS heralds a change in mortality risk from the 40% to 60% range to the 90% to 100% range. The current methodologies for risk assessment do not allow identification of the patients who will develop this problem (13). Current technologic methods of organ support, such as hemodialysis or its hemoperfusion variants, have also not been demonstrated to improve outcome (1,11).

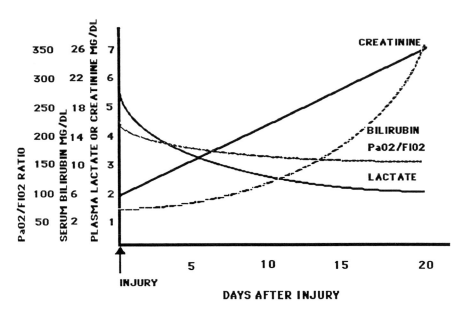

FIG. 2. The clinical manifestations of MOFS appear over time and are usually heralded by a progressive rise in serum bilirubin (secondary hepatic failure). It is probable that the propensity to develop MOFS occurs during shock-resuscitation and is enhanced by a persistent systemic inflammatory response.

Thus, the clinical characterization of MOFS is that of a defined injury associated with circulatory compromise followed by resuscitation. The postresuscitative response then depends on the severity of injury, the organ reserve of the patient at the time of injury, the time lapse before instituting effective treatment, the adequacy of the treatment instituted, and the number and severity of subsequent injuries and complications. This postresuscitative response and its associated primary organ failures manifests as SIRS. Secondary organ dysfunction then occurs, as in liver and kidney. The SIRS and secondary organ dysfunction may abate or may progress to organ failure and death (Table 1).

TABLE 1. *Characteristics of progressive MOFS.*

Progressive rise in serum bilirubin and creatinine
Falling or low plasma visceral protein levels that are nonresponsive to nutrition support
Elevated plasma lactate with a normal lactate/pyruvate ratio
Rising plasma triglyceride level and betahydroxybutyrate/acetoacetate ratio and an RQ >1 in the absence of excess glucose administration
Increased urinary nitrogen excretion with an inability to maintain nitrogen balance; usually associated with a picture of progressive prerenal azotemia when adequate renal blood flow appears present, and in the absence of nutrition support
Rising plasma levels of hepatically extracted amino acids such as phenylalanine
A plasma polyunsaturated fatty acid profile in the phospholipid fraction that resembles that of hepatic failure

---

PHYSIOLOGY AND METABOLISM

The physiology and metabolism of shock, resuscitation, SIRS, and MOFS have been described in a large number of research publications and reviews and are not discussed in this paper (1,2,10,11). Several aspects of these phenomena, however, are reviewed as they pertain to the current understanding of MOFS.

The onset of the postresuscitative systemic inflammatory response is usually heralded by pulmonary insufficiency, frequently requiring mechanical ventilation, and by a hyperdynamic physiologic response (1). The pneumonitis or the acute lung injury may become the persistent focus that is associated with the systemic inflammatory response and the risk of MOFS (14,15). A primary event in the systemic physiologic response seems to be an increase in demand for oxygen consumption. This demand must be met by an increase in supply. The inability to achieve this balance of oxygen delivery and demand is associated with an increased mortality risk (11,16–18).

In patients with low flow, flow-dependent oxygen consumption is observed during resuscitation (17–20). In a subgroup of patients, usually with sepsis, flow-dependent oxygen consumption cannot be successfully treated, and continued increases in oxygen delivery are met with increases in oxygen consumption (17,18). This group of patients is at very high risk to develop progressive MOFS. The origin of the phenomenon is unclear.

The decrease in systemic vascular resistance appears to be independent of flow and presumably is a response to the primary increase in tissue oxygen consumption demand (11). This reduction in vascular resistance, however, is not homogeneous in all vascular beds (21). In acute unresuscitated shock, vascular resistance in increased and flow is reduced in the visceral compartment. Restoration of visceral compartment perfusion appears to lag behind the skeletal muscle compartment where vascular resistance is reduced and flow is increased and may take several days before resuscitation is complete, even though the usual criteria of systemic resuscitation have been met (22). The clinical finding is one of delayed return of the plasma lactate to within a normal range in the presence of a normal lactate/pyruvate ratio.

An extraction failure of oxygen in the peripheral microcirculation also commonly occurs (2,11). Many consider that the elevated lactate frequently observed in MOFS confirms the extraction defect. This increased lactate, however, is not necessarily associated with the other metabolic characteristics of anaerobic metabolism and does not necessarily imply an energy deficit. In resuscitated patients it appears to reflect the presence of aerobic glycolysis as the dominant metabolism for energy production. Energy production per se does not appear to be a significant problem in patients who are adequately resuscitated (23).

Postresuscitative hypermetabolism occurs irrespective of the etiology of MOFS and is characteristic of SIRS and the organ dysfunction process (24). The metabolic responses are regulated and dependent on the degree of injury, type and severity of underlying disease, type and dose of medications, and the prior treatment received Table 2. The regulatory mechanisms serve to modulate basic cell functions such

TABLE 2. *Cytokine effects.**

Effects	Cell function (T and B cell)
	Parenchyme function (liver acute-phase protein)
	Vascular physiology (vasodilation)
	Systemic responses (fever, anorexia)
	Metabolic regulation (LPL, PDH)
	Injury protection
Regulation of effects	Single-agent and combination
	Dose-response
	Associated factors (LPS)
	Local and systemic

* Cytokines are regulatory molecules.
LPL, lipoprotein lipase; PDH, pyruvate dehydrogenase; LPS, lipopolysac-charide.

as energy production and distribution, the synthesis of structural and nonstructural compounds, biotransformation and detoxification reactions, and cell division.

A major clinical feature of the postresuscitative phase of organ dysfunction is the alteration in body composition (23,25–27). Systemic interstitial edema occurs and the skeletal muscle mass rapidly disappears, the latter process often being referred to as autocannibalism (23). The lean body mass (LBM) disappears at a rate that exceeds that anticipated from bedrest or as a result of the use of paralyzing agents and closely correlates with the net nitrogen loss, frequently exceeding 20 to 30 g/d in such injuries as burns or closed head trauma. The use of nutrition support can counter the nitrogen loss, but is unable to reclaim the LBM as long as the inflammatory process is active (23). The LBM is used for energy production, support of gluconeogenesis in liver in kidney, and to support protein synthetic functions in the visceral organs, wounds, the mononuclear cell mass, and areas of increased energy expenditure (2).

Energy expenditure is also increased proportionate to the degree of injury and is reflected in increased oxygen consumption and carbon dioxide production (2,27). The endogenous respiratory quotient (RQ) ranges from 0.78 to 0.85, reflecting mixed oxidation of carbohydrate, fat, and amino acids. This increased energy expenditure is supported by an oxidative process best described as aerobic glycolysis (2,11,23,24) (Table 3, Fig. 3). The production of adenosine triphosphate is efficiently maintained in the presence of adequate resuscitation, with a failure of energy production occurring

TABLE 3. *Observed characteristics of aerobic glycolysis.*

Reduction in oxidation of pyruvate
Increased use of fat and amino acids as oxidative substrate
Normal lactate/pyruvate ratio
Normal acetoacetate/betahydroxybutyrate ratio
Formation and release of large amounts of alanine (pyruvate + amino group) and glutamine
(from transamination of glutamate) in relationship with lactate and pyruvate

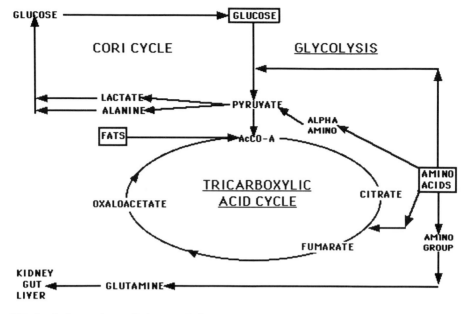

FIG. 3. In the postresuscitative metabolic response, energy production appears to occur by an altered form of aerobic metabolism best described as aerobic glycolysis. A mixture of carbohydrate, fat, and amino acids is oxidized for the production of high-energy phosphates in the tricarboxylic acid cycle.

primarily during perfusion shock and as a terminal event in MOFS (2,11,28). The metabolic parameters observed are not consistent with persistent microcirculatory hypoxia or vascular shunting of significant magnitude to effect adequate energy availability.

Within the limits of this regulated response, an excess of total calories or an excess of glucose calories can have a number of detrimental effects: fatty liver syndrome, hyperosmolar states, excess carbon dioxide production, increased oxygen consumption, stimulation of catecholamine release, increased lactate formation, a failure to suppress gluconeogenesis, and a failure to alter catabolic or synthetic rates (29–34). The turnover of short-, medium-, and long-chain fatty acids is also increased (35,36). The liver releases increased amounts of VLDL triglyceride and the peripheral clearance of triglyceride is reduced, in part reflecting a reduced lipoprotein lipase activity in skeletal muscle and adipose tissue. Tumor necrosis factor (TNF) has been implicated as one mechanism for this reduced lipase activity (37). The plasma polyunsaturated fatty acid profile comes to resemble that reported for hepatic failure. Administering long-chain fatty acid lipid can increase the metabolism of arachidonic acid with an increased production of its metabolites. Long-chain fatty acid triglyceride emulsions in doses exceeding 1.5 g/kg/d have been associated with increased bacteremia rates, acute hypoxemia, and suppression of in vitro tests of lymphocyte function (35,38). The catabolic rate is relatively unresponsive to exogenous amino acids

TABLE 4. *Summary overview.*

Clinical presence	Reduced microcirculatory perfusion	Resuscitation	Systemic inflammatory response	Progressive organ failure
Pathogenesis/ mechanisms of regulation and injury	Oxygen deprivation Activation of compliment, coagulation, PMNs, endothelial cell; eicosinoids Macrohormone release Mechanical effects of the injury	Local injury —oxygen radicals, cytokine, Pg Systemic injury— endothelial cells, macrophage, LPS release from gut, nitric oxide, eicosinoids	Macrohormone release Cell-cell communication— endothelial cell; fixed macrophage; cytokines, eicosinoids Molecular regulation	Dyshomeostatic organ cell regulation Molecularly mediated death
Therapy	Source control	Restore oxygen transport Antibody against LPS, cytokine effects	Nutrition support ω-3 PUFA, Arg, RNA Monoclonal/ polyclonal antibody	Prevention

(2,23,39). The total body synthetic rate, however, does respond. As the dose of exogenous amino acids is increased, the synthetic rate increases until it equals the catabolic rate, at which point, nitrogen equilibrium is achieved. Approximately 1.5 to 2.0 g/kg/d of protein (amino acids) is needed to achieve this relationship. The nitrogen retained, however, does not accrue in LBM (23,33).

PATHOGENESIS

The patients who develop MOFS sustain a period of reduced microcirculatory perfusion followed by a resuscitation intervention and then manifest a SIRS with progressive multiple organ dysfunction and failure in those patients who expire. The shock-resuscitation interval is associated with primary organ dysfunction; the persistent SIRS is associated with secondary organ dysfunction that results in death if SIRS becomes progressive. Time is a key variable in the manifestation of the clinical response (2). Thus, the response is a time continuum within which one can identify clusters of clinically recognizable constellations of symptoms, signs, and laboratory tests, e.g., shock, SIRS, MOFS. Even though the manifestations differ in each of the time-based clusters, pathogenic events in an earlier time most likely effect the pathogenic events in a later time. In addition, operator-dependent variables at all points in the course are also likely to effect both pathogenesis and responses. The pathogenesis must, then, explain the time course and the observed clinical manifestations. Table 4 presents a scheme that coordinates the clinical events and manifestations with potential pathogenic mechanisms. Given the uncertainties concerning pathogenesis, such a scheme would represent hypotheses to be tested. In addition, it would provide a framework within which to develop and test new therapies.

Interestingly, the same injury can be associated with death in shock, death following resuscitation, recovery, or progressive MOFS (10). Some of the explanations for this phenomenon include what organs are injured and how severely they are injured; preexisting disease as it effects the "reserve" of such response systems as the cardiovascular system and such operator-dependent variables as the time from injury to treatment; and the adequacy of the treatment received. The implication, however, is that there may be a genetic component to the response itself (10).

The clinical time course implies that the pathogenic mechanisms change over time (Table 4). The initial event is an injury to tissue followed by reduced microcirculatory perfusion in the area of injury, or reduced perfusion alone. Examples of the former would include trauma, a local infection, or pancreatitis; examples of the latter would include penetrating vascular trauma or a ruptured abdominal aortic aneurysm.

When the reduction in circulating volume is significant, not necessarily accompanied by a reduction in blood pressure, alterations in systemic perfusion occur. These alterations are regional and dependent on the degree and type of injury and adequacy of the cardiovascular response. Vasoconstriction occurs first in the splanchnic viscera and skin, then in the extremities with preservation of the cardiocerebral axis until the low perfusion state becomes severe, at which time cardiocerebral perfusion can also be reduced. Within individual organs in the areas of reduced flow, total volume flow is reduced and the distribution of flow may also be altered. This altered flow distribution may take the form of corticomedullary shunting in the kidney or capillary dilatation in the viscera. In endotoxemia, this altered microcirculatory regulation results in a very poor relationship between oxygen delivery and capillary recruitment. Endothelial injury occurs in the area of local trauma as well as in these areas of underperfusion (40–42). The injury results from direct effects of oxygen deprivation and/or products of infecting agents, from activation of the contact systems of the coagulation and compliment cascades, and from the release of eicosinoids, nitric oxide, endothelin, and the inflammatory mediators. Platelets and white cells become activated and adhere to endothelial cells, and endothelial cells release cytokine and eicosanoid (41–44). Thus, there is microcirculatory stagnation, coagulation, initiation of inflammation, and injury to endothelial cells and associated parenchymal cells both within the area of primary injury and in the systemic response areas (Fig. 4).

There is also activation of the neurohumoral system with increased autonomic tone, release of cortisol, catecholamine, aldosterone, antidiuretic hormone, glucagon, insulin, and other hormones (45–48). This neurohumoral response mediates the systemic physiologic response and initiates the flow of metabolic substrate to support that response.

Resuscitation restores perfusion in the microcirculation. With reperfusion, new mechanisms of injury occur, both in the area of injury and systemically. The degree of injury depends on how much shock occurred, how long it persisted, and on the kind and quality of resuscitation performed. There are a number of mediators of reperfusion injury: prostaglandins such as thromboxane/prostacycline; leukotrienes such as LTB_{4-6}; nitric oxide and endothelin; polymorphonuclear neutrophil (PMN) adhesion and transmigration with oxygen radical release; release of platelet-activating

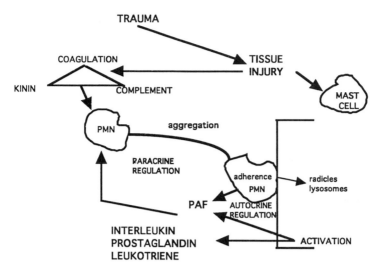

FIG. 4. Injury and reduced perfusion activate the contact system, promote platelet and polymorphonuclear leukocyte adhesion, and the transmigration of the leukocytes. A number of paracrine and autocrine regulatory systems promote the release of eicosinoids and cytokines.

factor (PAF) and of endothelially-released cytokine such as interleukin-1 (IL-1) (47–52).

In the gut, the sequence of ischemia-reperfusion alters the mucosal barrier. In animal models, this can result in translocation of bacteria into the regional lymph nodes and into the viscera (53,54). There is no evidence to date in humans, however, to indicate that translocation is a pathogenic mechanism. In patients sustaining major blunt trauma requiring laparotomy, the portal vein was aspirated for several days postinjury and did not demonstrate either the presence of microorganisms or lipopolysaccharide (LPS), even though SIRS was present (55,56). Intestinal permeability, however, is altered in both animal models and in humans, presumably reflecting the accompanying mucosal injury. This altered permeability barrier can result in the efflux of toxin from the gut into the local and systemic circulation.

With reperfusion, the local response products become systemic, as do the products of tissue injury, such as tissue and intravascularly derived peptides (Fig. 5). A systemic response appears, generally manifested by changes in temperature, blood pressure, skin perfusion, WBC count, and primary organ dysfunction such as acute lung injury. The effluent from the local injury site and visceral response areas appears to either cause or potentiate injury at distant organs. In severe cases of muscle underperfusion, the rhabdomyolysis that appears with reperfusion also contributes to the distant organ injury, as in myoglobin-induced renal dysfunction. The IL-1 released from the local site might induce systemic nitric oxide production from endothelial cells, either causing or potentiating a fall in systemic vascular resistance (50,51, 57–59). The PAF and IL-1 together with PMNs primed for adherence may injure pulmonary endothelium and result in acute lung injury (51). The leukotriene released

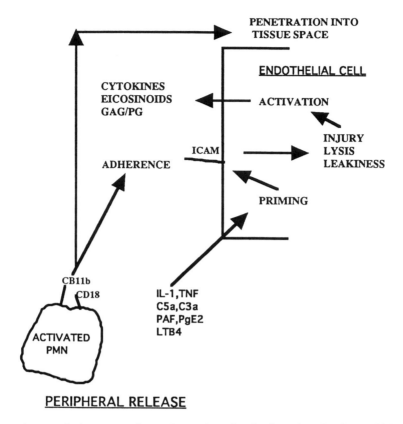

PERIPHERAL RELEASE

FIG. 5. As resuscitation occurs, the products released and cells activated at the local injury site are released into the systemic circulation. These products and activated cells can induce injury and response in distant sites such as the lung.

with liver reperfusion may also contribute to the pulmonary endothelial injury and the reduced contractile function and noncompliance of the ventricles of the heart. Tumor necrosis factor released systemically may also contribute to vasodilatation and parenchymal cell injury (37,60–62).

The macrophage populations become activated. A number of initiating mechanisms are present and include LPS, bacteria, cytokines, hypoxia, PAF, and interferon (63,64). This phenomena initiates and probably sustains the persistent systemic inflammatory response.

One of the major controversies in the SIRS response is whether inadequate microcirculatory perfusion persists after resuscitation has been completed. The data would suggest that some organs, particularly liver, do not have a return of normal perfusion for 2 to 3 days after resuscitation has been completed using systemic criteria (22). After adequate initiation and maintenance of resuscitation, however, oxygen delivery and subsequent energy production and availability appear to be adequate. The biochemical and metabolic studies indicate aerobic glycolysis as the basis for energy production. This altered form of substrate oxidation appears, at least in part, to be regulated by cytokine effects on the enzyme systems (posttranslation regulation), particularly the dehydrogenase enzymes that regulate the tricarboxylic acid cycle (37,50,62,65). Energy availability, even though proton transport may not be entirely normal, does not seem to become a clinically significant problem again until the late phase of progressive MOFS, as long as oxygen delivery is maintained at an appropriate level.

The activated macrophage populations modulate their associated parenchyme through autocrine/paracrine mechanisms (cell-cell interaction) (63,64,66,67). This phenomenon has been modeled in macrophage–liver cell cultures evaluating the regulation of hepatocellular protein synthesis (Figure 6). The activated macrophage releases cytokine (e.g., IL-1, IL-6, TNF) and prostaglandins (e.g., PGE2) that simulate total hepatocellular protein synthesis with a relative augmentation in acute-phase protein synthesis (e.g., C-reactive protein) (64). When enough mediator is released, total hepatocellular protein synthesis decreases, mainly due to a decrease in non-acute-phase protein synthesis (e.g., albumin, transferrin). This decrease in total protein synthesis is associated with reduced mitochondrial proton transport and strongly correlates with nitric oxide formation by the liver cell (68). The liver cell releases a number of mediators that maintain the release of Kupffer cell mediator (66,67). Thus, a paracrine-regulated system is present that amplifies itself once initiated. This process is also influenced by a number of other mechanisms. The high amino acid delivery rate drives the synthesis by direct substrate induction. Cortisol activates a soluble cell membrane receptor that then stimulates gene transcription for a number of acute-phase reactants. Interestingly, the stimulation ceases soon after the cortisol is removed from the system. Certain acute-phase proteins can be directly stimulated by LPS without macrophage mediation (63). It appears to act through the protein kinase C transduction system and directly modulate transcription. Cytokine activates the G-protein signal transduction system of the cell membrane and then modulates gene transcription through phosphorylation and protein kinase reactions. This mechanism

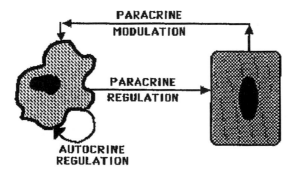

FIG. 6.   The Kupffer cells regulate liver cell function. The liver cells also modulate Kupffer cell function. These autocrine and paracrine mechanisms may serve to sustain the inflammatory response.

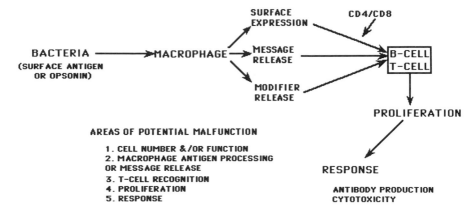

FIG. 7. The inflammatory state also modulates immune function. Two general manifestations of these effects are a reduced ability of macrophages to process and present antigens and a reduced capacity of lymphocytes to undergo proliferative responses.

produces a sustained effect on protein synthesis that lasts for days after removal of the cytokine.

These forms of metabolic regulation can explain a number of the observed metabolic-physiologic responses observed in SIRS. Another consequence of the inflammatory state is a compromised immune system and an increased susceptibility to infection. Hemorrhage and tissue injury result in a number of alterations in T cell function (69–72) (Figure 7). The ability of CD4 and CD8 cells to become activated by specific or nonspecific antigen is diminished. There is reduced release by CD4 Th1 cells of TNF, IL-2, and interferon (IFN), and an increased release by CD4 Th2 cells of IL-4, IL-5, and IL-10. In addition, there are excessive amounts of prostaglandin E2 in the cell-cell interaction milieu (73). The net result of this altered signaling is a reduced capacity of antigen processing and presentation function and reduced proliferative responses by the T cell system (69–73).

Nosocomial infections are acquired after an injury. The major sites are sinuses, lower respiratory tract, invasive lines or prosthetic devices, and urinary tract. Most of the epidemiology in this area documents that the organisms involved tend to be those harbored in the skin and gastrointestinal tract. Within a few days of injury, the enteral flora will have colonized the skin, upper gut, and respiratory tract in up to 80% of patients. Within 7 to 10 days of injury, up to 80% of those colonized will manifest a nosocomial infection. Infections with such organisms as *Pseudomonas* species, *Enterobacter* or *Klebsiella* species, *Candida* species or *Staphylococcus epidermis* are characteristic of the organ failure process (74–75). The precise pathogenesis of these nosocomial infections remains controversial, as does their role in the pathogenesis of MOFS. Because the infecting agents seem to arise, in part, from the gut, selective gut decontamination (SDD) has been employed as a method to control them. The technique is one of administering poorly absorbed antibiotics by the oral-nasogastric route, to selectively suppress the aerobic flora that reside in gut lumen without significant suppression of the anaerobes residing in the crypts. The results of the studies indicate a reduction of nosocomial infections by 50% to 80%, depending on the definitions used. However, there have been no significant alterations in the occurrence of organ failures, gross mortality, organ failure mortality, or infection-related mortality (76,77). Thus, a patient with MOFS may expire with a nosocomial infection and *not as a result of* a nosocomial infection.

The transition to progressive MOFS remains the most problematic area of investigation. While the cell-cell interaction mechanisms are homeostatic, it has been difficult to prove that they are capable of causing irreversible cell injury and dysfunction in a manner that reproduces the clinical syndrome of progressive MOFS. The mediator systems are also cytoprotective and promote tissue repair. It is possible that toxic substances might be present, although their existence remains elusive in this late form of the disease. Current thinking implicates molecular mechanisms as an explanation for the transition (78–80). There are two lines of experimentation.

The first is that the accumulated injuries reach a threshold at which gene-mediated self-destruction occurs (apoptosis). The second hypothesis takes into account the time-based pathogenesis of progressive MOFS. During the omeostatic response, pathways of protein synthesis become up-regulated and obligate the flow of energy and substrate away from the production of constitutive functions (e.g., structural components). When a threshold of injury occurs, the heat shock genes are expressed and further divert the flow of energy and substrate. The result is a reduced constitutive capacity of the cell and a progressive loss of cell integrity. This process appears to be initiated, at least in part, by oxygen radicals released early in the injury process (79,80). It is not necessary to hypothesize that individual cell death needs to occur in order to explain organ and systemic dysfunction. Rather, only enough cell dysfunction needs to be present to interfere with organ function or that upsets interorgan balance in ways that are not consistent with life.

THERAPEUTIC APPROACHES

Current therapy of MOFS focuses on prevention of organ injury and at supportive care; a cure for established MOFS does not exist at this time. Three types of therapy are emphasized: source control, restoration, and maintenance of microcirculatory perfusion and metabolic support (Fig. 8). Persistence of a source assures a high risk of both a developing MOFS and a high mortality from it. Whenever possible, complete control or removal of the cause of the inflammatory response is desirable, as in surgical control of bleeding, early drainage of an abscess, and full-thickness burn excision and skin grafting for third degree burns. In many cases, however, this is not possible, as in primary pneumonias, pancreatitis, soft-tissue injury, and hemorrhage into soft tissues. In these cases, efforts to minimize the cause should be rapidly

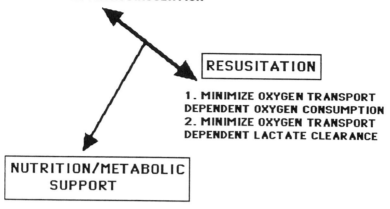

FIG. 8. The current approach to MOFS is one of prevention. The mainstays of prevention are source control, resuscitation of the microcirculation, and nutrition-metabolic support.

instituted, such as fracture fixation and appropriate antimicrobial agents. In iatrogenically immune-suppressed patients, minimizing the dose of immune suppressive agents during critical illness is also associated with improved survival.

The pulmonary events in MOFS are related to the primary lung injury or pathology, the development of acute lung injury, the mechanics of meeting the ventilatory demands of the systemic response, and the methods of mechanical ventilation (14,15). Primary lung injury is usually in the form of aspiration, lung contusion, or inhalation injury. Primary lung pathology usually occurs as a bacterial pneumonitis. The primary lung injury or pathology can trigger acute lung injury and can become the persistent inflammatory focus that drives the SIRS response. Nosocomial pneumonitis can also occur as a secondary infection during the course of MOFS; selective gut decontamination can significantly reduce its incidence.

Typically 15 to 20 liters of minute ventilation and an oxygen consumption index over 160 ml/min are necessary to meet the ventilatory and respiratory demands of the patient. The combination of the ventilatory demand and the intrinsic lung pathology usually necessitate mechanical ventilation. There is increasing recognition that the method of mechanical ventilation can prolong the mechanical ventilation interval, contribute to the lung pathology, and, perhaps, increase the overall mortality. Modes of ventilation that utilize high peak inspiratory pressures, high inspiratory plateau pressures, and high mean pressures are associated with these adverse outcomes. These observations have led to the development of alternate modes of ventilation that have minimized these pressure endpoints, modes such as pressure-limited and inverse ratio ventilation (81). Definitive demonstration that these new modes of ventilation improve outcome awaits clinical testing. An adverse effect of these modes of ventilation is also present. They usually require heavy sedation and neuromuscular paralysis to be effective. These latter modalities have been associated with increased wasting of LBM and neuromuscular injury. The neuromuscular injury is primarily motor in type, whereas that associated with the MOFS process appears to be both sensory and motor (82). In animal models, high inspired oxygen tensions are associated with pulmonary pathology similar to that seen in autopsy analysis of lungs from patients that have expired from ARDS. Evidence of inspired oxygen injury in humans has yet to be demonstrated. Because it has been demonstrated that ARDS is not a homogeneous disease and that there are areas of normal lung, the feeling remains that as low an inspired oxygen tension as possible should be maintained. Most patients with ARDS do not die from their pulmonary failure. It has become clear that in most cases, a systemic process is present and is the primary determinant of outcome (14,15).

Rapid and effective systemic resuscitation is a major therapeutic endpoint. The primary events in the systemic physiologic response seem to be both a reduction in systemic vascular resistance and an increase in demand for oxygen consumption. A critical level of oxygen delivery is present below which oxygen consumption becomes supply dependent. In addition, the extraction ratio at which supply dependency exists is reduced, a phenomenon that, along with the increase in oxygen demand, increases the risk of supply dependency being present. The usual clinical criteria of resuscitation (i.e., pulse, blood pressure, urine output, skin perfusion) do not appear sensitive enough to indicate when oxygen delivery is equal to oxygen demand in these clinical settings. Rather, invasive monitoring during the shock-resuscitation phase with measurements of oxygen delivery and consumption appear to be necessary (83–85).

The inability to achieve a balance of oxygen delivery and demand is associated with an increased mortality (2,11). This presence of supply dependency necessitates an increase in oxygen delivery. The inability to achieve the increased delivery generally occurs for one of four reasons: inadequate preload, preexisting cardiac disease, acquired cardiac dysfunction, or as a manifestation of the underlying metabolic dysfunction of the organ failure process. Preexisting cardiac disease that limits flow, such as valvular cardiac pathology, or that precludes an adequate muscle response, such as previous scarring from myocardial infarction or cardiomyopathy, necessitates interventional manipulation if there is to be adequate oxygen delivery. Acquired myocardial dysfunction is also common. The acquired dysfunction can result from reduced ventricular preload if there has been inadequate fluid resuscitation, probably the most common reason for inadequate cardiac performance. The acquired ventricular dysfunction causes either a reduction in contractile performance or a disorder of diastolic compliance (86,87). The compliance dysfunction has two components: ventricular dilation with an increase in end-diastolic volume and a decrease in ventricular wall compliance. In these settings, adequate function of the ventricles requires a higher than expected pulmonary capillary wedge pressure, increase volume administration, and inotropic support, frequently with the addition of a systemic unloading agent.

Clinically relevant, flow-dependent oxygen consumption is treated with a comprehensive approach. Arterial blood oxygen content is increased by oxygen tension that will maintain over 90% saturation of the hemoglobin in the presence of a hemoglobin concentration in the 11 to 12 gm% range. Oxygen delivery is then increased until there is no clinically relevant increase in oxygen consumption and the lactate pyruvate ratio or plasma lactate returns to a normal range. There is a subgroup of patients in whom this goal cannot be achieved; they usually develop progressive MOFS (83,84). Even though this approach can reduce morbidity and mortality, a significant percentage of patients will still develop SIRS and MOFS in the presence of the high flow state and in the absence of a demonstrable oxygen deficit or inadequacy of energy supply. The implication is that some other nutrient has become supply dependent, a hypothesis that is currently receiving experimental attention (27).

The use of fluids for resuscitation usually raises concerns about the occurrence of interstitial edema, particularly in the lungs. Indeed, the level at which the pulmonary capillary wedge pressure should be maintained is a great clinical controversy. Lower wedge pressures are associated with reduced lung water, and patients who manifest less systemic interstitial edema have improved outcomes. When this reduced level of wedge pressure is associated with reduced volume perfusion, however, an increased incidence of organ failure is present. Patients in whom the increase in extracellular water can be maintained appear to develop fewer infectious complications (88).

Within the confines of these observations, the type and volume of fluid and pharmacologic support can be chosen to allow reasonable microcirculatory perfusion while "trading one organ off against another." For example, in order to achieve adequate systemic resuscitation in the presence of a noncompliant ventricle, it may be necessary to use a capillary wedge pressure that promotes more lung water; the presence of an acute closed head injury may necessitate crystalloid restriction and the use of larger particle-based solutions to maintain blood volume and preload.

Starvation malnutrition is both a comorbidity-comortality, and acquired malnutrition is also a primary manifestation of persistent SIRS and of MOFS. It seems increasingly clear that current nutrition support does not alter the course of the disease process itself. Rather, standard nutrition support can effectively manage single nutrient and generalized nutrient deficiencies resulting in a small but significant reduction in morbidity and mortality. Research in this area also indicates that the enteral route of nutrition and metabolic support, although associated with equivalent, measured nutritional outcomes relative to parenteral nutrition, is associated with improved disease-related and patient-related outcomes. The findings include a reduction in acquired infectious complications, a reduced duration of infectious complications, an attenuation of the hormonal response to injury, a reduction in the length of stay in those patients who will survive the organ dysfunction process, and a more cost-effective use of resources. In addition, the earlier the enteral nutrition is initiated postinjury, the greater the outcome effects observed (89).

It has become quite clear that the metabolism of patients with SIRS and MOFS is quite different than that of nonstressed, fasting humans. Application of the nutrition support principles used in simple starvation can be detrimental to this group of patients. Thus, to minimize complications and to maximize the benefits, a different group of nutrient administration goals have been developed (2,89):

1. Avoid overfeeding by providing no more than 20 to 25 total calories/kg/d with 3 to 5 g/kg/d as glucose.
2. Avoid feeding with anything but glucose, vitamins, minerals, and trace elements during shock.
3. Begin enteral nutrients as soon as resuscitation is complete, even if full volume enteral feeding cannot be achieved.
4. Avoid administering long-chain, polyunsaturated ω-6 fatty acids (ω-3 PUFA) in doses that exceed 1.5 g/kg/d.
5. Start amino acids or protein at 1.5 g/kg/d. Promote nitrogen retention by adjusting the dose of amino acids every 5 to 7 days. Current clinical studies indicate that the modified amino acids are a more efficient protein source and can facilitate nitrogen retention with a higher rate of protein synthesis and less ureagenesis than the standard amino acid formulas (90).
6. Provide increased quantities of zinc and magnesium and vitamin E to prevent acute deficiencies and to maximize antioxidant potential.

There is also increasing data that the timing of initiation of enteral feeding is important in achieving the beneficial outcomes. Waiting until the inflammatory response is established to begin enteral nutrition appears to have no outcome benefit over total parenteral nutrition (TPN) (91). There appears to be no benefit in patient outcome with small peptide formulas. The role of mucosotrophic agents such as glutamine, ketone bodies, and bombesin remains to be clarified. As yet, clinical trials have not demonstrated nutritional or outcome efficacy relative to standard nutrition for these agents in patients who have sustained surgical trauma.

In spite of these approaches to prevention and treatment, the morbidity and mortality rates in patients with persistent SIRS and MOFS remain substantially elevated even in the younger age groups. With the concept that the response to injury may also contribute to the morbidity, mortality, and resource costs, new therapies are being directed at modulating the inflammatory response. These approaches are both specific and nonspecific. Specific therapy is targeted against a defined mediator, such as endotoxin, IL-1 receptors, or TNF. Nonspecific therapy is directed at altering the responses to the mediators of the metabolic response to injury at the cellular level, such as second messenger generation (Figs. 9, 10).

One of the most well-studied specific therapies is the use of antibodies directed against endotoxin from gram-negative bacteria (92,93). The rationale is that such agents would prevent or ameliorate direct cell injury from LPS and reduce the amount

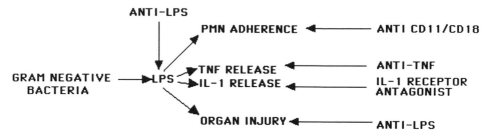

FIG. 9. The persistent inflammatory response may become a pathogenic mechanism for the development of progressive MOFS. One approach to the management of MOFS is to provide agents directed at specific mediators of that response.

of inflammatory response that occurs. In addition, it is becoming clear that lytic antibiotics may increase the endotoxin load; and it has been hypothesized that anti-endotoxin therapy may be useful in settings where lytic antibiotics have been administered. To date, the clinical trials have been disappointing and have generated a lot of new questions. At least two monoclonal antibodies targeted against LPS have not shown clinical efficacy and may have adverse effects in control populations. Experience with IL-1 receptor antagonist (IL-1ra) indicates that effectiveness is related to the mortality risk of the patient (94). Patients with a high mortality risk at the time of administration appear to have an outcome benefit; those with a low mortality risk appear to experience a greater risk of an adverse outcome. This may also be the case with antibodies directed against TNF. Many questions remain and are in stages of testing: How many doses; how much efficacy in the absence of gram-negative bacteremia but in settings where LPS is thought to be a significant mediator; what is the timing of administration relative to antibiotics and surgical intervention, and timing and dose relative to the onset of the inflammatory response?

Currently, either in testing or going into testing are a number of monoclonal antibodies targeted to interfere with PMN adherence and transmigration (anti–CD 18 or –CD 11). Data are not yet available for analysis. However, a number of questions and concerns are present and are related to dosing, the timing of their use, and

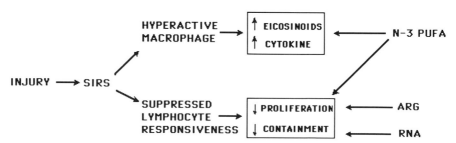

FIG. 10. Another approach to modulating the inflammatory response and restore immune function is to alter cellular responses to the mediators of inflammation. Nutrients have been identified that may have this capacity. These nutrients include fish oils, arginine, and uracil.

adverse reactions. This is true regardless of whether or not there will be reasonable efficacy because they are too well targeted, leaving many alternate mediator pathways available.

For those reasons, less-targeted therapies directed at the cells responding to the mediators of the metabolic response to injury are also being evaluated. Of great interest are nutrients whose use is designed to suppress the overactive macrophage and alter the output of interleukin, TNF, and eicosinoids such as PGE2 and LTB, and to stimulate lymphocyte proliferative responses. The former would include ω-3 PUFA such as eicosapentanoic acid (EPA) and docasahexanoic acid (DHA); and the latter would include arginine, uracil, RNA and ω-3 PUFA. Such an approach has been termed *nutrient pharmacology* (95–107).

Arginine is a nitrogen-dense amino acid and is considered conditionally essential in settings of prolonged metabolic stress. It is a potent endocrine secretogogue and has been observed to restore antigen-induced lymphocyte blastogenesis (95–97). Ribonucleotides are precursors of RNAs. Dietary nucleotides are effective in restoring macrophage activation of the T helper-inducer population. Uracil, unlike adenine, can restore delayed type hypersensitivity response to various foreign antigens reduce abscess formation in mice, and also reverse the immunosuppression associated with blood transfusion. The absence of dietary nucleotides, present in all forms of parenteral nutrition and in most commercially available formulations of enteral nutrients, results in suppression of cellular immune responses. Dietary nucleotides are also considered by many to be conditionally essential nutrients in settings of prolonged metabolic stress (98–100).

Lipid membrane composition is influenced by the type and quantity of exogenous lipid administration and can alter membrane fluidity, second messenger generation, and the pattern of eicosanoid synthesis and release (101–104). Generally, the products of ω-3 PUFA metabolism are less biologically potent than those of ω-6 PUFA. A relative excess of linoleic acid substrate stimulates PGE2 production, decreases cell membrane fluidity, and increased the melting point. The release of dienoic eicosinoids and TNF, and IL-1 release by macrophages, is directly related to the amount of ω-6 PUFA and the ω-3/n-6 PUFA ratio in the cell membrane. The incorporation of the n-3 PUFAs into cell membranes can occur within hours of ingestion and become stabilized within 2 to 4 days. In T lymphocytes, such incorporation is associated with enhanced proliferative responses to antigenic stimulation (105). In animal models utilizing cecal ligation and puncture peritonitis, ω-3 PUFA incorporation into cell membranes of liver cells and Kuppfer cells was associated with a reduction in mortality (35).

Clinical trials with these agents as part of an enteral nutrition regimen have demonstrated restoration and enhancement of the in vitro tests of immune function, improved nutritional outcomes, and significant reductions in length of hospital stay and complication rates (106,107). Unfortunately, in a recently completed multicenter trial, there was no effect on mortality and the incidence or severity of MOFS. These agents appeared to improve the ability of those patients who were going to survive, with little effect on those patients who were destined to expire (107).

Unquestionably, combination therapies will be tested. These therapies will be designed to effect multiple points of the inflammatory response concurrently and sequentially.

Tissue injury, whether from infection, volume loss, trauma, or inflammation as pancreatitis, induces local and systemic responses. The systemic responses include shock, reperfusion, systemic inflammation (hypermetabolism) with primary organ dysfunction, and secondary organ dysfunction that either becomes progressive and leads to death or from which the patient recovers and enters into a period of prolonged rehabilitation. In addition, there are operator-dependent variables during shock-resuscitation and during the postresuscitation treatment that can effect the development and severity of the SIRS and MOFS responses. Each of these time-related responses to injury has its respective dominant pathogenesis mechanisms that serially effect the subsequent responses. These pathogenic mechanisms have treatments that are appropriate and are at least partially effective. The research also indicates that the response(s), particularly the systemic inflammatory response, may contribute to the development of cell and organ injury and to progressive MOFS.

Current therapy is designed to remove the cause of injury, resuscitate the microcirculation, and institute nutrition-metabolic therapy to prevent single and generalized nutrient deficiencies and promote repair and healing without causing harm from the therapy itself. Newer therapies are designed to modulate the inflammatory response in order to minimize its injury potential and to promote tissue repair and recovery of the patient. The genetic regulation of metabolism also appears to be a pathogenic mechanism. Its role is just starting to be understood; new therapies will need to await this understanding. Nonetheless, significant survival rates are now occurring, with continued improvements expected in response to the newer therapeutic approaches. Professionals trained in critical care and in cellular and molecular biology provide the milieu within which continued improvements in prevention, therapy, and outcome will continue to occur.

REFERENCES

1. Barton R, Cerra FB. The hypermetabolism multiple system organ failure. *Chest* 1989;96:1153–1160.
2. Cerra F. Hypermetabolism, organ failure, and metabolic support. *Surgery* 1987;101(1):1–14.
3. Baue AE. Multiple, progressive or sequential systems failure: a syndrome of the 1970's. *Arch Surg* 1975;110:779–781.
4. Pine RW, Wertz MJ, Lennard ES, et al. Determinants of organ malfunction or death in patients with intraabdominal sepsis. *Arch Surg* 1983;118:242.
5. Tilney N, Bailey G, Morgan A. Sequential systems failure after rupture of abdominal aortic aneurysms. *Ann Surg* 1973;118:117.
6. Goris RJA, Draisma J. Causes of death after blunt trauma. *J Trauma* 1982;22:141.
7. ACCP–SCCM Consensus Conference. Definitions for sepsis and organ failure and guidelines for the use of innovative therapies in sepsis. *Chest* 101(6):864–874.
8. Cerra FB, Negro F, Eyer S. Multiple organ failure syndrome: patterns and effect of current therapy. In: Vincent JL, ed. *Update in Intensive Care and Emergency Medicine*. Berlin: Springer-Verlag, 1990;22–31.
9. Moyer ED, Border JR, Cerra FB, et al. Multiple systems organ failure VI: Death predictors in the trauma-septic state—the most critical determinants. *J Trauma* 1981;21(10):862–869.

10. Cerra FB. Multiple organ failure syndrome. *DM* December, 1992.
11. Siegel JH, Cerra FB, Border JR, et al. Physiological and metabolic correlation in human sepsis. *Surgery* 1979;806:409.
12. Moyer ED, Border JR, Cerra FB, et al. Multiple systems organ failure VI: Death predictors in the trauma-septic state—the most critical determinants. *J Trauma* 21(10):862–869, 1981.
13. Cerra FB, Abrams J, Negro F. APACHE II score does not predict MOFS or mortality in postoperative patients. *Arch Surg* 1990;125:519–522.
14. Petty PE. ARDS: definition and historical perspective. *Clin Chest Med* 1982;3:3.
15. Pepe PE, Porkin RT. Clinical predictors of ARDS. 1982;144:124.
16. Bihari D, Smithies M, Gimson A, et al. The effects of vasodilation with prostacyclin on oxygen delivery and uptake in critically ill patients. *N Engl J Med* 1987;317:397.
17. Gutierrez G, Pohil R. Oxygen consumption is linearly related to the oxygen supply in critically ill patients. *J Crit Care Med* 1986;1:45.
18. Danek S, Lynch J, Weg J, et al. The dependence of oxygen uptake on oxygen delivery in the adult respiratory distress syndrome. *Am Rev Respir Dis* 1980;122:387.
19. Cain SM. Physiologic and pathologic oxygen supply dependency. In: Gutierrez G, Vincent JL, eds. *Update in Intensive Care and Emergency Medicine: Tissue Oxygen Utilization.* Berlin: Springer-Verlag, 1991;114–124.
20. Thijs LG, Groenveld ABJ. Oxygen supply dependency in septic shock. In: Gutierrez G, Vincent JL, eds. *Update in Intensive Care and Emergency Medicine: Tissue Oxygen Utilization.* Berlin: Springer-Verlag, 1991;217–227.
21. Schlichtig R, Snyder JV, Pinsky MR. Multiple organ oxygen supply-demand relationships in redistributional flow. In: Gutierrez, Vincent JL, eds. *Update in Intensive Care and Emergency Medicine: Tissue Oxygen Utilization.* Berlin: Springer-Verlag, 1991;143–160.
22. Lange MS, Lobdell P, et al. Splanchnic and total body oxygen consumption in septic and injury patients. *Surgery* 1987;101:69.
23. Cerra FB, Siegel JH, Coleman B, et al. Septic autocannibalism, a failure of exogenous nutritional support. *Ann Surg* 1980;192:570–580.
24. Cerra FB, Siegel JH, Border JR, et al. Correlations between metabolic and cardiopulmonary measurements in patients after trauma, general surgery and sepsis. *J Trauma* 1979;19:621–629.
25. Cuthbertson D, Tilstone W. Metabolism during the post-injury period. *Adv Clin Chem* 1977;12:1–55.
26. Wilmore DW, Orlick L. Systemic responses to injury and the healing wound. *JPEN* 1980;4:147.
27. Giovannini I, Boldrini G, Castagnato M, et al. Respiratory quotient and patterns of substrate utilization in human sepsis and trauma. *JPEN* 1993;226–230.
28. Chaudry IH, Herkema JM, Dean RE. Alterations in energy production: a manifestation of cell injuries. In: Bihari DJ, Cerra FB, eds. *New Horizons: Multiple Organ Failure.* Fullerton, CA: Society of Critical Care Medicine, 1989;277–297.
29. Elwyn D, Kinney JM, Juvanandum M. Influence of increasing carbohydrate intake on glucose kinetics in injured patients. *Ann Surg* 1979;190:117–127.
30. Wolfe R, Allsop J, Burke J. Glucose metabolism in man: responses to intravenous glucose infusion. *Metabolism* 1979:28:210–220.
31. Long C, Kinney J, Geiger J. Nonsuppressability of gluconeogenesis in septic patients. *Metabolism* 1981;25:513–519.
32. Askanazi J, Rosenbaum H, Hyman A, et al. Respiratory changes induced by high glucose loads of total parenteral nutrition. *JAMA* 1980;243:1444–1447.
33. Shaw JHF, Wolfe RR. Glucose and urea kinetics in patients with early and advanced gastrointestinal cancer: the response to glucose infusion, parenteral feeding, and surgical resection. *Surgery* 1987;101:181–191.
34. White RH, Frayn KN, Little RA, et al. Hormonal and metabolic responses to glucose infusion in sepsis studies by the hyperglycemic glucose clamp technique. JPEN 1987;11:345–353.
35. Cerra FB, Alden PA, Negro F, et al. Sepsis and exogenous lipid modulation. *JPEN* 1988;12(6):63S–69S.
36. McGilvery RW, Goldstein G. The oxidation of fatty acids. In: *Biochemistry: A Functional Approach.* 2nd ed. Philadelphia: WB Saunders, 1979;434.
37. Tracey KJ. Tumor necrosis factor (cachectin) in the biology of septic shock syndrome. *Circ Shock* 1991;35:123–128.
38. Frases I, Neoptolemos J, Darby H, et al. Effects of intralipid and heparin on human monocyte and lymphocyte function. *JPEN* 1986;8:381.

39. Pearl RH, Clowes GHA, Hirsch EF, et al. Prognosis and survival as determined by visceral amino acid clearance in severe trauma. *J Trauma* 1985;25:777–783.
40. Snyder L, Cerra F. Shock. In: Greenfield LJ, ed. *Surgery: Scientific Principles and Practice*. Philadelphia: JB Lippincott, in press.
41. Burke JF, Gelfand JA. Events in early inflammation. In: Howard RJ, Simmons RL, eds. *Surgical Infectious Disease*. New York: Appleton-Century-Crofts, 1988;201–208.
42. Taylor AE, Adkins WK, Moore T. Ischemia-reperfusion lung injury: repair of endothelial damage by adenosine and cAMP. In: Vincent JL, ed. *Yearbook of Intensive Care and Emergency Medicine*. Berlin: Springer-Verlag, 1993;12–20.
43. Ward PA, Warren JS, Remick DG, et al. Cytokines and oxygen-radical–mediated tissue injury. In: Bihari DJ, Cerra FB, eds. *New Horizons: Multiple Organ Failure*. Fullerton, CA: Society of Critical Care Medicine, 1989;93–100.
44. Cook JA, Halushka PV. Arachidonic acid metabolism in septic shock. In: Bihari DJ, Cerra FB, eds. *New Horizons: Multiple Organ Failure*. Fullerton, CA: Society of Critical Care Medicine, 1989; 101–124.
45. Wilmore DW, Orlick L. Systemic responses to injury and the healing wound. *JPEN* 1980;4:147.
46. Goetz KL, Wang BC. Secretion of vasopressin during hemorrhage: Effects of receptors in the ventricles of the heart. In: *Vasopressin: Cellular and Integrative Functions*. New York: Raven Press, 1988;399.
47. Clowes GHA. Stresses, mediators, and responses of survival. In: Clowes GHA Jr, ed. *Trauma, Sepsis and Shock: The Physiological Basis of Therapy*. Marcel Dekker, 1988;1–53.
48. Davies CL, Newman RJ, Molyneux SG, Grahame-Smith DG. The relationship between plasma catecholamines and severity of injury in man. *J Trauma* 1984;24:99.
49. Garrison RN, Cryer HM. Role of the microcirculation to skeletal muscle during shock. In: Bond RF, Adams R, Chaudry IH, eds. *Perspectives in Shock Research: Progress in Clinical and Biological Research*. vol. 264. New York: Alan R. Liss, 1988;43–52.
50. Dinarello C. Interleukin-1 and the pathogenesis of the acute-phase response. *N Engl J Med* 1984; 311:341–344.
51. Chang S, Feddersen CO, Henson PM, et al. Platelet-activating factor mediates hemodynamic changes and lung injury in endotoxin-treated rats. *J Clin Invest* 1987;79:1498–1509.
52. Vilcek LEJ. Biology of disease TNF and IL-1: cytokines with multiple overlapping biological activities. *Lab Invest* 1987;56:234–248.
53. Deitch EA, Maejima K, Berg R. Effect of oral antibiotics and bacterial overgrowth on the translocation of the GI-tract microflora in burned rats. *J Trauma* 1985;25:385–392.
54. Wells CI, Maddaus MA, Simmons R. Proposed mechanism for the translocation of enteric bacteria. *Rev Infect Dis* 1988;10:958–979.
55. Pittsman AB, Udekwu A, Ochva J, Smith S. Bacterial translocation in trauma patients. *J Trauma* 1991;31:1083–1087.
56. Moore FA, Moore EE, Poggetti R. Gut bacterial translocation via the portal vein: a clinical perspective in patients with major torso trauma. *J Trauma* 1991;31:629.
57. Le J, Weinstein D, Gubler U, Vilcek J. Induction of membrane-associated interleukin-1 by tumor necrosis factor in human fibroblasts. *J Immunol* 1987;138:2137–2142.
58. Mortensen RF, Shapiro J, Lin BF, et al. Interaction of recombinant IL-1 and recombinant tumor necrosis factor in the induction of mouse acute phase proteins. *J Immunol* 1988;140:2260–2666.
59. Okusawa S, Gelfand JA, Ikejima T, et al. Interleukin-1 induces a shock-like state in rabbits. *J Clin Invest* 1988;81:1162–1172.
60. Munro JM, Pober JS, Cotran RS. Tumor necrosis factor and interferon-gamma induce distinct patterns of endothelial activation and associated leukocyte accumulation in skin of papio anubis. *Am J Pathol* 1989;135(1):121.
61. Meyer JD, Yurt RW, Duhaney R, et al. Tumor necrosis factor-enhanced leukotriene B4 generation and chemotaxis in human neutrophils. *Arch Surg* 1988;123(12):1454.
62. Beutler BA. Orchestration of septic shock by cytokines: The role of cachectin (tumor necrosis factor). In: Roth, Nielson, Mckee, eds. *Molecular and Cellular Mechanics of Septic Shock*. New York: Alan R. Liss, 1989;219–235.
63. Mazuski JE, Platt JL, West MA, et al. Direct effects of endotoxin on hepatocytes. *Arch Surg* 1988; 123:340–344.
64. West MA, Keller G, Hyland B, et al. Hepatocyte function in sepsis: Kupffer cells mediate a biphasic protein synthesis response in hepatocytes after endotoxin and killed *E. coli*. *Surgery* 1985;98: 388–395.

65. Vary TC, Siegel JH, Placko R, et al. Effect of dichloroacetate on plasma and hepatic amino acids in sterile inflammation and sepsis. *Arch Surg* 1989;124:1071–1077.
66. Bankey P, Fiegel B, Singh R, et al. Hypoxia and endotoxin induce macrophage-mediated suppression of fibroblast proliferation. *J Trauma* 1989;29(7):972–980.
67. Mazuski JE, Bankey PE, Carlson A, Cerra FB. Hepatocytes release factors that can modulate macrophage IL-2 secretion and proliferation. *Surg Forum* 1988;39:13–15.
68. Curran RD, Finari FK, Kispert PH, et al. Effects of endogenous nitric oxide on mitochondrial respiration of rat hepatocytes. *Arch Surg* 1991;126:186–191.
69. Abraham E. Effects of critical illness on macrophage, T and B cell functions. In: Vincent J, ed. *Yearbook of Intensive Care and Emergency Medicine.* Springer-Verlag, 1993;35–48.
70. Munster AM, Winchurch RA, Birmingham WJ, et al. Longitudinal assay of lymphocyte responsiveness in patients with major burns. *Ann Surg* 1980;192:772.
71. Abraham E, Chang Y-H. The effects of hemorrhage on mitogen-induced lymphocyte proliferation. *Circ Shock* 1985;15:171.
72. Abraham E, Regan RF. The effects of hemorrhage and trauma on interleukin 2 production. *Arch Surg* 1985;120:1341.
73. Kinsella J, Lakesh B, Boughton S. Dietary PUFA and eicosinoids potential effects on the modulation of inflammation and immune cells. *Nutrition* 1990;6:24–45.
74. Atherton ST, White DJ. Stomach as a source of bacteria colonising respiratory tract during artificial ventilation. *Lancet* 1983;2:968–969.
75. Driks M, Craven DE, Bartolome R, et al. Nosocomial pneumonia in intubated patients given sucralfate as compared with antacids or histamine type 2 blockers. *N Engl J Med* 1987;317:1376.
76. Blair PHB, Rowlands K, Lowry H, et al. A stratified randomized prospective study in a mixed ICU. *Surgery* (in press).
77. Tetteroo GWM, Qagenvoort JHT, Castelein A, et al. SDD to reduce gram-negative colonization and infections after esophageal resection. *Lancet* 1990;335:704–707.
78. Barke RA, Brady PS, Brady LJ. The effect of peritoneal sepsis on hepatic gene expression and hepatic mitochondrial long chain fatty acid oxidation in rats. *Surg Forum* 1991;42:62–64.
79. De Maio A, Buchman T. Molecular biology of circulatory shock. IV. Translation and secretion of HEP G2 cell proteins are independently attenuated during heat shock. *Surgery* 1991;34:329–335.
80. Buchman TG, Cabin DE, Vickers S, et al. Molecular biology of circulatory shock. II. Expression of four groups of hepatic genes is enhanced following resuscitation from cardiogenic shock. *Surgery* 1990;108:902–912.
81. Baum M, Mutz NJ, Hormann C: BIPAP, APRV, IMPRV: methodological concept and clinical impact. In: Vincent J, ed. *Yearbook of Intensive Care and Emergency Medicine.* Berlin: Springer-Verlag, 1993;514–526.
82. Bolton C, Young G. Sepsis and septic shock: central and peripheral nervous systems. In: Sibbald W, Sprung C, eds. *New Horizons: Perspectives in Sepsis and Septic Shock.* Fullerton, CA: Society of Critical Care Medicine, 1985;157–171.
83. Shoemaker WC. Hemodynamic and oxygen transport patterns in septic shock: physiologic mechanisms and therapeutic implications. In: Sibbald W, Sprung C, eds. *New Horizons: Perspectives in Sepsis and Septic Shock.* Fullerton, CA: Society of Critical Care Medicine, 1985;203–234.
84. Shoemaker W, Appel PL, Kram HB. Tissue oxygen debt as a determinant of lethal and nonlethal postoperative organ failure. *J Crit Care Med* 1989;16:1117–1121.
85. Tuchschmidt. 1992;102:216.
86. Stahl TJ, Alden PB, Ring WS, et al. Sepsis induced diastolic dysfunction in chronic canine peritonitis. *Am J Physiol* 1990;27(3):H625–633.
87. Natanson H, Eichenholm PW, Danner RI, et al. Endotoxin and TNF challenges in dogs simulates the cardiovascular profile of human septic shock. *J Exp Med* 1989;169:823–832.
88. Scheltingna MR, Young LS, Benfall K, et al. Glutamine enriched parenteral feedings attenuate extracellular fluid expansion after a standard stress. *Ann Surg* 1991;214:385–391.
89. Wilmore DW, Carpentier Y, eds. *Roundtable Conference on Metabolic Support.* Berlin: Springer-Verlag, in press.
90. Cerra FB, Hirsch J, Mullen K, et al. The effect of stress level, amino acid formula, and nitrogen dose on nitrogen retention in traumatic and septic stress. *Ann Surg* 1987;205:282–287.
91. Cerra FB, McPherson J, Konstantinides FN, et al. Enteral nutrition does not prevent multiple organ failure syndrome after sepsis. *Surgery* 1988;104(4):727–733.
92. Dunn DL, Ferguson RM. Immunotherapy of gram-negative sepsis: enhanced survival in a guinea pig model by use of rabbit antiserum to *Escherichia coli* J5. *Surgery* 1982;92:212.

93. Ziegler EJ, Fisher CJ, Sprung CL, the HA-1A Study Group. Treatment of gram-negative bacteremia and septic shock with HA-1A human monoclonal antibody against endotoxin: a randomized, double-blind, placebo-controlled trial. *N Engl J Med* 1991;324:429–436.

94. Fisher CJ. Administration of IL-1ra in patients with severe sepsis: results of a phase III trial. Presented at 13th International Symposium of Intensive Care and Emergency Medicine, Brussels, March 23–26, 1993.

95. Barbul A, Sisto DA, Wasserkrug HL, et al. Metabolic and immune effects of arginine in post-injury hyperalimentation. *J Trauma* 1981;21:970–974.

96. Barbul A, Wasserkrug HL, Sisto DA, et al. Thymic and immune stimulatory actions of arginine. *JPEN* 1980;4:446–449.

97. Reynolds JV, Thom AK, Zhang SM, et al. Arginine, protein calorie malnutrition and cancer. *J Surg Res* 1988;45:513–522.

98. Zollner N, Grobner W. In: *Purine and Pyrimidine Metabolism*. Amsterdam: Elsevier, 1977;165–178.

99. Kulkarni AD, Fanslow WC, et al. Effect of dietary nucleotides on response to bacterial infections. *JPEN* 1986;10:169–171.

100. Rudolph FB, Kulkarni AD, Fanslow WC, et al. Role of RNA as a dietary source of pyrimidines and purines in immune function. *Nutrition* 1990;6:45–52.

101. Spector AA, Yorek MA. Membrane lipid composition and cellular functions. *J Lipid Res* 1985;26:1015–1019.

102. Holman RT. Nutritional and metabolic interrelationships between fatty acids. *Fed Proc* 1964;23(5):1062–1067.

103. Holman RT. Control of polyunsaturated acids in tissue lipids. *J Am Coll Nutr* 1986;5:236–265.

104. Billiar TJ, Bankey PE, Svingen BA, et al. Fatty acid intake and Kupffer cell function alters eicosanoid and monopkine production to endotoxin stimulation. *Surgery* 1988;104:343–349.

105. Cerra FB, Lehman S, Konstantinides N, et al. Effect of enteral nutrient on in vitro tests of immune function in ICU patients: a preliminary report. *Nutrition* 1990;6:84–87.

106. Daly JM, Lieberman D, Goldfine MS, et al. Enteral nutrition with supplemental arginine, RNA, and omega 3 fatty acids in patients after operation: immunologic, metabolic, and clinical outcome. *Surgery* 1992;112:56–67.

107. Bower RH, Lavin PT, Cerra FB, et al. Early enteral administration of a formula supplemented with arginine, nucleotides and fish oil reduces length of stay of ICU patients: a randomized prospective trial. (Submitted for publication)

Organ Metabolism and Nutrition:
Ideas for Future Critical Care, edited by
J. M. Kinney and H. N. Tucker.
Raven Press, Ltd., New York © 1994.

24

Future Nutritional Goals in the Intensive Care Unit

Jan Wernerman and Hugh N. Tucker

Department of Anesthesiology and Intensive Care, Karolinska Institute, Huddinge University Hospital, S-141 86 Huddinge, Sweden; and Department of Scientific and Medical Affairs, Clintech Nutrition Company, Deerfield, Illinois 60015

The development of nutrition support techniques for patients during intensive care periods have evolved rapidly over the last two decades; however, knowledge of metabolic regulating mechanisms and pathophysiology has increased only very slowly. As in other areas of medical practice, there has been frequent overenthusiasm regarding the application of some of the newer concepts in nutrition. New therapies have been adapted without enough critical thinking or adequate experience to demonstrate efficacy through clinically relevant parameters. Consequently, several reports have now been presented in the literature describing complications or possible adverse effects of nutrition that could outweigh the beneficial effects (1,2). Individualized assessment of requirements and more relevant indicators of improvement in clinical outcome for critically ill patients will be required in the future. Principles of care have evolved that reflect the incremental knowledge gained from past experience.

ENERGY REQUIREMENT

When indirect calorimetry was first used to estimate the resting energy expenditure of critically ill patients, relatively high expenditures were reported (3). There is no reason to believe that these measurements were erroneous, but it should be realized that treatment of patients was very different 12 to 15 years ago than it is today. Current treatment of polytrauma, complicated postsurgical patients, and extensive burn patients includes the use of potent antibiotics, a better understanding of fluid and electrolyte balance, and improved circulatory and ventilatory monitoring and other techniques that, when combined with modern energy expenditure measurement techniques, have refined the recommendations for energy requirements. The result has been that energy expenditure estimates during critical illness are now much closer to the basal levels of normal subjects (4). With the exception of extensive thermal injury, it is rare that patients exhibit increases in energy demand over basal energy expenditures greater than 15% to 25%. Consequently, the number of these patients with energy requirements exceeding 2,200 kcal/24 h is relatively small. Extensive thermal injury may increase energy expenditure by 35% or more and represent the highest energy consumers.

Several factors affect the accuracy of energy requirements estimated across patient groups when calculated basal energy expenditure is used as the mathematical standard. The considerable variability in energy expenditure between individuals was previously pointed out in the classic work of Harris and Benedict (5). The impact of age on basal energy metabolism was also recognized, although the number of elderly individuals in the original investigation was comparatively small. The impact of age and individual variability is frequently ignored when standardized estimates for energy supply are given. It should be obvious that regimens based on standard kcal/kg bw dosing have limited applicability to patients in intensive care. Accurate current body weight, which is difficult to obtain in the critical care environment, may not reflect usual weight due to previous rapid weight loss, body fluid changes related to the status of resuscitation, and fluid gain or loss.

Several simplified methods for estimating energy expenditure based on increments over basal energy expenditure determined by "stress factors" have been published. The subjective methods of clinical assessment used to estimate the incremental degree of stress sometimes creates an overestimate of the value for the risk factor multiplier for patients due to the apparent degree of illness as viewed in the critical care setting (6). In a recent paper, calculated energy expenditures derived by multiplying basal energy expenditure by several factors based on trauma scores, injury severity scores and APACHE II scores were compared with measured expenditures by indirect calorimetry (Table 1). The measured energy expenditure was 14.1% below the calculated energy expenditure for patients with sepsis and 16.1% below the measured energy expenditure for multiple trauma patients (7). The most common reason for the error was variable clinical impressions. These data confirm a tendency to overestimate energy requirements if measurements are not performed.

Frequent monitoring of requirements is important to success in the critical care setting. There have been several reports in the literature of overfeeding to the extent

TABLE 1. *Estimation of energy expenditure versus measuring energy expenditure.*

	TS	SSS	ISS	APACHE II	BEE (kcal)	CEE (kcal)	MREE (kcal)
Sepsis (n = 15)		32 ± 3		15 ± 1	1139 ± 34	2189 ± 65	1882 ± 126
Multiple trauma (n = 15)	14 ± 1		29 ± 3	10 ± 1	1466 ± 83	2640 ± 83	2216 ± 100

Adapted from Hwang T-L, et al. (7).
SSS, septic severity score; APACHE II, Acute Physiology and Chronic Health Evaluation II scoring system; BEE, basal energy expenditure; CEE, calculated energy expenditure; MREE, measured energy expenditure; TS, trauma score; ISS, injury severity score.

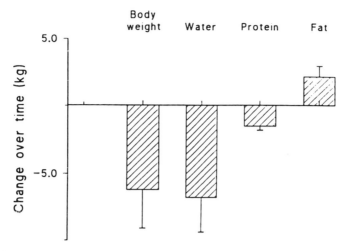

FIG. 1. Body composition measurements of critically ill patients show a reduction in body water during 10 days following resuscitation, while TPN resulted simultaneously in a gain of body fat. Data from Streat et al. (10).

of difficulty in weaning from the ventilator (8), elevated body temperature (9), and lipogenesis (10). In addition, many of the adverse effects attributable to excess carbo-hydrates or excess fat, such as fatty infiltration of the liver, suppression of immune function, and so on, are related frequently to caloric overfeeding (Fig. 1).

During critical illness, the risk of overfeeding the patient must be considered larger than the risk of underfeeding. Various techniques of intravenous nutritional support are associated intrinsically with morbidity and mortality risks in postsurgical patients (Fig. 2). Screening for protein-calorie malnutrition linked with careful selection is key to treating those patients who benefit the most from nutritional support. These must be differentiated from well-nourished patients with a very similar clinical condition and demographic data if efficacy of nutrition support is to be found (1). Appropriate nutrition support requires careful and continuous nutrition and metabolic assessment, including measurement of energy expenditure, where possible, and monitoring of clinical and laboratory parameters (11).

MIXED FUEL SUBSTRATES

Glucose

Emphasis has been placed on adjusting the parenteral and enteral macronutrient rations provided during nutrition support of the critical care patient. It was learned early that patients who were provided glucose alone in large quantities had several physiologic abnormalities. The first was the increase of carbon dioxide production from the exclusively carbohydrate fuel. Those experiences produced the recommendation for glucose to provide no more than 70% of the nonprotein calories. Obviously

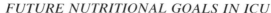

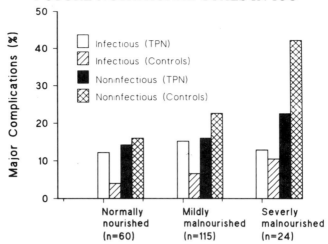

FIG. 2. Patients were divided into three categories based on their nutrition status. Within each group, patients were randomized to receive perioperative TPN or not. Complications were recorded and classified as infectious (e.g., cases related to the intravenous feeding catheter) or noninfectious (e.g., cases related to the nutritional status of the patient). The results show a high rate of infectious complications in normally nourished and mildly malnourished patients on TPN, while the noninfectious complications were lower in severely malnourished patients on TPN. The data point out the possibility that the adverse effects related to intravenous nutrition may not justify such treatment perioperatively in nonmalnourished patients. Data from The Veterans Affairs Total Parenteral Nutrition Cooperative Study Group (1).

other calorie sources were needed to provide the remainder of the energy requirement.

Lipid Emulsions

Intravenous lipid emulsions were designed to provide an alternative caloric substrate. The composition of the fat emulsions has traditionally been a mixture of long-chain fatty acids in the form of triglycerides (LCT) derived from soya bean oil. Standard emulsions provide the source for essential fatty acids during long-term parenteral support and are utilized well as calorie sources. The possible disadvantage of the carnitine requirement during transport across the mitochondrial membrane for beta-oxidation has been debated. Carnitine deficiency in critically ill patients has been described (12), but it is relatively rare (13). Limiting the use of LCT emulsions solely due to patients with carnitine deficiency does not seem justifiable.

It is, however, becoming an increasing concern that the choice of the oil for the lipid source may be more important in the critical care setting than originally envisioned. Supplying an excess of certain "essential" fatty acids has been questioned because they play major roles in the intricately balanced inflammatory and immune response systems responding to trauma and sepsis. Results from animal experiments suggest that higher concentrations of polyunsaturated fatty acids may induce enhanced inflammatory reactions as well as increased production of free radicals and a depression of the immune defense (14). The alternative to soya bean oil emulsions containing a high proportion of ω-6 (e.g., linoleic acid) are fat emulsions containing medium-chain triglycerides (MCT), oils high in monounsaturated fatty acids (e.g., olive oil) or the provision of a more balanced ω-6 to ω-3 content with canola oil or marine oil.

MCT Emulsions

Several enteral and parenteral products have been formulated with increased proportions of MCT. The MCT component is oxidized more rapidly, is not elongated for adipose tissue deposition, and is not dependent on carnitine for mitochondrial transport (15). In preclinical studies, advantages in improved protein metabolism, improved function of the immune system as well as the reticulo-endothelial system (RES) (16), and better stability of cellular membranes have been suggested (17). The administration of fat as MCT may enable metabolism of lipid emulsion without RES dysfunction and may be of particular benefit in critically ill or septic patients (18) (see Chapter 17). At the present time, adequately controlled clinical trials have not been completed that delineate the appropriate therapeutic application for MCT fuel substrates in critical illness.

Omega-3

Lipid emulsions containing higher concentrations ω-3 fatty acids (usually from marine oil sources) are being investigated. In clinical states with acute inflammation, a higher intake of ω-3 fatty acids is clearly shown to attenuate the inflammatory response. Additionally, an increased antioxidant (vitamin E) supply has been recommended during administration of highly reactive polyunsaturated fatty acids (19). The modulation of the immune response by manipulating the ratio of ω-3 to ω-6 fatty acid content of the nutrition is a controversial matter. A down-regulation of the cytokine response to trauma or sepsis may be achieved, but simultaneously a decrease in liver protein synthesis may be induced (20). As with other therapies, care should be exercised when introducing these new concepts to ensure that adequate trials are conducted utilizing relevant clinical parameters to evaluate the inclusion of the new lipid component.

NITROGEN REQUIREMENTS

The distinguishing characteristic of the amino acid and protein structure is the presence of the nitrogen molecule. This nitrogen can be used as a marker for the qualitative and quantitative fate of the amino acid. The benefit of any nutrition support regimen to the body's protein compartment may be estimated by calculating the effect on nitrogen homeostasis. In most cases, the nitrogen content of any nutrition intake is quantitatively related to the protein and amino acid intake.

The metabolism of amino acids is associated with a facultative thermogenic effect corresponding to 30% of the caloric value of the ingested amino acids (21); for example, if 10 g of nitrogen may correspond to 70 g of a specific amino acid mixture and approximately 280 kcal (~4 kcal/g). The corresponding facultative heat production (the energy converted into heat without any option of storage) would be around 84 kcal for each 70 g of amino acid administered. Fat and glucose may be used or stored at a comparatively low cost in terms of energy. One practical consequence of this is that an overload of amino acids increases heat production and urea excretion, thus increasing the metabolic burden. In the critical care setting, nitrogen dosing should provide sufficient quantities of a high-quality amino acid mixture, to offset any negative nitrogen balance without compromising the flux of free amino acids to the splanchnic area. This goal, as with caloric supply, should be reached without overfeeding the patient. Excessive amino nitrogen supply has not been shown to have incremental beneficial effects on whole-body nitrogen economy (22). Our current recommendations are to provide no more than 0.15 to 0.20 g N/kg bw/24 h.

THE COMPOSITION OF AMINO ACID SUPPLY

Requirements for certain amino acids that cannot be synthesized by normal human volunteers have been established. These "essential" or "indispensable" amino acids are well known for normal humans. It is frequently ignored that altered metabolic processes may greatly change the relationships between these essential nutrients, as well as alter the processes that allow the synthesis of sufficient amino acids that at other times are considered "nonessential."

The minor differences in the composition of the amino acid profiles of parenteral and enteral feeding regimens have not been shown to be of crucial importance. In critical illness, as in health, a well-balanced solution, consisting of essential as well as nonessential amino acids, seems to be appropriate. However, a great deal of emphasis has been (and continues to be) placed on determining which nutrients, if any, become rate limiting at specific times during the care of the critically ill (see Chapter 16) and if supplementing any or a group of amino acids during specific clinical situations will alter outcome.

Branched-chain Amino Acids

Over the years, increasing the proportions of branched-chain amino acids (BCAA) has been investigated in specific patient subsets—primarily trauma, stress, and hepatic encephalopathy. The evidence supporting clinical benefit has not been convincing (23). One rationale for supplementing BCAA has been to mimic blood concentrations. During the postprandial period, blood leaving the splanchnic area following a balanced meal contains a higher proportion of BCAA after hepatic clearance of the other amino acids. It was suggested that parenterally fed patients would benefit from an amino acid profile that reflected the splanchnic flow because the normal gastrointestinal modification was eliminated by the route of administration. Experimental studies have shown a stimulatory effect of BCAA on in vitro muscle protein synthesis in preparations from young animals (24). These data, combined with data that suggested that skeletal muscle has an increased demand for utilization of amino acid and fatty acid fuel during stress and trauma, were the theoretical foundations for consideration of BCAA optimization. The clinical results, however, have been not impressive in terms of nitrogen economy, protein metabolism, morbidity improvement, and mortality reduction (25,26). Positive nitrogen balance has been attained more rapidly with BCAA-supplemented parenteral regimens during the first 4 days after major insult, but common clinical outcome measures did not change (27). Concentration of free BCAA in muscle is increased; however, in critical illness these concentrations are already almost twice that of the basal state (28). The benefit of further elevation has not been observed.

On the other hand, BCAA enrichment has been reported to be of special importance for patients with hepatic encephalopathy, from whom nutritional support was frequently withheld. These patients are often malnourished and therefore they are likely to benefit from nutritional support. The introduction of BCAA-enriched nutrition improved the tolerance of patients to intravenous feeding. Improvement in encephalopathy was noted but clinical outcome parameters remained unchanged.

Current BCAA inclusion of 18% to 22% of protein intake seems to be adequate to meet the requirements of the critical care patient when total protein requirements can be met.

Glutamine

More recently, the inclusion of glutamine or glutamine peptides during amino acid support has been discussed extensively. Experimental and clinical data show a correlation between muscle protein synthesis and the concentration of glutamine in muscle (29,30). In addition, glutamine has been shown to be an important substrate for rapidly dividing cell populations (31).

In humans, glutamine is by far the most abundant free amino acid, and it serves to transport ammonia and amino groups between peripheral tissues and the splanchnic area (32). More than one third of the amino acid efflux from peripheral tissue is represented by glutamine. Blood reaching the splanchnic area from the periphery is enriched with glutamine. If mimicking the normal supply of amino acids to the tissues of the splanchnic area is an important goal of nutritional therapy, inclusion of glutamine would be appropriate. Additionally, depletion of glutamine in muscle during critical illness and injury is well known (33,34). Documentation of clinical effectiveness of this type of supplement has been limited to alterations in nitrogen economy, amino acid turnover, and protein metabolism of skeletal muscle (28,29). The effects are similar to standard amino acid control solutions. A reduction of infectious parameters and of hospital stay has also been demonstrated in patients undergoing bone marrow transplant when receiving glutamine supplemented parenteral feedings (35).

The appropriate daily dosage for glutamine remains a matter of debate. Clinical trials used 20 g of glutamine in addition to approximately 100 g of a standard amino acid mixture (15% to 20% of the total amino acids). This is twice the concentration of glutamine found in dietary proteins, but a lower fraction than that released from peripheral tissues. Case reports have indicated a better glutamine retention in muscle when the supply of glutamine is elevated (36). The inclusion of glutamine in nutritional support remains logical; however, much more evidence of improvement in morbidity needs to be provided, especially if the routine inclusion increases the overall cost of patient care and regulatory approval is to be sought.

Currently glutamine is not included in current parenteral amino acid solutions due to chemical instability during terminal sterilization. Investigations are being conducted to determine the comparative efficacy of alternative forms of glutamine that are more stable. Clinical investigations are ongoing with several more stable molecules, including glycyl-glutamine and alanyl-glutamine. An alternative way to provide glutamine may be to give alpha-ketoglutarate (25), which would provide the carbon skeleton of glutamine but would not add to the nitrogen burden. When given on an equimolar basis, alpha-ketoglutarate has been shown to have a more pronounced effect on muscle free glutamine than glutamine itself (37,38). Alpha-ketoglutarate, a constituent of Kreb's cycle in the mitochondria, also may influence directly the energy status of the cells.

Arginine

The possibility of positive effects by the provision of extra L-arginine on immune system, lymphocytes, and other tissues with rapid turnover has been discussed based on animal experiments (39). The experimental evidence from in vitro studies favors this concept, but definitive clinical or in vivo studies involving human subjects are not yet available. Adding to this interest is the current work centering around arginine as the precursor of nitric oxide (NO), which has become a new therapeutic modality in airway obstruction (40) and possibly in the resolution of pneumonia (41). Inhalation of NO in cases of airway obstruction has been proposed as an elegant way to obtain local smooth muscle relaxation. However, the supply of arginine by the enteral and intravenous route has not yet been shown to exert similar effects. To the contrary, there is no evidence of a generalized deficiency of arginine but, rather, a localized depletion of NO precursor in the airway epithelium. The link between the supplementation or restriction of dietary arginine will continue to be an exciting area of investigation and controversy until more definitive information is available on its role as an NO precursor is elucidated. This is becoming especially interesting in the critical care patient at risk for hypotensive septic shock because intravenous arginine has been shown to release sufficient NO to reduce total peripheral resistance in humans (42).

ADJUVANT THERAPIES

A growing number of substances are being proposed for possible beneficial effect when given in conjunction with nutrition support.

Insulin

Among hormones with a potentially anabolic effect, insulin is most widely used. Because of the insulin resistance frequently present in critical illness, high doses of insulin have been advocated (43). However, the exact role of insulin in protein metabolism is not without controversy. In muscle, insulin seems to affect the rate of protein degradation (44). Whether this has any therapeutic implication in critical illness is not known. Furthermore, insulin has been suggested to increase muscle protein synthesis, especially when given with BCAA. The experimental data to support these therapeutic suggestions are, however, very sparse. In the case of young, fast-growing animals, there are several reports of such effects, but these effects have not been reproduced in adult animals or humans (45). In critically ill patients, insulin is frequently used to control blood glucose concentrations, but the amounts used for this purpose are much lower than the dose required to affect protein metabolism. Very high levels of insulin may be a disadvantage in carbohydrate and fat metabolism. These effects should be evaluated before any recommendations for more enthusiastic use of high-dose insulin are made.

Growth Hormone

Growth hormone (GH) is now available in a recombinant form. It has long been recognized that GH supplementation in critically ill or postoperative patients improves nitrogen economy (46). This seems to be mediated by a lower rate of synthesis of urea and a consequent lowering of the serum urea concentrations (47). Similarly, effects have been reported on whole-body protein metabolism (48), peripheral tissue amino acid exchange (49), muscle amino acid content (50), and muscle protein synthesis (44). The mechanism behind these potentially beneficial effects is still obscure.

There remain questions to resolve regarding the use of GH. One important issue is the redistribution of substrates during any reported improvement in nitrogen economy. If substrates of importance for the splanchnic tissue are retained in the periphery, improved whole-body nitrogen economy may not be beneficial. Such interference with the usual metabolism of critically ill patients could be detrimental when response to a complication is required. Available data also indicate that some critically ill patients, as well as postoperative patients, respond to GH treatment, while others do not. It is important to identify possible GH resistance, to note it as a contraindication to treatment, and to use these experiences as possible ways of understanding the mechanisms of GH action. Although there have been some enthusiastic case reports involving dramatic effects of GH in critically ill patients, there many unanswered questions must be resolved before recommendations for clinical use may be made.

Beta-stimulators

Beta-stimulators are now used in animal meat production to improve growth and meat production. The use of a substance such as chlembuterol among athletes is banned by doping-control authorities. The use of beta-stimulators in the clinical practice of critical care is widespread for circulatory support. Beneficial effects on protein metabolism have been reported in that context. Experimental studies have also addressed the question of whether exercise-induced protein synthesis is mediated by beta-stimulators such as catecholamines (51). The area is open and the beneficial effects of treatment, as well as possible adverse effects, are unknown. When the larger doses of catecholamines are given in combination with cortisol and glucagon, the traditional depression of protein synthesis (52) as well as negative nitrogen balance (53) and loss of muscle amino acids is seen (54).

PRINCIPLES FOR NUTRITION SUPPORT DURING CRITICAL CARE

The Purpose of Nutrition Support

Nutrition therapy has no potential nor is it intended to cure critical illnesses per se, but is the way of preventing loss of important lean body mass and the way to maintain the energetics of the patient through the required lengths of hospital stay for other curative treatments to be instituted. Nutrition support, by maintenance of adequate nutrition status, may also improve the outcome of care, reduce complications, and shorten length of stay.

Use of Specific Substrates and Adjuvant Therapies to Enhance Nutrition Support

So far, substances suggested to have any possible positive effects on the metabolism of critically ill patients are constituents or imitation of constituents of the human body. This is true of specific substrates as well as of adjuvant substances. Looking to the future, there is very little hope of any "wonder drugs" that will have dramatic effects on the outcome for critically ill patients. In some respects, modern antibiotics are such wonder drugs, but the proposed metabolic substrates or adjuvant substances are not likely to revolutionize intensive care therapy. Instead, a more professional use of available nutrition products may improve the care for many critically ill patients. A better knowledge of the pathophysiology of metabolism in critical illness will give a sound basis for the use of specific substrates in nutritional treatment.

Early Enteral Intervention

In many patients, nutritional and metabolic support via the enteral route is an alternative (or additive) to parenterally administered nutritional support. Of course, enteral feedings require that the patient's gastrointestinal tract be functional, at least to some degree, and that the patient's clinical condition does not contraindicate enteral nutrition support. Potential contraindications to enteral nutrition support include upper gastrointestinal hemorrhaging, gastrointestinal obstruction, severe vomiting, or diarrhea. The rationale for enteral nutrition support in the immediate postinjury period is based on animal studies comparing early enteral nutrition versus early parenteral nutrition (55) and immediate (i.e., less than 12 to 24 hours postinjury) versus delayed enteral nutrition support (56).

Monitoring nutrition status using parameters such as nitrogen balance indicate that the route of administration seems to be of little importance in critical illness (57). However, the use of the gastrointestinal tract has a number of potentially beneficial effects for the critically ill patients. A better proliferation of the intestinal mucosa is seen (58). Rather than state that parenteral nutrition is not beneficial, it is perhaps better to say that the absence of enteral nutrition is the disadvantage. For patients in which all enteral access is contraindicated, the lack of enteral stimulation may, at least partially, be counteracted by intravenous glutamine (59). The presence of nutrients in the intestinal lumen has a direct "trophic" effect on the mucosa and on the stimulation of gastrointestinal hormone secretion. This may prevent translocation of bacteria through the intestinal epithelium (60). The presence of bacterial translocation in humans is a controversial issue, but convincing data are available from animal experiments. In burned patients, beneficial effects on the course of illness are reported (61), and although the reports from trauma patients are less conclusive, the advantage in economic terms is obvious. The enteral nutrition should be started as early as possible in the ICU, preferably by a feeding catheter placed in the upper part of the jejunum. Even if the total nutrition support is not possible by this route initially, any fraction of the intake as enteral nutrition must be considered an advantage. If patients are able to receive enteral nutrition, withholding of enteral support and institution of intravenous nutrition must be considered unethical, especially in critical illness.

Customized Nutrition for Individual Patient Variability

Nutritional support in critical illness must be given under the motto, "Above all else, do no harm." To attain this goal, an individualized nutrition program should be developed. Critically ill patients are a heterogeneous group with great variability in metabolism. Although the basic underlying mechanisms of altered metabolism are shared by specific subsets of patients, the degree of expression in each individual case is unpredictable. Recent studies covering large groups of critically ill patients underline this variability and the difficulty of prediction (2). Customizing the regimen and components of nutrition support must not be neglected because patients will have varying severity of underlying disease, malnutrition, and advanced age. Differentiating the patients who will benefit from treatment and those that are at higher risk of suffering from adverse effects of techniques or therapies is impossible. The entire group of critically ill patients must be provided nutrition support with care. Conservative treatment includes close monitoring of biochemical as well as clinical parameters and measurements of the energy expenditure by indirect calorimetry. Most of the noncatheter-related adverse effects of nutrition support are due to over-feeding.

Long-Term Consequences of Short-term Action

In healthy well-nourished patients who become acutely ill for short periods, the composition of nutritional support does not seem to be important (Fig. 3). However, the lack of ability to identify acute changes does not exclude the possibility of an effect on the length of the convalescent period after the acute episode has been resolved. Follow-up studies designed to measure differences in the return to full functionality after the acute illness are needed. Comparing patients with and without nutrition support during the acute illness after several months of recuperation may provide more insight regarding appropriate prescriptions during the critical care period.

Bearing these principles in mind, what are the future goals for nutrition support in ICU? It is definitely the "long-timers" in intensive care that are the challenge. For this group of patients, nutritional care is crucial. Today, the goal of the conventional nutrition support is to slow down the autocannibalism of body proteins. Meeting this goal must be attained by avoiding excessive calories that increase the risk of adverse effects but do not counteract the protein catabolism. New substrates and adjuvant therapies may have a potential to slow down these processes and improve the efficiency of nutrition support. Improved diets and equipment for administering enteral

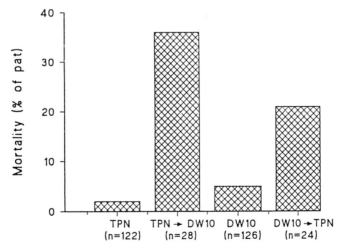

FIG. 3. Patients undergoing major general surgery were randomized to receive TPN or 10% intravenous glucose postoperatively. The majority of patients (80%) tolerated this regimen without any adverse effects. Some patients did not start to eat after 14 days of treatment (DW 10 → TPN) or did not tolerate the TPN (120% of BEE) given (TPN → DW 10). Among these subgroups of patients, the complication rate and the mortality was high. It was not possible to identify these patients preoperatively. Data from Sanström et al. (2).

feedings may be as important to attain these goals as new growth factors. Combination of enteral and parenteral feeding should be considered to ensure that the patients have both sufficient intake and maintain gastrointestinal integrity during long periods in the critical care environment. Refinement of substrates for nutrition support may modify the metabolic response to trauma and sepsis and provide new tools for the management of these patients. Clearer understanding of the metabolic response to illness and implementation of individualized patient care plans during the course of the critical care will create the clinical setting in which to meet the goals of better care in the ICU.

REFERENCES

1. The Veterans Affairs Total Parenteral Nutrition Cooperative Study Group. Perioperative total parenteral nutrition in surgical patients. *N Engl J Med* 1991;325:525–532.
2. Sanström R, Drott C, Hyltander A, et al. The effect of postoperative intravenous feeding (TPN) on outcome following major surgery evaluated in a randomized study. *Ann Surg* 1993;217(2):185–195.
3. Wilmore DW. In: Thomas K, Reemtsma K, ed. *The Metabolic Management of the Critically Ill.* New York and London: Plenum Medical Book Company, 1977.
4. Foster GD, Knox LS, Dempsey DT, Mullen JL. Caloric requirements in total parenteral nutrition. *J Am Coll Nutr* 1987;6:231–254.
5. Harris JA, Benedict FG. *Biometric Studies of Basal Metabolism in Man.* Carnegie Institution of Washington, Publication No. 279, 1919.
6. Cortez V, Nelson L. Errors in estimating energy expenditure in critically ill surgery patients. *Arch Surg* 1989;124:287.
7. Hwang T-L, Huang S-L, Chen M-F. The use of indirect calorimetry in critically ill patients—The relationship of measured energy expenditure to injury severity score, septic severity score, and APACHE II score. *J Trauma* 1993;34:247–251.
8. Carlsson M, Burgerman R. Overestimation of caloric demand in a long-term critically ill patient. *Clin Nutr* 1985;4:91–93.
9. Henneberg S, Sjölin J, Stjernström H. Over-feeding as a cause of fever in intensive care patients. *Clin Nutr* 1991;10:266–271.
10. Streat SJ, Beddoe AH, Hill GL. Aggressive nutritional support does not prevent protein loss despite fat gain in septic intensive care patients. *J Trauma* 1987;27:262–266.
11. Wernerman J. Nutrition for intensive therapy patients. In: Wilmore DW, Carpentier YA, eds. *Update in Intensive Care and Emergency Medicine 15—Metabolic Support.* Berlin: Springer Verlag, 1993; 215–235.
12. Bremer J. Carnitine-metabolic and function. *Physiol Rev* 1983;63:1420–1480.
13. Wennberg A, Hyltander A, Sjöberg Å, et al. A descriptive study of the carnitine status in critically ill patients, which provides valuable background information necessary for the evaluation of the new medium-chain triglyceride and long-chain triglyceride lipid emulsions. *Metabolism* 1992;41:165–171.
14. Carpentier YA, Van Gossum A, Dubios DY, Deckelbaum RJ. Lipid metabolism. In: Rombeau JL, Caldwell MD, eds. *Clinical Nutrition: Parenteral Nutrition.* 2nd Ed. Philadelphia: Saunders, 1993; 35–74.
15. Hill JO, Peters JC, Yang D, et al. Thermogenesis in humans during overfeeding with medium-chain triglycerides. *Metabolism* 1989;38:641–648.
16. Hamawy KJ, Moldawer LL, Georgieff M, et al. The effect of lipid emulsions on reticuloendothelial system function in the injured animal. *JPEN* 1985;9:559–565.
17. Bach AC, Frey A, Lutz O. Clinical and experimental effects of medium-chain triglyceride-based fat emulsions—A review. *Clin Nutr* 1989;8:223–235.
18. Jensen GL, Mascioli EA, Seidner DL, et al. Parenteral infusion of long- and medium-chain triglycerides and reticuloendothelial system function in man. *JPEN* 1990;14:467–471.
19. Traber MG, Carpentier YA, Kayden HJ, et al. Alterations in the distribution of alpha- and gamma-tocopherols in human lipoproteins in response to intravenous infusion of triglyceride-rich emulsions. *Metabolism* 1993;42:701–709.

20. Grimble RF, Modulation of cytokine biology by dietary fat. In: Vincent JL, ed. *Yearbook of Intensive Care and Emergency Medicine*. Berlin: Springer Verlag: 1993;212–221.
21. Thörne A, Wahren J. Diet-induced thermogenesis in welltrained-subjects. *Clin Physiol* 1989;9: 295–305.
22. Larsson J, Lennmarken C, Mårtensson J, et al. Nitrogen requirements in severely injured patients. *Br J Surg* 1990;77:413–416.
23. Brennan MF, Cerra F, Faly JM, et al. Report of research workshop: branched-chain amino acids in stress and injury. *JPEN* 1986;10:446–452.
24. Adibi SA, Fekl W, Langenbeck U, Schauder P. *Branched Chain Amino and Keto Acids in Health and Disease*. Basel: S. Karger, 1984.
25. Lennmarken C, Skullman S, Wirén M, et al. The impace of leucine infusion on skeletal muscle amino acid and energy metabolism in severely traumatized patients. *Clin Nutr* 1992;11:140–146.
26. Vente JP, von Meyenfeldt MF, van Eijk HMH, et al. Effects of infusion of branched chain amino-acids enriched TPN solutions on plasma amino-acid profiles in sepsis and trauma patients. *Clin Nutr* 1990;9:241–245.
27. Cerra FB, Mazuski JE, Chute E, et al. Branched chain metabolic support. A prospective, randomized, double-blind trial in surgical stress. *Ann Surg* 1984;199(3):286–291.
28. Vinnars E, Bergström J, Fürst P. Influence of the postoperative state on the intracellular free amino acids in human muscle tissue. *Ann Surg* 1975;182:665–671.
29. Jepson MM, Bates PC, Broadbent P, et al. Relationship between glutamine concentration and protein synthesis in rat skeletal muscle. *Am J Physiol* 1988;255:E166–E172.
30. Wernerman J, Hammarqvist F, Vinnars E. Alpha-ketoglutarate and postoperative muscle catabolism. *Lancet* 1990;335:701–703.
31. Häussinger D, Sies H. *Glutamine Metabolism in Mammalian Tissues*. Berlin: Springer-Verlag, 1984.
32. Souba WW, Smith RJ, Wilmore DW. Glutamine metabolism by the intestinal tract. *JPEN* 1985; 608–617.
33. Stehle P, Mertes N, Puchstein C, et al. Effect of parenteral glutamine peptide supplements on muscle glutamine loss and nitrogen balance after major surgery. *Lancet* 1989;i:231–233.
34. Hammarqvist F, Wernerman J, Ali MR, et al. Addition of glutamine to total parenteral nutrition after elective abdominal surgery spares free glutamine in muscle, counteracts the fall in muscle protein synthesis, and improves nitrogen balance. *Ann Surg* 1989;209:455–461.
35. Ziegler TR, Young LS, Benefell K, et al. Clinical and metabolic efficacy of glutamine-supplemented parenteral nutrition after bone marrow transplantation. *Ann Intern Med* 1992;116:821–828.
36. Roth E, Winkler S, Hölzenbein T, et al. High load of alanylglutamine in two patients with acute pancreatitis. *Clin Nutr* 1992;11(Spec Suppl):82.
37. Hammarqvist F, Wernerman J, von der Decken A, Vinnars E. Alpha-ketoglutarate preserves protein synthesis and free glutamine in skeletal muscle after surgery. *Surgery* 1991;109:28–36.
38. Petersson B, Gamrin L, Hammarqvist F, et al. Alpha-ketoglutarate given together with TPN improves the free glutamine-levels in glutamine-depleted intensive care patients. *Clin Nutr* 1992;11(Spec suppl): 26.
39. Barbul A, Wasserkrug HL, Youshimura N, et al. High arginine levels in intravenous hyperalimentation abrogate post-traumatic immune suppression. *J Surg Res* 1984;36:620–624.
40. Frostell CG, Fratacci MD, Wain JC, Zapol WM. Inhaled nitric oxide: a selective pulmonary vasodilator reversing hypoxic pulmonary vasoconstriction. *Circulation* 1991;83:2038–2047.
41. Blomqvist H, Wickerts CJ, Andreen M, et al. Enhanced pneumonia resolution by inhalation of nitric oxide? *Acta Anesth Scand* 1993;37:110–114.
42. Nakaki T, Hishikawa K, Suzuki H, et al. L-Arginine-induced changes in haemodynamics in man. In: Moncada S, Marletta MA, Hibbs JB, Higgs EA, eds. *The Biology of Nitric Oxide. I. Physiological and Clinical Aspects*. London: Portland Press, 1992;351–352.
43. Haider WJ. High dose insulin therapy in the critically ill patient. In: Kleinbergh G, Deutsch E, eds. *New Aspects of Clinical Nutrition*. Basel: Karger, 1983;271–282.
44. Millward DJ. The hormonal control of protein turnover. *Clin Nutr* 1990;9:115–126.
45. Garlick PJ, Wernerman J, McNurlan MA, Heys SD. Organ-specific measurements of protein turnover in man. *Proc Nutr Soc* 1991;50:217–225.
46. Liljedahl S-O, Gemzell C-A, Plantin L-O, Birke G. Effect of human growth hormone in patients with severe burns. *Acta Chir Scand* 1961;122:1–14.
47. Wernerman J. The effect of growth hormone on muscle and proteins in critically ill patients. *Acta Endocrinol* 1993;2:19–22.

48. Ward HC, Halliday D, Sim AJW. Protein and energy metabolism with biosynthetic human growth hormone after gastrointestinal surgery. *Ann Surg* 1987;206:56–61.
49. Jiang Z-M, He G-Z, Zhang S-Y, et al. Low-dose growth hormone and hypocaloric nutrition attenuate the protein-catabolic response after major operation. *Ann Surg* 1989;210:513–525.
50. Hammarqvist F, Strömberg C, von der Decken A, et al. Biosynthetic growth hormone preserves both muscle protein synthesis, the decrease in muscle free glutamine and improves whole body nitrogen economy postoperatively. *Ann Surg* 1992;216:184–191.
51. Nie ZT, Wallberg-Henriksson H, Johansson S, Henriksson J. Effects of adrenaline and prior exercise on the release of alanine, glutamine and glutamate from incubated rat skeletal muscle. *Acta Physiol Scand* 1989;136:395–401.
52. Wernerman J, Botta D, Hammarqvist F, et al. Stress hormones given to healthy volunteers alter the concentration and configuration of ribosomes in skeletal muscle, reflect changes in protein synthesis. *Clin Sci* 1989;77:611–616.
53. Bessey PQ, Watters JM, Aoki TT, Wilmore DW. Combined hormonal infusion simulates the metabolic response to injury. *Ann Surg* 1984;200:264–281.
54. Wernerman J, Hammarqvist F, Botta D, Vinnars E. Stress hormones alter the pattern of free amino acids in human skeletal muscle. *Clin Physiol* 1993;13:309–319.
55. Saito H, Trocki O, Alexander JW, et al. The effect of route of nutrient administration on the nutritional state, catabolic hormone secretion, and gut mucosal integrity after burn injury. *JPEN* 1987;11:1–7.
56. Mochizuki H, Trocki O, Dominioni JW, et al. Mechanism of prevention of post burn hypermetabolism and catabolism by early enteral feeding. *Ann Surg* 1984;200:297–310.
57. Cerra FB, Shronts EP, Raup S, Konstantinides N. Enteral nutrition in hypermetabolic surgical patients. *Crit Care Med* 1989;17:619–622.
58. Wilmore DW, Smith RJ, O'Dwyer ST, et al. The gut: a central organ after surgical stress. *Surgery* 1988;104:917–923.
59. O'Dwyer ST, Smith RJ, Hwang TL, Wilmore DW. Maintenance of small bowel mucosa with glutamine-enriched parenteral nutrition. *JPEN* 1989;13:579–585.
60. Alverdy JC, Aoys E, Moss G. Total parenteral nutrition promotes bacterial translocation from the gut. *Surgery* 1988;104:185–190.
61. Chiarelli A, Enzi GE, Casadei A, et al. Very early nutrition supplementation in burned patients. *Am J Clin Nutr* 1990;51:10035–10039.

*Organ Metabolism and Nutrition:
Ideas for Future Critical Care,* edited by
J. M. Kinney and H. N. Tucker.
Raven Press, Ltd., New York © 1994.

Overview

Peter A. Ward

*Department of Pathology, University of Michigan Medical School,
Ann Arbor, Michigan 48109–0602*

The contributions to this section provide a comprehensive analysis of the complex issues of gas exchange, metabolism and nutritional support in surgical patients, mechanisms of ischemia-reperfusion injury, and the role of inflammatory mediators, all in the context of the response to injury and the extent to which interventional approaches can be employed in order to hasten recovery and prevent or successfully treat multiorgan failure (MOF), adult respiratory distress syndrome (ARDS), and related abnormalities. What is evident from the material presented and reviewed is the lack of adequate information to understand the pathophysiology of developing MOF. Although a great deal of promise came about as a result of studies in mice suggesting that anti–tumor necrosis factor α (anti-TNFα) was highly effective in preventing lethality after infusion of lipopolysaccharide (LPS), clinical trials in human patients with sepsis and shock in which anti-LPS or anti-TNFα has been employed have been very disappointing. This has suggested that either LPS and/or TNFα are not important in the shock-sepsis syndrome or there has been inadequate selection of patient cohorts for treatment. Again, this emphasizes our lack of adequate knowledge regarding the sequence of pathophysiologic events responsible for development of MOF. An alternative possibility also exists: Because it is well known that inflammatory mediators have overlapping activities, which appear to be part and parcel of the inflammatory system, selective targeting of a mediator such as TNFα may result in an inadequate blockade, especially since interleukin-1 (IL-1) shares with TNFα many of the same biological properties (e.g., signal transductions of phagocytic cells, induction of endothelial cell adhesion molecules, etc.). In order to try to explain why, with all the rapid scientific advances, we still seem mired in a morass of conflicting and contradictory information, some general scientific principles gleaned from our own research efforts as well as those from several other groups in the area of inflammation may be appropriate.

THE RELATIONSHIP BETWEEN PRIMARY AND SECONDARY ORGAN INJURY

Understanding of MOF addresses the issue as to whether or not involvement of various organs is sequential and related. Alternatively, as has been suggested elsewhere in this publication, it is possible that multiorgan involvement progressing to failure may be the result of cumulative effects on organs, with the varying times of onset for individual organ dysfunction reflecting the "resistance" of that organ to repetitive insults. Such differences in organ resistance could, for instance, be associated with variations in constitutive or induced levels of antioxidants (e.g., glutathione, superoxide dismutase, catalase, etc.). An alternative explanation for MOF appearing in sequential fashion, with lung failure heralding subsequent hepatic and renal failure, might be due to the fact that inflammatory activation products generated as the result of single-organ failure gain access to the circulation and begin to affect adversely other organs. Support for this possibility is established in experimental studies. What has been proven experimentally is that damage of one organ can lead to injury of another. Following thermal injury to skin or after cerulein-induced pancreatitis in rats, lung injury develops slowly and progressively (1,2). The same type of phenomenon has been found in the case of hindlimb ischemia followed by local reperfusion (3,4). By whatever mechanism, the lung becomes injured in a manner that depends on the availability of complement as well as blood neutrophils. Lung injury has been defined by the extravascular leakage of ^{125}I-albumin and extravasation of ^{51}Cr-RBC. Complement-depletion (induced by serial infusions of cobra venom factor [CVF]) or complement blockade (induced by infusion of soluble complement receptor-1 [sCR-1]) is highly protective as is neutrophil depletion (induced with antibody or by treatment with cyclophosphamide). In addition, the use of antioxidants (catalase, superoxide dismustase, dimethylsulfoxide, or dimethylthiourea) has proven to be protective, as has been pretreatment with the iron chelator defcrroxamine. The last finding suggests that hydroxyl radical (HO·) generation from H_2O_2 in an iron-dependent manner may be the ultimate product of the activated neutrophil responsible for the lung vascular endothelial cell injury. The enigma is how, under these experimental conditions, neutrophil activation within the vasculature has occurred. The most logical conclusion is that perfusion of the injured tissue results in activation of plasma complement. It has been known for some time that cell debris, such as cell membranes, will activate complement via the alternative pathway. This could then lead to formation of C5a, which will not only activate neutrophils (causing enzyme release and O_2^- production) but will also cause up-regulation of neutrophil CD11b/CD18 (Mac-1, Mo-1), the result of which would be increased adhesive interactions with endothelial cells via interaction of neutrophils with endothelial intercellular adhesion molecule-1 (ICAM-1).

The rat model of ischemia-reperfusion of hindlimb, with resultant secondary injury to lungs (as noted), has provided additional information on mediators involved in lung injury. During the course of reperfusion of hindlimbs, there is evidence of systemic consumption of complement, with CH50 levels falling by 50% within 2 hours (3). Not surprisingly, because complement activation products would be expected to appear in parallel with consumption depletion of complement blood, blood neutrophils show up-regulation of CD11b and CD18 but not CD11a. Simultaneously, there is the appearance in plasma of TNFα, IL-1, and IL-6, which are first evident approximately 90 minutes after reperfusion and peaking at 2.5 hours. The relevance of TNFα ischemia/reperfusion injury of hind limbs

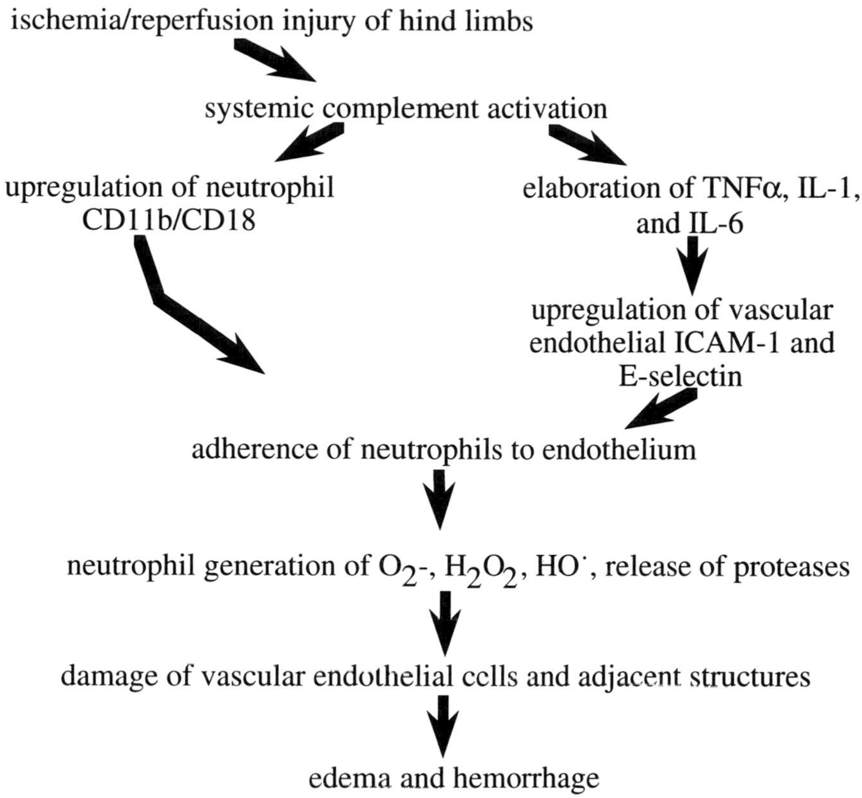

systemic complement activation

upregulation of neutrophil
CD11b/CD18

elaboration of TNFα, IL-1,
and IL-6

upregulation of vascular
endothelial ICAM-1 and
E-selectin

adherence of neutrophils to endothelium

neutrophil generation of O_2^-, H_2O_2, $HO^{\cdot}$, release of proteases

damage of vascular endothelial cells and adjacent structures

edema and hemorrhage

FIG. 1. Mechanism of local and remote vascular injury after ischemia/reperfusion.

and IL-1 to local (skeletal muscle) and remote (lung) injury has been demonstrated by the protective effects achieved by the blocking of these cytokines (5). The most likely explanation for the requirement for these cytokines in tissue injury may be in their abilities to up-regulate endothelial ICAM-1 and E-selectin (6). The proposed pathophysiologic events are summarized in Fig. 1. Complement activation leads directly to up-regulation of neutrophil β2-integrin (Mac-1) within the vascular compartment. Although it is unproven, complement activation products may somehow also trigger production of IL-1, IL-6, and TNFα, and perhaps other cytokines. The presence in plasma of IL-1 and TNFα sets the stage for endothelial up-regulation of ICAM-1 and E-selectin, leading to selectin-mediated "rolling" along the endothelial surface, followed by β2-integrin–dependent firm attachment. The presence of complement activation products would also induce the neutrophils to exhibit a respiratory burst, productive of O_2^- and H_2O_2. Granule-bound proteases would simultaneously be released from activated neutrophils. The composite effects would be vascular injury, resulting in edema and hemorrhage. The source of the cytokines is entirely unknown. Whether these cytokines arise from macrophages or other cellular sources in the injured extremity that is being reperfused, or whether elsewhere but due to products of the ischemically infused extremity, is entirely unknown. Although this body of information is incomplete, it at least provides the conceptual basis to understand how injury of one organ can lead to damage of another organ. Such information may be vital in developing interventional strategies to block the inexorable progression in MOF, provided early treatment is employed.

MECHANISMS FOR INJURY OF ENDOTHELIAL CELLS BY ACTIVATED NEUTROPHILS

Because the reviews in this volume underscore the evidence that products of activated phagocytic cells are responsible for injury of the vascular endothelium in a variety of conditions, including shock and sepsis, and because it has been suggested that neutrophils play an important role in MOF and ARDS (see previous section), understanding the nature of this injurious interaction is important. Our current knowledge is summarized in Fig. 2. Unexpectedly, interactions leading to endothelial cell injury by neutrophils indicate a mutual interaction between activated neutrophils and endothelial cells, leading to selective destruction of the latter in a manner that requires the ''cooperation'' of endothelial cells (7).

As discussed here and elsewhere in this book, complement activation causes up-regulation of the neutrophil $\beta2$ integrin CD11a/CD18, whose ''counterligand'' is endothelial ICAM-1. This up-regulation will greatly facilitate the adhesive interactions between neutrophils and endothelial cells and will enhance the effector function of activated neutrophils. If endothelial ICAM-1 up-regulation has also occurred, as would be expected when TNFα or IL-1 is present, the adhesive interactions would be all the more enhanced. Because it is known that $\beta2$ integrin/ICAM-1 in vivo also require selectin engagement under conditions of shear stress (8), both selectin as well as ICAM-1 engagement are important. Activated neutrophils that are adherent to the endothelial cell monolayer then release constituents of granules to the exterior, elastase being the major neutral proteinase of the human neutrophil. Simultaneously, neutrophils generate both O_2^- and H_2O_2, the former requiring entry to the endothelial cell via an anionic channel (resulting in slow entry), the latter being freely diffusible (thus gaining rapid entry into the endothelial cell). The presence of elastase within the endothelial cell results in limited proteolysis of cytoplasmic xanthine dehydrogenase, converting it to xanthine oxidase (XO). Xanthine oxidase uses as its substrates xanthine (X) and hypoxanthine (HX), converting them to uric acid and transferring a single electron to O_2, resulting in superoxide (O_2^-) formation. O_2^- apparently has two functions. The first is to reduce endothelial Fe^{3+} to Fe^{2+}. This electron transfer reoxidizes O_2^- to O_2. Additional O_2^- undergoes dismutation to form H_2O_2. Endothelial Fe^{2+} then reacts with H_2O_2, transferring an electron which regenerates Fe^{3+}. H_2O_2 is reduced, resulting in the formation of HO·. The source of H_2O_2 within the endothelial cell appears to be the activated neutrophil. The production of HO· within the endothelial cell results in cytotoxicity, although the target(s) of the injury is(are) unclear. This sequence of events has been deduced by the protective roles of catalase,

Events Related to Neutrophil-Mediated Injury of Endothelial Cells

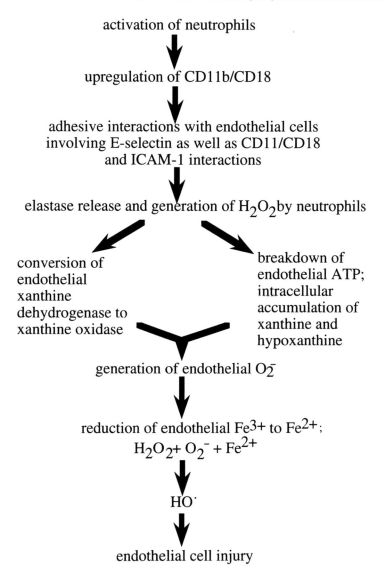

activation of neutrophils

upregulation of CD11b/CD18

adhesive interactions with endothelial cells
involving E-selectin as well as CD11/CD18
and ICAM-1 interactions

elastase release and generation of H_2O_2 by neutrophils

conversion of
endothelial
xanthine
dehydrogenase to
xanthine oxidase

breakdown of
endothelial ATP;
intracellular
accumulation of
xanthine and
hypoxanthine

generation of endothelial O_2^-

reduction of endothelial Fe^{3+} to Fe^{2+};
$H_2O_2 + O_2^- + Fe^{2+}$

$HO^{\cdot}$

endothelial cell injury

FIG. 2. Events related to neutrophil-mediated injury of endothelial cells.

deferroxamine, and the XO inhibitor, allopurinol, as well as by the protective effects of inhibitors of elastase (7,9,10). In addition, it has been shown that preloading of endothelial cells with superoxide dismutase (SOD), such that the intracellular levels are approximately tenfold above basal levels, is highly protective (11), substantiating the intracellular role of O_2^- in events leading to endothelial cell injury or death by activated neutrophils. Thus, endothelial cell injury by activated neutrophils is a complex array of events in which complement activation products, cytokines, proteases, and toxic derivatives of oxygen all come into play. This also reveals how complement products and cytokines appear to play central roles in tissue and organ injury that results from triggering of the inflammatory system.

Another recent, interesting observation suggests that endothelial cells can be directly activated by C5a to generate O_2^- (12). In a dose-dependent manner, incubation of C5a with endothelial cells causes both human umbilical vein and rat pulmonary artery endothelial cells to generate O_2^-. The response is unlike the respiratory burst in stimulated neutrophils in suspension, the result of which is rapid but prolonged (>20 minutes). Endothelial cells (which have been studied as cell suspensions) respond to C5a with a prolonged (>30 minutes) generation of O_2^-. As would be expected, C5a desarg has no similar effect. In addition, TNFα (but not IL-1) also induces O_2^- generation by endothelial cells. The presence of constitutive SOD in the endothelial cell affects the outcome. If endothelial SOD is inactivated by chemical means, the amount of O_2^- generated either by C5a or TNFα is correspondingly enhanced. These data imply that complement activation products and/or TNFα can directly activate endothelial cells to generate O_2^-, putting the endothelial cell at risk of injury by the presence of activated neutrophils. As has already been suggested, the presence of TNFα will further exacerbate the situation by inducing endothelial up-regulation of adhesion molecules, facilitating interactions between neutrophils and endothelial cells. Finally, if the endothelium has been subjected to conditions leading to a loss of SOD activity, it is put at further risk of injury. These data begin to demonstrate the complex and inimical interactions between neutrophils and endothelial cells.

SELECTIVE CYTOKINE INVOLVEMENT IN INFLAMMATORY INJURY

It is clear from the various contributions to this book that inflammatory cytokines are important participants in inflammatory injury, at least with respect to in vitro and in vivo experimental models. As indicated elsewhere in this book, the detection of TNFα and IL-1 in the plasma of patients with shock-sepsis and MOF has suggested that these cytokines may be related to the progressive clinical deterioration of these patients. The relevance of plasma cytokine presence to human shock-sepsis and MOF is not clearly defined. However, emerging evidence from experimental studies has suggested that both IL-1 and TNFα have important biological functions that link directly to the inflammatory response. As emphasized elsewhere, these cytokines directly stimulate phagocytic cells and indirectly facilitate their effector function by altering the endothelium to bring about up-regulation of adhesion molecules. What has recently become apparent is the fact that IL-1 and TNFα may participate conjointly or disparately in inflammatory reactions and that there are clear-cut differences in cytokine participation which are organ-related (see next page). This concept has important implications for the understanding of inflammatory injury in humans and in the construction of therapeutic interventions.

The conclusions referred to previously derive from several experimental observations emerging from our laboratories in which inflammatory models of tissue injury (lung, skin, and renal glomerular) have been employed in rats, using IgG immune complexes as the most common trigger of the inflammatory response. A summary of data is shown in Fig. 1. Four models involving immunologic triggers have been employed.

The first is intrapulmonary deposition of IgG immune complexes, induced with rabbit polyclonal IgG antibody to bovine serum albumin (BSA), which is instilled into the airway. BSA is then injected intravenously. This results, in 4 hours, in acute lung injury is manifested by influx of neutrophils, intraalveolar hemorrhage, and fibrin deposition. As will be discussed further, this injury is TNFα and IL-1 dependent and requires the participation of E-selectin as well as CD11a/CD18 and ICAM-1 (12–14). Cytokine up-regulation of endothelial adhesion molecules appears to be the major function of TNFα and IL-1 in this model. In the dermal vasculature, IgG immune complex deposition has also been induced by the local injection of anti-BSA and the systemic infusion of BSA. The resulting acute vasculitis is complement and neutrophil dependent and, as in the case of the lung, is E-selectin dependent (13). As in the lung, injury in the dermis peaks 4 hours after deposition of immune complexes.

The second model of injury involves intraalveolar of IgA immune complexes. This deposition, similar to the model of IgG immune complex-induced injury, occurs after airway instillation of IgA protein and intravenous administration of the antigen trinitrophenol, covalently linked to BSA. Lung injury in this model is neutrophil independent, complement dependent, peaks at 4 hours, and appears to involve generation from residential lung macrophages of toxic products of L-arginine and oxygen (15). Very little TNFα and IL-1 are found in the bronchoalveolar lavage (BAL) fluids of these animals (16). Injury is E-selectin independent (15) but requires participation of both CD11a/CD18 and CD11b/CD18 (14). As would be expected, injury is also ICAM-1 dependent.

The third model of injury involves infusion of polyclonal sheep IgG antibody to glomerular basement membrane into rats. Glomerular injury is associated with extensive damage and destruction of endothelial and epithelial cells, resulting in hematuria and proteinuria. Proteinuria at 24 hours is the quantitative endpoint of injury. Damage is complement and neutrophil dependent, independent of a requirement for E-selectin, but dependent on the roles of both CD11a/CD18 and CD11b/CD18 (as well as ICAM-1) (17).

The fourth model of injury is related to the intravascular infusion of CVF, which induces systemic activation of complement, resulting in activation of neutrophils, their aggregation, and neutrophil adherence to the pulmonary vascular endothelium (18). Vascular injury, the intensity of which peaks at 30 minutes, is associated with

TABLE 1. *Contrasting cytokine requirements in immunologic tissue injury.*

Organ	Tissue	Cytokine requirements[a]		
		TNFα	IL-1	MCP-1
Lung	IgG immune complex	65	67	<5
Skin	IgG immune complex	<5	60	ND
Lung	IgA immune complex	<5	<5	67
Kidney	IgG immune complex	76	<5	27
Lung	CVF	<5	<5	ND

[a] Data from references 20, 39; numbers represent permeability or hemorrhage changes and how blocking of a cytokine reduces tissue injury (shown as %).
ND, not determined; CVF, cobra venom factor.

focal destruction of the pulmonary capillary wall and extensive intraalveolar hemorrhage and fibrin deposition. As would be expected, the outcome is neutrophil and complement dependent. Recent studies revealed the participation of both CD11a/CD18 and CD11b/CD18 as well as ICAM-1 (19).

The requirements for three cytokines (IL-1, TNFα and monocyte chemotactic protein-1 [MCP-1]) in the development of vascular injury in each of these four models have been defined by the use of blocking antibodies. The results are shown in Table 1. In the IgG immune complex model of lung injury, both TNFα and IL-1 contribute significantly to the injury. Blocking of either cytokine with antibody reduces lung injury by 65% to 67% (20). These results have also been confirmed by the use of IL-1 receptor antagonist (IL-1ra) and by the use of soluble TNFα receptor-1 (sTNFR-1). Blocking of MCP-1 by antibody produces no protection in this model. In this model, alveolar macrophages demonstrate immunohistochemical evidence for the presence of both TNFα and IL-1. In striking contrast to findings in the lung, BSA–anti-BSA complexes in the skin induce injury that is IL-1 dependent but TNFα independent. Immunohistochemical analysis of the dermal reactions reveals the presence in what appears to be mast cells of IL-1 but not TNFα, suggesting that under the conditions employed, immune complexes preferentially cause expression of IL-1 but not TNFα in the rat dermis, whereas in the lung the same immune complexes cause coexpression of TNFα as well as IL-1. These findings do not imply that the dermal vasculature of the rat is refractory to the effects of TNFα, because addition of either TNFα or IL-1 to the anti-BSA (which was injected intradermally) results in increased accumulation of neutrophils and, correspondingly, intensified injury as measured by permeability and hemorrhage indices (20). These data suggest important organ differences in the expression and roles of inflammatory cytokines, depending on the vascular bed under study.

In the case of IgA immune complex–induced lung injury, BAL fluids contain little measurable TNFα or IL-1 but abundant amounts of MCP-1 (21). With the use of blocking antibodies, only anti–MCP-1 results in substantial protection (67%) against lung injury. Neither anti–TNFα nor anti–IL-1 is protective in this model of injury.

The reason for the dramatic differences in cytokine requirements for IgG and IgA immune complex–induced lung injury remains unexplained. The data indicate that, within the same organ, dramatically different patterns of cytokine engagement occur, depending in the nature of the inflammatory trigger.

When acute nephrotoxic nephritis is induced with sheep antiglomerular basement membrane (anti-GBM) and proteinuria (at 24 hours) is employed as the endpoint of injury, the profile of cytokine requirements is also unique: Blocking of IL-1 has no protective effects, while blocking of TNFα reduces injury by 76%, and blocking of MCP-1 reduces injury by 27% (17). By immunohistochemical analysis of glomeruli, TNFα but not IL-1 is present in mesangial cells. Renal artery infusion of TNFα causes up-regulation in glomeruli of vascular cell adhesion molecule-1 (VCAM-1) and E-selectin, while infusion of IL-1 fails to induce up-regulation of either protein. These data suggest that, under the experimental conditions employed, glomeruli respond to the immune complex stimulus with up-regulation of TNFα but not IL-1. The reasons for this specificity are not known. However, the inability of IL-1 (in contrast to TNFα) to cause up-regulation of glomerular vascular endothelial adhesion molecules suggests that the rat glomerulus not only fails to generate IL-1 but also is refractory to the effects of IL-1, in contrast to the dermal vasculature where immune complexes cause expression of IL-1 but not TNFα. In contrast to the kidney, in the rat dermis it has been shown that the vasculature is reactive to both cytokines that have been added extrinsically. Finally, CVF-induced lung injury, which is related to intravascular generation of complement activation products and neutrophil participation, shows the lack of requirements for either TNFα or IL-1. As described, this finding is not surprising in as much as the endpoint for assessment of injury is 30 minutes after infusion of CVF.

DISCREPANT IN VIVO DATA RELATED TO ROLES OF CYTOKINES IN SHOCK-SEPSIS

As has been emphasized elsewhere in this book, experiments to define the role of TNFα in the shock-sepsis syndrome have largely emphasized the intravenous infusion of LPS into rodents or the intravenous injections of gram-negative living bacteria into rodents or into subhuman primates.

As described elsewhere in this publication, the initial reports claiming that antibody either to LPS or to TNFα is highly protective against LPS-induced shock in mice gave rise to a great deal of excitement and anticipation that an effective therapeutic intervention for the sepsis-shock in humans was at hand. Assuming that the majority of cases of shock-sepsis in humans is linked to gram-negative septicemia, and assuming that the pathophysiologic effects of LPS are due to the appearance in plasma of either TNFα or IL-1 (or both), the strategy to block these cytokines either with antibody or with natural antagonists seems reasonable. In vivo blocking of cytokines can be achieved either by the use of monoclonal antibodies to TNFα or by IL-1, provided the binding is of sufficient affinity and the bioreactive sites on the cytokines are sterically blocked. Given the resolution of these problems, the concerns regarding the use of monoclonal antibodies are twofold: the duration of the blocking effects and the immunogenicity of the murine antibody. The latter problem, to the extent clinically that it represents a real obstacle, can be overcome by the use of "humanized antibodies" (in which segments of the constant regions of the IgG molecule are replaced with those contained in human IgG) or by the use of a single clinical application of the antibody. While the half-life (t 1/2) of murine IgG_1 in humans is several days, this is a "mixed blessing." Although the prolonged half-life would appear to be desirable, there exists the possibility that prolonged blockade (for several days) of TNFα or IL-1 may lead to undesirable effects. While the early plasma peak of cytokines would likely be negated by the presence of antibody, the antibody could also block cytokine in the extravascular compartment. In such locations, TNFα and IL-1 may play an important role in host-defense mechanisms. In the context of animal models, support for this concern is described next.

The other approach to the blocking of cytokines avoids the problems with use of monoclonal antibodies and involves the use of naturally occurring antagonists. To date, the most well described natural antagonists are IL-1ra and sTNFR-1. IL-1ra has a binding affinity for the IL-1 receptor similar to that for IL-1. sTNFR-1 has been generated in chimeric form, with sTNFR-1 being linked to the Fc region of IgG, conferring a relatively long half-life in vivo to this molecule. Whether in its native form or in the chimeric version, sTNFR-1 binds with TNFα, effectively preventing it from binding to a cell surface receptors for TNFα. As indicated here, both IL-1ra and sTNFR-1 are highly effective in blocking cytokine-dependent inflammatory reactions in experimental animals. Since the initial experimental reports, clinical trials in humans with antibody to LPS or with IL-1ra have failed to meet clinical expectations.

What accounts for these discrepancies? To begin with, in most animal models featuring the bolus infusion of LPS, only a transient and early appearance in plasma TNFα has been demonstrated (22–28). Furthermore, anti-TNFα monoclonal antibody has effectively protected rodents from LPS-induced lethality (29,30). In mice, infusion of *Escherichia coli* alone or with *Bacillus fragilis* in the face of anti-TNFα has enhanced the survival rates (31,32). However, anti-TNFα decreases survival in mice infused with *Salmonella typhimurium* (33) or with *Listeria monocytogenes* (34,35). Thus, it must be concluded that TNFα plays a role that is dependent on the type of microorganism injected. Tumor necrosis factor α also affects the outcome in a manner that can be adverse or beneficial to survival, depending on the microorganism. Another indication of the complexity of the issue is found in the cecal ligation and perforation model. This model induces a peritonitis and a progressive bacteremia that is fatal within a week or so, a seemingly good experimental equivalent of sepsis and shock occurring in humans after polytrauma. When such animals have been pretreated with anti-TNFα, the survival times have actually decreased (36). This would suggest that, under the conditions employed, TNFα plays an important role in bolstering host defenses (e.g., by priming phagocytic cells for an enhanced respiratory burst or inducing endothelial up-regulation of adhesion molecules). Accordingly, the interception of TNFα may compromise natural host defenses.

Primate models of shock-sepsis have revealed that anti-TNFα enhances survivals of baboons infused intravenously with *E. coli* (37,38), although the ultimate outcome in these animals as well as the onset of multiorgan failure has not been convincingly alleviated by treatment with anti-TNFα. What is unknown at present is whether simultaneous blocking of IL-1 might significantly affect the longer term complications in the primate models of shock-sepsis after infusion of *E. coli*.

This body of information provides a compelling note of caution in the extrapolation of data from experimental models (and the manipulation of these models) to mechanisms of shock-sepsis occurring in humans. It may be that the animal models are too artificial, especially when bolus infusions of LPS or living bacteria are employed, because this almost assuredly does not duplicate events occurring in humans. Furthermore, differences in biological responses to LPS are known to be notoriously variable between species, with rabbits exhibiting approximately the same reactivity to LPS as humans, while rats and mice are highly resistant to the adverse effects of bolus infusion of LPS. To what extent these differences may reflect variable biological functions of cytokines in different species remains to be determined. This information implies that caution must be observed in the generalization of data derived from experimental models of shock-sepsis and the extent to which this information is relevant to humans. It is also quite likely that the "cytokine alphabet" is as yet incomplete and that it is premature to be absolute in defining the biological role of cytokines in adverse human states.

THE FUTURE FOR ANTIINFLAMMATORY INTERVENTIONS IN SHOCK-SEPSIS STATES

Antiinflammatory interventions in the treatment of shock-sepsis states hold great promise, and, at the same time, represent a tremendous challenge. The most perplexing problems involve patient selection and agreement on the endpoints of measurement. As the clinical trials involving the use of anti-LPS have suggested, it may be that the selection of patients has not been adequately discriminating and that within the large cohorts of patients studied to date differences in the outcomes involving relatively limited subsets of patients have been disguised by the large numbers of subjects in the overall study. Another problem may relate to insufficiently sensitive endpoints. Reliance on survival rates as the endpoints may not have sufficient sensitivity of measurement and discrimination, even though the ability to demonstrate that survival rates have been significantly improved remains the gold standard for interventional approaches.

Another problem relates to the definition of shock-sepsis, especially the meaning of *sepsis*. Is it sufficient to have hyperpyrexia and leukocytosis, or is the demonstration of LPS or bacteria in the blood the desirable endpoint? The dilemma is further complicated by the fact that abdominal sepsis (i.e., presence of bacteria in the peritoneal cavity) may occur in the absence of detectable bacteremia. Until there is a clearly understood and agreed upon definition of *sepsis,* inadequate patient selection and the attendant skewing of clinical outcome may be unavoidable.

Another dilemma is the decision on what inflammatory mediator or product should be blocked or neutralized. It is obviously not affordable to conduct a series of clinical trials in sequence in which multiple candidate mediators are individually the subjects of clinical investigation. Another problem is linked to evidence of redundancy of inflammatory mediators, the best examples being TNFα and IL-1. Each cytokine has pleiotropic biological properties that are very similar. There is little evidence to support the concept that these cytokines appear in sequence, resulting in a situation in which the expression of one governs expression of the other. Most experimental studies suggest that both cytokines appear in parallel, indicating that blocking of one cytokine may not be especially effective in preventing the biologic effect of the other. Aside from the evidence for selective cytokine participation that is organ-dependent (as described here), this raises this issue as to whether or not "cocktails" of cytokine blocking agents may have to be considered for clinical trial. Obviously, such a strategy would have complex implications due to federal regulatory control of clinical trials. As also indicated here, protocols for the various interventional strategies will have to be designed in accord with the t 1/2 values of the agents being administered. Of course, this also implies that there are reliable endpoints of measurement and that one also knows how, when, and for how long to administer the interventional agents. If there is discord on any of these points, construction of protocols for clinical trials will be difficult. This underscores how insufficient is our understanding of the shock-sepsis syndrome and our incomplete knowledge about the cytokine networks and other relevant mediators. Until additional basic knowledge is attained, our strategies for interventional treatment of shock-sepsis in humans will be based more on empiricism and guesswork than on predictions that rest on solid scientific foundations.

REFERENCES

1. Till GO, Beauchamp C, Menapace D, et al. Oxygen radical dependent lung damage following thermal injury of rat skin. *J Trauma* 1983;23:269–277.
2. Guice KS, Oldham KT, Johnson KJ, et al. Pancreatitis-induced acute lung injury: an ARDS model. *Ann Surg* 1988;208:71–77.
3. Seekamp A, Mulligan MS, Till GO, et al. Role of β2-integrins and ICAM-1 in hind limb ischemia/reperfusion injury and remote lung injury. *Am J Pathol* (in press).
4. Welbourn CRB, Goldman G, Paterson IS, et al. Neutrophil elastase and oxygen radicals: synergism in lung injury after hindlimb ischemia. *Am J Physiol* 1991;269:H1852–H1856.
5. Seekamp A, Warren JS, Remick DG, et al. Requirements for TNFα and IL-1 in limb ischemia/reperfusion injury and associated lung injury. *Am J Pathol* (in press).
6. Mulligan MS, Vaporciyan AA, Miyasaka M, et al. TNFα regulates in vivo intrapulmonary expression of ICAM-1. *Am J Pathol* 1993;142:1.
7. Ward PA. Mechanisms of endothelial cell killing by H_2O_2 or products of activated neutrophils. *Am J Med* 1991;91:89S–94S.
8. Lasky LA, Rosen SD. The selectins: carbohydrate-binding adhesion molecules of the immune system. In: Gallin JI, Goldstein IM, Snyderman R, eds. *Inflammation: Basic Principles and Clinical Correlates.* New York: Raven Press, 1992;407–412.

9. Varani J, Bendelow MJ, Sealey DE, et al. Tumor necrosis factor enhances susceptibility of vascular endothelial cells to neutrophils-mediated killing (brief communication)). *Lab Invest* 1988;59:292–295.
10. Stubbs EB Jr, Walker BAM, Owens CA, et al. Formyl peptide stimulates and ATPγS potentiates [³H]cytidine 5'-diphosphate diglyceride accumulation in human neutrophils. *J Immunol* 1992;148: 2242–2247.
11. Markey BA, Phan SH, Varani J, et al. Inhibition of cytotoxicity by intracellular superoxide dismutase supplementation. *Free Rad Biol Med* 1990;9:307–314.
12. Murphy HS, Shayman JA, Till GO, et al. Superoxide responses of endothelial cells to C5a and TNFα: divergent signal transduction pathways. *Am J Physiol* 1992;263:L51–L59.
13. Mulligan MS, Varani J, Dame MK, et al. Role of endothelial-leukocyte adhesion molecules-1 (ELAM-1) in neutrophil-mediated lung injury in rats. *J Clin Invest* 1991;88:1396–1406.
14. Mulligan MS, Wilson GP, Todd RF, et al. Role of β1, β2 integrins and ICAM-1 in lung injury after deposition of IgG and IgA immune complexes. *J Immunol* 1993;150:2407–2417.
15. Mulligan MS, Warren JS, Smith CW, et al. Lung injury after deposition of IgA immune complexes: requirements for CD18 and L-arginine. *J Immunol* 1992;148:3086–3092.
16. Warren JS, Barton PA, Jones ML. Contrasting roles for tumor necrosis factor in the pathogenesis of IgA and IgG immune complex lung injury. *Am J Pathol* 1991;138:581–590.
17. Mulligan MS, Johnson KJ, Todd RF III, et al. Requirements for leukocyte adhesion molecules in nephrotoxic nephritis. *J Clin Invest* 1993;91:577–587.
18. Till GO, Johnson KJ, Kunkel R, Ward PA. Intravascular activation of complement and acute lung injury. Dependency on neutrophils and toxic oxygen metabolites. *J Clin Invest* 1982;69:1126–1135.
19. Mulligan MS, Smith CW, Anderson DC, et al. Role of leukocyte adhesion molecules in complement-induced lung injury. *J Immunol* 1993;150:2401.
20. Mulligan MS, Ward PA. Immune complex–induced lung and dermal vascular injury: differing requirements for TNFα and IL-1. *J Immunol* 1992;149:331–339.
21. Jones ML, Mulligan MS, Flory CM, et al. Potential role of monocyte chemoattractant protein 1/JE in monocyte/macrophage–dependent IgA immune complex alveolitis in the rat. *J Immunol* 1992;149: 2147–2154.
22. Remick DG, Strieter RM, Eskandari MK. Role of tumor necrosis factor-alpha in lipopolysaccharide-induced pathologic alterations. *Am J Pathol* 1990;136:49–60.
23. Mozes T, Ben-Efraim S, Tak CJ, et al. Serum levels of tumor necrosis factor determine the fatal or nonfatal course of endotoxic shock. *Immunol Lett* 1991;27:157–162.
24. Kolsterhalfen B, Horstmann-Jungemann K, Vogel P, et al. Time course of various inflammatory mediators during recurrent endotoxemia. *Biochem Pharmacol* 1992;43:2103–2109.
25. Fong Y, Tracey KJ, Moldawer LL, et al. Antibodies to cachectin/tumor necrosis factor reduce interleukin 1 beta and interleukin 6 appearance during lethal bacteremia. *J Exp Med* 1989;170: 1627–1633.
26. Ulich TR, Guo KZ, Irwin B, et al. Endotoxin-induced cytokine gene expression in vivo. II. Regulation of tumor necrosis factor and interleukin-1 alpha/beta expression and suppression. *Am J Pathol* 1990; 137:1173–1185.
27. Creasey AA, Stevens P, Kenney J, et al. Endotoxin and cytokine profile in plasma of baboons challenged with lethal and sublethal *Escherichia coli*. *Circ Shock* 1991;33:84–91.
28. Redl H, Schlag G, Bahrami S, et al. Plasma neutrophil-activating peptide-1/interleukin-8 and neutrophil elastase in a primate bacteremia model. *J Infect Dis* 1991;164:383–388.
29. Zanetti G, Heumann D, Gerain J, et al. Cytokine production after intravenous or peritoneal gram-negative bacterial challenge in mice. Comparative protective efficacy of antibodies to tumor necrosis factor-alpha and to lipopolysaccharide. *J Immunol* 1992;148:1890–1897.
30. Beutler B, Milsark IW, Cerami AC. Passive immunization against cachectin/tumor necrosis factor protects mice from lethal effect of endotoxin. *Science* 1985;229:869–871.
31. Evans T, Carpenter A, Silva A, Cohen J. Differential effects of monoclonal antibodies to tumor necrosis factor alpha and gamma interferon in induction of hepatic nitric oxide synthase in experimental gram-negative sepsis. *Infect Immun* 1992;60:4133–4139.
32. Sawyer RG, Adams RB, May AK, et al. Anti-tumor necrosis factor antibody reduces mortality in the presence of antibiotic-induced tumor necrosis factor release. *Arch Surg* 1993;128:73–77 (discussion).
33. Mastroeni P, Arena A, Costa GB, et al. Serum TNF alpha in mouse typhoid and enhancement of a *Salmonella* infection by anti-TNF alpha antibodies. *Microb Pathol* 1991;11:33–38.

34. Havell EA. Evidence that tumor necrosis factor has an important role in antibacterial resistance. *J Immunol* 1989;143:2894–2899.
35. Nakane A, Minagawa T, Kato K. Endogenous tumor necrosis factor (cachectin) is essential to host resistance against *Listeria monocytogenes* infections. *Infect Immun* 1988;56:2563–2569.
36. Echtenacher B, Falk W, Mannel DN, Krammer PH. Requirement of endogenous tumor necrosis factor/cachectin for recovery from experimental peritonitis. *J Immunol* 1990;145:3762–3766.
37. Tracey KJ, Fong Y, Hesse DG, et al. Anti-cachectin/TNF monoclonal antibodies prevent septic shock during lethal bacteraemia. *Nature* 1987;330:662–664.
38. Hinshaw LB, Tekamp-Olson P, Chang AC, et al. Survival of primate in LD100 septic shock following therapy with antibody to tumor necrosis factor (TNF alpha). *Circ Shock* 1990;30:279–292.

Subject Index

Note: Page numbers in italics indicate figures; page numbers followed by t indicate tables.